# Manual of Clinical Problems in Infectious Disease
## FOURTH EDITION

# Manual of Clinical Problems in Infectious Disease
## FOURTH EDITION

### Nelson M. Gantz, M.D., F.A.C.P.
*Chairman, Department of Medicine, Chief, Division of Infectious Diseases, Pinnacle Health Hospitals, Harrisburg, Pennsylvania; Clinical Professor of Medicine, MCP Hahnemann School of Medicine, Philadelphia, Pennsylvania*

### Richard B. Brown, M.D.
*Chief, Infectious Diseases Division, Baystate Medical Center, Springfield, Massachusetts; Professor of Medicine, Tufts University School of Medicine, Boston, Massachusetts*

### Steven L. Berk, M.D.
*Professor and Chairman, Department of Medicine, East Tennessee State University, James H. Quillen College of Medicine, Johnson City, Tennessee*

### Anthony L. Esposito, M.D.
*Chief, Department of Medicine, Director, Division of Infectious Diseases, St. Vincent's Hospital, Worcester, Massachusetts; Associate Professor of Medicine, University of Massachusetts School of Medicine, Worcester, Massachusetts*

### Richard A. Gleckman, M.D.
*Chairman, Department of Medicine, Chief, Infectious Diseases, St. Joseph's Hospital and Medical Center, Paterson, New Jersey*

00-1669

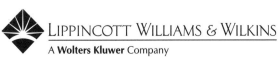

LIPPINCOTT WILLIAMS & WILKINS
A **Wolters Kluwer** Company
Philadelphia · Baltimore · New York · London
Buenos Aires · Hong Kong · Sydney · Tokyo

Acquisitions Editor: Jonathan Pine
Developmental Editor: Ellen DiFrancesco
Manufacturing Manager: Kevin Watt
Production Manager: Robert Pancotti
Production Editor: Jeff Somers
Indexer: Pam Edwards
Compositor: Circle Graphics
Printer: RR Donnelly–Crawfordsville

Printed in the United States of America

9  8  7  6  5  4  3  2  1

---

**Library of Congress Cataloging-in-Publication Data**

Manual of clinical problems in infectious disease / edited by Nelson
    M. Gantz . . . [et al.]. — 4th ed.
        p.      cm.
    Includes bibliographical references and index.
    ISBN 0-7817-1910-0 (alk. paper)
    1. Communicable diseases—Handbooks, manuals, etc. I. Gantz,
Nelson Murray, 1941–   .
    [DNLM: 1. Communicable Diseases handbooks.      WC 39 M294 1999]
    RC111.M265    1999
    616.9—dc21
    DNLM/DLC
    for Library of Congress                                        98-46884
                                                                        CIP

---

# CONTENTS

## I.  UPPER RESPIRATORY TRACT

## II.  LOWER RESPIRATORY TRACT

## III.   CARDIOVASCULAR SYSTEM

## IV.   GASTROINTESTINAL SYSTEM

## XI.  FEVER

## XII.  IMMUNITY

## XIII.  NOSOCOMIAL INFECTIONS

## XIV.  ZOONOSES

## XV.  NEWLY APPRECIATED INFECTIONS

## XVI.  PROPHYLAXIS OF INFECTION IN TRAVELERS

## XVII.  TUBERCULOSIS

## XVIII.  SELECTED LABORATORY PROCEDURES

## XIX.  ANTIMICROBIAL, ANTIVIRAL, ANTIPARASITIC, AND ANTIFUNGAL AGENTS

## XX.  AIDS

# PREFACE

In 1979, at the request of our students and house officers, we prepared the first edition of *Manual of Clinical Problems in Infectious Disease*. At that time, our aim was to provide medical students, house officers, and practitioners with a contemporary approach to selected problems in infectious disease; key annotated references supported the text.

In 1986, with the help of two additional authors, Drs. Richard Brown and Anthony Esposito, the second edition of *Manual of Clinical Problems in Infectious Disease* was published and covered a list of new subjects.

Since that time, numerous new infectious agents have been recognized, new concepts have evolved, and new treatments have emerged. For the third edition, to satisfy the need for a contemporary text addressing this information, we prepared a new list of subjects and added Dr. Steven Berk to our team.

The fourth edition of *Manual of Clinical Problems in Infectious Disease* is not simply an updated version of the three earlier books: it reexamines some older material and explores new subjects such as Hepatitis C and VRE. Every effort has been made to add contemporary references to the text to enhance the accuracy of the manual and to provide a springboard for further reading; all references are annotated.

Like the three previous editions, this manual is not meant to be all-inclusive. Numerous major texts that fulfill this mission have already been published. The fourth edition of *Manual of Clinical Problems in Infectious Disease* represents an attempt to provide contemporary, scientifically accurate, and readable material on topics of concern to the practicing physician, house officer, and medical student. All of the editors are clinicians who see patients on a regular basis, and have written chapters based on a "real world" approach to patient care while keeping with a scientific basis of management. Chapters have been added, removed, or revised in keeping with changes in infectious diseases over the past five years. We are proud of our effort, and feel that this book will prove valuable to the clinician in the day-to-day management of patients with infections.

*N.M.G.*
*R.B.B.*
*S.L.B.*
*A.L.E.*
*R.A.G.*

## ACKNOWLEDGMENTS

We would like to express appreciation to those who have assisted us in the preparation of this book. We thank Libby Coldsmith at the Pinnacle Health System library for her invaluable assistance in searching the literature. We are grateful to Sandy Weaver who did an excellent job typing, proofreading, and organizing the manuscript. We also appreciate the secretarial support of Theresa Podurgiel. Special thanks to Donna Forrester for assistance with the library research and preparing the manuscript.

# Manual of Clinical Problems in
# Infectious Disease
**FOURTH EDITION**

# I. UPPER RESPIRATORY TRACT

# 1. TONSILLOPHARYNGITIS IN ADULTS

Tonsillopharyngitis (more simply, pharyngitis) is a common complaint characterized by inflammation of the mucous membranes of the throat. Erythema is generally present, but exudate is variably noted. Less commonly, ulceration or a membrane can be seen. Up to 40 million office visits are made annually by persons of all ages because of this illness, primarily during colder seasons, and it may account for up to 100 million days lost from work each year. Many patients and clinicians are aware of the importance of group A β-hemolytic streptococci (*Streptococcus pyogenes*) as a cause of pharyngitis, and concern for this pathogen must be a major focus in the management of sore throat. It is also felt to be the only commonly encountered pathogen for which treatment is clearly indicated. However, numerous other potentially treatable causes of this illness exist, and most cases of pharyngitis in adults are not caused by *S. pyogenes*. Table 1-1 lists some etiologies that need to be considered in the differential diagnosis of pharyngitis in adults. Patients who are immunosuppressed may be infected with additional pathogens—for example, enteric gram-negative bacilli or mixed anaerobes (granulocytopenia) and *Candida albicans* (T cell-mediated immunosuppression, HIV infection). Furthermore, HIV itself may be a cause of pharyngitis.

The clinical presentation of pharyngitis is usually a soreness in the throat. Dysphagia may also be noted, and if the uvula is involved, a rather discomforting feeling of a "lump" when swallowing may be felt. A major responsibility of all clinicians is to distinguish treatable from untreatable disease and to recognize potential complications. An important component of this process is the history. As an example, a sexual history may help define the likelihood of *Neisseria gonorrhoeae* pharyngitis, whereas an immunization history will help define the possibility of diphtheria. Risk factors for HIV infection should always be assessed. A patient's inability to manage secretions or severe dysphagia should alert the clinician to epiglottitis or abscess. Constitutional symptoms are variable. In many instances, initial assessment will not allow differentiation among etiologies. Streptococcal and adenoviral pharyngitis are commonly accompanied by significant fever; chills may also be present. The onset is generally abrupt, and patients are ill. Physical examination reveals pharyngeal erythema, and exudate is noted in at least 50% of cases. Exudate is uncommon in rhinovirus, coxsackievirus, and herpes simplex virus pharyngitis. Anterior cervical adenopathy often exists with streptococcal infection. Alternatively, the presence of posterior cervical adenopathy, laryngitis, diarrhea, or rhinorrhea generally indicates a viral etiology, and these symptoms have a negative predictive value of about 80% for disease caused by *S. pyogenes*. Infectious mononucleosis is often associated with severe pharyngitis, but other evidence of this disease is often present.

Gram's stain of pharyngeal exudate is an underemployed test that may be useful in determining the etiology of pharyngitis. In trained hands, groupable streptococci can be identified. The presence of polymorphonuclear leukocytes suggests bacterial or adenoviral infection. Additionally, although little literature exists, experience should allow differentiation of *Neisseria* species, *Haemophilus influenzae,* and *Corynebacterium* species (*C. diphtheriae* or *C. hemolyticum*). Infection with Epstein-Barr virus (EBV) is often associated with exudative pharyngitis; however, Gram's stain demonstrates only mixed organisms and no polymorphonuclear leukocytes. In the presence of EBV, Gram's stain demonstrating polymorphonuclear leukocytes suggests a confounding bacterial infection, usually with *S. pyogenes*.

A complete physical examination may help to identify the infection; splenomegaly or generalized lymphadenopathy with EBV, *S. pyogenes* with scarlet fever, *C. hemolyticum* with scarlatiniform or urticarial rash, adenovirus with conjunctivitis, *N. gonorrhoeae* with rectal or genital disease or disseminated infection, and *Mycoplasma pneumoniae* with pneumonia.

An immediate goal in the evaluation of pharyngitis is to detect cases caused by *S. pyogenes*. Although culture for *S. pyogenes* remains the gold standard for diagnosis, antigen testing of material from the tonsillopharyngeal area is the most expeditious means of identifying the organism. It is sensitive (80% to 90%) and specific (>95%) and

Table 1-1. Notable causes of pharyngitis in adults and percentages of cases

| Bacterial/treatable | Viral/untreatable (42) |
| --- | --- |
| *Streptococcus pyogenes* (5–20) | Rhinovirus |
| Other "groupable" streptococci (6) | Adenovirus (19) |
| *Haemophilus influenzae* | Epstein-Barr virus (7–15) |
| *Arcanobacterium hemolyticum* (0.4–2) | Cytomegalovirus |
| *Corynebacterium diphtheriae* (rare) | Respiratory syncitial virus (2) |
| *Neisseria gonorrhoeae* (rare) | Myxovirus (10) |
| *Mycoplasma pneumoniae* (10–13) | |
| *Chlamydia pneumoniae* | |

* Adapted from Carroll K, Reimer L. Microbiology and laboratory diagnosis of upper respiratory tract infections. *Clin Infect Dis* 1996; 23:442–448.

provides information while the patient is still in the office. The test results may be adversely affected if performed by unskilled personnel. A positive test result should prompt therapy. A negative test result should be followed by formal culture for this and possibly other bacterial pathogens, based on epidemiologic information. The easiest method is to swab the throat simultaneously with two swabs. If the first swab (for antigen detection) is negative, the second can be formally cultured. It is extremely important to sample the posterior pharynx and tonsils because yields from the tongue, gums, buccal mucosa, and other areas are far lower. *H. influenzae, C. hemolyticum,* and *N. gonorrhoeae* require special media and will not be identified by standard culture techniques or antigen-detection systems. Thus, when they are suspected, the clinician must communicate directly with the microbiology laboratory to access appropriate media and techniques.

A recent survey of board-certified pediatricians was conducted to determine actual practice patterns for the management of presumed streptococcal pharyngitis. Rapid tests were employed by about 64% of respondents, whereas 85% employed cultures. Only 42% of physicians in the survey employed the protocol of rapid test followed by culture if the result of the rapid test was negative. A third of physicians routinely discontinued antibiotics if studies for *S. pyogenes* were negative. Patients who are known to be immunosuppressed by virtue of underlying disease or therapy should be evaluated for other potential pathogens. Alternatively, persons who are demonstrated to have unusual etiologies or fail to respond to standard therapy may require evaluation for underlying diseases. For example, a patient with oral thrush should be evaluated for infection with HIV unless another risk factor is known. Similarly, when a patient has severe, unresolving pharyngitis, a CBC should be performed to assess for EBV or granulocytopenia.

### Specific Etiologies of Pharyngitis
*Groupable Streptococci*
Streptococci remain the most commonly identified cause of sore throat. *S. pyogenes* is the most common and important of these organisms, but other groupable streptococci, including groups C and G, have been implicated. These may be associated with large food-borne or respiratory droplet outbreaks. However, only *S. pyogenes* is associated with rheumatic fever. Group C streptococcal pharyngitis has also been associated with glomerulonephritis. Reasons to treat *S. pyogenes* pharyngitis include (a) relief of symptoms, (b) prevention of spread, (c) prevention of immunologic sequelae, and (d) prevention of local suppurative complications. Rheumatic fever complicates *S. pyogenes* infections of the throat and can be prevented by administration of an appropriate antimicrobial agent within 8 to 9 days of disease onset. There is no evidence that poststreptococcal glomerulonephritis is preventable by use of antimicrobial agents. The most common local suppurative complication is peritonsillar abscess. Typical presentation is that of ongoing, generally unilateral pharyngitis and constitutional symptoms, often associated with dysphagia and the presence of a mass on digital palpation

around the tonsil. In adults, retropharyngeal abscess is uncommon because lymphatic drainage from the tonsils does not flow in this direction. Peritonsillar abscess requires drainage for cure. If employed early, antimicrobial agents shorten the course of pharyngitis caused by *S. pyogenes* but have not been shown to alter that of group C or G streptococcal infection.

Penicillin remains the agent of choice for streptococcal pharyngitis, and a single dose of IM benzathine penicillin (1.2 million U) often suffices and ensures compliance. However, this regimen may be sensitizing and is accompanied by a bacteriologic failure rate of up to 20%. Thus, many clinicians prefer penicillin V potassium. Current recommendations for this agent are 250 to 500 mg thrice daily. Numerous studies demonstrate, however, that compliance with a regimen of this length is poor. Some data demonstrate that only 8% of patients continue to take medication by day 9. Treatment for less than 10 days is associated with fewer bacteriologic cures. Other agents that can be employed include first-generation cephalosporins, erythromycin, and clindamycin. Agents that include azithromycin, cefuroxime, cefpodoxime, and cefixime have been successfully employed for less than 10 days of treatment, but the author continues to recommend a full therapeutic course. Antimicrobial agents that should not be used for streptococcal pharyngitis include trimethoprim-sulfamethoxazole (TMP-SMX), sulfonamides, quinolones, and tetracyclines; their activity against *S. pyogenes* is less favorable.

Routine reculturing of the throat following therapy is not indicated, except perhaps in patients with prior rheumatic fever or rheumatic heart disease. After therapy, approximately 10% of patients continue to harbor *S. pyogenes* (representing asymptomatic carriage), and in the absence of symptoms this should not be a reason to repeat therapy or for the physician or patient to panic ("streptomania"). Reasons for ongoing or rapidly recurrent illness despite apparently appropriate therapy with penicillin include (a) deep-seated infection within tonsillar crypts, (b) simultaneous presence of a β-lactamase-producing organism (e.g., *Staphylococcus aureus*) that antagonizes penicillin therapy, and (c) noncompliance. If rapid recurrence or lack of response is demonstrated, repeated treatment with a β-lactamase-stable agent for up to 3 weeks usually suffices. Appropriate choices include clindamycin or amoxicillin-clavulanate.

Infection caused by group G streptococci is clinically indistinguishable from that associated with *S. pyogenes*. The likelihood of suppurative complications is unknown, and the impact of therapy on spread has not been formally established. Therapy has not been demonstrated to alter symptomatology. Group C streptococci may cause endemic or epidemic disease and may be associated with up to 6% of cases of sore throat. Symptoms associated with group C streptococci are similar to but generally less severe than those seen with *S. pyogenes* infection. Occasional cases of poststreptococcal glomerulonephritis have been associated with these organisms, and elevations of antistreptolysin O titer occur. Need for therapy is undetermined, but clinicians generally treat in a manner similar to that used for *S. pyogenes* pharyngitis.

### Haemophilus influenzae

Pharyngitis associated with *H. influenzae* has been reported infrequently but is probably underdiagnosed. A recent review suggests that it may be the second most commonly noted bacterial cause of pharyngitis. Most cases are probably associated with nontypeable, nonencapsulated strains. In adults, clinical presentation is generally subacute, with throat soreness predominating over constitutional symptoms. Examination reveals mild pharyngeal erythema, usually without exudate or cervical adenopathy, and the clinician may initially suspect viral disease. Suppurative complications are rare. In the absence of therapy, symptoms linger for weeks. Therapy with an agent active against *H. influenzae* (e.g., second-generation cephalosporins, doxycycline, or TMP-SMX) results in rapid resolution of symptoms. The need to employ an agent with activity against β-lactamase-producing strains is uncertain. Throat cultures need to be plated specifically for *H. influenzae* because neither rapid antigen-detection tests nor routine cultures on blood agar can identify this organism.

### Corynebacterium hemolyticum

*C. hemolyticum* accounts for approximately 2% of cases of pharyngitis, and infection with this organism occurs primarily in teenagers and young adults. Occasionally, it may be isolated in association with groupable streptococci. The organism is susceptible to penicillin and erythromycin, but data fail to demonstrate its routine eradication following therapy. Clinically, disease typically is associated with tonsillopharyngitis. Exudates or membranes may be noted, and the disease may mimic diphtheria in this regard. Several days after throat complaints, a rash develops in 40% to 50% of patients that may be urticarial or scarlatiniform and can also be confused with a drug eruption. A toxin produced by *C. hemolyticum* is thought to be the cause of rash. Relapse may occur, and optimal therapy is unknown.

*Neisseria gonorrhoeae*
Gonococcal pharyngitis is an important consideration in all persons who are sexually active and is statistically correlated with oral sex. It has been best described in prostitutes, service men, and male homosexuals. In high-risk populations, positive cultures may be noted in up to 6% of patients. Documentation requires culturing on special media under carbon dioxide; thus, routine cultures for group A β-hemolytic streptococci will fail to isolate this pathogen. Disease is often asymptomatic but may be associated with erythema or exudate. Lymphadenitis and constitutional symptoms are uncommon. However, the pharynx may still serve as a nidus for disseminated disease. Therapy with 250 mg of ceftriaxone IM as a single dose is effective and should usually be accompanied by therapy for chlamydial infection. Spectinomycin may not be effective for pharyngeal gonococcal infection.

*Corynebacterium diphtheriae*
Currently, fewer than five cases of diphtheria are reported in the United States annually. In several outbreaks noted in the 1970s, disease occurred almost entirely in nonimmunized populations. The organism is noninvasive, and most morbidity and mortality is associated with complications resulting from toxin production. The disease should be suspected in patients representing populations unlikely to have been immunized: selected religious sects, immigrants from Third World countries, and people of lower socioeconomic status. Clinical presentation generally involves the upper respiratory tract. Seropurulent nasal discharge may be noted in the absence of pharyngeal complaints. Pharyngitis may occur and is associated with exudative or membranous changes that involve the soft palate and uvula. Onset is often rapid and in the early stage resembles other forms of exudative pharyngitis. Within days, a membrane forms, which turns from white to dark. Extent of membrane correlates with severity of disease, which may involve the larynx and trachea.

Antimicrobial therapy with penicillin or erythromycin is preferred and probably limits the spread of disease and aids in terminating toxin production. Standard doses of antimicrobial agents are employed for 14 days, and patients require strict isolation until cultures are proved negative on several occasions. Patients identified as carriers should also be treated, although eradication may be difficult.

The mainstay of therapy is diphtheria antitoxin, a horse-derived hyperimmune antiserum. It should be administered early in management, generally in doses of 20,000 to 100,000 U IM or IV, depending on the extent, severity, and duration of disease.

*Nonbacterial Potentially Treatable Pathogens*
*Mycoplasma pneumoniae* and *Chlamydia pneumoniae* have been associated with pharyngitis, although it is generally unlikely that the clinician will make a specific etiologic determination. A recent investigation suggests that almost 10% of patients with sore throat will harbor *M. pneumoniae,* and a similar percentage (8%) was associated with *C. pneumoniae.* Infections with both were more common than infection with *S. pyogenes.* Cases of *M. pneumoniae* and *C. pneumoniae* infection could not be clinically differentiated from those caused by *S. pyogenes,* and about 33% demonstrated pharyngeal exudates. Although lower respiratory infection, such as pneumonia, has been associated with both *M. pneumoniae* and *C. pneumoniae,* pharyngitis may be the sole manifestation of disease. Antibiotics active against these pathogens include the newer quinolones, erythromycin, clarithromycin, azithromycin, and tetracyclines. However, clinical experience is limited, and these agents may not affect the length of disease or likelihood of complications. Additionally, quinolones should generally not

be employed in patients less than 18 years old, and quinolones and tetracyclines may not be satisfactory agents for disease associated with *S. pyogenes.*

*Viral Pathogens*
Viruses, including EBV, cytomegalovirus (CMV), HIV, adenovirus, herpes simplex virus, coxsackievirus, and respiratory syncytial virus, have been implicated in tonsillopharyngitis in adults. In most instances, the diagnosis becomes one of exclusion. EBV and adenovirus are often associated with pharyngeal exudate, and infection with these agents can mimic bacterial disease. EBV may be associated with other clinical manifestations, and a CBC can provide useful information. In up to 50% of cases, EBV pharyngitis can be complicated by infection with *S. pyogenes,* and in the presence of EBV infection, many clinicians associate severe pharyngitis with the presence of both pathogens. Gram's stain and culture of pharyngeal exudate often can clarify the situation. When EBV or CMV is considered, neither ampicillin nor amoxicillin should be employed because of the risk for severe dermatitis. This feature is the result of a toxic rather than an allergic reaction to the antimicrobial agents. Thus, use of these products after clinical recovery is not contraindicated.

Herpes simplex virus and coxsackievirus are often associated with oral vesicular or ulcerative eruptions. The former most commonly involves the anterior mouth, whereas the latter is more commonly located posteriorly. Ulcerative or vesicular lesions are uncommon with bacterial infections, and their presence should make the clinician suspect a virus or another process, such as oral erythema multiforme.

## Summary of Evaluation and Treatment
Adults who present with a complaint of sore throat should undergo a thorough history and physical examination to identify epidemiologic features that may help identify etiology. Risk factors for HIV and a sexual history should be obtained. Information about outbreaks of streptococcal disease may be available from local health departments. Acute onset associated with pharyngeal exudates, anterior cervical adenopathy, and fever is commonly associated with *S. pyogenes* infection, and therapy based on these findings is reasonable. When available, a Gram's stain of pharyngeal exudate can provide immediate practical information to guide initial antimicrobial decision making. In the consideration of *S. pyogenes* pharyngitis, a rapid strep test should be performed. If the result is negative, a specimen should be sent for cultural confirmation. Patients with risk factors for *N. gonorrhoeae* infection should be appropriately cultured. Adolescents and young adults may be infected with EBV, *M. pneumoniae,* or *C. pneumoniae.* The first can be assessed by CBC or monospot, or both, whereas consideration of the other two agents (generally suspected by failure to respond to penicillin and lack of other identified pathogen) may necessitate empiric antimicrobial therapy. (R.B.B.)

## Bibliography
Bisno AI, et al. Diagnosis and management of group A streptococcal pharyngitis: a practice guideline. *Clin Infect Dis* 1997;25:574–583.
   *This document represents a comprehensive guide to the diagnosis and treatment of* S. pyogenes *pharyngitis. Recommendations for testing, choices of test, and therapeutic alternatives are provided. A comprehensive table depicting etiologic agents for pharyngitis is provided. The authors favor 10-day courses of therapy, despite the availability of data recommending shorter ones.*
Carroll K, Reimer L. Microbiology and laboratory diagnosis of upper respiratory tract infections. *Clin Infect Dis* 1996; 23:442–448.
   *The authors review the preferred methods for the diagnosis of several upper respiratory infections, including group A β-hemolytic streptococcal pharyngitis. They point out the pitfalls of diagnosis, which can include sampling error. They also review the indications and limitations of the rapid tests for detection of* S. pyogenes. *The usual laboratory is not geared for the routine diagnosis of unusual pathogens, and the clinician needs to communicate directly with laboratory personnel if these are suspected to be present.*
Crawford G, Brancato F, Holmes KK. Streptococcal pharyngitis: diagnosis by Gram stain. *Ann Intern Med* 1979;90:293–297.

*In the hands of persons experienced in interpreting Gram's stains, this method provided excellent early information for the diagnosis of streptococcal pharyngitis. The authors note that patients with other diagnoses (C. hemolyticum, Vincent's angina) can also be identified in a similar manner. This inexpensive and rapid test should be utilized in patients with exudative pharyngitis, as it can provide useful information for a variety of etiologies.*

Hofer C, Binns HJ, Tanz RR. Strategies for managing group A streptococcal pharyngitis. A survey of board-certified pediatricians. *Arch Pediatr Adolesc Med* 1997; 151:824–829.

*The authors received responses to a survey of 510 pediatricians. Only 42% routinely employed both a rapid strep test and culture, and fewer than 30% routinely discontinued antibiotics if results of tests for S. pyogenes were negative. Penicillin or a derivative was employed as standard therapy by the vast majority of respondents.*

Krober MS, Bass JW, Michels GN. Streptococcal pharyngitis. Placebo-controlled double-blind evaluation of clinical response to penicillin therapy. *JAMA* 1985;253:1271–1274.

*Although penicillin treatment for group A β-hemolytic streptococcal pharyngitis has been recommended for many years, its efficacy in producing clinical improvement has been debated. This well-performed study in children is one of just a few in the literature documenting that early administration of penicillin is associated with enhanced clinical improvement when compared with placebo.*

Miller RA, Brancato F, Holmes KK. *Corynebacterium hemolyticum* as a cause of pharyngitis and scarlatiniform rash in young adults. *Ann Intern Med* 1986;105:867–872.

*In this investigation, 0.4% of throat cultures yielded C. hemolyticum (compared with 8.3% for S. pyogenes). Most cases occurred in patients 10 to 20 years old, and about 50% of cases were associated with bilateral cervical lymphadenopathy. Most patients demonstrated a rash that was often pruritic. Gram's stain of pharyngeal exudate often allowed a presumptive diagnosis, but ancillary tests were generally of little value. Penicillin or erythromycin appeared to accelerate clinical improvement.*

Pichichero ME, Cohen R. Shortened course of antibiotic therapy for acute otitis media, sinusitis, and tonsillopharyngitis. *Pediatr Infect Dis J* 1997;16:680–695.

*The authors review available data regarding courses of therapy considered shorter than standard for three common upper respiratory infections. For tonsillopharyngitis, numerous studies have compared various agents with classic 10-day penicillin treatment. Although many are associated with equivalent clinical outcomes, penicillin treatment for less than 10 days does not satisfactorily eradicate the organism. Several cephalosporins and macrolides do appear to be equivalent in both clinical and microbiologic outcomes.*

---

## 2. SINUSITIS

---

Sinusitis presents a number of diagnostic and therapeutic problems to the clinician. The classic features of the disease—fever, purulent nasal discharge, facial pain and tenderness—may be absent. It is often difficult to differentiate a viral upper respiratory infection from a superimposed bacterial sinusitis requiring antimicrobial therapy. There are no simple diagnostic tests available to establish the diagnosis, and the sinus radiographs may be confusing at times. Laboratory confirmation of the etiologic agent is also difficult to obtain without an invasive procedure. Because the throat or nasal swab cultures are generally misleading in a patient with sinusitis (sinus aspirations are not routinely performed), empiric antimicrobial therapy is usually initiated.

Sinusitis is a common disorder, occurring from the first year of life. About 11.6 million office visits are made for sinusitis yearly in the United States. Infection occurs most often in the maxillary sinus and rarely in the sphenoid sinus. The opening of the maxillary sinus is located on the upper part of the medial wall of the sinus, and as a result, the maxillary sinus does not drain by gravity in the upright position. The close relationship of the sinuses to the orbits, frontal and maxillary bones, and intracranial structures easily explains the potentially life-threatening complications that can result from either contiguous spread or hematogenous dissemination of infection from the sinuses. Complications of sinusitis include orbital cellulitis, subperiosteal abscess, orbital abscess, frontal (Pott's puffy tumor) and maxillary osteomyelitis, subdural abscess, cavernous sinus thrombosis, meningitis, and brain abscess. The most common complication is periorbital swelling resulting from impaired venous drainage, which can occur with maxillary or ethmoid sinusitis.

Obstruction of the sinus ostia by anatomic causes, such as a nasal foreign body or vascular congestion secondary to a viral upper respiratory infection, or by allergic rhinitis can result in an alteration of the local flora and sinusitis. Sinusitis can also occur when local host defenses are impaired, as in patients with the immotile cilia syndrome. About 10% of adult patients have maxillary sinusitis with a dental source—the extension of a periapical abscess of an upper tooth directly to the maxillary sinus. Sinusitis can be caused by diving into a pool or by barotrauma. In a hospitalized patient with a nasotracheal or nasogastric tube, sinusitis should be considered as a possible occult source of unexplained fever. One small series noted sinusitis in about 25% of patients who underwent nasotracheal intubation for 5 days or longer. In the majority of patients in whom sinusitis develops, however, a preceding viral upper respiratory infection or, less often, a history of allergic rhinitis can be elicited.

The etiologic agents involved in acute sinusitis are similar to those in acute otitis media. Aspiration of the maxillary sinuses has shown that *Streptococcus pneumoniae* and *Haemophilus influenzae* are responsible for just over half of the cases. The *H. influenzae* strains are usually nontypeable, and 17% to 68% produce β-lactamase. About 20% or more of the cases in children, depending on the cultural methods, are caused by *Moraxella (Branhamella) catarrhalis,* an organism that is almost always β-lactamase-positive. Other organisms recovered from the sinuses of patients with acute infection include anaerobes, *Staphylococcus aureus,* and *Streptococcus pyogenes* (group A). Viruses account for about 10% to 20% of the cases. Gram-negative rods, such as *Pseudomonas* species, are the most frequent cause of nosocomial sinusitis. Anaerobes are isolated more often in patients with associated dental disease and in those with chronic sinusitis. A variety of anaerobes, such as anaerobic streptococci and *Bacteroides* species, can be found in half of the patients with chronic sinusitis. *Pseudomonas aeruginosa* and *H. influenzae* are the predominant organisms found in patients with acute maxillary sinusitis and cystic fibrosis. The possibility of fungal infection caused by *Mucor* species, *Aspergillus* species, or *Pseudoallescheria boydii* should be considered when a diabetic patient, a renal transplant recipient, or patient with acute leukemia presents with acute illness, usually maxillary or ethmoid sinusitis. Rhinocerebral mucormycosis results from extension of the fungi from the sinuses to the orbit, meninges, and frontal lobes of the brain.

The presenting features of maxillary sinusitis can include nasal discharge, which is usually purulent; facial pain; impaired sense of smell; and sense of fullness of the sinus. Only half of children and adults with maxillary sinusitis will be febrile, but a nasal discharge is generally present. In children, a cough, nasal discharge, and fetid breath are frequently present. Facial pain and headache are major complaints in older children. Patients can have pus in the sinuses and still be asymptomatic. A clue to the diagnosis of acute sinusitis is an unusually severe or protracted "cold" (persisting beyond 10 days). Sphenoid sinusitis is frequently misdiagnosed and should be considered in patients with a severe headache, fever, purulent nasal discharge, and paresthesias of cranial nerve V. Facial tenderness, periorbital swelling, and pus on rhinoscopy may be present, but in the majority of patients, the physical examination is not helpful in establishing the diagnosis of acute sinusitis.

A variety of diagnostic tests are available to help confirm the diagnosis of sinusitis: transillumination, radiography, ultrasonography, computed axial tomography (CAT), magnetic resonance imaging (MRI), and sinus endoscopy. Routine sinus radiographs are obtained most often, and the presence of an air-fluid level, complete opacification, or 4 mm or more of mucosal thickening correlates with a positive sinus aspirate in 75% of patients. Sinus x-ray studies are of value in persons over 1 year of age, but findings are often abnormal in those under 1 year of age without a history to suggest acute sinusitis. CT is the noninvasive modality of choice to evaluate the sinuses. A limited

CT scan (5-mm slices) of the sinuses is a cost-effective study comparable in price with plain sinus radiography. Sinus endoscopy is recommended for patients with recurrent acute and chronic sinusitis. Determination of the bacteriology of sinusitis requires that sinus secretions be obtained directly from the sinus by needle aspiration. Unfortunately, nose, throat, and nasopharyngeal cultures do not predict the etiology of the sinusitis well in comparison with sinus aspiration cultures. Indications for sinus aspiration are (a) nosocomial sinusitis, (b) sinusitis in an immunocompromised host, (c) sinusitis in a severely ill patient, and (d) failure of the sinus infection to respond to several courses of antimicrobial therapy. Aspiration of the maxillary sinus can be performed safely in patients 2 years of age or older. The presence of a normal sinus flora is controversial. One small study recovered both anaerobic and aerobic organisms by obtaining sinus aspirates from normal sinuses.

Sinusitis should be considered as a cause of unexplained fever in patients with acute leukemia or HIV disease. The clinical presentation is often subtle. *Aspergillus* is a frequent pathogen in patients with acute leukemia. Approximately 75% of patients with HIV disease have a diffuse sinus infection with a median of six sinuses affected. The etiology of the sinus disease in patients with HIV infection remains unclear. For patients with a presumed sinus infection who fail to respond to conventional antimicrobial therapy, consideration should be given to aspirating the sinus. If the aspirate is nondiagnostic, a mucosal biopsy is indicated. Further information from a prospective study is needed to define the etiology better and determine an appropriate treatment of sinusitis in patients with HIV infection.

Because sinus aspirates are not routinely performed, antimicrobial therapy of this disease is usually empirically based on the bacteriology from previous studies. The antimicrobial agents selected should be at least adequate for *S. pneumoniae* and *H. influenzae. M. catarrhalis* appears to have an increasing role in this disease. Ampicillin, amoxicillin, amoxicillin-clavulanic acid, azithromycin, cefaclor, cefuroxime axetil, cefprozil, ciprofloxacin, clarithromycin, doxycycline, levofloxacin, loracarbef, and trimethoprim-sulfamethoxazole (TMP-SMX) are acceptable and show comparable efficacy.

There is no antimicrobial agent of choice for the therapy of acute sinusitis. The presence of a penicillin allergy, the prevalence of penicillin-resistant *H. influenzae* and *M. catarrhalis,* the frequency and nature of adverse effects, and drug cost are important factors to consider. Amoxicillin appears to be the preferred drug to initiate treatment of a patient with acute sinusitis. Amoxicillin-clavulanic acid, azithromycin, cefaclor, cefprozil, cefuroxime axetil, ciprofloxacin, clarithromycin, doxycycline, levofloxacin, loracarbef, and TMP-SMX are suitable alternative therapeutic agents. TMP-SMX is ineffective in patients with group A streptococcal infections. The optimal duration of therapy is unknown, but 10 to 14 days is conventional for acute disease.

Although controlled studies are lacking, establishing drainage with topical or oral decongestants is important. The best decongestant is steam. Decongestants, however, inhibit ciliary motion, an important local defense mechanism. Antihistamines should be avoided; they tend to thicken sinus secretions and impair drainage. Topical corticosteroids help reduce edema and are useful for patients with allergic rhinitis and chronic sinusitis. Guaifenesin has a limited role in thinning secretions. Analgesics are indicated, and any underlying predisposing factors should be corrected. Irrigation and surgical drainage are usually reserved for patients who fail to respond to conventional therapy. It is reasonable to try an alternative antimicrobial agent, such as amoxicillin-clavulanic acid, azithromycin, cefaclor, cefuroxime axetil, clarithromycin, cefprozil, ciprofloxacin, doxycycline, levofloxacin, or loracarbef, if a patient fails to respond to a course of amoxicillin.

The optimal therapy for chronic sinusitis is unknown, but amoxicillin and clindamycin are reasonable drugs with which to initiate therapy. If the patient fails to respond to therapy, then other disorders, such as Wegener's granulomatosis or neoplastic disease, should be investigated. (N.M.G.)

## Bibliography

Axelsson A, Runze U. Comparison of subjective and radiological findings during the course of acute maxillary sinusitis. *Ann Otol Rhinol Laryngol* 1983;92:75.
   *Radiographic improvement lags the clinical course.*

Bert F, Lambert-Zechovsky N. Sinusitis in mechanically ventilated patients and its role in the pathogenesis of nosocomial pneumonia. *Eur J Clin Microbiol Infect Dis* 1996;15:533–544.
*Sinusitis is a cause of occult fever in intubated ICU patients.*
Bluestone CD, Steiner RE. Intracranial complications of acute frontal sinusitis. *South Med J* 1965;58:1.
*Classic description of neurologic complications of acute frontal sinusitis.*
Brook I. Bacteriology of chronic maxillary sinusitis in adults. *Ann Otol Rhinol Laryngol* 1989;98:426.
*Anaerobes were isolated in 88% of adults with chronic sinusitis.*
Chandler JR, Langenbrunner DJ, Stevens ER. The pathogenesis of orbital complications in acute sinusitis. *Laryngoscope* 1970;80:1414.
*Orbital complications with vision loss may result from sinusitis.*
DeShazo RD, Chapin K, Swain RE. Fungal sinusitis. *N Engl J Med* 1997;337:254.
*Aspergillus is the most common cause of fungal sinusitis. Noninvasive disease (e.g., allergy or mycetoma) must be distinguished from invasive disease.*
Evans FO Jr, et al. Sinusitis of the maxillary antrum. *N Engl J Med* 1975;293:735.
*Results of nasal swab cultures correlated poorly with those of direct sinus aspirate cultures.*
Ferguson MA, Todd JK. Toxic shock syndrome associated with *Staphylococcus aureus* sinusitis in children. *J Infect Dis* 1990;161:953.
*A possible site for* S. aureus *infection in a patient with toxic shock syndrome.*
Frederick J, Braude AI. Anaerobic infection of the paranasal sinuses. *N Engl J Med* 1974;290:135.
*Classic article. Anaerobes are an important cause of chronic sinusitis.*
Giebink GS. Criteria for evaluation of antimicrobial agents and current therapies for acute sinusitis in children. *Clin Infect Dis* 1992;14 (Suppl 2):S212.
*Criteria for clinical and microbiologic evaluation are presented.*
Godofsky EW, et al. Sinusitis in HIV-infected patients: a clinical and radiographic review. *Am J Med* 1992;93:163.
*MRI or CT was more sensitive than plain radiography. Half of the patients had persistent or recurrent disease.*
Gwaltney JM Jr. Acute community-acquired sinusitis. *Clin Infect Dis* 1996; 23:1209–1225.
*Review. About 60% of cases of acute sinusitis are caused by bacteria; in 15% of cases, viruses are isolated.*
Gwaltney JM Jr, Sydnor A Jr, Sande MA. Etiology and antimicrobial treatment of acute sinusitis. *Ann Otol Rhinol Laryngol* 1081;90:68.
*The presence of an air-fluid level on x-ray film correlates with a positive culture in 89% of patients; with opacity, the yield is 56%.*
Hamory BH, et al. Etiology and antimicrobial therapy of acute maxillary sinusitis. *J Infect Dis* 1979;139:197.
S. pneumoniae *and* H. influenzae *accounted for 64% of the isolates.*
Humphrey MA, Simpson GT, Grindlinger GA. Clinical characteristics of nosocomial sinusitis. *Ann Otol Rhinol Laryngol* 1987;96:687.
*In 90% of patients, the infection was polymicrobial. (For a discussion noting that the infection is often clinically obscure in the ICU setting, see also Caplan ES, Hoyt NJ. Nosocomial sinusitis.* JAMA *1982;247:639.)*
Kennedy DW, Senior BA. Endoscopic sinus surgery. A review. *Otolaryngol Clin North Am* 1997;30:313–330.
*A favorable outcome was noted in 85% of patients having endoscopic sinus surgery for infection.*
Lawson W, Reino A. Isolated sphenoid sinus disease: an analysis of 132 cases. *Laryngoscope* 1997;107:1590–1595.
*Isolated sphenoid sinus disease had an infectious etiology in 61% and was caused by a benign or malignant tumor in 29%. Cranial nerve defects were noted in 12% of infectious cases and 60% of neoplasms.*
Lehrer RI, et al. Mucormycosis. *Ann Intern Med* 1980;93:93.
*Ketoacidotic diabetics are predisposed to rhinocerebral mucormycosis.*

Lew D, et al. Sphenoid sinusitis. *N Engl J Med* 1983;309:1149.
*Often unsuspected. An intense unilateral, frontal, or occipital headache occurs. Neurologic complications such as cavernous sinus thrombosis and meningitis can be life-threatening.*

McAlister WH, Lusk R, Muntz HR. Comparison of plain radiographs and coronal CT scans in infants and children with recurrent sinusitis. *AJR Am J Roentgenol* 1989; 153:1259.
*CT scans are superior to plain radiographs in establishing the diagnosis.*

Mofenson LM, et al. Sinusitis in children infected with human immunodeficiency virus: clinical characteristics, risk factors, and prophylaxis. *Clin Infect Dis* 1995; 21:1175–1181.
*Sinusitis in HIV-infected children is most often subacute and recurrent, with nasal discharge and cough common. Fever is usually absent.*

Nord CE. The role of anaerobic bacteria in recurrent episodes of sinusitis and tonsillitis. *Clin Infect Dis* 1995;20:1512–1524.
*Most cases of chronic sinusitis are caused by anaerobes.*

Remmler D, Boles R. Intracranial complications of frontal sinusitis. *Laryngoscope* 1980;90:1814.
*Subdural empyema is the most frequent complication of frontal sinusitis.*

Savage DG, et al. Paranasal sinusitis following allogeneic bone marrow transplant. *Bone Marrow Transplant* 1997;19:55–59.
*Sinusitis occurred in more than one third of patients after an allogeneic bone marrow transplant.*

Senior BA, et al. Long-term results of functional endoscopic sinus surgery. *Laryngoscope* 1998;108:151–157.
*At the 7-year follow-up, most (98%) patients after endoscopic sinus surgery were improved and did not require further surgery.*

Shapiro ED, et al. Bacteriology of the maxillary sinuses in patients with cystic fibrosis. *J Infect Dis* 1982;146:589.
*P. aeruginosa was isolated most commonly.*

Talmor M, Li P, Barie PS. Acute paranasal sinusitis in critically ill patients: guidelines for prevention, diagnosis, and treatment. *Clin Infect Dis* 1997;25:1441–1446.
*Nosocomial sinusitis occurs in 18% to 32% of endotracheally intubated patients and is usually caused by gram-negative bacilli or is polymicrobial.*

vanBuchem FL, et al. Primary-care-based randomised placebo-controlled trial of antibiotic treatment in acute maxillary sinusitis. *Lancet* 1997;349:683–687.
*In patients with mild acute maxillary sinusitis, amoxicillin was not better than placebo in improving the outcome of the disease.*

Wald ER. Sinusitis in children. *N Engl J Med* 1992;326:319.
*Review.*

Wald ER. Chronic sinusitis in children. *J Pediatr* 1995;127:339–347.
*Chronic sinusitis caused by infection is uncommon in children; persistent nasal symptoms are often caused by allergy.*

Wald ER, et al. Acute maxillary sinusitis in children. *N Engl J Med* 1981;304:749.
*Classic study in children. Cough and nasal symptoms occur most often. Only half of children had fever initially.*

Wald ER, et al. Subacute sinusitis in children. *J Pediatr* 1989;115:28.
*Similar clinical presentation (nasal discharge, cough), etiology, and radiographic findings as in acute disease.*

Wald ER, et al. Treatment of acute maxillary sinusitis in childhood: a comparative study of amoxicillin and cefaclor. *J Pediatr* 1984;104:297.
*Approximately 80% cure rates with amoxicillin or cefaclor when 40 mg/kg per day was administered in three divided doses.*

Williams JW Jr, et al. Clinical evaluation for sinusitis. *Ann Intern Med* 1992;117:105.
*Best predictors of sinusitis include maxillary toothache, abnormal transillumination, poor response to nasal decongestants, colored nasal discharge, and mucopurulence on examination.*

Williams JW Jr, Holleman DR Jr, Samsa GP. Randomized controlled trial of 3 vs 10 days of trimethoprim/sulfamethoxazole for acute maxillary sinusitis. *JAMA* 1995; 273:1015–1021.
*A 3-day course of TMP-SMX plus oxymetazoline was as effective as a 10-day course of the same drug in patients with mild sinusitis.*
Zurlo JJ, et al. Sinusitis in HIV1 infection. *Am J Med* 1992;93:157.
*Sinusitis is often (25%) asymptomatic in patients with HIV infection.*

## 3. INFECTIOUS MONONUCLEOSIS: MANY FACES OF A COMMON DISEASE

Infectious mononucleosis caused by the Epstein-Barr virus (EBV) is a common disease, most commonly noted in children and adolescents. Presentation is age-dependent. Clinical expression is most often seen in adolescents or young adults, whereas subclinical disease occurs frequently in younger children. Older persons may have subtle, primarily constitutional presentations. Recent advances in serologic testing for infectious mononucleosis have demonstrated an enlarging spectrum of disease caused by this virus. For instance, 5% to 10% of patients with typical illness test negatively for heterophil antibodies but have positive EBV-specific test results. The classic syndrome of infectious mononucleosis includes fever, atypical lymphocytosis, lymphadenopathy, pharyngitis, and heterophil positivity in the adolescent and generally poses few clinical difficulties. However, many unusual presentations of EBV-related disease exist that may pose difficult diagnostic problems. These can be seen primarily in young children and adults. The following discussion focuses on atypical manifestations of this disease, summarized in Table 3-1, which also provides an overview of many of the uncommon presentations. An understanding of these syndromes can prevent both unnecessary diagnostic evaluations and the unneeded prescription of medications.

### Serologic Testing for Epstein-Barr Virus
Because approximately 90% to 95% of cases of infectious mononucleosis can be diagnosed by standard heterophil antibody testing, more specific serologic evaluations are needed infrequently. EBV-specific testing is indicated mainly when infectious mononucleosis is clinically suspected but results of heterophil antibody testing are negative, or when the presentation is atypical and the diagnosis of infectious mononucleosis is suspected. IgM antibodies to viral capsid antigen appear early in the course of disease and persist for only several months. Thus, a positive test result, combined with the presence of IgG and the absence of EBV nuclear antigens, confirms acute disease. IgG antibodies to the same antigen peak early in the course of disease, and therefore it may be difficult to demonstrate a change in titer. Because of lifelong persistence of this antibody, positivity on a single test does not imply acute disease. Antibodies to Epstein-Barr nuclear antigen appear late in the course of infectious mononucleosis and persist indefinitely. This test is most useful as an epidemiologic tool and cannot define acute disease.

### Hematologic Manifestations
Up to 3% of patients with infectious mononucleosis manifest hematologic abnormalities that can involve any primary marrow component. In most instances, problems arise during weeks 2 to 4 of illness and thus complicate a more classic presentation. However, occasional patients present with primarily hematologic complaints; more usual components of infectious mononucleosis have either not occurred or have been overlooked. Hemolytic anemia is the most commonly recognized abnormality and is usually caused by the presence of IgM cold agglutinins with anti-i specificity. Hemolysis may be severe and life-threatening and may require administration of corticosteroids. Thrombocytopenia may also be noted but rarely reaches critical levels. However, cases with platelet levels below 1,000/mm$^3$ have been reported, and bleeding complications may occur. In

Table 3-1.  Unusual manifestations of infectious mononucleosis

| Hematologic | Neurologic |
|---|---|
| Hemolytic anemia | Guillain-Barré syndrome |
| Neutropenia | Cranial nerve palsy |
| Thrombocytopenia | Radiculopathy |
| **Gastrointestinal** | Encephalitis |
| Hepatitis | Aseptic meningitis |
| Jaundice | Transverse myelitis |
| Splenomegaly | **Cardiopulmonary** |
| Splenic rupture | Interstitial pneumonitis |
| **Rheumatologic** | Myocarditis |
| Arthralgia | Pericarditis |
| Arthritis | **Renal** |
| Myalgia | Acute oliguric renal failure |
| **Dermatologic** | Interstitial nephritis |
| Maculopapular rash | |
| Petechiae | |

most instances, thrombocytopenia is caused by peripheral destruction of platelets rather than primary marrow hypoproduction, and both corticosteroids and splenectomy have been used therapeutically. Neutropenia and absolute granulocytopenia have been reported. Clinical problems related to this are rare, and counts generally return to normal within 5 to 21 days. However, the absence of granulocytes has occasionally proved fatal. In most cases, bone marrow evaluation reveals maturation arrest, possibly caused by a toxic effect of the virus. Recent investigations of aplastic anemia and agranulocytosis have demonstrated an unexpected, statistically important relationship between a history of infectious mononucleosis at least 1 year previously and the presence of agranulocytosis (but not aplastic anemia). Reasons for this are unclear at the present.

## Gastrointestinal Manifestations

Subclinical elevations of hepatic enzymes occur in at least 50% of patients with infectious mononucleosis and can be considered part of the normal course of this illness. Severe jaundice that may be associated with icteric hepatitis can be the presenting complaint. Recent anecdotal reports demonstrate cases that have progressed to fulminant hepatic failure. Other cases of jaundice with clinically milder disease probably represent a combination of hemolysis and hepatitis. Maximum levels of serum bilirubin reported have been 38.5 mg/dL. Prompt response to corticosteroids was noted. Clinical and laboratory manifestations mimicking viral hepatitis may also denote this disease, making other viral diseases the major diagnostic considerations. Cases of acute hepatitis secondary to EBV infection are usually associated with complete recovery. Cases progressing to chronicity have been documented. Hepatitis caused by EBV should be suspected when alternative diagnoses have been ruled out.

Splenomegaly occurs regularly in uncomplicated infectious mononucleosis and rarely poses clinical problems. Rupture of this organ is well documented and represents the most common cause of death from EBV infection. Rupture most often occurs during weeks 2 and 3 and may be the primary manifestation of infectious mononucleosis. Abdominal pain may herald this complication and probably represents the presence of subcapsular hematoma. Rupture secondary to bleeding may also be a consequence of severe thrombocytopenia but more commonly is associated with trauma. Initial presentation of rupture may be hypovolemic shock, but abdominal pain and a more subacute course are the rule. If rupture is suspected, emergent splenectomy is generally recommended.

Patients with significant splenomegaly should be cautioned about injury.

**Rheumatologic Manifestations**

Vague arthralgias and myalgias may be noted during the course of uncomplicated infectious mononucleosis but rarely are of clinical significance. True arthritis is rare, but at least one review demonstrated polyarthritis in up to 50% of patients studied. Disease was always self-limited.

**Neurologic Manifestations**

Neurologic dysfunction may be noted either as a primary manifestation of EBV disease or as a complication of classic infectious mononucleosis. Common syndromes include (a) aseptic meningitis, (b) Guillain-Barré syndrome, (c) transverse myelitis, (d) Bell's palsy, (e) cerebellar meningoencephalitis, and (f) other focal cranial nerve palsies. In general, patients who present with manifestations such as these and have no other diagnosis should be evaluated for infectious mononucleosis. Recent retrospective investigations of EBV disease in children also demonstrate the clinical presentations of combative behavior, seizures, and severe headache. Clinical manifestations of these may be noted at any time during the course of EBV infection. In up to 7% of cases of EBV-related infection, a neurologic syndrome may either herald or be the sole sign of disease. More often, however, central nervous system manifestations occur in conjunction with more characteristic forms of disease, but clinical documentation may prove elusive. Historically, most authorities have felt that complete neurologic recovery could be anticipated. However, recent investigations in children suggest that approximately 40% may demonstrate neurologic sequelae at long-term follow-up. These include global impairment, autistic behavior, and limb paresis.

Aseptic meningitis is the most common central nervous system abnormality associated with infectious mononucleosis and has been reported in up to 25% of patients. Often, the patient is free of central nervous system-related complaints. Lymphocytic pleocytosis with normal cerebrospinal fluid glucose levels is most commonly noted, and atypical lymphocytes may be seen.

In a prospective investigation designed to assess the role of EBV in neurologic diseases, 7 of 24 persons with Guillain-Barré syndrome and 3 of 16 with Bell's palsy demonstrated serologic evidence of acute infection with EBV. This study also demonstrated that many of these persons had no other evidence of infectious mononucleosis and that several had negative results on heterophil agglutination tests.

A number of investigations have depicted the role of EBV as a cause of meningoencephalitis and have documented its capacity to cause primarily an acute cerebellar syndrome. More global forms of encephalitis may also be noted, and seizures have been described. In some instances, routine heterophil agglutination test results have been negative, with atypical lymphocytes present at nondiagnostic levels.

**Dermatologic Manifestations**

Skin disorders in infectious mononucleosis are noted in fewer than 5% of patients. A severe maculopapular eruption with hemorrhage may be noted in 60% to 80% of patients with infectious mononucleosis who receive ampicillin or amoxicillin. This response is toxic rather than allergic and does not contraindicate the future use of these agents. A single case of solitary penile ulcer has been reported with infectious mononucleosis, but the relationship is uncertain.

**Cardiopulmonary Manifestations**

Symptomatic cardiac disease with infectious mononucleosis is unusual. However, both myocarditis and pericarditis have been demonstrated, usually in association with more classic presentations of the disease. The most commonly observed cardiac disturbance is nonspecific ST-T wave changes on electrocardiogram, noted in up to 6% of persons. Deaths are unusual.

Chronic interstitial pulmonary infiltrates associated with fever have been recently described in two patients following recovery from acute infectious mononucleosis. Both persons demonstrated continued viral replication and had a clinical response to acyclovir.

## Otorhinolaryngologic Manifestations

Ear, nose, and throat complaints in infectious mononucleosis are well documented. In one series of patients hospitalized with this disease, 55% had such problems. Findings included airway obstruction, peritonsillar abscess, sinusitis, and periorbital cellulitis. The latter two were more likely to have been secondary to bacterial complications than to EBV infection itself. Tonsillopharyngitis is commonly seen in classic infectious mononucleosis and must be differentiated from numerous other causes of this syndrome. A recent retrospective investigation of infectious mononucleosis in children demonstrated that approximately 50% of 60 patients with infectious mononucleosis complicated by tonsillopharyngitis had severe airway obstruction. Three required surgical intervention, and the remainder responded to systemic corticosteroids.

A common presentation of mononucleosis is tonsillopharyngitis, treated with ampicillin or amoxicillin, with resultant severe rash. Dramatic illness with dysphagia and "touching tonsils" should make the clinician consider streptococcal pharyngitis, even if the diagnosis of infectious mononucleosis has been confirmed. Most cases of airway obstruction are related to hypertrophy of the tissue comprising Waldeyer's ring. The cause of such obstruction was thought to be EBV-induced. If this and other ear, nose, and throat complications occur, a bacterial process should always be ruled out by suitable laboratory studies.

## Renal Manifestations

Involvement of the kidneys with infectious mononucleosis has been reported infrequently, and infectious mononucleosis generally has not been associated with symptomatic renal disease. A recent investigation reviewed 27 cases of infectious mononucleosis with symptomatic renal involvement and reported a case that resulted in oliguric renal failure requiring hemodialysis. Interstitial nephritis was seen on renal biopsy specimens. Recovery was associated with the use of corticosteroids and acyclovir.

## Epstein-Barr Virus in Older Patients

Although cases of infectious mononucleosis in adults over 30 years of age have historically been felt to comprise less than 3% of cases, recent investigations suggest that this is an underestimate. Infectious mononucleosis may be overlooked in older persons because of its historic association with younger people and the higher likelihood of atypical presentation. Disease in older persons is well described and may be acquired either parenterally (e.g., blood transfusions) or by less obvious means. Fever and fatigability may be the sole clinical manifestations. Splenomegaly, lymphadenopathy, and pharyngitis occur much less frequently than in younger persons. The time course of disease in older persons may be more prolonged, perhaps related to a higher degree of hepatic dysfunction. Fever may be substantially more prolonged (13 days in adults vs. 7 days in adolescents), and peak WBC counts may be lower ($6,600/mm^3$ in adults vs. $11,000/mm^3$ in adolescents). Usually, typical serologic manifestations and atypical lymphocytosis are noted, although the latter may be demonstrable only on serial testing. Infectious mononucleosis in patients over 40 years of age should be suspected when individuals present with fever and malaise even if other classic features are absent.

## Chronic Epstein-Barr Viral Syndrome

The role of EBV in patients suffering from chronic fatigue remains controversial. Although data have surfaced concerning the presence of chronic fatigue syndrome and its relationship to EBV infection, most recent studies fail to provide support for a relationship. Therapeutic trials with antiviral medications such as acyclovir have been unrewarding. Treatment remains primarily supportive.

## Therapy

The mainstay of management of infectious mononucleosis is supportive care coupled with careful observation for the occasional bacterial complication, primarily streptococcal pharyngitis. The role of corticosteroids remains controversial, and these agents are not indicated for the usual case. However, these agents, generally administered as 60 to 80 mg of prednisone daily for short periods, may be beneficial for the occasional patient with severe tonsillopharyngeal complications of EBV infection. A recent investigation suggests that this may preclude the need for surgical intervention. Rebound may occasionally be noted. Secondary infection with *Streptococcus pyogenes* must be ruled out. Corticosteroids are also occasionally utilized for severe thrombocytopenia. Acyclovir has been studied, with mixed results. Most patients did not demonstrate clinical or laboratory improvement when treated with this agent in comparison with those treated with placebo. A double-blinded, placebo-controlled trial of acyclovir plus prednisolone versus placebo demonstrated that EBV shedding was significantly reduced in the drug group, but that no clinical variables were favorably influenced. As noted above, a recent case of acute oliguric renal failure was successfully treated with acyclovir plus corticosteroids.

A recent double-blinded, placebo-controlled trial of ranitidine compared with placebo demonstrated only that liver enzymes returned to baseline more quickly in the drug-treated group ( $p = .03$ ). No other variables were influenced in a statistically significant manner. (R.B.B.)

## Bibliography

Andersson J, et al. Effect of acyclovir on infectious mononucleosis; a double-blind, placebo-controlled study. *J Infect Dis* 1986;153:283–290.
  *Thirty-one patients with infectious mononucleosis of short duration were randomized to receive acyclovir or placebo. Therapy reversibly inhibited oropharyngeal viral shedding but generally had no effect on individual symptoms or laboratory parameters. However, the authors conclude that cumulatively, patients who received acyclovir fared better. Acyclovir is not indicated for the usual patient with this disease; other studies may uncover a subset of severely ill patients who may benefit.*
Carter J, Edson RS, Kennedy CC. Infectious mononucleosis in the older patient. *Mayo Clin Proc* 1978;53:146–150.
  *In an early report of six patients over the age of 60 years with infectious mononucleosis, presentation was often primarily constitutional, without exudative pharyngitis. An awareness of the subtle presentation may disallow unnecessary diagnostic studies.*
Cheeseman S. Infectious mononucleosis. *Semin Hematol* 1988;25:261–268.
  *This excellent recent overview of the classic syndrome of infectious mononucleosis also contains brief discussions of issues related to diagnosis and treatment.*
Comachowske JB, et al. Acute manifestations and neurologic sequelae of Epstein-Barr virus encephalitis in children. *Pediatr Infect Dis J* 1997;16:871–875.
  *This retrospective analysis of 11 cases of infectious mononucleosis-associated encephalitis demonstrates the diversity of clinical presentations that may occur. Classic accompanying features are infrequently observed. Long-term sequelae are noted in about 40% of cases.*
Farley DR, et al. Spontaneous rupture of the spleen due to infectious mononucleosis. *Mayo Clin Proc* 1992;67:846–853.
  *This report reinforces the possibility of spontaneous nontraumatic splenic rupture as a life-threatening complication of infectious mononucleosis. Presentation is often one of acute abdominal pain, and emergent splenectomy remains the treatment of choice.*
Ghosh A, et al. Infectious mononucleosis hepatitis: report of two patients. *Indian J Gastroenterol* 1997;16:113–114.
  *Two patients in whom icteric hepatitis was associated with infectious mononucleosis are presented. One case was complicated by fulminant hepatic failure, and the patient died. Infectious mononucleosis-associated hepatitis should be suspected if other causes have been ruled out.*
Halevy J, Ash S. Infectious mononucleosis in hospitalized patients over forty years of age. *Am J Med Sci* 1988;295:122.
  *This investigation compares the clinical presentation of infectious mononucleosis in patients over the age of 40 years with that of a similar number of adolescents. The older persons were more likely to run a prolonged febrile course and have lower total WBC counts, and splenomegaly, lymphadenopathy, and pharyngitis were less likely to develop in these patients.*
Kirov SM, Marsden KA, Wongwanich S. Seroepidemiological study of infectious mononucleosis in older patients. *J Clin Microbiol* 1989;27:356–358.

*This Australian report documents a higher likelihood of noted infectious mononucleosis in older patients than is generally considered.*

Levy M, et al. Risk of agranulocytosis and aplastic anemia in relation to history of infectious mononucleosis: a report from the International Agranulocytosis and Aplastic Anemia Study. *Ann Hematol* 1993;67:187–190.

*A retrospective analysis of patients with either agranulocytosis or aplastic anemia was performed. Among those with agranulocytosis, 4% had a history of prior infectious mononucleosis. This was significantly different from controls. No association with aplastic anemia was identified.*

Madigan NP, et al. Intense jaundice in infectious mononucleosis. *Mayo Clin Proc* 1973;48:857–862.

*This represents a clinical report of the association of severe jaundice with infectious mononucleosis. Hemolysis plus hepatitis is the likely explanation. The presence of jaundice does not rule out infectious mononucleosis as the source of the problem.*

Mayer HB, et al. Epstein-Barr virus-induced infectious mononucleosis complicated by acute renal failure: case report and review. *Clin Infect Dis* 1996;22:1009–1018.

*A case of acute oliguric renal failure associated with Epstein-Barr virus is presented, and the related literature is reviewed. Twenty-seven cases of symptomatic renal disease have been published. Disease is generally self-limited. Severe cases appear to respond to treatment that includes corticosteroids and acyclovir.*

Schooley RT, Dolin R. Epstein-Barr virus (infectious mononucleosis). In: Mandell GL, Douglas RG, Bennett JE, eds. *Principles and practice of infectious diseases,* 3rd ed. New York: Churchill Livingstone, 1990:1172–1184.

*This chapter summarizes much information on the presentation and complications of infectious mononucleosis and provides a reasonable presentation of the entire clinical and virologic picture of the disease.*

Silverstein A, Steinberg G, Nathanson M. Nervous system involvement in infectious mononucleosis. *Arch Neurol* 1972;26:353–358.

*This investigation reports on 15 patients with documented infectious mononucleosis whose initial clinical presentation or heralding feature was neurologic. In six of these, the neurologic finding was the sole manifestation of illness. Findings included severe headache, seizures, paresis, cranial nerve palsies, and radiculopathy.*

Snyderman NL. Otorhinolaryngologic presentations of infectious mononucleosis. *Pediatr Clin North Am* 1981;28:1011–1016.

*This review focuses on ear, nose, and throat presentations of infectious mononucleosis. In many instances, the process may represent complications rather than the EBV infection itself.*

Straus SE, et al. Epstein-Barr virus infections: biology, pathogenesis, and management. *Ann Intern Med* 1993;118:45–58.

*This National Institutes of Health conference represents an excellent overview of many issues related to infection with EBV. It provides information concerning EBV serology, clinical manifestations, and molecular biology. Regarding management, the authors reinforce the need for supportive care and hedge on the role of corticosteroids. These agents may be of benefit for persons with severe tonsillopharyngeal symptoms caused by EBV, however.*

Tynell E, et al. Acyclovir and prednisolone treatment of acute infectious mononucleosis: a multi-center, double-blind, placebo-controlled study. *J Infect Dis* 1996;174:324–331.

*In a randomized placebo-controlled study of acute infectious mononucleosis, acyclovir plus prednisolone was used in the therapy arm. Ninety-four patients were identified. Therapy resulted in no clinical benefit but did inhibit oropharyngeal EBV replication. No effect was noted on later cellular immunity.*

# II. LOWER RESPIRATORY TRACT

# 4. ACUTE BRONCHITIS

Acute bronchitis, an inflammatory condition of the bronchi, refers to a clinical syndrome whose most distinctive hallmark is the recent onset of cough, which is usually productive. This disorder, occurs more frequently in the winter, is often preceded by headache, sore throat, and coryza, and is on occasion accompanied by fever and chest discomfort. Bronchitis is usually, but not exclusively, caused by a respiratory pathogen, predominantly a virus (rhinovirus, coronavirus, adenovirus, influenza virus) and less frequently a bacterium (*Mycoplasma pneumoniae, Chlamydia pneumoniae, Bordetella pertussis, Bordetella parapertussis, Legionella* species, *Streptococcus pneumoniae,* and *Haemophilus influenzae*). Neither the appearance of the sputum (purulence) nor the measurement of the white cell count is a reliable indicator of the cause of the acute bronchitis (viral vs. bacterial).

When wheezing, shortness of breath, and tightness of the chest occur, the disease can resemble an acute attack of asthma. In fact, when these symptoms of bronchospasm develop, patients often display spirometric evidence of reversible airway obstruction, and these cases are referred to as "adult acute asthmatic bronchitis." The symptoms of acute infectious bronchitis, when consisting of fever, chest discomfort, cough, and shortness of breath, can imitate those of infectious pneumonia, and chest radiography would then be required to distinguish precisely between acute bronchitis and pneumonia. The absence of fever and focal crackles suggests bronchitis rather than pneumonia.

The preponderance of evidence indicates that most healthy persons experience spontaneous resolution of bronchitis and do not sustain any sequelae. With rare exceptions (such as disease caused by influenza virus), the disease in these patients does not progress to pneumonia or cause irreversible anatomic abnormalities of the respiratory tract. In contrast, patients with HIV infection are at risk for having their disease evolve into bronchiectasis.

Neither blood nor sputum analyses appear to be indicated for the management of immunocompetent patients. There is also no convincing need to prescribe an antibiotic. For the nonpregnant patient with "presumed" influenza A bronchitis and symptoms for less than 48 hours, either amantadine (Symmetrel) or rimantadine (Flumadine) should be prescribed. Patients who experience insomnia from "bouts" of coughing can obtain symptomatic improvement from an antitussive, codeine-containing medication, and patients who have symptoms consistent with "adult acute asthmatic bronchitis" are candidates for inhaled bronchodilator therapy with albuterol. Studies have demonstrated the superiority of albuterol in comparison with erythromycin. The value of increasing fluid intake remains unknown.

Most physicians feel pressured to prescribe an antibiotic, as the public has the expectation of receiving a "magic bullet" to hasten the resolution of infection. Patients should be reassured that most infections are viral and will not respond to an antibiotic. In addition, physicians are concerned that some of these episodes of acute bronchitis are precipitated by *potentially* treatable organisms (*M. pneumoniae, C. pneumoniae, B. pertussis*), so that although there are no rapid, readily available ways, either clinical or laboratory-based, to distinguish among these etiologies, and although there are no convincing data that antibiotic treatment accelerates the resolution of symptoms of acute bronchitis caused by *M. pneumoniae* or *C. pneumoniae*, clinicians often elect to administer a course of an antimicrobial agent, such as erythromycin, clarithromycin, azithromycin, doxycycline, cefaclor, cefuroxime, loracarbef, or trimethoprim-sulfamethoxazole (TMP-SMX). That approach has no scientific foundation, adds to medical costs, fosters the emergence of resistant organisms, and contributes to drug toxicity, manifested as skin eruptions and gastrointestinal adverse events.

Many patients, with or without antimicrobial therapy, will cough for weeks. If a patient fails to improve within 4 to 5 days, efforts should be made to confirm the diagnosis, exclude alternative disorders, including pneumonia, and attempt to identify specific offending pathogens, such as *B. pertussis*. Patients infected with this bacterium, who serve as a reservoir of infection for nonimmune children and adults, merit antibiotic treatment (erythromycin or TMP-SMX). Pertussis is characterized by paroxysmal, nonproductive cough that worsens at night. In contrast to children, adults with pertussis do not have absolute lymphocytosis. Patients symptomatic for more than 3 weeks require additional investigations to exclude tuberculosis, drug-induced disorders, BOOP (bronchiolitis obliterans–organizing pneumonia), sarcoid chronic eosinophilic pneumonia, Wegener's granulomatosis, and cancer.

Acute bronchitis is the most frequent lower respiratory tract illness in HIV-infected patients. These patients typically present with cough, purulent sputum, and low-grade fever. Their sputum culture often grows *S. pneumoniae, H. influenzae,* or *Pseudomonas aeruginosa.* They should receive an antibiotic. Unfortunately, however, they are prone to recurrences. When HIV-infected patients with acute bronchitis manifest cough and shortness of breath unaccompanied by purulent sputum, an effort needs to be made to distinguish this disease from roentgenographically negative *Pneumocystis carinii* pneumonia and tuberculosis.

## Acute Exacerbation of Chronic Bronchitis

When a patient with known chronic bronchitis experiences a syndrome consisting of the abrupt development of fatigue, chest tightness, worsening cough, and dyspnea, accompanied by an increased volume and/or purulence of sputum, an "exacerbation" has occurred. Definition of the syndrome does not require all these elements to be present, and although infections precipitate some exacerbations, most are not associated with fever. An exacerbation not only produces uncomfortable and disabling symptoms, but can also result in lost work time, significant financial costs, and hospitalization. The 7.5 million Americans with chronic bronchitis are not a homogenous group. Some of these people escape exacerbations, some have one or two winter exacerbations, and others have numerous episodes each year. Certainly not all exacerbations are precipitated by an infectious event. Those organisms most frequently associated with the exacerbation of chronic bronchitis include viruses, *M. pneumoniae, H. influenzae, S. pneumoniae,* and *Moraxella (Branhamella) catarrhalis.* Limited data suggest a role for *Haemophilus parainfluenzae* and, rarely, *C. pneumoniae.*

As a general rule, there is no compelling need to analyze the blood or sputum or to obtain a chest x-ray study during the first encounter with a patient who does not appear seriously ill. A blood gas determination would be appropriate for patients experiencing insomnia, agitation, or increasing dyspnea.

For more than 50 years, physicians have prescribed antimicrobial agents to patients with chronic bronchitis experiencing an exacerbation, but the efficacy of this treatment has remained a subject of controversy. It has been difficult to assess the value of administering an antimicrobial agent to these patients because there is no precise definition of an exacerbation, not all exacerbations are caused by a bacterial infection, patients' symptoms are often relieved by co-medications, and meaningful endpoints of treatment are difficult to identify. In addition, there are few published clinical trials, and the available investigations have some design defects. The randomized trials suggest that antibiotic treatment effects a modest but statistically significant clinical improvement. Antimicrobial agents appear to have their greatest impact in the therapy of the patient experiencing a more "severe" exacerbation—not simply an increase or change in the appearance of sputum, but both of these features plus increased shortness of breath. Antimicrobials have accelerated the rate of clinical resolution and reduced the need for additional medication, return visits, and hospitalization, and they have caused negligible toxicity.

Table 4-1 lists the macrolides, aminopenicillins, cephalosporins, carbacephem, fluoroquinolones, TMP-SMX combination, and tetracyclines that clinicians prescribe for patients experiencing an exacerbation of chronic bronchitis. There are no convincing scientific data to indicate that any one of these oral agents produces enhanced clinical resolution when compared with the others. Features of the host and antimicrobial agent that would influence drug selection include the following: patient history of drug allergy; track record of the drug; its potential to initiate untoward events or undesirable drug-drug interactions; its spectrum of activity; ease of compliance; and cost of the drug.

TMP-SMX and doxycycline appear to be appealing drugs. They inhibit the growth of the majority of bacteria incriminated in the exacerbation of chronic bronchitis. Addi-

Table 4-1. Antimicrobial agents

| Macrolides | Aminopenicillins | Tetracyclines |
|---|---|---|
| Erythromycin | Ampicillin | Doxycycline |
| Clarithromycin | Amoxicillin | Minocycline |
| Azithromycin | Amoxicillin-clavulanate | Tetracycline |
| Dirithromycin | Bacampicillin | |
| | | Trimethoprim-sulfamethoxazole |
| **Cephalosporins** | **Flouroquinolones** | |
| Cefaclor | Ciprofloxacin | |
| Cefuroxine | Ofloxacin | |
| Cefixime | Lomefloxacin | |
| Cefprozil | Levofloxacin | |
| Cefpodoxime | Sparfloxacin | |
| proxetil | Grepafloxacin | |
| Ceftibuten | Trovafloxacin | |
| Cefdinir | | |
| **Carbacephem** | | |
| Loracarbef | | |

tionally, they are an appropriate selection for penicillin-allergic patients, can be taken twice a day, and are relatively safe and inexpensive compounds with an established track record. However, some patients experience hypersensitivity reactions (fever, rash) or gastrointestinal untoward events with TMP-SMX, and there is a risk for interaction when it is coadministered with warfarin, cyclosporine, phenytoin, methotrexate, or oral hypoglycemic agents. In addition, older patients are at greater risk for TMP-SMX–induced blood dyscrasias and hyperkalemia. Doxycycline has a potential to cause gastrointestinal toxicity. This antibiotic has also produced esophageal ulcerations and strictures (particularly in elderly patients) and, rarely, hepatitis, rashes, and photosensitivity. The drug should not be prescribed for patients who are taking antacids, ferrous sulfate, or cimetidine. Treatment with either of these compounds can be restricted to approximately 1 week.

Ancillary treatment consists of encouraging smoking cessation. The use of a bronchodilator, such as ipratropium or a β-adrenergic sympathomimetic agent, may confer some additional benefit. The value of drinking copious fluids or taking an expectorant is undocumented. Patients usually improve clinically within 4 days and achieve complete resolution of the exacerbation within 2 weeks.

When a patient fails to demonstrate any improvement within 5 days, the clinician should consider the following: incorrect diagnosis (perhaps pneumonia, neoplasm, or congestive heart failure); noncompliance; inappropriate antimicrobial selection (organism resistant to the medication prescribed); diminished antimicrobial bioavailability (concomitant administration of iron, antacids, didanosine, and multivitamins with zinc decreases the absorption of tetracyclines and fluoroquinolones); and excessive bronchospasm and bronchial secretions.

Patients with chronic bronchitis are candidates for an annual immunization with influenza vaccine, as well as pneumococcal vaccine, although the value of pneumococcal vaccine for these patients is controversial. Another potential preventive measure is to offer the patient antibiotic prophylaxis with an agent such as tetracycline, ampicillin, amoxicillin, or TMP-SMX prescribed once a day either four times a week or every day during the winter. The published scientific data are very "soft" here, however. Antibiotic prophylaxis should be restricted to the patient who experiences four or more exacerbations per year.

Researchers have recently examined the role of oral immunization with bacterial extracts as an approach to stimulating respiratory tract immune defenses and reducing exacerbations of chronic bronchitis. Limited data suggest that this approach may have some merit. The basis for oral immunization is that stimulation of gut-associated lymphoid tissue can prime bronchial tube-associated lymphoid tissue, presumably through cell traffic between these two systems. (R.A.G.)

**Bibliography**

Ball P, et al. Acute infective exacerbations of chronic bronchitis. *Q J Med* 1995;88: 61–68.
  *Fever is not a common manifestation of the exacerbation.*
Ball P, Make BP. Acute exacerbations of chronic bronchitis. *Chest* 1998;113:199S–204S.
  *Reviews of the guidelines for management of acute exacerbation of chronic bronchitis, as developed in the United States, Canada, and Europe.*
Cherry JD. Pertussis in adults. *Ann Intern Med* 1998;128:64–66.
  *Pertussis as a cause of chronic nonproductive cough in adults who do not demonstrate absolute lymphocytosis.*
Crimin N, Mastruzzo C, Vancheri C. The long-term antimicrobial prophylaxis of chronic bronchitis exacerbations. *J Chemother* 1995;7:307–310.
  *Use of oral administration of bacterial extracts to stimulate immune defenses and reduce recurrent respiratory infections.*
Gump DW. Chronic bronchitis: common and controversial. *Infect Dis Clin Pract* 1996;5:227–231.
  *A review of chronic bronchitis.*
Isada CM. Pro: antibiotics for chronic bronchitis with exacerbations. *Semin Respir Infect* 1993;8:243–253.
  *An attempt to make the case for the use of an antibiotic to manage the exacerbation.*
Leiner S. Acute bronchitis in adults: commonly diagnosed but poorly defined. *Nurse Pract* 1997;22:104–115.
  *A contemporary review of the clinical manifestations, etiology. and management of acute bronchitis.*
MacKay DN. Treatment of acute bronchitis without underlying lung disease. *J Gen Intern Med* 1996;11:557–562.
  *Antibiotics should not be routinely prescribed to healthy adults who experience acute bronchitis.*
Roessingh PH, et al. Viral and atypical pathogens as causes of type 1 acute exacerbations of chronic bronchitis. *Clin Microb Infect* 1997;3:513–514.
  *An attempt to identify the infectious causes of the exacerbation of chronic bronchitis.*

---

## 5. ANTIBIOTIC-RESISTANT PNEUMOCOCCI

---

*Streptococcus pneumoniae* causes more cases of community-acquired pneumonia than any other pathogen. The pneumococcus is responsible for more than half of all community-acquired pneumonia deaths. Particular populations are very vulnerable to pneumococcal pneumonia, including the elderly, patients with chronic obstructive lung disease and congestive heart failure, and patients with asplenia, sickle cell anemia, and multiple myeloma. It is estimated that 500,000 cases of pneumococcal pneumonia occur annually in the United States.

Within the past several years, some strains of pneumococci have developed resistance to penicillin and other antibiotics. Although penicillin was always recommended as the antibiotic of choice for pneumococcal infection, this recommendation is now not always appropriate, and the management of pneumococcal infection is much more complex. The problem is exacerbated by the common practice of using empiric antibiotic therapy for the treatment of community-acquired pneumonia without efforts to determine a particular etiologic agent. This type of empiric therapy is much more difficult in areas where resistant pneumococci have emerged.

The development of resistance to penicillin has been well recognized in Australia and New Guinea for 20 years. Resistance in South Africa has also been well appreciated, with early efforts for vaccine development sparked by concerns about antibiotic resistance. The resistance of the pneumococcus to penicillin and erythromycin was carefully tracked in the 1980s with increasing concern in Spain and other European countries. In 1994, a multicenter surveillance study in the United States showed that 24% of pneumococcal isolates had reduced sensitivity to penicillin, and 10% had high-level resistance. These percentages have been found to vary dramatically from one region of the country to another, and they can change rapidly in any one region.

The majority of penicillin-resistant pneumococci are of a few specific serotypes, and these serotypes are included in the 23-valent pneumococcal vaccine. Penicillin resistance has developed through chromosomally mediated genetic mutations that have caused changes in penicillin-binding proteins. The affinity of penicillin for these binding proteins is weakened, resulting in less antibiotic activity.

Classification of penicillin activity in regard to pneumococci can be confusing, as different authors have set up somewhat different categories. *S. pneumoniae* with minimal inhibitory concentrations (MIC) of less than 0.06 µg/mL are always considered penicillin-susceptible. Penicillin resistance is defined as intermediate when the MIC falls between 0.1 and 1 µg/mL. High-level resistance is usually defined as greater than 1 µm/mL, but sometimes as greater than 2 µm/mL. These breakpoints are most useful in understanding the treatment of meningitis, in that the breakpoints were determined based on antibiotic levels in cerebrospinal fluid.

Because alterations in penicillin-binding proteins will influence the binding of other β-lactam antibiotics, some pneumococci have developed multiple drug resistance. Resistance to cephalosporins generally develops in association with penicillin resistance, particularly when penicillin-binding proteins 2x and 1a are affected. However, different β-lactams bind to different proteins, and some antibiotics may retain their activity even when penicillin-binding protein changes have occurred. Hence, some β-lactams, such as ceftriaxone and cefotaxime, may be active against penicillin-intermediate and even penicillin-resistant strains.

With the development of resistance to penicillin, there has been a parallel rise in the incidence of resistance to other antibiotics, particularly the macrolides. In a recent drug susceptibility study sponsored by the Centers for Disease Control, most penicillin-resistant isolates were also resistant to at least one additional group of antibiotics, suggesting that penicillin resistance serves as a marker for other types of antibiotic resistance.

Resistance to erythromycin is an issue of particular importance because the most popular empiric regimen for community-acquired pneumonia continues to be the macrolide group. The resistance to erythromycin of pneumococci in the United States has been reported to be as high as 19%, too high to justify empiric treatment of community-acquired pneumonia with this antibiotic group. Erythromycin resistance is more likely to occur with penicillin-resistant organisms, although, of course, the mechanism of resistance is different. Erythromycin resistance usually emerges through changes in the ribosome or development of a macrolide efflux system.

Fluoroquinolones continue to show activity to both penicillin-sensitive and penicillin-resistant pneumococci. However, the older quinolones have not been recommended for pneumococcal disease because of well-documented cases of treatment failures. Newer quinolones, such as sparfloxacin and levofloxacin, exhibit good *in vitro* activity against most pneumococcal isolates, including penicillin-resistant strains; they have good penetration into pulmonary tissue and a good safety profile in adults.

Antibiotic susceptibility studies should be performed on all isolates of pneumococci that have been obtained from patients who are suspected of having pneumococcal disease. For patients at high risk for penicillin-resistant organisms, these studies must be carried out as quickly as possible. High-risk patients include those who are at the extremes of age, have previously received antibiotic therapy, have been recently hospitalized or institutionalized, or are attending day care or respite care centers.

The 1-µg oxacillin disk is used for screening of nonsusceptible strains. The disk will detect more than 99% of nonsusceptible strains with 80% specificity. These nonsusceptible strains should then be tested for susceptibility to vancomycin, ceftriaxone, fluoroquinolones, and other agents, depending perhaps on local susceptibility data.

The E test is a new, simpler method for MIC determination. A calibrated, antibiotic-impregnated strip is applied to the surface of an inoculated plate. An antibiotic gradient is produced that results in an elliptic zone of inhibition. The test correlates well with microdilution methods for determining MICs to the pneumococcus.

Even if adequate sputum samples and blood cultures are obtained from all patients with pneumococcal pneumonia, culture results will not be available for several days, and initial antibiotic regimens must be chosen without the benefit of this information. In addition, clinical studies are not yet available to settle fully controversy about the importance of in vitro sensitivity testing in treating penicillin-resistant pneumococci. At least one study could not show any difference in mortality among patients with sensitive versus resistant pneumococci as long as meningitis was not present and corrections were made for other predictors of mortality. Another study found that success of treatment was no different for penicillin-sensitive and penicillin-intermediate strains. Nevertheless, the Infectious Disease Society of America, in its guidelines for the management of community-acquired pneumonia, has made the following recommendations for the treatment of pneumococcal pneumonia:

1. For penicillin-susceptible strains of pneumococci: Penicillin or ampicillin is recommended (as always in the past before the emergence of resistant pneumococci).
2. For isolates that are intermediately resistant to penicillin (MICs between 0.1 and 1 μg/mL): Parenteral penicillin, ceftriaxone or cefotaxime, amoxicillin, or fluoroquinolones are recommended.
3. For highly resistant strains of pneumococci (MIC >2 μg/mL): Fluoroquinolones or vancomycin is recommended. Other agents can then be chosen based on results of susceptibility tests.
4. For empiric therapy: Fluoroquinolones are recommended. Penicillin can be used when the rate of penicillin resistance in the community is low and the patient is low risk for penicillin-resistant pneumococci.

Although these recommendations have been reviewed by many infectious disease experts, some will be concerned about the lack of data regarding clinical success with high-dose penicillin for intermediately resistant strains. There are also only preliminary data regarding the success of fluoroquinolones for highly resistant pneumococci. Whether the pneumococcus will develop resistance to fluoroquinolones as they become drugs of choice for this organism is also not known.

Slightly different recommendations have been published by others. Some have recommended ceftriaxone for intermediately resistant pneumococci if the MIC of ceftriaxone is less than 2 μg/mL. This would be the recommendation for a patient with pneumococcal pneumonia and possible or documented meningitis. Others have suggested that vancomycin and not fluoroquinolones be considered the initial drug of choice for highly resistant pneumococci in debilitated patients.

Immunization also becomes of increasing importance in the era of higher mortality from pneumococcal infection. The currently available pneumococcal vaccine includes the major serotypes in which resistance has developed. Newer, more immunogenic vaccines will be used in children. These vaccines may decrease the colonization rate in day care centers and decrease the spread of resistant organisms from children to adults.

Reynolds and others have recommended that the use of performed specific antibody be reevaluated for life-threatening pneumococcal infection in preparation for the possibility of increasing antibiotic resistance. (S.L.B.)

## Bibliography

Aubier M, et al. Once-daily sparfloxacin versus high-dosage amoxicillin in the treatment of community-acquired, suspected pneumococcal pneumonia in adults. *Clin Infect Dis* 1998;26:1312.
   *Sparfloxacin treatment was successful in patients with pneumococcal pneumonia, including 20 of 24 patients with bacteremia.*
Austrian R. The enduring pneumococcus: unfinished business and opportunities for the future. *Microb Drug Resist* 1997;3:111.
   *Essay puts penicillin resistance in historical perspective and emphasizes the value of the pneumococcal vaccine.*
Bartlett JG, et al. Community-acquired pneumonia in adults: guidelines for management. *Clin Infect Dis* 1998;26:811.
   *Practice guidelines for pneumonia developed by the Infectious Disease Society of America. The article emphasizes the importance of specific diagnosis and provides*

*antibiotic recommendations for pneumococcal pneumonia based on whether organism is susceptible to penicillin, intermediately resistant, or completely resistant. The use of fluoroquinolones is recommended for penicillin-resistant pneumococci.*

Breiman RF, et al. Emergence of drug-resistant pneumococcal infections in the United States. *JAMA* 1994;271:1831.
   *Surveillance study found that 6.6% of all pneumococcal isolates from 13 hospitals in 12 states were penicillin-resistant. Most of the resistant isolates were serotypes present in the 23-valent pneumococcal vaccine.*

Campbell GD, Silberman R. Drug-resistant *Streptococcus pneumoniae. Clin Infect Dis* 1998;26:1188.
   *Includes discussion of risk factors for antibiotic-resistant pneumococci. These include extremes of age, recent antimicrobial therapy, coexisting illness, HIV infection, attendance at day care centers, and recent hospitalization or institutionalization.*

Guillemot D, et al. Low-dosage and long-term treatment duration of β-lactam. Risk factors for carriage of penicillin-resistant *Streptococcus pneumoniae. JAMA* 1998;279:365.
   *Low-dose and long-duration therapy with β-lactam antibiotics promotes pharyngeal carriage of penicillin-resistant pneumococci.*

Klugman KP. Pneumococcal resistance to antibiotics. *Clin Microbiol Rev* 1990;3:171.
   *Detailed review of the prevalence and mechanism of resistance of pneumococci to penicillin, erythromycin, tetracycline, chloramphenicol, and other agents.*

Musher DM. Infections caused by *Streptococcus pneumoniae:* clinical spectrum, pathogenesis, immunity, and treatment. *Clin Infect Dis* 1992;14:801.
   *Summarizes data on the clinical features of pneumococcal pneumonia and approach to diagnosis. Predicted the increasing use of quinolones in the treatment of penicillin-resistant pneumococci.*

Nuorti JP, et al. An outbreak of multidrug-resistant pneumococcal pneumonia and bacteremia among unvaccinated nursing home residents. *N Engl J Med* 1998;338:1861.
   *A multidrug-resistant (type 23F) pneumococcus caused an outbreak of pneumonia in a nursing home. None of the patients had received the pneumococcal vaccine. After vaccination, there were no additional cases and the colonization rate decreased.*

Pallares R, et al. Risk factors and response to antibiotic therapy in adults with bacteremic pneumonia caused by penicillin-resistant pneumococci. *N Engl J Med* 1987;317:18.
   *Patients with penicillin-resistant pneumococci had a higher mortality rate than patients with penicillin-sensitive organisms. Sixty-five percent of patients with resistant pneumococci had previously received β-lactam antibiotics.*

Reynolds HY. Respiratory infections: community-acquired pneumonia and newer microbes. *Lung* 1996;174:207.
   *Detailed review of newer pathogens in community-acquired pneumonia provides recommendations for management of pneumococcal pneumonia, including long-term strategies of immunotherapy.*

---

# 6. FEVER AND PLEURAL EFFUSIONS

---

Pleural effusions associated with fever constitute a common medical problem. The clinician must have a thorough understanding of the pathophysiology of pleural effusions and a realistic approach to diagnosis and treatment if optimal treatment is to be provided.

## Anatomy and Pathophysiology of the Pleural Space
The pleural space, truly a "potential space" formed at the interface of the parietal and visceral pleurae, acts as a lubricant and normally contains only 7 to 14 mL of fluid. The area becomes a true space in disease states, when it may fill with air or fluid.

Blood supply to the parietal pleura comes primarily from branches of the intercostal and superior phrenic arteries, whereas the visceral pleura is supplied by both pulmonary and pericardiophrenic arteries. Venous drainage of the parietal pleura is via the intercostal veins; the visceral pleura is drained primarily by pulmonary veins.

Pleural lymphatics, located in the connective tissues that underlie the mesothelial cells of the pleural surfaces, freely interconnect with those below the diaphragm. Materials placed in subdiaphragmatic lymphatics drain into the intercostal and mediastinal nodes. Drainage is extremely important for removal of erythrocytes and proteins from the pleural space. Gases and liquids are rapidly cleared from the pleural space. Particulate matter, including erythrocytes and proteins, is removed primarily through the lymphatics. Normally, 250 to 500 mL of fluids and contained materials can be removed daily in this fashion. Pleural effusions develop when discrepancies develop between the rates of production and absorption of fluid. Causes include disorders of hydrostatic or colloid oncotic pressure, lymphatics, and capillary permeability.

Pleural fluid is normally sterile, but it easily supports growth of pathogens. This is in part related to the fluid basis of effusion, which allows extreme mobility of bacteria and thus impairs early phagocytosis before the arrival of opsonins. Recently, reviews have documented the pathophysiology of empyema. The presence of bacteria within pleural effusions initiates a variety of host responses that involve cytokines. If the response fails to inhibit bacterial growth, opsonins and complement become deficient, and the fluid becomes hypoxic and acidic. The inflammatory process typical of empyema releases components capable of bacterial inhibition. In such a state, bacterial reproduction slows and may be reduced to every 24 hours. This may explain in part why antibiotics need to be administered for prolonged periods in patients treated for undrained empyema.

### Evaluation of Pleural Effusions

History and physical examination provide important clues for both presence and etiology. Questions regarding the presence of pneumonia, subdiaphragmatic illness, or malignancy, and medicine use and epidemiology (e.g., travel and tuberculosis exposure) are indicated. Specific risks for HIV infection should be assessed, as recent literature has summarized some characteristic experiences with pleural effusions in this disease. Physical examination should be comprehensive. Patients housed in adult critical care units are often identified to have pleural effusions. Most are small and need not be sampled unless infection or another specific diagnosis is strongly suspected.

The chest roentgenogram is often insensitive (even with lateral decubitus views) until at least 500 mL of fluid is present. Ultrasonography may reveal as little as 5 to 50 mL, whereas computed tomography has the advantage of additionally revealing details of the pulmonary parenchyma and mediastinum and is better at differentiating pleural thickening from fluid. Either study may be employed to guide thoracentesis in selected cases.

Thoracentesis is indicated to assess the cause of most effusions and provides a diagnosis in about 75% of cases. There are no absolute contraindications, although bleeding tendencies, poor patient cooperation, and mechanical ventilation are considered relative contraindications. Well-documented congestive heart failure or generalized anasarca may be managed without this study. Occasionally, because of small size or difficult location, thoracentesis employing either ultrasound or computed tomographic guidance may be indicated. Recent prospective studies demonstrate that this procedure provides useful information more than 90% of the time but may be associated with both technical problems and adverse reactions. Table 6-1 lists studies to be considered once fluid has been obtained.

*Biochemical Tests*

Pleural effusions may be exudative or transudative. The latter type tends to be benign and occurs when mechanical factors alter pleural fluid formation or resorption. Thus, the identification of transudative fluid generally truncates the evaluation. Patient position may modify fluid characteristics. An upright position may result in documentation of exudates, whereas borderline transudates may have been noted while the patient is supine. Exudates result from inflammation or malignancy that inter-

Table 6-1. Common tests useful in evaluating thoracentesis fluid

| | |
|---|---|
| **Microbiologic** | Gram's stain |
| | Aerobic/anaerobic culture |
| | Acid-fast smear/culture* |
| | Fungal smear/culture* |
| | *Legionella* culture* |
| **Hematologic** | Cell count/differential |
| | Cytology* |
| **Biochemical** | pH |
| | Glucose |
| | Lactate dehydrogenase |
| | Protein |
| | Amylase |
| **Tests of occasional value** | Counterimmunoelectrophoresis |
| | Rheumatoid factor, antinuclear antibody |
| | Adenosine deaminase |
| | Neutrophil elastase, $\alpha_1$-proteinase inhibitor |
| | Flow cytometry with immunochemistry |
| | Cholesterol |

* Performed on stored fluid aliquots or unstained slides if initial assessment is nondiagnostic.

feres with pleural surfaces or lymphatic drainage. Differentiation is important because of the broad types of illness that fall into the two categories. Some diagnostic categories may be either; significant diuresis may alter pleural fluid protein and lactate dehydrogenase (LDH) levels so that the fluid mimics exudate. Simultaneous measurements of serum and pleural fluid LDH and protein content allow for more accurate assessment. A pleural fluid-to-serum LDH ratio above 0.6 or protein ratio above 0.5, or a pleural fluid LDH level above 200 IU/L, generally documents an exudate. Virtually all exudates exhibit at least one of these characteristics, and transudates typically lack all three. Pleural fluid cholesterol above 45 mg/dL appears specific for exudative effusion but may not be as sensitive as the prior criteria. The combination of pleural fluid cholesterol above 45 mg/dL and LDH above 200 IU/L appears to be both highly sensitive and specific for exudate and does not require simultaneous blood sampling.

Pleural fluid glucose levels below 40 mg/100 mL are generally seen in effusions caused by bacterial infection, tuberculosis, malignancy, or rheumatoid arthritis. The value of low glucose levels lies more in documenting the need for further evaluation than in providing a specific diagnosis. Pleural fluid amylase levels are elevated in pancreatitis and esophageal rupture, and with amylase-producing tumors. Amylase may be further divided into that of salivary or pancreatic origin. Markedly elevated levels of pancreatic origin almost always result from pancreatitis and are usually associated with a pleural fluid-serum amylase ratio above 1. Esophageal rupture may be suspected by the presence of amylase of salivary origin.

Pleural fluid pH is useful in defining parapneumonic effusions that must be treated by tube thoracostomy. Low pleural fluid pH values occur primarily in malignancy, tuberculosis, and bacterial infections. Pleural fluid acidosis is defined by a pH below 7.3 or (if acidemia is present) by a value more than 0.15 below that of blood pH. Some authors now recommend immediate chest tube drainage for parapneumonic effusions associated with pH below 7.1, glucose below 40 mg/dL, LDH above 1,000 IU/L, or evidence of loculation. Parapneumonic effusions with pH values above 7.1, especially if accompanied by glucose levels above 40 mg/100 mL, may be successfully treated without tube placement. Repeated thoracentesis to document trends is recommended

*Cell Type*
Exudates often contain more than 1,000 cells per milliliter, but this parameter is not as useful as LDH and protein ratios for distinguishing between exudates and transudates.

An elevated percentage of polymorphonuclear leukocytes, seen primarily in bacterial infections, is also noted in pancreatitis, connective tissue disease, and pulmonary infarction. Tuberculosis of short duration has been associated with this cell type as well. A predominance of lymphocytes is seen in more than 80% of tuberculous and malignant pleural effusions. Tuberculosis is also associated with a relative absence of mesothelial cells in the differential count. Newer tests to define lymphocyte type further may be important in defining the etiology of pleural effusions. As an example, recent studies have demonstrated elevated levels of helper T cells in a patient with pleural effusion resulting from sarcoidosis.

Eosinophilic pleural effusions contain more than 10% eosinophils and may account for 2% to 9% of all pleural effusions. A recent investigation documented only idiopathic cases and effusions following thoracic surgery as statistically correlated with eosinophilia, and survivorship was longer in patients with eosinophilic effusions.

Erythrocytes are common but of uncertain importance. Historically, the presence of blood-tinged fluid was considered indicative of tuberculosis, pulmonary infarction, or malignancy. However, less than 2 mL of blood per 1,000 mL of fluid in an effusion creates this appearance. An RBC level of more than 100,000/mL is generally associated with malignancy, trauma, and pulmonary infarction.

Malignant cells should be sought in exudative effusions not otherwise diagnosed. Cytologic examination establishes a diagnosis in about 50% of malignant pleural effusions. Fresh samples must be used, and several techniques may be necessary to demonstrate malignant cells.

*Bacteriologic Studies*

All pleural effusions should be analyzed by Gram's stain and aerobic and anaerobic culture. Although only 5% of bacterial pneumonias are complicated by infected pleural fluid, laboratory information is valuable. Not all effusions need to be evaluated for tuberculosis or fungal infection. Smears for acid-fast bacilli (AFB) and fungal smears and cultures should be obtained with lymphocytic exudative effusions or when the diagnosis of an exudate is elusive. Smears for AFB are positive in fewer than 25% of cases and increase both patient and laboratory costs.

*Tests of Occasional Value*

Pleural effusions in systemic lupus erythematosus may be associated with antinuclear antibody titers above 1 : 160 and pleural fluid-to-serum antinuclear antibody ratios of more than 1. Positive lupus erythematosus preparations are noted in at least 85% of cases. Determination of levels of both complement and rheumatoid factor in pleural fluid may help diagnose rheumatoid arthritis. Measurement of adenine deaminase has become an effective means of diagnosing tuberculous pleural effusion, and in the presence of a lymphocytic effusion, an elevation is virtually pathognomonic. Investigators have considered an elevation in pleural effusion to levels above 45 to 55 U/L to be highly suggestive of tuberculosis.

Tests for the detection of bacterial antigens may document a bacterial etiology in the absence of viable organisms. Thus, partially treated infections may be diagnosed despite negative results on cultures. Organisms detectable include *Haemophilus influenzae* type b, *Streptococcus pneumoniae*, and several types of *Neisseria meningitidis*. Results with these techniques have been comparable to those of routine cultures. Other studies of occasional value include neutrophil elastase and $\alpha_1$-proteinase inhibitor (malignancy) and flow cytometry with immunochemistry (malignancy).

*Pleural Biopsy and / or Thoracoscopy*

Thoracoscopy, often with pleural biopsy, should be performed in difficult cases of exudative pleural effusion. Thoracoscopy has become increasingly popular and now can be performed under video guidance, which allows better visibility and fewer complications. Most authors will employ it if routine pleural biopsy findings are nondiagnostic. A recent review demonstrated that more than 90% of cases of elusive exudative effusions can be diagnosed by the use of this procedure. It is especially useful for finding nodular pleural lesions, which can then be sampled. Biopsy specimens should be submitted for bacteriology (aerobic/anaerobic, mycobacteriology, and mycology) and histopathology.

Despite best efforts, for some patients (especially those with exudative pleural effusions), an etiologic diagnosis cannot be made. Most of these cases are benign and remain undiagnosed. The mean time to resolution is 5 to 6 months; however, some cases relapse. Etiologies eventually discovered in a minority of these patients include asbestosis, rheumatoid arthritis, congestive heart failure, cirrhosis, and adenocarcinoma.

## Types of Pleural Effusion
Table 6-2 lists some of the common causes of fever and pleural effusion. Selected ones are discussed below.

*Parapneumonic Effusion*
Parapneumonic effusion is that associated with pneumonia, lung abscess, or bronchiectasis. Between 30% and 70% are associated with positive results on pleural fluid cultures. Regarding bacterial pneumonia, the likelihood of encountering parapneumonic effusions is as follows: *Staphylococcus aureus,* 75%; *S. pneumoniae,* 57%; viruses, 15% to 25%; *H. influenzae,* 50% to 75%; and *Streptococcus pyogenes,* 90%. The yield may be related to the duration of effusion, as organisms such as *S. pneumoniae* may undergo autolysis. *Mycoplasma pneumoniae* may be associated with parapneumonic effusions in up to 20% of cases. The relative frequency with *Legionella* species or gram-negative enteric bacilli remains unknown.

The management of parapneumonic effusions includes thoracentesis and antimicrobials. β-Lactams penetrate the pleural space well and achieve therapeutic levels early in therapy. Levels of parenteral aminoglycosides are decreased in the face of empyema in comparison with other effusions. As mentioned earlier, characteristics of the fluid help determine the need for tube or other forms of drainage.

*Pleural Empyema*
Pleural empyema is defined as pus in the pleural space and can be demonstrated only by direct sampling. Often, pH values below 7 and glucose levels under 40 mg/100 mL are observed. The presence of pleural empyema requires parenteral antimicrobials and definitive drainage. Although tube thoracostomy has been traditionally employed, some persons may now benefit from thoracoscopy with repeated irrigations. Anaerobes may be noted in up to 40% of cases. Gram's stain, culture, and other standard tests usually provide information sufficient to initiate therapy. Antimicrobial doses higher than those commonly used for uncomplicated pneumonia are necessary to ensure adequate drug levels. Length of therapy is variable, but generally therapy should be continued until the patient is afebrile, the peripheral WBC count approaches

Table 6-2. Common pleural effusions associated with fever

| Condition | Effusion type | Cells | Glucose (mg/dl) | pH |
|---|---|---|---|---|
| Empyema | Exudate | PMNs >50,000 | <30 | <7.0 |
| Parapneumonic effusion | Exudate | PMNs often <50,000 | >30 | >7.2 |
| Tuberculosis | Exudate | Lymphocytes | 30–60 | 7.0–7.3 |
| Systemic lupus erythematosus | Exudate | PMNs, lymphocytes | Variable | Variable |
| Malignancy | Exudate | Generally lymphocytes | Variable | Variable, generally >7.2 |
| Pulmonary infarction | Variable (usually exudate) | Variable; RBCs >100,000 | Variable, generally >30 | Variable |

PMNs, polymorphonuclear leukocytes.

normal, and tube thoracostomy drainage is meager. If complicated pneumonia or lung abscess is simultaneously present, prolonged therapy may be needed. Patients who fail to defervesce with appropriate antimicrobials and closed tube thoracostomy should be evaluated for loculated pus. Either ultrasound or computed tomography can be used, and open surgical drainage or thoracoscopy may be indicated.

*Tuberculous Pleurisy*
Involvement of the pleural space occurs in about 4% of patients diagnosed with tuberculous and most commonly is noted as an early complication of primary disease. Presentation may be acute and mimic bacterial pneumonia, or more chronic, in which case it is characterized by weight loss and anorexia. Approximately 75% to 80% of patients with tuberculous pleurisy are febrile. Thirty percent have simultaneous pulmonary parenchymal involvement. For obscure reasons, pleural effusions most commonly involve the right hemithorax and almost invariably are unilateral. Lymphocytes generally predominate; however, early in the course of disease polymorphonuclear leukocytes may be noted. Glucose levels may be normal or low, and AFB smears are generally negative. Cultures of pleural effusion are positive in about 50% of cases. Diagnosis should be suspected in lymphocyte-predominant exudative effusions, and pleural biopsy is generally the procedure of choice if the AFB smear of fluid is initially negative. Recommendations are for submission of three biopsy specimens, as yield from a pleural fluid increases from about 70% to above 90% with additional specimens. Adenosine deaminase has been recommended as a test for tuberculous pleurisy. In some hands, levels above 50 U/L were more than 90% sensitive and specific for tuberculosis, whereas levels below 45 U/L were 100% specific and sensitive for alternative diagnoses. This test should be performed when tuberculous pleurisy is suspected.

*Pulmonary Infarction*
Fever occurs in up to 68% of angiographically documented cases of pulmonary thromboembolic disease, may reach levels of 39°C, and can last for many days. Observations suggesting pulmonary thromboembolic disease include (a) a history of embolic events, (b) fever, and (c) phlebitis. Pleural fluid evaluation is often nondiagnostic. In 33% of cases, fluid is transudative and contains fewer than 10,000 RBCs per milliliter. RBC counts above 100,000/mL suggest this diagnosis if trauma and malignancy can be excluded. WBC counts can reach 70,000/mL. Early on, polymorphonuclear leukocytes predominate, and lymphocytes are noted after several days.

*Iatrogenic Pleural Effusions*
Causes of iatrogenic pleural effusions include drugs (e.g., heparin, hydralazine, sulfa drugs, nitrofurantoin, albumin, ionic contrast dye) and procedures (e.g., sclerotherapy, surgery, misadventures with central intravascular lines, and peritoneal dialysis). All can be associated with fever. The diagnostic approach is similar to that with other effusions, and discontinuation of an offending medication often results in clinical improvement.

## Conclusions
Pleural effusions associated with fever are a common problem and may have many causes. The physician should have a working knowledge of the mechanisms involved in the formation of fluid and be comfortable using tests available for diagnosis. In selected situations, small effusions that have been incidentally identified may be observed. When pleural fluid has been sampled, hematologic, chemical, and microbiologic studies generally provide a diagnosis. Occasionally, cases prove more frustrating, and biopsy or other analyses may be indicated. The cause of the effusion may remain elusive on occasion, and repeated assessments may be necessary. Fortunately, many cases of chronic exudative undiagnosed effusion appear to be benign. (R.B.B.)

## Bibliography
Bartter T, et al. The evaluation of pleural effusion. *Chest* 1994; 106:1209–1214.
  *The authors present an excellent review of the roles of imaging, thoracentesis, and other studies in the evaluation of pleural effusions. They also provide a good frame-*

work for differentiating exudates from transudates and for the management of exudative pleural effusions.

Black LF. The pleural space and pleural fluid. *Mayo Clin Proc* 1972;47:493–506.
*This article, now more than two decades old, is a superb review of the anatomy and physiology of the pleural space. Although somewhat technical, it provides an excellent basis for the understanding of pleural disease.*

Bryant RE, Salmon CJ. Pleural empyema. *Clin Infect Dis* 1996;22:747–764.
*This article is an excellent in-depth review of the history, pathophysiology, anatomy, diagnosis, and management of pleural empyema. It contains contemporary information about the role of intrapleural thrombolysis and video-assisted thoracoscopy. Recommendations regarding antibiotic therapy are basic and do not really address the role of newer agents, which may have a role for prolonged oral therapy in selected cases.*

Collins TR, Sahn SA. Thoracentesis: clinical value, complications, technical problems, and patient experience. *Chest* 1987;91:817–822.
*Eighty-nine patients undergoing 129 consecutive thoracenteses were evaluated. Ninety-two percent of procedures provided useful information. Twenty percent of procedures were associated with complications that included pneumothorax and cough. Subjective patient discomfort was seen in more than 20% of cases, and technical problems were encountered in more than 20% of cases.*

Ferrer SJ. Pleural tuberculosis: incidence, pathogenesis, diagnosis and treatment. *Opin Pulmon Med* 1996;2:327–334.
*The author presents an excellent overview of issues related to pleural tuberculosis and deals with the issue in patients with HIV/AIDS as well. Therapy is primarily with antituberculous agents, with very limited roles for either corticosteroids or repeated thoracenteses.*

Ferrer JS, et al. Evolution of idiopathic pleural effusion. *Chest* 1996;109:1508–1513.
*This report of 40 patients followed for as much as 10 years demonstrates that many patients with exudative pleural effusions and no specific diagnosis did well. Mean time to resolution was less than 6 months, and the course of most patients was benign. One of the entry criteria for this study was an adenosine deaminase level below 43 IU/L, which in the opinion of the authors was valuable for ruling out pleural tuberculosis. Despite long-term follow-up, in 80% a diagnosis was never obtained; most of the remainder had nonmalignant conditions.*

Harris RJ, et al. The diagnostic and therapeutic utility of thoracoscopy. *Chest* 1995;108:828–841.
*An excellent review of the historical and current uses of thoracoscopy as a modality for diagnosing and treating pleural disease. This technique is actually not new, but it has undergone a renaissance in part because of the addition of video assistance, which allows easier imaging of the pleural space. The use of this technique needs to be studied better in controlled trials so that overuse will be avoided. However, it does appear to be extremely valuable as a tool to recognize specific intrapleural lesions.*

Henschke CI, et al. Pleural effusions: pathogenesis, radiographic evaluation, and therapy. *J Thorac Imaging* 1989;4:49–60.
*This excellent overview of the radiographic evaluation of pleural effusions describes clinical conditions that mimic effusions, difficulties with loculated collections, and clues to the presence of empyema. The roles of ultrasound, computed tomography, and magnetic resonance imaging are also discussed. The latter modalities are useful in distinguishing pleural from parenchymal disease, and magnetic resonance imaging may prove beneficial in distinguishing etiologies of effusions.*

Leslie WK, Kinasewitz GT. Clinical characteristics of the patient with nonspecific pleuritis. *Chest* 1988;94:603–608.
*This retrospective analysis of 119 patients who underwent pleural biopsy identifies variables associated with malignant or granulomatous disease. Patients with a diagnosis of nonspecific pleuritis can be managed conservatively if weight loss, a positive tuberculin test result, lymphocytosis above 95%, and a fluid level above half of the hemithorax are not demonstrated.*

Light RW, et al. Parapneumonic effusions. *Am J Med* 1980;69:507–512.
*The authors prospectively assessed 90 patients with parapneumonic effusion. A glucose level below 40 mg/100 mL or a pH below 7 predicted complicated effusions and*

*indicated the need for tube thoracostomy. Patients with a pH above 7.2 and a pleural fluid LDH level below 1,000 mg/100 mL only rarely have a complicated course.*

Mattison LE, et al. Pleural effusions in the medical ICU: prevalence, causes, and clinical implications. *Chest* 1997;111: 1018–1023.

*The investigators assessed 100 patients admitted to a medical ICU. Of these, 62% were documented to have pleural effusions; about two thirds of these were present on admission. Most were small and of no clinical significance. Most were present on chest roentgenograms. If not clinically suspected to be infected, the authors feel that most of these can be observed prospectively without thoracentesis.*

Poe RH, et al. Utility of pleural fluid analysis in predicting tube thoracostomy/ decortication in parapneumonic effusions. *Chest* 1991;100:963–967.

*The authors retrospectively evaluated 133 patients at three hospitals who underwent thoracentesis. Assessment included laboratory data from effusions and ultimate need for surgical drainage or decortication. They concluded that Light's standard criteria for drainage (purulence, glucose <40 mg/100 mL, LDH >1,000 IU/L, pH <7) are specific but not sensitive in predicting the need for eventual chest tube drainage and decortication. Patients who do not meet the criteria must still be carefully followed.*

Rubins JB, Rubins HB. Etiology and prognostic significance of eosinophilic pleural effusions. *Chest* 1996;110:1271–1274.

*This is an interesting brief report of more than 470 patients with pleural effusions, of which almost 10% were eosinophilic. The authors conclude that the only statistical significance of eosinophilia in pleural effusions was either after thoracic surgery or in idiopathic cases. No correlations with malignancy were noted, and eosinophilic effusions generally resulted in more prolonged survival than others.*

Sahn SA. The differential diagnosis of pleural effusions. *West J Med* 1982;13:99–108.

*This excellent basic article by one of the giants in the field of pleural effusion reviews physiology, thoracentesis, and analysis of pleural effusion. Charts are provided to distinguish among causes of pleural effusion based on laboratory characteristics.*

Trejo O, et al. Pleural effusion in patients infected with the human immunodeficiency virus. *Eur J Clin Microbiol Infect Dis* 1997;16:807–815.

*A cohort of HIV-positive patients with pleural effusions was compared with a similar number of patients without HIV infection but with documented pleural effusion— either parapneumonic effusion or tuberculosis. Most HIV-positive persons were intravenous drug users, and this population had a high incidence of infection as a cause of the effusion. Tests demonstrated similar results between the two groups for a given diagnosis.*

## 7. PNEUMONIA IN THE INTENSIVE CARE UNIT

Pneumonia is the leading cause of death from nosocomial infection in the United States. The incidence of nosocomial pneumonia in community hospitals and general medicine wards is about 10 cases per 1,000 admissions but is 10- to 20-fold higher in the ICU. The overall mortality rate of pneumonia in the ICU in one study was 50%. Factors such as ventilator-associated pneumonia and development of adult respiratory distress syndrome significantly worsen the prognosis.

### Pathogenesis

In the normal host, various defense mechanisms, such as filtration of inspired air by the upper respiratory tract, intact cough reflex, secretion of mucus in the tracheobronchial tree, intact humoral immunity, and pulmonary macrophage clearing of bacteria, keep the lower respiratory tract sterile. When these defenses break down or are overwhelmed by a large inoculum of a virulent organism, pneumonia can occur. Compromise of host defenses is common in the typical ICU patient, who is often debilitated or traumatized. Indeed, stroke, seizure, and drug intoxication (common ICU admitting diagnoses) compromise epiglottic closure and cough, resulting in aspiration of oropharyngeal bacteria. Endotracheal intubation or tracheostomy bypasses upper respiratory filtration defenses. The duration of endotracheal intubation is also important as a risk factor in nosocomial pneumonia, having an estimated additive risk of 1% for each day of mechanical ventilation. Impaired pulmonary macrophage function occurs in hypoxemia, uremia, malnutrition, and heart failure. One study also implicates nasogastric tubes, upper abdominal and thoracic surgery, and bronchoscopy as independent risk factors.

In the ICU, bacteria may gain access to the lung by one of these mechanisms: (a) hematogenous spread (e.g., *Staphylococcus aureus* may cause pneumonia when an infected intravenous line results in bacteremia and pulmonary seeding); (b) aerosolization, as may occur during respiratory therapy, particularly with reservoir nebulizers (e.g., *Pseudomonas aeruginosa* pneumonia); and (c) aspiration of endogenous bacteria colonizing the oropharynx.

## Microbiology

Whereas pneumonia acquired in the community is typically caused by pathogens such as *Streptococcus pneumoniae, Haemophilus influenzae, Moraxella (Branhamella) catarrhalis, Legionella pneumophila,* and *Mycoplasma pneumoniae,* pathogens causing pneumonia in the ICU are somewhat different. Most nosocomial, and particularly ICU-acquired, pneumonia is caused by gram-negative bacilli or *S. aureus.* These bacteria can be found colonizing the oropharynx of most ICU patients, and the prevalence of gram-negative colonization increases with severity of illness. Factors that have been shown to increase colonization include coma, hypotension, acidosis, azotemia, and endotracheal intubation.

The spectrum of microorganisms known to cause nosocomial pneumonia has increased rapidly to include several low-virulence organisms, such as *Staphylococcus epidermidis, Corynebacterium,* nontypeable *H. influenzae,* and *M. catarrhalis.* However, the etiologic agents responsible for pneumonia in the ICU have remained predominantly *P. aeruginosa* and other gram-negative bacilli, such as *Klebsiella, Enterobacter, Escherichia coli, Proteus,* and *Serratia,* with *S. aureus* a close second. Table 7-1 summarizes these and other agents that cause pneumonia in an intensive care setting.

There are some pathogens and circumstances worth special mention. *S. pneumoniae,* the common community-acquired pathogen, is known to cause pneumonia in the ICU occasionally, and superinfection with gram-negative bacilli is not uncommon. Severe community-acquired pneumococcal pneumonia may frequently result in ICU admission, particularly if the organism is penicillin-resistant and inappropriate therapy has been started. *S. pneumoniae* is by far the most common organism to cause severe, life-threatening pneumonia in elderly patients. Other streptococci, particularly group A and group B β-hemolytic streptococci, as well as enterococci (group D streptococci), can cause pneumonia in the ICU. Predisposing factors for these pathogens include preceding viral infections, coinfection with *S. aureus,* and previous treatment with broad-spectrum antimicrobials. *H. influenzae,* usually nontypeable, is an important respiratory pathogen in patients with chronic obstructive pulmonary disease and can lead to bronchopneumonia causing respiratory failure. *M. catarrhalis,* now clearly recognized as an important respiratory pathogen, also tends to occur in those with underlying lung disease, many of whom are receiving corticosteroids. *Legionella* species have also been implicated in hospital- and ICU-acquired pneumonia; spread of *L. pneumophila* by aerosol from hospital cooling or hot water systems can potentially make this a serious consideration, especially when sputum Gram's stain and culture are unrevealing.

Hantavirus is an additional cause of life-threatening pneumonia, first described in 1993 when an outbreak was reported in New Mexico. Hantavirus pulmonary syndrome is characterized by a flulike illness followed by noncardiogenic pulmonary edema. Symptoms of fever, myalgia, nausea, and diarrhea are accompanied by tachycardia, tachypnea, and hypotension.

Finally, the nonbacterial opportunistic pathogens such as *Candida albicans, Pneumocystis carinii, Aspergillus,* Phycomycetes, herpes simplex virus, cytomegalovirus, and varicella-zoster virus occur in a selected population of patients (i.e., the immunosuppressed) and have been associated with poor outcome.

Table 7-1. Frequency of etiologic agents in ICU pneumonia

| | Intubated patients, TA (Salata et al., 1987)* (%) | All medical ICU patients, TA (Craven et al., 1988) (%) | ICU intubated, PSB (Fagan et al., 1989) (%) | ICU intubated, PSB (Chastre et al., 1984) (%) | ICU with ARDS, TA (Seidenfeld et al., 1986) (%) |
|---|---|---|---|---|---|
| *Pseudomonas aeruginosa* | 27 | 16 | 19 | 24 | 17 |
| Other gram-negative bacilli | 52 | 69 | 28 | 44 | 39 |
| *Staphylococcus aureus* | 19 | 16 | 20 | 8 | 11* |
| *Staphylococcus epidermidis* | 8 | — | — | — | —* |
| Streptococci | — | 18 | 13 | 10 | 20** |
| *Candida* | 4 | 2 | — | 6 | — |
| *Haemophilus influenzae* | — | 9 | 6 | 2 | — |
| *Legionella* | — | — | 6 | — | — |
| *Moraxella catarrhalis* | — | — | 6 | — | — |
| Anaerobes | — | — | 2 | — | 5 |

TA = tracheal aspirate; PSB = protected sterile brush; ARDS = adult respiratory distress syndrome.
* No distinction was made between *S. aureus* and *S. epidermidis.*
** More than 15% were *Enterococcus.*

## Complications

Pneumonia, especially in the debilitated, critically ill patient, can be complicated by several life-threatening conditions. For instance, when a response to appropriate antimicrobial therapy cannot be obtained, empyema should be considered. When pleural fluid is noted on physical examination or chest x-ray films in the patient with pneumonia, thoracentesis is necessary to rule out infection of the pleural space. Patients with a pleural fluid pH of 7 or less, a glucose level below 40 mg/dL, or gross pus in the pleural space usually require chest tube placement. The organism most prone to cause pleural space infection is *S. aureus.* However, gram-negative bacilli, anaerobes, *H. influenzae, S. pneumoniae,* and β-hemolytic streptococci can all produce empyema. Purulent pericarditis, a common complication of pneumococcal pneumonia in the era before antimicrobial therapy, is now rarely seen as a complication of pneumonia. When encountered, purulent pericarditis is most likely to be associated with *S. aureus* or gram-negative bacilli and to occur in the critically ill patient, particularly after thoracic surgery. The diagnosis of purulent pericarditis should be considered in the pneumonia patient who has not responded to antimicrobial therapy and has signs of an expanding cardiac silhouette or cardiac tamponade, atrial arrhythmias, and chest pain. Echocardiography will demonstrate pericardial fluid, and prompt drainage is almost always required.

An equally important complication of pneumonia in the ICU is meningitis. In patients with pneumonia, abnormal mental status or coma is sometimes attributed to hypoxia or sepsis, and central nervous system infection is not considered. Lumbar puncture must be performed in the patient with pneumonia who is comatose or shows a rapid change in mental status, even if meningeal signs are absent. Initial treatment with vancomycin and ceftriaxone is required if resistant pneumococci are suspected.

Superinfection is likely to occur in ICU patients being treated for pneumonia, especially those on broad-coverage antimicrobials. When an ICU patient deteriorates after initial improvement or becomes febrile, or if a new pulmonary infiltrate develops, one must consider the possibility of pneumonia with a secondary organism.

## Diagnosis

The diagnosis of pneumonia in the ICU should be entertained in the patient who has (a) a new or progressive asymptomatic infiltrate, (b) fever, (c) leukocytosis or leukopenia, and (d) purulent tracheal secretions. However, nosocomial pneumonia may be a subtle illness, and the usual clinical criteria for the diagnosis may lead to false-negative rates as high as 66%. The explanation for such potential misdiagnosis includes confusion of atelectasis and pulmonary edema with infectious infiltrate on chest x-ray films, lack of febrile response to infection from the critically ill (especially the elderly), inability to mount an effective WBC response, and poor-quality sputum samples.

The most convincing argument for accurate diagnosis before treatment is the potential for development of superinfection and increased mortality with antimicrobial-resistant organisms. Furthermore, empiric antimicrobial treatment compromises efforts to document infection and recover a causative organism. Also, there is a risk for drug reactions, drug-drug interactions, and *Clostridium difficile* infection, which can lead to increased morbidity and mortality. Finally, treating all suspected cases of pneumonia in the ICU with a long course of empiric antimicrobials is an unnecessary and inefficient use of financial resources. Streamlining antibiotic therapy—that is, the practice of converting a broad-spectrum regimen to a more specific regimen on the second or third day of therapy—can help reduce the risk for superinfection and emergence of resistance.

When pneumonia is suspected in the ICU, the physician's quest to obtain a "good" sputum sample (i.e., one with <10 epithelial cells and >25 WBCs per high-power field) should be relentless. Sputum examined by Gram's stain for bacteria, potassium hydroxide for fungi, Ziehl-Neelsen stain for acid-fast bacilli, and, when appropriate, silver methenamine stain for *P. carinii* may be all that is needed, along with culture results to establish the cause of pneumonia. Often, sputum cannot be expectorated by the critically ill patient because of extreme weakness, poor cough, the presence of an endotracheal or tracheostomy tube, or unresponsiveness. Thus, the nasotracheal suction catheter is often used to obtain a sputum sample. When introduced through an endotracheal tube, the aspiration catheter is capable of obtaining samples representative of true lower respiratory secretion. Often, the critically ill patient cannot tolerate deep suctioning (e.g., because of face or head trauma or induction of oxygen desaturation), and a more invasive technique for obtaining a sample of lower respiratory tract secretion is needed. Transtracheal aspiration is rarely used today because the procedure is not commonly taught, and it is risky when performed by an unskilled operator. Furthermore, the procedure cannot be carried out in an intubated patient.

Percutaneous needle aspiration can be accurate in the diagnosis of a peripheral cavitary lesion or an anaerobic lung abscess. However, it provides a small inoculum of a small sampling area (and is thus prone to yield a high false-negative rate), is contraindicated in the mechanically ventilated patient, and has a high rate of complications, such as pneumothorax and hemorrhage.

Bronchial washings have been of little use in the diagnosis of pneumonia in the ICU. Transbronchial biopsy is helpful in the diagnosis of a central mass lesion, but its diagnostic utility is unproved with pneumonic infiltrates, and it also is associated with the problems of limited sample area and risk for pneumothorax. Bronchoalveolar lavage of samples of more than 1 million alveoli has been shown to be safe and is the method of choice at many institutions. Although some investigators believe that the rate of contamination of bronchoalveolar lavage cultures with colonizing bacteria is high, bronchoalveolar lavage sampling is attractive because it is easily performed at bedside, allows immediate results (Gram's stain and cell count), and has a low element of risk (only a rare episode of hemoptysis or pneumothorax). Protected specimen bronchoscopy (protected brush) allows collection of lower respiratory specimens protected from contamination by secretions that may pool on the outside of the bronchoscope. With much lower cutoffs for the number of colony-forming units per milliliter to indicate infection ($10^3$ for protected brush versus $10^5$ for expectorated sputum), excellent results can be obtained with essentially no false-negatives, suggesting a very high sensitivity. Disadvantages to the use of protected specimen bronchoscopy include reduced accuracy after prior use of antimicrobials, delay before obtaining culture results, concern that protected specimen bronchoscopy samples only a small area of lung, cost, and concern that many centers are not yet equipped to perform these procedures. In general, the role of bronchoscopy in the diagnosis of pneumonia in the ICU patient remains controversial among pulmonologists.

Finally, open lung biopsy, the most invasive procedure, has long been regarded as the gold standard in the diagnosis of pneumonia. Open lung biopsy has been found to have 97% accuracy and a complication rate of 9.6%. Furthermore, the results frequently lead to antimicrobial changes. Despite the accuracy of this procedure, it cannot be performed quickly and easily in most patients (especially ventilated ICU patients), and the complication rate of 10% is too high to justify its use on a routine basis. Open lung biopsy should be reserved for patients in whom other methods of specimen recovery have failed.

## Treatment

Supportive measures in the treatment of pneumonia in the ICU include physiotherapy and postural drainage, percussion, and tracheal suctioning to mobilize purulent secretions. These measures may improve gas exchange in the patient with thick, copious secretions. Other supportive measures include intermittent positive pressure breathing, supplemental oxygen therapy, adequate analgesics, and antipyretics. Intermittent positive pressure breathing is used to increase lung inflation in many types of lung disease, including pneumonia. However, its utility in pneumonia is unproved, and its routine use is not recommended in the treatment of pneumonia. Oxygen therapy is critical in patients with pneumonia and documented hypoxemia. Indiscriminate use of oxygen and oxygen toxicity must be avoided. Codeine or parenteral meperidine for analgesia is sometimes needed to allow deeper breathing and coughing. Finally, if antipyretics are used, they should be given around the clock; sporadic use can increase the patient's discomfort by causing periods of heavy sweating.

The first step in choosing an antimicrobial agent is to obtain a thorough history and physical examination in conjunction with a Gram's-stained smear of respiratory secretions. In patients ill enough to require ICU admission, bronchoscopy or protected brush is often necessary to determine an etiologic agent. If a good expectorated sputum sample can be obtained and a presumptive diagnosis made on the basis of a Gram's-stained smear, further diagnostic study is usually not pursued. The treatment of gram-negative pneumonia depends in part on the antimicrobial sensitivity patterns of a particular hospital. Treatment of gram-negative bacillary pneumonia in the extremely ill patient requires initial antipseudomonal coverage. Ticarcillin or piperacillin plus an aminoglycoside is the commonly used regimen for the ICU patient. Ceftazidime, cefepime, aztreonam, and imipenem plus cilastatin have been used successfully as monotherapy, again depending on known susceptibility patterns. When staphylococci are suspected in a Gram's-stained smear, the incidence of methicillin-resistant staphylococci becomes a critical issue. Suspicion of methicillin-resistant staphylococci requires initial therapy with vancomycin. When *H. influenzae* or *M. catarrhalis* is suspected, initial therapy with a second- or third-generation cephalosporin is begun. When sputum reveals an abundance of polymorphonuclear leukocytes but no staining organisms, *Legionella* must be considered and initial therapy with erythromycin begun.

Recently, the Infectious Disease Society of America published guidelines for the treatment of community-acquired pneumonia. For treatment of the patient hospitalized in an ICU, the panel recommended erythromycin, azithromycin, or a fluoroquinolone plus cefotaxime, ceftriaxone, or a β-lactamase inhibitor.

Table 7-2 lists the most common causes of pneumonia in ICU patients and the treatments of choice. (S.L.B.)

Table 7-2. Drug regimens of choice for etiologic agents in pneumonia

| Agent | Drug of choice | Alternate |
|---|---|---|
| *Streptococcus pneumoniae;* | | |
| penicillin susceptible (MIC <0.1ug/mL) | Penicillin G, amoxicillin parenteral penicillin G, ceftriaxone, fluoroquinolone | Erythromycin Clindamycin, doxycycline |
| penicillin intermediately resistant (MIC .1–1ug/mL) highly penicillin resistant (MIC >2 ug/mL) | Fluoroquinolone or vancomycin-based on in vitro susceptibility results. | |
| *Haemophilus influenzae* | Cephalosporin second generation (cefuroxime, cefonicid, cefamandole) or third generation (cefotaxime, ceftizoxime, ceftriaxone) Ampicillin-sulbactam | Ampicillin (if beta-lactamase negative) |
| *Staphylococcus aureus* Methicillin-sensitive | Oxacillin, nafcillin, cephalosporin first generation | Vancomycin |
| Methicillin-resistant | Vancomycin | Imipenem-cilastalin (for some strains) |
| Gram-negative bacilli | | |
| *Klebsiella pneumoniae* | Cephalosporin third generation with or without aminoglycoside | Aztreonam, Imipenem |
| *Pseudomones aeruginosa* | Antipseudomonal penicillin plus aminoglycoside Ceftazidime plus aminoglycoside | Ceftazidime, Aztreonam, Imipenem (depends on hospital sensitivity pattern) Cefepime |
| *Serratia marcescens* | Cephalosporin third generation plus aminoglycoside | Imipenem, Aztreonam |
| *Legionella* | Erythromycin; may add rifampin | Fluoroquinolone |
| *Pneumocystis carinii* | Trimethoprim-sulfamethoxazole (steroids may be indicated for life-threatening infection) | Pentamidine |

MIC, minimum inhibitory concentration.

## Bibliography

American Thoracic Society. Hospital-acquired pneumonia in adults: diagnosis, assessment of severity, initial antimicrobial therapy, and preventive strategies. A consensus statement. *Am Rev Respir Crit Care Med* 1996;153:1711.
*Defines severe, hospital-acquired pneumonia requiring admission to ICU. The role of bronchoscopy in diagnosis of pneumonia in ICU remains controversial among pulmonologists.*

Andrews CP, et al. Diagnosis of nosocomial bacterial pneumonia in acute, diffuse lung injury. *Chest* 1981;80:3.
*The diagnosis of bacterial pneumonia in the setting of acute respiratory distress syndrome is particularly difficult.*

Ashbaugh DG, Petty TL. Sepsis complicating the acute respiratory distress syndrome. *Surg Gynecol Obstet* 1972;135:865.
*Mortality is high in patients with acute respiratory distress syndrome and concurrent pulmonary infection.*

Baigelman W, et al. Bacteriologic assessment of the lower respiratory tract in intubated patients. *Crit Care Med* 1986;14:864.
*Routine nasal suctioning compared well with flexible fiberoptic bronchoscopy.*

Bartlett JG, et al. Bacteriology of hospital-acquired pneumonia. *Arch Intern Med* 1986;146:868.
*Pathogens causing nosocomial pneumonia include, in order of decreasing prevalence, gram-negative bacilli, anaerobic bacteria,* S. aureus, *and* S. pneumoniae.

Bartlett JG, et al. Community-acquired pneumonia in adults. *Clin Infect Dis* 1998; 26:811.
*Infectious Disease Society of America guidelines on the treatment of community-acquired pneumonia. For patients hospitalized in an ICU, the panel recommends erythromycin, azithromycin, or a fluoroquinolone plus cefotaxime, ceftriaxone, or a β-lactamase inhibitor.*

Berk SL, Verghese A. Emerging pathogens in nosocomial pneumonia. *Eur J Clin Microbiol Infect Dis* 1989;8:11.
*Gram-negative bacilli have become the most common etiologic agents in nosocomial pneumonia, but some gram-positive cocci, such as enterococci, group B streptococci, staphylococci, and pneumococci, have taken on new significance.*

Bryan CS, Reynolds KL. Bacteremic nosocomial pneumonia. Analysis of 172 episodes from a single metropolitan area. *Am Rev Respir Dis* 1984;129:668.
*Bacteremic nosocomial pneumonia causes a 58% mortality rate.*

Bryant LR, et al. Misdiagnosis of pneumonia in patients needing mechanical respiration. *Arch Surg* 1973;106:286.
*Bacterial pneumonia is often overdiagnosed in the ICU setting.*

Celis R, et al. Nosocomial pneumonia. A multivariate analysis of risk and prognosis. *Chest* 1988;93:319.
*Identification of predisposing factors to nosocomial pneumonia ("high risk" microorganisms, bilateral pneumonia, respiratory failure, inappropriate antibiotics, age over 60 years, and presence of an ultimately or rapidly fatal underlying disease) may improve prognosis.*

Chastre J, et al. Prospective evaluation of the protected specimen brush for the diagnosis of pulmonary infections in ventilated patients. *Am Rev Respir Dis* 1984; 130:924.
*Quantitative cultures obtained from protected specimen brush bronchoscopy are useful in the diagnosis and treatment of pulmonary infections in ventilated patients.*

Chastre J, et al. Diagnosis of nosocomial bacterial pneumonia in intubated patients undergoing ventilation: comparison of the usefulness of bronchoalveolar lavage and the protected specimen brush. *Am J Med* 1988;85:499.
*Quantitative cultures from protected brush specimen were sensitive and specific in the diagnosis of ICU pneumonia.*

Craven DE, et al. Risk factors for pneumonia and fatality in patients receiving continuous mechanical ventilation. *Am Rev Respir Dis* 1986;133:792.
*The presence of an intracranial pressure monitor, treatment with cimetidine, hospitalization during fall-winter seasons, and ventilator circuit changes every 24 hours*

*were found to be significant risk factors for nosocomial pneumonia in the ventilated patient.*

Craven DE, et al. Nosocomial infection and fatality in medical and surgical intensive care unit patients. *Arch Intern Med* 1988;148:1161.
*Identifies nine variables significantly associated with fatality in nosocomial infection.*

Ekenna O, et al. Isolation of β-hemolytic streptococci from the respiratory tract: serotypic distribution and clinical significance. *Am J Med Sci* 1988;295:94.
*Group B streptococci were found to cause pneumonia in patients with mean age of 68.1 years. There was a 34% incidence of S. aureus coinfection.*

Fagan JY, et al. Detection of nosocomial lung infection in ventilated patients. Use of a protected specimen brush and quantitative culture techniques in 147 patients. *Am Rev Respir Dis* 1988;138:110.
*Protected specimen brush bronchoscopy was used in evaluating patients with pulmonary infiltrates and purulent tracheal secretions, the majority of whom did not have bacterial pneumonia.*

Fagan JY, et al. Nosocomial pneumonia in patients receiving continuous mechanical ventilation. Prospective analysis of 52 episodes with use of a protected specimen brush and quantitative culture techniques. *Am Rev Respir Dis* 1989;139:877.
*P. aeruginosa and S. aureus were involved in 33% of ventilator-associated pneumonias studied by protected specimen brush bronchoscopy.*

Fang GD, et al. New and emerging etiologies for community-acquired pneumonia with implications for therapy. A prospective multicenter study of 359 cases. *Medicine* 1990;69:307.
*Prospective study of community-acquired pneumonia defines etiologic agents well. Mortality is determined by etiologic agent.*

Gaussorgues P, et al. Comparison of nonbronchoscopic bronchoalveolar lavage to open lung biopsy for the bacteriologic diagnosis of pulmonary infections in mechanically ventilated patients. *Intesive Care Med* 1989;15:94.
*A cuffed catheter blindly guided through an endotracheal tube can be used for bronchoalveolar lavage in the diagnosis of pneumonia.*

Graybill JR, et al. Nosocomial pneumonia: a continuing major problem. *Am Rev Respir Dis* 1973;108:1130.
*Gram-negative nosocomial pneumonia, often following oropharyngeal colonization, is a common and frequently catastrophic event with high morbidity and mortality rates despite new antimicrobial agents.*

Hitt CM, et al. Streamlining antimicrobial therapy for lower respiratory infections. *Clin Infect Dis* 1997;24(Suppl 2):S231.
*The authors emphasize an approach to antibiotic therapy in lower respiratory infection in which a broad-spectrum empiric regimen is switched to a narrower-spectrum antibiotic based on culture results and other data.*

Johanson G, et al. Bacteriologic diagnosis of nosocomial pneumonia following prolonged mechanical ventilation. *Am Rev Respir Dis* 1988;137:259.
*Bronchoalveolar lavage provides the best reflection of the pulmonary bacterial burden in intubated patients.*

Johanson WG. Ventilator-associated pneumonia. Light at the end of the tunnel? *Chest* 1990;97:1027.
*Concise overview of methods for diagnosing ventilator-associated pneumonia.*

Johanson WR, et al. Nosocomial respiratory infections with gram-negative bacilli. The significance of colonization of the respiratory tract. *Ann Intern Med* 1972;77:701.
*Colonization of the respiratory tract with gram-negative bacilli is extremely common in the ICU patient, and respiratory tract infection occurs in 23% of such colonized patients.*

Joshi N, Localio AR, Hamory BH. A predictive risk index for nosocomial pneumonia in the intensive care unit. *Am J Med* 1991;93:135.
*Factors that lead to high risk for pneumonia in the ICU include endotracheal intubation, upper abdominal thoracic surgery, bronchoscopy, and presence of a nasogastric tube.*

Kappstein I, et al. Incidence of pneumonia in mechanically ventilated patients treated with sucralfate or cimetidine as prophylaxis for stress bleeding: bacterial colonization of the stomach. *Am J Med* 1991;91(Suppl 2A):125S–131S.

*Increased gastric pH may lead to a higher incidence of retrograde colonization of the oropharynx from the stomach with Enterobacteriaceae.*

Karnad A, Alvarez S, Berk SL. Pneumonia caused by gram-negative bacilli. *Am J Med* 1985;79:63.
*In pneumonia caused by gram-negative bacilli, associated bacteremia is most commonly seen with* P. aeruginosa *or* Serratia marcescens, *and outcome is poor.*

Meduri GU, Baselski V. The role of bronchoalveolar lavage in diagnosing nonopportunistic bacterial pneumonia. *Chest* 1991;100:179.
*Bronchoalveolar lavage is a simple and relatively safe technique with an expanding role in the diagnosis of nonopportunistic pulmonary infection.*

Miller KS, Sahn SA. Chest tubes: indications, technique, management and complications. *Chest* 1987;91:259.
*Current standards in critical care often require invasive procedures such as bronchoscopy and pulmonary biopsy. The potential for pneumothorax is significant, and those performing invasive procedures should be comfortable with chest tube insertion.*

Rello J, et al. Severe community-acquired pneumonia in the elderly: epidemiology and prognosis. *Clin Infect Dis* 1996;23:723.
S. pneumoniae *is the most common organism—seen in about half of all cases—to cause life-threatening pneumonia in the elderly.*

Salata RA, et al. Diagnosis of nosocomial pneumonia in intubated intensive care unit patients. *Am Rev Respir Dis* 1987;135:426.
*In intubated ICU patients, serial examination of endotracheal aspirates for elastin fibers, graded Gram's stain, and bacterial colony counts are useful in the diagnosis of pneumonia.*

Sanderson PJ. The sources of pneumonia in ICU patients. *Infect Control* 1986;7:104.
*Describes rates of colonization and pneumonia in ICUs in Great Britain.*

Scheld WM, Mandell GL. Nosocomial pneumonia: pathogenesis and recent advances in diagnosis and therapy. *Rev Infect Dis* 1991;13(Suppl 9):S743.
*Pneumonia is the leading cause of death from nosocomial infections, with a mortality rate of 20% to 50%.*

Seindenfeld JJ, et al. Incidence, site, and outcome of infections in patients with the adult respiratory distress syndrome. *Am Rev Respir Dis* 1986;134:12.
*Bacterial pathogens, the majority of them gram-negative organisms, account for most infections in patients with adult respiratory distress syndrome, and mortality rate can reach as high as 70% to 80%.*

Stevens RM, et al. Pneumonia in an intensive care unit. A 30-month experience. *Arch Intern Med* 1974;134:106.
*Established the high incidence and mortality rate of ICU pneumonia.*

Winterbauer RH, et al. The use of quantitative cultures and antibody coating of bacteria to diagnose bacterial pneumonia by fiberoptic bronchoscopy. *Am Rev Respir Dis* 1983;128:98.
*Quantitative cultures and immunofluorescent demonstration of antibody-coated bacteria are used to differentiate colonizing from infecting bacteria in lower respiratory tract secretions obtained by fiberoptic bronchoscopy.*

Young LS. Treatment of respiratory infections in the patient at risk. *Am J Med* 1984;76(Suppl 5A):61.
*Includes review of treatment response among patients with gram-negative pneumonia.*

---

## 8. COMMUNITY-ACQUIRED PNEUMONIA IN THE GERIATRIC PATIENT

---

Most elderly patients in whom community-acquired pneumonia (CAP) develops have an identifiable risk factor. Predisposing factors include chronic obstructive lung disease, lung cancer, alcoholism, influenza, congestive heart failure, multiple myeloma, chronic lymphocytic leukemia, esophageal disease, neurologic disorders that affect cough and swallowing reflexes (such as basal ganglia stroke), and immunosuppressive medication. Table 8-1 lists some of the relationships between predisposing illnesses and specific organisms that cause CAP in geriatric patients. *Streptococcus pneumoniae* is the most common bacterial pathogen. Mycobacteria often causes a chronic clinical disorder, unassociated with fever or night sweats, that resembles a pulmonary neoplasm. *Mycoplasma pneumoniae* is a rare cause of CAP in elderly patients, but polymicrobic infections, *Chlamydia pneumoniae* pneumonia, and respiratory syncytial virus pneumonia may be more common than initially believed. *Legionella* pneumonia very rarely is mild enough to permit management in the outpatient setting.

Manifestations of CAP in elderly patients are variable, ranging from septic shock or adult respiratory distress syndrome to altered mental status (acute confusion or a deterioration from baseline) with cough. Cough occurs more commonly than dyspnea. Some, although not all, patients experience pleuritic pain, sputum production, and fever.

A technically good chest x-ray film, even if the patient is dehydrated, should reveal an infiltrate. Rare exceptions include *Pneumocystis carinii* pneumonia in the HIV-infected patient and tuberculosis. A number of disorders can produce similar clinical and radiologic abnormalities and resemble pneumonia. The list includes both infectious (bronchitis) and noninfectious [heart failure, pulmonary embolism, lung cancer, aspiration of gastric contents, and BOOP (bronchiolitis obliterans–organizing pneumonia)] disorders. Rarely, pneumonia can be the initial manifestation of lung cancer.

Many elderly patients with pneumonia can be effectively treated without hospitalization. Hospitalization would be indicated for the patient who is immunocompromised (by disease or treatment) or disoriented, or who has concomitant unstable

Table 8-1. Microbiologic associations

| Disorders | Pathogen |
|---|---|
| Chronic obstructive lung disease | *Streptococcus pneumoniae* <br> *Haemophilus influenzae* <br> *Moraxella* (*Branhamella*) *catarrhalis* <br> *Legionella* species |
| Obstructive neoplasm | Polymicrobic (anaerobes/aerobes) |
| Alcoholism | *S. pneumoniae* <br> *H. influenzae* <br> *Klebsiella* species <br> *Mycobacterium tuberculosis* <br> Anaerobes |
| HIV infection | *Pneumocystis carinii* <br> *S. pneumoniae* <br> *H. influenzae* <br> *M. tuberculosis* |
| Central nervous system depression/ esophageal disease | Anaerobes |
| Multiple myeloma/chronic lymphocytic leukemia | *S. pneumoniae* <br> *H. influenzae* <br> Gram-negative bacilli |
| Hodgkin's disease/steroid treatment | Gram-negative bacilli <br> *Pneumocystis carinii* <br> *S. pneumoniae* <br> *M. tuberculosis* <br> Fungi |
| Granulocytopenia | Gram-negative bacilli <br> *Aspergillus* species <br> *Staphylococcus aureus* |

medical disorder(s), an obstructive neoplasm, or infection beyond the lung (concomitant empyema, meningitis, endocarditis, pericarditis, septic arthritis). Patients should also be admitted to the hospital when they are noncompliant or have an inadequate support system, the disease is caused by a bacterium other than *S. pneumoniae, Haemophilus influenzae,* or *Branhamella (Moraxella) catarrhalis,* or there is a need for immediate intervention (as in shock, respiratory failure, electrolyte abnormalities, or failure of initial outpatient treatment). This listing is not complete, however, and additional social, ethical, economic, and medical considerations can influence the decision for hospitalization.

Candidates for admission to the ICU include patients who require mechanical ventilation or who have a respiratory rate greater than 30 breaths per minute, multiple lobe involvement, shock that fails to respond to intravenous fluid challenge, or concomitant life-endangering events (myocardial ischemia, meningitis).

The hospitalized patient merits a CBC count, arterial blood gas analysis, electrocardiogram, tests for renal and hepatic function, and measurement of serum electrolytes (including calcium, phosphate, and magnesium). Hypokalemia and hypomagnesemia can precipitate digitalis-related arrhythmias. Hypophosphatemia impairs the contractile properties of the diaphragm during acute respiratory failure, and hypocalcemia, which can occur during gram-negative infections, impairs cardiac contractility, causing arrhythmias and contributing to hypotension.

Although its value is debated, I feel that a properly performed and interpreted Gram's stain of valid expectorated sputum is a useful guide to direct initial antibiotic selection, and that blood cultures should be obtained before antibiotic treatment is begun. Additional laboratory studies that on occasion provide invaluable microbiologic information include the following: sputum culture, acid-fast bacilli stain/culture, urine *Legionella* antigen testing, and analysis of pleural fluid.

Fiberoptic bronchoscopy is usually reserved for patients who are immunocompromised and critically ill and for those who have a nonresolving pneumonia. Bronchoscopy can be useful to identify endobronchial pathology (tumors, foreign bodies), polymicrobic infections, and unusual or drug-resistant organisms.

Computed tomography of the lungs is particularly useful when the plain film shows a questionable finding or an obstructive mass, when there is a need to differentiate between a parenchymal lung abscess and empyema, and when interventional diagnostic and therapeutic procedures, such as guided transthoracic biopsy, aspiration, or drainage, are indicated.

Therapy consists of antibiotic treatment, adequate oxygenation, fluid/electrolyte administration, patient positioning, nutritional support, drainage of empyema, and, in the case of patients who will experience prolonged inactivity, prophylaxis for deep venous thrombosis. Patients who experience delirium should be assessed for meningitis, hypoxemia, hypoglycemia, and overmedication. Ancillary treatments that have not proved efficacious include vigorous hydration, postural drainage (in the absence of a lung abscess), and administration of an antipyretic.

Guidelines for the initial empiric administration of an antibiotic to the nonimmunocompromised elderly patient have been published. Selection of an empiric antibiotic would take into account the following: drug allergy history, occupational/exposure history, renal function, immune status, the probable organism, and the potential for drug-drug interaction. For a patient who is not penicillin-allergic and does not meet the criteria for management in the medical ICU, ceftriaxone would be an appropriate selection. For a patient who merited admission to an ICU, I would consider prescribing levofloxacin, as this fluoroquinolone has demonstrated efficacy in patients with pneumonia caused by the traditional bacterial pathogens, and also in patients infected with *Legionella* species and *Staphylococcus aureus.* The antimicrobial should be administered as soon as possible.

When a patient fails to respond to therapy, the clinician should consider the following reasons: The disease is of noninfectious origin; the infection is caused by an unusual organism or is polymicrobic; the respiratory pathogen is resistant to the antibiotic selected; unrecognized/undrained empyema is present; an endobronchial lesion is present; host defenses are deficient, or the cardiovascular system is deteriorating concomitantly (arrhythmia, congestive heart failure, or compromised cardiac blood flow). In the case of an outpatient receiving an oral antibiotic, an additional consideration of drug failure is lack of compliance.

Selected hospitalized elderly patients are candidates for oral antibiotic treatment after 72 hours of intravenous therapy. Candidates for this "switch" ("step-down," "follow-on," "sequential") therapy must be immunocompetent and clinically improving, have no impairment of absorption of oral medication, and have an appropriate support system on discharge. Appropriate drugs for switch therapy include amoxicillin-clavulanate, doxycycline, trimethoprim-sulfamethoxazole, cefuroxime, and levofloxacin, as they are well absorbed, have excellent bioavailability, and provide therapeutic tissue concentrations that inhibit the majority of strains of the two traditional bacterial respiratory pathogens, *S. pneumoniae* and *H. influenzae*.

Some measures that appear to enhance drug compliance among geriatric patients include the following: oral and written instructions, the establishment of a daily routine for taking the medication, a simplified medication program, and assistance from family and friends. Patient compliance is also enhanced when oral antibiotic treatment is prescribed no more frequently than twice a day.

The optimum treatment duration for geriatric patients with uncomplicated CAP caused by *S. pneumoniae* or *H. influenzae* has never been firmly established. There are data to indicate, however, that a 7- to 10-day treatment course is appropriate. Recovery of premorbid physical health often exceeds 30 days, and complete radiographic resolution often takes 3 to 4 months after the onset of antimicrobial therapy. Malignancy and neurologic disease are associated with a high risk for death within 30 days of the recognition and management of pneumonia. (R.A.G.)

## Bibliography

Bartlett JG, et al. Community acquired pneumonia in adults: guidelines for management. *Clin Infect Dis* 1998;26:811–838.
*Recommended guidelines issued by the Infectious Disease Society of America.*
Beck SL. Justifying the use of blood cultures when diagnosing community-acquired pneumonia. *Chest* 1995;108:891–892.
*Editorial underscores the value of blood cultures in the evaluation of the hospitalized patient.*
Gleckman R, DeLaRosa G. In-hospital management of pneumonia in the elderly. *J Crit Illness* 1997;12:163–171.
*A review of microbiology, clinical and laboratory features, and treatment.*
Houston M, Silverstein MD, Surman VJ. Risk factors for 30-day mortality in elderly patients with lower respiratory tract infection. *Arch Intern Med* 1997;157:2190–2195.
*Malignancy and neurologic disease are associated with a high risk for death within 30 days of pneumonia.*
Meehan TP, et al. Quality of care, process and outcomes in elderly patients with pneumonia. *JAMA* 1997;278:2080–2084.
*Administering antibiotics within 8 hours of admission is associated with improved survival.*
Niederman MS, et al. Guidelines for the initial management of adults with community-acquired pneumonia: diagnosis, assessment of severity, and initial antimicrobial therapy. *Am Rev Respir Dis* 1993;148:1418–1426.
*A statement adopted by the American Thoracic Society.*
Reimer LG, Carroll KC. Role of the microbiology laboratory in the diagnosis of lower respiratory tract infections. *Clin Infect Dis* 1998;26:742–748.
*Use of body fluids to define the etiology of CAP.*
Rhew DC, et al. The clinical benefit of in-hospital observation in "low-risk" pneumonia patients after conversion from parenteral to oral antimicrobial therapy. *Chest* 1998;113:142–146.
*Conversion from intravenous to oral antibiotic therapy does not require a day of observation in the hospital.*
Siegel RE, et al. A prospective randomized study of inpatient IV antibiotics for community-acquired pneumonia. *Chest* 1996;110:965–971.
*Demonstrates the safety, efficacy and cost savings from a shortened course of IV antibiotic treatment.*

## 9. DISEASE CAUSED BY *LEGIONELLA PNEUMOPHILA* AND *CHLAMYDIA PNEUMONIAE*

*Legionnella*

An unrecognized bacterial genus until 1977, *Legionella* was isolated by the Centers for Disease Control during the investigation of an explosive outbreak of pneumonia among American Legion conventioneers in Philadelphia. More than 25 species of *Legionella* have subsequently been isolated, and 14 serotypes of *Legionella pneumophila* have been identified. About 90% of human infections are caused by *L. pneumophila;* other species recovered from patients include *L. micdadei, L. bozemanii, L. dumoffii, L. gormanii,* and *L. feeleii. Legionella* is usually associated with community-acquired and nosocomial pneumonia; however, members of this genus have been recovered from a variety of extrapulmonary infections.

*L. pneumophila,* the etiologic agent of Legionnaires' disease, can be isolated from water found in nature (e.g., lakes, creeks), heat-exchange units (e.g., cooling towers), and domestic supplies (e.g., taps, showers), and most epidemics of Legionnaires' disease have been traced to contaminated water from one of these sources. On the basis of the epidemiologic observations, investigators have assumed that Legionnaires' disease develops after a person inhales aerosols containing the organism; however, contemporary studies have suggested that aspiration may play a prominent role in the pathogenesis of the infection. Person-to-person transmission has not been documented.

A facultative, intracellular pathogen, *L. pneumophila* is capable of persisting and multiplying within pulmonary alveolar macrophages. Thus, an intact cellular immune system is essential for preventing and controlling infection by the organism. Not surprisingly, many patients who experience Legionnaires' disease are immunosuppressed. Optimal antimicrobial treatment includes drugs that penetrate macrophages (macrolides, rifampin, fluoroquinolones), and relapses have occurred following short courses of therapy.

The risk for Legionnaires' disease is increased in men, persons over the age of 50 years (mean age, 56 years), and smokers. Risk is also increased among patients who receive corticosteroids or cytotoxic agents, who are alcoholic, or who have diabetes mellitus, cancer, chronic obstructive pulmonary disease, or renal failure requiring dialysis or transplantation. Case-control studies have also found a significant association between Legionnaires' disease and the occupation of construction worker, the presence of excavation sites near the home, and a history of travel within the preceding 2 weeks.

The onset of Legionnaires' disease is typically abrupt. The initial symptoms are usually nonspecific and include fever, anorexia, malaise, myalgias, and headache. Recurrent chills or rigors are experienced by most patients. The fever may increase in a stepwise fashion, and temperatures above 40°C are seen in more than half of cases. Pulmonary symptoms appear 2 to 3 days after the onset of illness, and they may progress within a few hours to include dyspnea and cyanosis. The cough is initially dry but becomes productive of nonpurulent secretions and, subsequently, frankly purulent sputum; hemoptysis occurs in up to one third of cases. Chest pain, which is usually pleuritic, is common. Diarrhea, which consists of the passage of three to four loose or watery stools daily, occurs in about one half of all cases, and this symptom may precede or follow the respiratory complaints.

The physical examination typically reveals an acutely ill patient with tachypnea and an unremitting fever above 38.4°C; a relative bradycardia is found in two thirds of patients. Auscultation of the chest reveals moist crackles and rhonchi; evidence of consolidation or a pleural effusion may appear later in the course. An abnormal neurologic evaluation is recorded in up to one third of patients; changes in mental status include emotional lability, confusion, delirium, hallucinations, lethargy, and stupor. The neurologic examination may also reveal fine or coarse tremors, hyperactive reflexes, and signs of cerebellar dysfunction, such as dysarthria or ataxia.

A total WBC count of more than 10,000/mm$^3$ is found in three fourths of patients, and immature granulocytes are common; however, the leukocyte count rarely exceeds 20,000/mm$^3$. Thrombocytopenia and disseminated intravascular coagulation occur infrequently. The urinalysis may demonstrate proteinuria or hematuria. Evidence of acute renal failure may be present; the kidney dysfunction is usually a consequence of shock, disseminated intravascular coagulation, immune complex glomerulonephritis, interstitial nephritis, hemoglobinuria, or myoglobinuria. A number of nonspecific biochemical abnormalities have been noted in patients with Legionnaires' disease, including modest elevations in bilirubin and hepatic enzymes, hypoalbuminemia, hypophosphatemia, and hyponatremia. Cerebrospinal fluid is almost always normal. The initial chest radiograph characteristically reveals a patchy, unilobar infiltrate; any area of the lungs may be involved, although lower lobe disease is most common. The pulmonary infiltrate usually progresses to complete consolidation, and occasionally cavitation may occur; patients who are receiving corticosteroids are at greater risk for development of a lung abscess. The pulmonary process can spread to involve adjacent lobes or the opposite lung. Pleural effusions are typically small.

A number of laboratory methods are available for diagnosing Legionnaires' disease. A serologic assay, the indirect fluorescent antibody (IFA) test, represents the most commonly employed diagnostic procedure. A fourfold increase in IFA titer to at least 1:128 between acute and convalescent phases of the disease is considered confirmatory. Unfortunately, an interval of 6 to 8 weeks is often required to detect a diagnostic rise in IFA titers. A single acute-phase IFA titer of 1:256 or above in a patient with an illness compatible with Legionnaires' disease has been believed to represent strong presumptive evidence of the infection; however, recent studies have cast doubt on the predictive value of a single antibody titer in the patient with sporadic legionellosis. The urinary antigen assay has become commercially available; this technique is 80% to 90% sensitive in patients infected with *L. pneumophila* serogroup 1, which is responsible for about 80% of the sporadic cases of Legionnaires' disease. Direct fluorescent antibody (DFA) staining is a rapid means of diagnosing the disease. This technique can be used to examine expectorated sputum, transtracheal aspirates, pleural fluid, and lung or extrapulmonary tissues for the presence of *L. pneumophila*. In laboratories with extensive experience with the procedure, DFA staining of sputum is about 70% sensitive and 95% specific. The existence of multiple serogroups of *L. pneumophila* contributes to the difficulty of DFA staining. *L. pneumophila* can be recovered from primary cultures of sputum, pleural fluid, blood, lung biopsy specimens, and other clinical material. Special media, such as buffered charcoal yeast extract agar and biphasic blood culture broth, are required for isolation. It usually requires 3 to 7 days to detect the growth of *L. pneumophila*. Occasionally, *Legionella* organisms can be seen on the Gram's stain of clinical material; they appear as faintly staining, small, gram-negative bacilli. Special stains (e.g., DFA, Dieterle silver impregnation) are usually required to detect the organism in pathologic specimens. Finally, DNA amplification through the use of the polymerase chain reaction (PCR) has been shown to be very sensitive and highly specific, and the technique has been used to detect *Legionella* in bronchoalveolar lavage specimens and throat swabs; PCR for the diagnosis of Legionnaires' disease will likely become widely available.

The overlap in the clinical manifestations of sporadic legionellosis and other pneumonias is usually sufficient to obscure the correct diagnosis early in the patient's course. The presence of a progressive pneumonic disease associated with multisystem abnormalities; a paucity of sputum; the absence of a predominant organism on Gram's stain or culture; and the persistence of prostration, unremitting fever, and recurrent rigors despite therapy with penicillins, cephalosporins, or aminoglycosides should raise the possibility of Legionnaires' disease. Infection with *Mycoplasma pneumoniae* and *Chlamydia pneumoniae* can resemble disease caused by *L. pneumophila;* however, patients with *M. pneumoniae* and *C. pneumoniae* infection tend to be healthy younger adults, and they usually experience an illness that is more insidious in onset and less intense in severity. Psittacosis, tularemia, and Q fever can produce clinical syndromes that parallel those associated with Legionnaires' disease; these alternative diagnoses can usually be excluded by a detailed epidemiologic history. Because patients with Legionnaires' disease are often immunocompromised hosts, they are at risk to experience either concurrent or sequential infection with other pathogens, including common pyogenic bacteria, such as *Streptococcus pneumoniae* and *Mycobacterium tuberculosis*.

Under laboratory conditions, *L. pneumophila* demonstrates susceptibility to a large number of antimicrobial agents, including macrolides/azalides, tetracyclines, and fluoroquinolones. Clinical experience during the past two decades has supported the use of erythromycin as the drug of choice for the therapy of Legionnaires' disease; similarly, observations made during the initial outbreak of Legionnaires' disease in Philadelphia 1976 and subsequent reports indicate that tetracycline or doxycycline is also effective. In generally small, noncomparative studies, azithromycin, clarithromycin, ciprofloxacin, ofloxacin, and perfloxacin have all been shown to be curative. At present, some experts recommend that a fluoroquinolone be utilized as initial therapy. The use of ciprofloxacin or ofloxacin eliminates some of the nettlesome problems associated with high-dose erythromycin therapy, including phlebitis at the infusion site, gastrointestinal intolerance, a number of potential drug-drug interactions, and the need to infuse the macrolide with large volumes of fluid.

In general, high doses of antimicrobials should be administered to patients with suspected or confirmed Legionnaires' disease. For patients with a milder clinical illness and without significant underlying diseases, some experts recommend clarithromycin or azithromycin as initial therapy; for immunosuppressed or critically ill patients, a fluoroquinolone might be selected. If erythromycin or doxycycline is employed and if the patient appears seriously ill, rifampin should also be administered. Of note, all antimicrobial regimens have been associated with treatment failures, and if the patient fails to demonstrate some improvement within 48 to 72 hours, an alternate therapy should be considered.

The response to appropriate antimicrobial therapy is characteristically prompt, and most patients show substantial improvement within 24 to 48 hours. Occasionally, the chest radiograph will demonstrate a progression of the infiltrate during the first few days of treatment; however, some clearing of the pneumonia usually occurs within the first 2 weeks of therapy. Complete resolution of pulmonary infiltrates may take 4 to 8 weeks. With clinical improvement, patients may be given oral antimicrobials. A 3-week course of antimicrobial therapy should be completed to reduce the likelihood of relapse; patients with lung abscesses require more prolonged therapy.

The prognosis among patients with Legionnaires' disease is correlated with the severity of underlying disease and the use of appropriate antimicrobials. The overall case fatality rate for sporadic legionellosis ranges from 6% to 25%; however, among patients who are immunosuppressed and who do not receive appropriate antimicrobial therapy, mortality rates of up to 80% have been noted. Persistent malaise, fatigue, and problems with memory are common complaints among patients who experience Legionnaires' disease.

Pontiac fever represents the second most common syndrome associated with *L. pneumophila*. Although the etiology remained obscure until *Legionella* was isolated, the disease was first observed in 1968 among employees in a county health department building in Pontiac, Michigan. Since that time, a limited number of epidemics have been reported. Aerosolized contaminated water has been implicated as the source of these outbreaks. Pontiac fever is a nonpneumonic form of legionellosis that affects previously healthy adults. The illness is remarkable for a short incubation period (24 to 48 hours) and a high attack rate (up to 95% of exposed persons). Clinically, Pontiac fever is characterized by fever of up to 40°C, chills, myalgias, headache, fatigue, a dry cough, and vague neurologic symptoms, such as dizziness. A leukocytosis is frequently noted among hospitalized patients. The acute illness usually resolves within 48 to 96 hours without specific therapy. Residual complaints are common, and these symptoms include lassitude, forgetfulness, and an inability to concentrate. Neither secondary cases nor deaths have been reported. Other *Legionella* species, including *L. feeleii,* have been identified as causes of outbreaks of Pontiac fever.

Resulting from hematogenous dissemination, extrapulmonary infections with *L. pneumophila* usually occur as a complication of Legionnaires' disease. Pericarditis and hemodialysis fistula infections have been described in association with Legionnaires' disease. A few other localized infections, such as pyelonephritis and myocarditis, have been identified at postmortem examination. On occasion, infections with *Legionella* species can occur in the absence of obvious lung involvement; *L. pneu-*

*mophila* has been identified as the cause of bacterial endocarditis in a patient with prosthetic valves, and *Legionella* has been implicated as a cause of granulomatous hepatitis, fever of unknown origin, and postoperative wound infections.

### Chlamydia pneumoniae

*C. pneumoniae* (TWAR agent) was first isolated from the conjunctivae of a Taiwanese child in 1965 and subsequently associated with acute respiratory tract infections in humans in 1983. Following the recognition that the microbe can cause sinusitis, pharyngitis, bronchitis, and pneumonia, epidemiologic studies demonstrated that infections with *C. pneumoniae* are prevalent; for example, approximately 50% of all adults and 75% of aged individuals have serologic evidence of prior infection, and the microbe has been implicated in about 5% of episodes of sinusitis and 10% of cases of community-acquired pneumonia.

Like other chlamydial species, *C. pneumoniae* is an obligate intracellular pathogen. In contrast to *C. psittaci,* which can also cause pneumonia in adults, *C. pneumoniae* does not have a zoonotic reservoir, and all disease is believed to result from human-to-human transmission via respiratory tract secretions. The incubation period seems to last several weeks. Although outbreaks of disease among close contacts, such as family members, have been reported, transmission appears inefficient, and most cases are likely the consequence of acquisition from asymptomatic carriers. Finally, *C. pneumoniae* can remain viable on environmental surfaces for hours, raising the possibility that fomites play a role in transmission.

Infection with *C. pneumoniae* leads to both cellular and serologic immune responses; the latter includes IgM and IgG antibodies, and those immunoglobulins serve as important markers for the diagnosis of acute infection and for epidemiologic studies. Of note, the seroprevalence studies have demonstrated that epidemics of infection occur in 4- to 6-year cycles and that attack rates are highest in children 5 to 14 years of age. The seroepidemiologic investigations have also suggested that immunity is not long-lived and that many people are infected repeatedly throughout life.

The symptoms and signs of bronchitis and pneumonia caused by *C. pneumoniae* do not appear to be unique. As in other nonpyogenic respiratory tract infections, the onset of disease is usually insidious. Often, the illness is biphasic; initially, the patient experiences pharyngitis that may be associated with hoarseness, and after the upper respiratory tract symptoms abate, the patient notes fever and a nonproductive cough. The most notable physical examination finding may be a relative bradycardia; focal rales on chest auscultation are usually present in patients with pneumonia. Relevant laboratory test results include a normal WBC count and a focal, usually subsegmental lower lobe infiltrate on chest radiograph; among older patients and persons with underlying diseases, the infiltrates can be extensive. Occasionally, patients may have coinfection with *S. pneumoniae* and, of course, these patients can be very ill. Case fatality rates for relatively fit persons with pneumonia are extremely low; however, cough and malaise can persist for weeks following resolution of the infection.

The isolation of *C. pneumoniae* requires tissue culture systems. Accordingly, serologic testing represents the usual method of diagnosis. The *C. pneumoniae*-specific microimmunofluorescence test appears to be the most reliably sensitive and specific assay. The serologic response to infection is variable and occurs slowly; accordingly, acute and convalescent phase sera should be secured 3 to 4 weeks apart, and the paired specimens should be submitted for testing. Because patients can experience either an acute primary infection or an acute reinfection, the patterns of serologic response will vary. In general, in acute primary infection, IgM antibodies appear about 2 to 3 weeks following the onset of illness, and IgG antibodies become detectable 6 to 8 weeks after the onset of disease; a fourfold antibody rise, an IgM titer at or above 1:16, or an IgG titer at or above 1:512 is considered diagnostic. In patients with reinfection, IgM antibodies may not appear, and a fourfold titer rise, which can occur in 1 to 2 weeks, is considered diagnostic. Finally, although employed primarily as a research tool, PCR has been utilized successfully to detect *C. pneumoniae* in clinical specimens, such as pharyngeal swabs and sputum.

Controlled trials concerning the therapy of lower respiratory tract infections caused by *C. pneumoniae* remain limited. *In vitro,* the microbe is susceptible to erythromycin, azithromycin, clarithromycin, doxycycline, and some of the fluoroquinolones; limited clinical data suggest that the macrolides and the azalide (azithromycin) possess comparable efficacy. The course of therapy should be 14 to 21 days; some authorities suggest that if cough or malaise persists, a second course of antimicrobials be administered, and in the absence of contraindications, doxycycline or tetracycline is recommended. Like other chlamydial organisms, the agent is not susceptible to beta-lactam antibiotics, such as amoxicillin.

C. pneumoniae has also been identified as a cause of other acute illnesses; these include pharyngitis, sinusitis, otitis media, and rarely, a systemic sepsis-like syndrome. Of special note is the fact that the microbe has been associated with several chronic conditions, most notably asthmatic bronchitis and coronary artery disease. The relationship between C. pneumoniae and coronary artery disease is based on seroprevalence studies, which have demonstrated that patients with coronary artery disease are more likely to have serologic evidence of prior infection, and on morphologic and immunologic investigations, in which the microbe has been visualized by electron microscopy or detected by PCR or immunocytochemical staining in atheromatous plaques from coronary arteries and other vessels. Although C. pneumoniae has been definitively associated with atheromatous lesions, the role of the microbe in the pathogenesis of vascular disease remains to be defined. Finally, a number of reports have indicated that reinfection may precipitate the onset of acute myocardial infarction. (A.L.E.)

## Bibliography
*Legionnella*
Alexiou SD, et al. Isolation of *Legionella pneumophila* from hotels in Greece. *Eur J Epidemiol* 1989;5:47.
> Legionella *was recovered from water samples taken from hotels located in different areas of Greece that were associated with cases of Legionnaires' disease.*
Ampel NM, Rubin FL, Norden CW. Cutaneous abscess caused by *Legionella micdadei* in an immunosuppressed patient. *Ann Intern Med* 1985;102:630.
> *A patient receiving immunosuppressive drugs had a leg abscess complicate* Legionella pneumonia.
Arnow PM, Boyko EJ. Perirectal abscess caused by *Legionella pneumophila* and mixed anaerobic bacteria. *Ann Intern Med* 1983;98:184.
> Legionella pneumophila *and anaerobic bacteria were cultured from a perirectal abscess in an immunosuppressed patient with* Legionella pneumonia.
Bangsborg JM, et al. Legionellosis in patients with HIV infection. *Infection* 1990; 18:342.
> *Based on observations in 180 patients, the authors conclude that Legionnaires' disease is uncommon in HIV-infected patients. They did identify, however, two patients infected concurrently with* Legionella *and* Pneumocystis carinii.
Blatt SP, et al. Nosocomial Legionnaires' disease: aspiration as a primary mode of disease acquisition. *Am J Med* 1993;95:16.
> *In this prospective, case-control study of 14 patients with nosocomial Legionnaires' disease, the authors found evidence that the infections were caused by aspiration.*
Dorman SA, Hardin NJ, Winn WC Jr. Pyelonephritis associated with *Legionella pneumophila* serogroup 4. *Ann Intern Med* 1980;93:186.
> *The authors report the isolation of* Legionella *from the lungs and kidneys of a patient with metastatic bladder cancer and fatal pneumonia.*
Dowling JN, Saha AK, Glew RH. Virulence factors of the family Legionellaceae. *Microbiol Rev* 1992;56:32.
> *An excellent review of the molecular mechanisms that enable* Legionella *to persist and replicate within phagocytic cells.*
Dowling JN, et al. Pneumonia and multiple lung abscesses caused by dual infection with *Legionella micdadei* and *Legionella pneumophila*. *Am Rev Respir Dis* 1983;127:121.
> *A patient immunosuppressed by medications and a splenectomy experienced a nearfatal infection caused by two distinct species of* Legionella.

Edelstein PH. Antimicrobial therapy for Legionnaire's disease: a review. *Clin Infect Dis* 1995;21 (Suppl 3):S265.

*Based on an exhaustive review of the laboratory and clinical data concerning the activity and efficacy of macrolides, tetracyclines, and other classes of antimicrobials, this expert recommends that patients with Legionnaires' disease who are immunocompromised or severely ill be treated with a fluoroquinolone rather than erythromycin.*

Evans CP, Winn WC. Extrathoracic localization of *Legionella pneumophila* in Legionnaires' pneumonia. *Am J Clin Pathol* 1981;76:813.

*In 6 of 12 cases of fatal Legionnaires' disease, the bacterium was isolated from extrapulmonary sites, including the spleen, liver, and kidney.*

Fang GD, Yu VL, Vickers RM. Disease due to Legionellaceae (other than *Legionella pneumophila*). *Medicine* 1989;68:116.

*An extensive review of the epidemiology, microbiology, and clinical diseases associated with this family of bacteria.*

Fraser DW, et al. Legionnaires' disease: description of an epidemic of pneumonia. *N Engl J Med* 1977;297:1189.

*In the summer of 1976, American Legion conventioneers in Philadelphia experienced an outbreak of disease that was associated with pneumonia in 90% of those affected and with a case fatality rate of 16%.*

Glick TH, et al. Pontiac fever: an epidemic of unknown etiology in a health department. I. Clinical and epidemiologic aspects. *Am J Epidemiol* 1978;107:149.

*Serologic studies confirmed that the acute febrile illness experienced by 95 of the 100 persons employed in the county health department facility in Pontiac, Michigan, was caused by the bacterium responsible for Legionnaires' disease.*

Hamedani P, et al. The safety and efficacy of clarithromycin in patients with *Legionella* pneumonia. *Chest* 1991;100:1503.

*A role for the use of clarithromycin in treating patients with Legionnaires' disease is suggested by the results of this study.*

Heath CH, Grove DI, Looke DFM. Delay in appropriate therapy for *Legionella* pneumonia associated with increased mortality. *Eur J Clin Microbiol Infect Dis* 1996;15:286.

*In this retrospective review of 39 cases of Legionnaires' disease, the mortality rate was correlated with delays in initiating therapy with erythromycin.*

Jaulhac B, et al. Detection of *Legionella* spp. in bronchoalveolar lavage fluids by DNA amplification. *J Clin Microbiol* 1992;30:920.

*Polymerase chain reaction was more sensitive than bacterial cultures or serologic assays in detecting the presence of Legionella.*

Kalweit WH, Winn WC. Hemodialysis fistula infections caused by *Legionella pneumophila*. *Ann Intern Med* 1982;96:173.

*In two patients receiving long-term hemodialysis, infections developed at fistula sites as complications of Legionnaires' pneumonia.*

Lake KB, et al. Legionnaires' disease and pulmonary cavitation. *Arch Intern Med* 1979;139:485.

Legionella *has the potential to produce lung abscesses.*

Lowry PW, et al. A cluster of *Legionella* sternal wound infections due to postoperative topical exposure to contaminated tap water. *N Engl J Med* 1991;324:109.

*The authors describe three patients in whom sternal wound infections with* Legionella *developed as the result of contact with contaminated tap water.*

Marrie TJ, et al. Control of endemic nosocomial Legionnaires' disease by using sterile potable water for high-risk patients. *Epidemiol Infect* 1991;107:591.

*Although Legionnaires' disease is considered inhalation-based in origin, the authors' data indicate that the infection can be aspiration-based in etiology. Immunosuppressed patients exposed to contaminated potable water through mechanical ventilation or nasogastric tubes were at greatest risk for the infection.*

Maycock R, Skale B, Kohler B. *Legionella pneumophila* pericarditis proved by culture of pericardial fluid. *Am J Med* 1983;75:534.

Legionella pneumophila *was isolated from the pericardial fluid of a patient with pericarditis complicating pneumonia.*

Milder JE, Rough RR. Concurrent Legionnaires' disease and active pulmonary tuberculosis. *Am Rev Respir Dis* 1982;125:759.
*An elderly patient infected with* Mycobacterium tuberculosis *and* Legionella pneumophila *is described.*

Passi C, Maddaluno R, Pastoris MC. Incidence of *Legionella pneumophila* infection in tourists: Italy. *Public Health* 1990;104:183.
*Legionella was isolated from the water systems of 10 Italian hotels that were associated with cases of Legionnaires' disease.*

Plouffe JF, et al. Reevaluation of the definition of Legionnaires' disease: use of the urinary antigen assay. *Clin Infect Dis* 1995;20:1286.
*A single acute-phase titer above 1:256 did not discriminate between adults with Legionnaires' disease and those with pneumonia caused by other microbes. The urinary antigen assay rarely gave a false-positive result (<1%), and results of the assay were positive in 56% of all cases of Legionnaire's disease and 80% of the cases in which* L. pneumophila serogroup 1 was isolated.

Ramirez JA, et al. Diagnosis of *Legionella pneumophila, Mycoplasma pneumoniae* or *Chlamydia pneumoniae* lower respiratory tract infection using the polymerase chain reaction on a single throat swab. *Diagn Microbiol Infect Dis* 1996;24:7.
*A single throat swab was 88% sensitive and 100% specific in detecting the presence of* L. pneumophila, M. pneumoniae, *or* C. pneumoniae *in patients with infection caused by one of those microbes.*

Ruf B, et al. The incidence of *Legionella* pneumonia: a 1-year prospective study in a large community hospital. *Lung* 1989;167:11.
*In this study of 476 patients,* Legionella *pneumonia was identified in 5% of the 240 cases of community-acquired infection and in 6.8% of the 236 cases of nosocomial disease.*

Tompkins LS, et al. *Legionella* prosthetic-valve endocarditis. *N Engl J Med* 1988;318:530.
*The authors of an epidemiologic investigation of seven patients with* Legionella *prosthetic valve endocarditis concluded that the infections were acquired nosocomially.*

Warner CL, Fayad PB, Heffner RR Jr. *Legionella* myositis. *Neurology* 1991;41:750.
*The authors provide evidence of direct muscle infection by* Legionella.

*Chlamydia pneumoniae*

Blasi F, et al. A possible association of *Chlamydia pneumoniae* infection and acute myocardial infarction in patients younger than 65 years of age. *Chest* 1997;112:309.
*This retrospective seroprevalence study confirmed an association between infection by* C. pneumoniae *and coronary artery disease and acute myocardial infarction.*

Grayston JT, et al. A new respiratory tract pathogen: *Chlamydia pneumoniae* strain TWAR. *J Infect Dis* 1990;161:618.
*The authors summarize the initial clinical and epidemiological observations concerning* C. pneumoniae.

Gupta S, et al. Elevated *Chlamydia pneumoniae* antibodies, cardiovscular events, and azithromycin in male survivors of myocardial infarction. *Circulation* 1997;96:404.
*In this prospective investigation, patients with acute myocardial infarctions and high titers (>1:64) of antibodies to* C. pneumoniae *experienced a fourfold greater risk for an adverse cardiovascular event during follow-up than did patients without increased titers.*

Gurfinkel E, et al. Randomised trial of roxithromycin in non–Q-wave coronary syndromes: ROXIS Pilot Study. *Lancet* 1997;350:404.
*In this prospective, double-blinded study of patients with unstable angina or non–Q-wave myocardial infarction, the use of roxithromycin, a macrolide antibiotic, was associated with a reduction in the rates of recurrent ischemic events, including infarction and death.*

Kuo CC, et al. *Chlamydia pneumoniae* (TWAR). *Clin Microbiol Rev* 1995;8:451.
*An excellent review that focuses on the microbiology, epidemiology, and laboratory diagnosis of disease caused by* C. pneumoniae.

Laurila AL, von Hertzen L, Saikku P. *Chlamydia pneumoniae* and chronic lung diseases. *Scand J Infect Dis Suppl* 1997;104:34.

C. pneumoniae *has been associated with several chronic pulmonary diseases, including asthma, chronic obstructive pulmonary disease, sarcoidosis, and even lung cancer.*

Mazzoli S, et al. *Chlamydia pneumoniae* antibody response in patients with acute myocardial infarction and their follow-up. *Am Heart J* 1998;135:15.

*In contrast to healthy and matched controls, patients with acute myocardial infarction had high titers of antichlamydial antibodies and elevated levels of interleukin 6.*

Troy CJ, et al. *Chlamydia pneumoniae* as a new source of infectious outbreaks in nursing homes. *JAMA* 1997;277:1214.

*In this retrospective investigation of three nursing homes, the authors found that attack rates for respiratory tract infections caused by* C. pneumoniae *were high among residents and workers and that pneumonia in the debilitated patient was often fatal.*

)

# III. CARDIOVASCULAR SYSTEM

# 10. INFECTIVE ENDOCARDITIS: DIAGNOSTIC CRITERIA

The diagnosis of bacterial endocarditis has long been based on a constellation of history, physical examination findings, laboratory data, including blood cultures, and an assessment of the patient's risk factors and underlying diseases. Many patients complain only of fever and fatigue and are found to have a new cardiac murmur. The disease, however, presents in a myriad of ways. Friable vegetations may result in embolic features, such as stroke, meningitis, blindness, myocardial infarction, or arterial occlusion. Some patients will initially appear septic, some will present with autoimmune disease, and others with congestive heart failure secondary to rapid destruction of a heart valve. Embolic signs on physical examination, such as Osler's nodes, Janeway lesions, Roth's spots, and splinter hemorrhages are less often seen today because of the rapid institution of antibiotic therapy in most patients. Although positive results on blood cultures are very helpful in diagnosis, some patients with endocarditis will have persistently negative cultures. Other patients with positive blood cultures may appear to have endocarditis but be found to have some other focus of infection instead. For these reasons, standardized diagnostic criteria for endocarditis have long been sought.

In 1981, von Reyn et al. published criteria for the diagnosis of endocarditis based on clinical-pathologic criteria. These criteria were helpful particularly because of the wider spectrum of presentation of the disease in recent decades, including the more subtle presentation that often occurs in the elderly. The von Reyn criteria are listed in Table 10-1. Endocarditis is categorized as definite only when the characteristic histology is demonstrated on a surgical specimen or at autopsy, or when bacteria are cultured from a heart valve or peripheral embolus. Cases are further categorized as probable endocarditis, possible endocarditis, or diagnosis rejected.

During the past several years, the von Reyn classification of diagnosis has become less useful for several reasons. Most importantly, the use of transthoracic echocardiography has become a major tool in the diagnosis of endocarditis, and results of this test need to be included in the overall assessment of the likelihood of endocarditis. Echocardiography is not part of the von Reyn diagnostic criteria. The von Reyn criteria were not studied prospectively, but recent reports suggest that some patients in whom the diagnosis is rejected by these criteria do in fact have the disease. The von Reyn criteria do not emphasize the importance of intravenous drug abuse as an extremely important predisposing factor.

In 1992, Lukes et al. proposed an endocarditis classification system that has come to be known as the Duke criteria. This classification system was published in 1994 and included an analysis of 67 patients with pathologically proven endocarditis, in whom the system proved to be very sensitive. The original article did not study the specificity of the classification method. Prospective studies have come to prove that this system is more sensitive and specific than the von Reyn system. The Duke approach classifies cases as definite, possible, or rejected on the basis of a scoring system of major and minor criteria (Table 10-2). For endocarditis to be diagnosed definitively by the system, a patient must show either histologic or pathologic evidence of the disease or exhibit definitive clinical criteria. Two major criteria, one major and three minor criteria, or five minor criteria provide sufficient evidence for a definitive diagnosis. Table 10-3 delineates the definitions of major and minor criteria.

Much like the von Reyn system, the Duke system classifies as definite any case of endocarditis for which there is evidence based on histology from surgery or autopsy or on direct culture from a vegetation or peripheral embolus. Unlike the von Reyn system, the Duke system can be used to make a definite diagnosis of endocarditis even without direct histologic or culture evidence. This definitive diagnosis requires either two major criteria, one major and three minor criteria, or five minor criteria. It should be noted that major criteria are related either to blood culture data or echocardiographic data. Positive results on blood cultures are not considered major criteria *per se*. Typical microorganisms, such as α-hemolytic streptococci, isolated from two separate cultures stand as a major criterion. Persistently positive blood cultures with an organism that can cause endocarditis would also count as a major criterion. Three

Table 10-1. The von Reyn criteria for diagnosis of infective endocarditis

Definite
  Direct evidence of infective endocarditis based on histology from surgery or
  autopsy, or on bacteriology (Gram's stain or culture) of valvular vegetation or
  peripheral embolus
Probable
  (A)  Persistently positive blood culture* plus one of the following:
       (1)  New regurgitant murmur
       (2)  Predisposing heart disease** *and vascular phenomena*‡
  (B)  Negative or intermittently positive blood cultures§ plus three of the following:
       (1)  Fever
       (2)  New regurgitant murmur, and
       (3)  Vascular phenomena
Possible
  (A)  Persistently positive blood cultures plus one of the following:
       (1)  Predisposing heart disease, or
       (2)  Vascular phenomena
  (B)  Negative or intermittently positive blood cultures with all three of the
       following:
       (1)  Fever
       (2)  Predisposing heart disease, and
       (3)  Vascular phenomena
  (C)  For *viridans* streptococcal cases only: at least two positive blood cultures
       without an extracardiac source, and fever
Rejected
  (A)  Endocarditis unlikely, alternative diagnosis generally apparent
  (B)  Endocarditis likely, empiric antibiotic therapy warranted
  (C)  Culture-negative endocarditis diagnosed clinically, but excluded by
       postmortem

* At least two blood cultures were obtained, with two of two or three of three positive, or at least
70% of cultures positive if four or more cultures obtained.
** Definite valvular or congenital heart disease, or a cardiac prosthesis (excluding permanent
pacemakers).
‡ Petechiae, splinter hemorrhages, conjunctival hemorrhages, Roth's spots, Osler's nodes,
Janeway lesions, aseptic meningitis, glomerulonephritis, and pulmonary, central nervous
system, coronary, or peripheral emboli.
§ Any rate of blood culture positively that does not meet the definition of persistently positive.

other major criteria are based on data available from echocardiography. They are
(a) an oscillating intracardiac mass in the absence of an alternative anatomic explanation (i.e., other than endocarditis); (b) abscess; and (c) a new partial dehiscence of a
prosthetic valve or new valvular regurgitation. Hence, the definitive diagnosis of endocarditis in more easily made in the Duke system than in the von Reyn system because
of the use of echocardiographic data.
    The sensitivity and specificity of transesophageal echocardiography for the diagno-
sis of endocarditis was established between 1981 and 1994, when the two classification schemes were established. The Duke system, unlike the von Reyn, can accept a
definitive diagnosis based on clinical criteria as long as enough clinical criteria are
available. Five minor criteria establish the diagnosis as definitive, whereas the same
clinical data would result only in a classification of possible endocarditis by the von
Reyn system. Hence, according to the Duke system, a patient having blood cultures
positive for a characteristic organism and positive findings on echocardiogram would
fulfill two major criteria and be given a definitive diagnosis. Similarly. a patient with
*Staphylococcus aureus* in the bloodstream (with no other focus of infection) and new
valvular regurgitation by echocardiography would also fulfill two major criteria and
be given a definitive diagnosis. Five minor criteria—such as fever, Janeway lesion,

Table 10-2. Proposed new criteria for diagnosis of infective endocarditis (Duke University)

Definite infective endocarditis
  Pathologic criteria
    Microorganism: demonstrated by culture or histology in a vegetation, or in a vegetation that has embolized, or in an intracardiac abscess, or
    Pathologic lesions: vegetation or intracardiac abscess present and confirmed by histology showing active endocarditis
  Clinical criteria, as specifically defined in Table 10-3
    Two major criteria or
    One major and three minor criteria, or
    Five minor criteria
  Possible infective endocarditis
    Findings consistent with infective endocarditis that fall short of "Definite," but not "Rejected"
  Rejected
    Firm alternate diagnosis explaining evidence of infective endocarditis, or
    Resolution of infective endocarditis syndrome, with antibiotic therapy for 4 days or less, or
    No pathologic evidence of infective endocarditis at surgery or autopsy, with antibiotic therapy for 4 days or less

Table 10-3. Definition of terms used in the proposed diagnostic criteria (Duke University)

Major criteria
  (A) Positive blood culture for infective endocarditis: typical microorganisms for infective endocarditis from two separate blood cultures
    (1) *Streptococcus viridans, Streptococcus bovis,* HACEK group, or
    (2) Community-acquired *Staphylococcus aureus* or enterococci, in absence of a primary focus, or
  (B) Persistently positive blood culture, defined as a microorganism consistent with infective endocarditis, from
    (1) Blood cultures drawn more than 12 h apart, or
    (2) All of three, or a majority of four or more separate blood cultures, with first and last drawn at least 1 h apart
  (C) Evidence of endocardial involvement: positive echocardiogram for infective endocarditis
    (1) Oscillating intracardiac mass, on valve or supporting structure, or in the path of regurgitant jets, or on iatrogenic devices, in the absence of an alternative anatomic explanation, or
    (2) Abscess, or
    (3) New partial dehiscence of prosthetic valve, or new valvular regurgitation (worsening or changing or preexisting murmur not sufficient)
Minor criteria
  (A) Predisposing heart condition or intravenous drug use
  (B) Fever: 38°C or higher
  (C) Vascular phenomena: arterial embolism, septic pulmonary infarcts, mycotic aneurysm, intracranial haemorrhage, Janeway lesions
  (D) Immunologic phenomena: glomerulonephritis, Osler's nodes, Roth's spots
  (E) Echocardiogram consistent with infective endocarditis but not meeting major criterion as noted previously, or serologic evidence of active infection with organism consistent with infective endocarditis

HACEK, *Haemophilus, Actinobacillus, Cardiobacterium, Eikenella, Kingella* species.

intravenous drug abuse, Osler node, and glomerulonephritis—would also be a basis for a definitive diagnosis.

Because at least some patients will be available for study who have definitive evidence for infective endocarditis by surgical or autopsy material, the sensitivity of the von Reyn and Duke criteria can be assessed in these cases. At least six studies have compared the Duke criteria with the von Reyn criteria prospectively. By the Duke criteria, 83% of the confirmed cases were considered definitive. None of the confirmed cases was rejected. By the von Reyn methodology, 48% of the confirmed cases were classified only as probable. Twenty-one percent of the confirmed cases would have been rejected by this system.

The usefulness of the Duke criteria was evaluated by reviewing cases during a 3-year period at 54 hospitals in the Philadelphia area. The clinical judgment of three infectious disease experts who reviewed the records of 410 patients was compared with classification that would be generated by the Duke system. There was excellent agreement (91%) for possible and probable cases. However, the experts found 36 cases that they did not feel were likely to be endocarditis but that would have been classified as definite or probable by the Duke criteria. The authors warn that although the Duke criteria are very sensitive, they may result in overdiagnosis of infective endocarditis.

The percentage of endocarditis cases in patients with prosthetic heart valves is increasing. The Duke criteria were studied in 25 patients with pathologically confirmed prosthetic valve endocarditis. Seventy-six percent of these cases were classified as definitive by Duke criteria, and none were rejected. The von Reyn criteria rejected five cases, or 20% of the confirmed cases.

Additional prospective studies will be required to confirm the validity of the Duke diagnostic criteria. The specificity of the system, in particular, needs further evaluation. The sensitivity of the methodology seems certain. Standardized systems for the diagnosis of endocarditis will be extremely important in prospective clinical studies evaluating new diagnostic or treatment methods. However, for the diagnosis of endocarditis in any particular patient, no standardized methodology can replace a clinician's skills and judgment. (S.L.B.)

## Bibliography

Bayer AS, et al. Evaluation of new clinical criteria for the diagnosis of infective endocarditis. *Am J Med* 1994;96:211.

*Sixty-three febrile patients with suspected infective endocarditis who had open heart surgery were evaluated, and the von Reyn and Duke criteria for endocarditis were compared. The Duke criteria were superior predominantly because of the use of transthoracic echocardiographic data.*

Cecchi E, et al. New diagnostic criteria for infective endocarditis. A study of sensitivity and specificity. *Eur Heart J* 1997;18:1149.

*Italian study in which 143 patients with suspected endocarditis had long-term follow-up. The sensitivity and specificity of the von Reyn and Duke criteria were compared. The Duke criteria were more sensitive and specific than the von Reyn criteria.*

Durack DT, et al. New criteria for the diagnosis of infectious endocarditis: utilization of specific echocardiographic findings. *Am J Med* 1994;96:200.

*Establishes the Duke criteria and uses the system to classify 400 patients as definite, possible, or rejected. The system was 80% sensitive in classifying 69 proven cases. No attempt to determine specificity was made.*

Hoen B, et al. The Duke criteria for diagnosing endocarditis are specific: analysis of 100 patients with acute fever or fever of unknown origin. *Clin Infect Dis* 1996;23:298.

*In a study of patients with acute fever admitted to medical wards, the Duke criteria were 99% specific (i.e., cases of acute fever were not misdiagnosed as endocarditis when the Duke criteria were used).*

Nettles RE, et al. An evaluation of the Duke criteria in 25 pathologically confirmed cases of prosthetic valve endocarditis. *Clin Infect Dis* 1997;25:1401.

*The authors used 25 cases of pathologically confirmed prosthetic valve endocarditis to compare the von Reyn and Duke criteria for diagnosis. When the Duke method was used, 76% of confirmed cases were considered definite. No cases were rejected. The von Reyn method would have rejected five cases or 20% of the total.*

Sekeres MA, et al. An assessment of the usefulness of the Duke criteria for diagnosing active infective endocarditis. *Clin Infect Dis* 1997;24:1185.
*Infectious disease experts reviewed the charts of 410 patients with suspected endocarditis for 3 years at 54 hospitals in Philadelphia. Cases were classified as definite, probable, or possible, and then results were compared with the Duke method of classification. The sensitivity of the Duke method was good to excellent, but some concern about specificity is expressed by the authors.*

von Reyn, et al. Infective endocarditis: an analysis based on strict case definitions. *Ann Intern Med* 1981;94:505.
*Established case definitions for endocarditis that have been widely used, especially for clinical studies. The system was not tested prospectively and was developed before breakthroughs in diagnosis by transesophageal echocardiography.*

## 11. CULTURE-NEGATIVE ENDOCARDITIS

Blood cultures are the critical element in the diagnosis of bacterial endocarditis. Endocardial vegetations exude bacteria into the bloodstream, causing continuous bacteremia and positive results on blood cultures in most patients. However, in all endocarditis series, some patients are found to have the disease despite negative cultures. The percentage of negative blood cultures varies among studies from 2% to 30%. The mean percentage appears to be about 10%, but with existing methods, probably fewer than 5% of cases of endocarditis will be culture-negative. High rates of culture-negative endocarditis from early studies probably reflect suboptimal technique and less rigorous criteria for diagnosis.

The most common cause of culture-negative endocarditis is prior antimicrobial therapy. In one large study, antimicrobial therapy reduced the incidence of positive blood cultures from 97% to 91%. Duration of antimicrobial therapy correlates with the likelihood of negative cultures. When antimicrobial therapy has been continued for several days, blood cultures usually remain negative for weeks or longer.

Several laboratory methods may be helpful when endocarditis is suspected in a patient already on antimicrobial therapy. Antimicrobial removal devices that bind antimicrobials in the serum to a resin are available. Blood must also be cultured by a routine system, as the antimicrobial removal device bottle may actually reduce the yield of some organisms.

Some studies have suggested that in patients already treated with antimicrobials, more frequent cultures should be taken. One recommendation is to obtain blood cultures every 8 to 12 hours for 3 days. Using 10 to 30 mL of blood (rather than the usual 5 mL) has also been recommended to increase culture positivity. If endocarditis is suspected in a patient who has received antimicrobial therapy, the microbiology laboratory should be asked to incubate blood cultures for at least 2 weeks.

A lysis centrifugation method has also been used to increase sensitivity in low-grade bacteremia. RBCs are lysed, and the organisms released are centrifuged. The method increases the incidence of contamination and may be less sensitive for anaerobes and streptococci.

Another important reason why some cases of endocarditis are culture-negative is that some organisms are fastidious and require special culture techniques. A group of slow-growing, gram-negative bacilli, including *Haemophilus aphrophilus, Actinobacillus actinomycetemcomitans, Cardiobacterium hominis, Eikenella corrodens,* and *Kingella* species (called as a group the HACEK bacteria), are particularly difficult to grow by standard method. These organisms require prolonged incubation and subculturing to chocolate agar.

Vitamin B and other nutritionally deficient streptococci cause about 5% of episodes of endocarditis. These organisms may fail to grow unless the medium is supplemented with pyridoxal hydrochloride or cysteine. These organisms will grow on blood agar streaked with staphylococci as satellite colonies. Nutritionally deficient streptococci show turbid growth in conventional media, so that subculturing can then be initiated (such culture methods are now routine in laboratories when endocarditis is suspected). Other unusual bacteria implicated in culture-negative endocarditis include *Brucella* species. The diagnosis is usually suspected by history. Culture requires special media and a carbon dioxide atmosphere. *Legionella,* an unusual cause of culture-negative endocarditis, has occurred almost exclusively in patients with prosthetic heart valves.

Fungal endocarditis frequently presents with negative blood cultures. *Mucor* species, *Aspergillus,* and *Histoplasma* can rarely cause endocarditis. Fungal endocarditis is often right-sided and may occur in drug users or patients with prosthetic valves. Vegetations are usually large, and major embolic complications are frequent. Hypertonic media and the use of arterial cultures have been recommended to improve laboratory diagnosis, but these recommendations are unproved.

*Coxiella burnetii* can cause Q-fever endocarditis in patients who have inhaled infected material from domesticated animals. Cultures of blood are negative. Serologic diagnosis using complement-fixing antibody is specific but not sensitive in making this diagnosis. Blood cultures must be obtained before antibiotic therapy is begun if the organism is to be isolated.

Shapiro et al. have reported a particularly well-documented case of *Chlamydia psittaci* endocarditis. Cultures of blood and pharyngeal specimens were positive, and *Chlamydia* was demonstrated in tissue by immunofluorescent stain. Unusual organisms such as the murine typhus agent and *Brucella* have also been diagnosed by serologic methods. The diagnosis of culture-negative enterococcal endocarditis was made in seven patients by using an immunoblotting technique directed against specific enterococcal antigen extracts.

*Bartonella quintana* has received increasing attention as a potentially important cause of culture-negative endocarditis. Several investigators have used polymerase chain reaction (PCR) to identify the organism in excised valves. In a multicenter international study, 22 cases of culture-negative endocarditis were reported to be caused by *Bartonella* species. Diagnostic studies included determination of antibody titers to *Bartonella* species by microimmunofluorescence, blood and vegetation culture, and amplification of *Bartonella* DNA from valvular tissue by PCR. Of the 22 patients studied, 13 had preexisting valvular heart disease, 11 were alcoholic, and only four owned cats.

In samples of resected heart valves from patients with culture-negative endocarditis made available at surgery, molecular techniques will be increasingly useful in determining an etiologic agent. In one study, broad-range PCR amplification of the 16S rRNA gene followed by single-stranded sequencing allowed detection of rare organisms that could not be cultured.

In patients with culture-negative endocarditis of native valves, a combination of ampicillin and aminoglycoside has been recommended as empiric therapy. This combination is effective against streptococci, including enterococci, and bacteria of the HACEK group. In patients with prosthetic heart valves and culture-negative endocarditis, both coagulase-positive and coagulase-negative staphylococci may cause the disease. Vancomycin plus aminoglycoside becomes the regimen most often recommended. Rifampin may be added as well. In patients who do not respond to antimicrobial therapy, a reassessment of etiologic agents, including fungi, *Chlamydia, Coxiella,* and other organisms indicated by history and epidemiology, should be pursued. Optimal antibiotic therapy for *Bartonella* endocarditis has not been well established. (S.L.B.)

## Bibliography

Abraham AK, et al. Culture-negative infective endocarditis. *Aust N Z J Med* 1984;14:223.
  *Among 265 endocarditis cases, 7% were culture-negative. All had received prior antimicrobial therapy.*
Agarwal AK. Culture-negative infective endocarditis. *Postgrad Med* 1982;72:123.
  *Summary of basic principles of diagnosis and treatment.*
Breathnach AS, et al. Culture-negative endocarditis: contribution of *Bartonella* infections. *Heart* 1997;77:474.
  *Describes two cases of* Bartonella *endocarditis: one in a homeless man, the other in a patient exposed to fleas. PCR of the excised valves was used to identify the organism.*

Burnie JP, et al. Role of immunoblotting in the diagnosis of culture-negative and ente-
rococcal endocarditis. *J Clin Pathol* 1987;40:1149.
*Describes antibody response to antigenic extracts of four enterococcal species.*
*Immunoblotting was used to diagnose seven cases of culture-negative enterococcal*
*endocarditis.*
Cannady PB Jr, Sanford JP. Negative blood cultures in infective endocarditis: a
review. *South Med J* 1976;69:1420.
*Good summary of the incidence of culture-negative endocarditis in different series.*
Ellner JJ, et al. Infective endocarditis caused by slow-growing fastidious gram-negative
bacteria. *Medicine (Baltimore)* 1979;58:145.
*Gives case reports and microbiologic characteristics of fastidious gram-negative*
*organisms, including* Cardiobacterium, Actinobacillus, *and* Haemophilus *species.*
Goldenberger D, et al. Molecular diagnosis of bacterial endocarditis by broad-range
PCR amplification and direct sequencing. *J Clin Microbiol* 1997;35:2733.
*A promising method for diagnosis of culture-negative endocarditis. Allows identifi-*
*cation of unusual, nongrowing organisms such as* Tropheryma whippelii.
Jalava J, et al. Use of the polymerase chain reaction and DNA sequencing for detection of *Bartonella quintana* in the aortic valve of a patient with culture-negative
endocarditis. *Clin Infect Dis* 1995;21:891.
*The patient described had negative blood cultures and negative bacterial cultures of*
*the resected valve. The authors used PCR and bacterial primers combined with DNA*
*sequencing from the aortic valve vegetation. PCR was used to amplify bacterial 16S*
*rDNA from a template of the vegetation.*
Kiehn TE, et al. Comparative recovery of bacteria and yeasts from lysis-centrifugation
and a conventional blood culture system. *J Clin Microbiol* 1983;18:300.
*The lysis centrifugation system was better than broth for detecting fungi and gram-*
*negative bacilli but was less likely to detect streptococci.*
McCabe RE, et al. Prosthetic valve endocarditis caused by *Legionella pneumophila*.
*Ann Intern Med* 1984;100:525.
*A case report of endocarditis caused by* Legionella pneumophila. *This organism is a*
*potential cause of culture-negative endocarditis in patients with prosthetic valves.*
Marrie TJ, et al. Culture-negative endocarditis probably due to *Chlamydia pneumo-*
*niae*. *J Infect Dis* 1990;161:127.
Chlamydia *endocarditis diagnosed by serology.*
Musso D, Raoult D. *Coxiella burnetii* blood cultures from acute and chronic Q-fever
patients. *J Clin Microbiol* 1995;33:3129.
*Diagnosis was made by positive blood cultures and serology. Blood cultures must be*
*obtained before the initiation of antibiotic therapy, or results will be negative.*
Pesanti EL, Smith IM. Infective endocarditis with negative blood cultures. An analysis of 52 cases. *Am J Med* 1979;66:43.
*Compares clinical features of 52 patients having culture-negative endocarditis with*
*those who are culture-positive. Culture-negative patients tend to respond less dra-*
*matically to antimicrobial therapy.*
Raoult D, et al. Diagnosis of 22 new cases of *Bartonella* endocarditis. *Ann Intern Med*
1996;125:646.
*Multicenter, international study suggests that* Bartonella *species are an important*
*cause of culture-negative endocarditis. Amplification of* Bartonella *DNA by PCR*
*was performed by using tissue from heart valve. Of the 22 patients, 13 had predis-*
*posing valvular heart disease, and 11 were homeless. There was a high level of cross-*
*reacting antibody to* Chlamydia, *making cross-adsorption necessary for proper*
*diagnosis.*
Shapiro DS, et al. Brief report: *Chlamydia psittaci* endocarditis diagnosed by blood
culture. *N Engl J Med* 1992;326:1192.
*A very well-documented case of* C. psittaci *endocarditis. The patient had been exposed*
*to her sister's sick parakeet.*
Tunkel AR, Kaye D. Endocarditis with negative blood cultures. *N Engl J Med*
1992;326:1215.
*An editorial accompanying a case report of* Chlamydia *endocarditis provides an update*
*on etiologic agents and the diagnostic approach to culture-negative endocarditis.*

Van Scoy RE. Culture-negative endocarditis. *Mayo Clin Proc* 1982;57:149.
*Describes an approach to culture-negative endocarditis. Survival is 92% if patient responds to therapy within 1 week.*

Walterspiel JN, Kaplan SL. Incidence and clinical characteristics of "culture-negative" infective endocarditis in a pediatric population. *Pediatr Infect Dis* 1986;5:328.
*Ten-year pediatric experience with culture-negative endocarditis.*

Washington JA II. The role of the microbiology laboratory in the diagnosis and antimicrobial treatment of infective endocarditis. *Mayo Clin Proc* 1982;57:22.
*Describes the approach to the diagnostic microbiology of endocarditis, including technique of blood culture, media to use, duration of incubation, and problems with fastidious organisms.*

Wright AJ, et al. The antimicrobial removal device. A microbiological and clinical evaluation. *Am J Clin Pathol* 1982;78:173.
*An antimicrobial removal device was of little value in 87 bacteremic patients. Bacteria from 8% of patients grew bacteria in the antimicrobial removal device bottles alone.*

## 12. SURGERY IN ACTIVE INFECTIVE ENDOCARDITIS

Infective endocarditis (IE) often results in death if not diagnosed and treated. Since the advent of effective bactericidal antimicrobials, mortality has declined from almost 100% to 20%-50%, depending on pathogen, host, and complications. Congestive heart failure (CHF) represents a common cause of death in these patients. The most common cause of CHF is valvular insufficiency. Surgery plays a major role in patients with complications of IE. Goals of surgery are to remove infected tissue, reestablish valve function, and restore normal cardiac mechanics.

### Preoperative Assessment of the Patient with Infective Endocarditis

Many patients with IE suffer no significant complications and can be managed successfully with appropriate antimicrobials and no surgical intervention. For all persons in whom this condition is diagnosed, routine laboratory data should be obtained to use as a baseline, monitor therapy, and assess for complications. Standard blood tests include CBC, urinalysis, determination of hepatic and renal function, and sedimentation rate; the role of serum bactericidal testing is controversial. Additionally, patients should have an electrocardiogram and echocardiography performed early in the course of disease. These are obtained to establish a baseline against which to compare future changes and look for abnormalities that could portend complications. The electrocardiogram can document conduction abnormalities that might represent extension of infection into the conducting system. Bundle blocks and first- and third-degree heart block have been reported as complications of IE, most commonly in aortic valve disease. The former is rather common and may indicate only inflammation. However, prolongations of the PR interval may also be associated with a high risk for complete heart block and the probability of deep abscess formation. Thus, patients with prolonged PR intervals should be closely monitored. Complete heart block complicates about 4% of cases of IE. Ischemia or acute myocardial infarction documented by electrocardiogram may represent coronary embolization from an infected aortic vegetation rather than primary coronary artery disease.

Most authorities now recommend that transesophageal echocardiography (TEE) be performed on most patients with IE, although absolute indications are not known. In competent hands, a positive study result can demonstrate vegetations (and thus define the presence of IE) and identify complications. TEE is superior to transthoracic echocardiography (TTE) in the visualization of both vegetations and complications, which can be anatomic or hemodynamic in nature. Examples of such complications include valve perforation, abscesses, and pericardial effusion. Hemodynamic complications may include valve incompetence, fistulae, and intracardiac thrombi. TEE is now considered the most reliable noninvasive test for defining this disease. However, it may not differentiate between active and healed vegetations and may not be able to discriminate between thickened valves or valvular nodules and vegetations. Thus, it should be utilized primarily in patients whose risk for IE is considered significant. Recent data prove the capacity of TEE to document IE and demonstrate valve ring abscesses not noted by other echocardiographic studies. Authorities now feel that TEE is at least 90% sensitive and specific in the diagnosis of IE. As an example, patients with abscess complicating IE were identified on only 13 of 44 TTE studies, compared with 40 of 44 by TEE. Both sensitivity and specificity were dramatically increased. Alternatively, a technically comprehensive TEE demonstrating no changes of IE virtually rules out that disease. Doppler should be employed in such clinical situations as (a) follow-up of patients with staphylococcal bacteremia (not considered to have IE) before discontinuation of antimicrobials, (b) assessment of patients with IE who remain febrile or persistently bacteremic, and (c) assessment of patients with IE plus conduction defects, CHF, or other potential intracardiac complications. It is the opinion of the author that selected patients with IE documented clinically, who show a prompt response to antibiotics and have no evidence of complications, may be managed without echocardiography.

Although many cardiologists appear reluctant to perform cardiac catheterization in patients with IE, it is occasionally useful when TEE has not provided adequate diagnostic or anatomic information. Cardiac catheterization can identify site of infection, assess for fistulae and abscesses, and evaluate hemodynamic status. Risk for complications is similar to that seen with cardiac catheterization in other groups, and thus it is not contraindicated because of the presence of active IE. Controlled studies of TEE versus cardiac catheterization to identify complications of IE have not been performed.

## Surgery in Patients with Native Valve Infective Endocarditis
Several studies demonstrate improved outcome of patients with IE who have undergone surgery after medical failure. Surgery should be performed when clinically indicated and should not be based on duration of effective antibiotic therapy. Benefits may be long-term. Table 12-1 lists reasons for valve replacement in patients with IE.

*Congestive Heart Failure*
CHF accounts for more than 80% of valve replacements in IE. Most commonly, it is a complication of aortic valve endocarditis with resultant cusp perforation, but it may also occur in association with mitral valve infection. CHF may also occur as a result of myocardial abscesses, pericardial effusion, fistulae, and other hemodynamic complications of IE. Significant CHF (defined as that requiring more than minimal therapy) results in death in 50% to 90% of patients treated medically, whereas up to 60% survive with surgery. Patients with severe CHF resulting from valve perforation should undergo early valve replacement regardless of duration of antibiotic therapy or continued positive blood cultures. For patients with diseased mitral valves, recent studies suggest that valve repair rather than replacement offers a better clinical outcome. Patients who survive the procedure have a good prognosis. Persons with mild CHF may be treated medically with careful observation. Those with moderate CHF may have

Table 12-1. Infective endocarditis: major indications for surgery

| Native valve IE | Prosthetic valve IE |
| --- | --- |
| Progressive congestive heart failure | Prosthetic valve dysfunction |
| Recurrent major vessel embolization | Most cases of early PVE |
| Resistant organisms (including fungi) | Duration of fever > 10 days |
| Lack of bactericidal agent | Sustained bacteremia |
| Extravalvular extension of infection | Indications listed under native valve IE |
| Failure of clinical response | |
| Vegetation >1.5–2.0 cm? | |

IE, infective endocarditis; PVE, prosthetic valve endocarditis.

higher-than-expected death rates from coronary artery embolization. A common procedure at the time of valve replacement is to obtain a Gram's stain and culture of the valve and possibly other removed tissues. A positive Gram's stain is common and is related to the duration of antibiotic therapy. However, no relationship exists with outcome.

*Infection with Resistant Organisms*
Treatment of IE requires an effective bactericidal agent. Those most commonly employed are β-lactams, aminoglycosides, and vancomycin. Unusual cases of IE caused by organisms such as *Chlamydia psittaci, Legionella pneumophila, Coxiella burnetii,* and *Brucella* species may not be treatable with such compounds. Endocarditis caused by *Pseudomonas aeruginosa* or fungi should generally be managed with early surgical intervention. Although many cases of enteric gram-negative IE will require surgery, each case should be assessed individually. Patients should receive high-dose bactericidal agents, serum bactericidal levels should be monitored, and patients should undergo surgery if persistent bacteremia, CHF, or clinical deterioration occurs.

*Extravalvular Extension of Infection*
Extension of infection beyond the valve generally represents surgical disease and is best defined by TEE. Examples include (a) pericarditis, (b) valve ring abscess, (c) invasion of the conducting system, (d) myocardial abscess, and (e) fistulae. These complications occur most often in aortic valve disease. Clues include persistent fever, repeatedly positive blood cultures, pericarditis (although friction rubs are infrequently noted), and CHF not accounted for by overt valvular insufficiency. In unusual circumstances, cardiac catheterization can also be used to obtain quantitative blood cultures from different areas of the heart in an attempt to define the lesion anatomically.

*Other Reasons for Operative Intervention*
Embolization commonly complicates IE and can be associated with major morbidity and mortality. Recent data obtained from studies with 2-D echocardiography demonstrate that first embolic events occurred at a rate of more than 6/1,000 patient-days and did not depend on the presence of vegetations. Risk for emboli decreased with increased length of antimicrobial therapy. Classically, fungi and fastidious gram-negative organisms of the HACEK group (species of *Haemophilus, Actinobacillus, Cardiobacterium, Eikenella, Kingella*) have been associated with large emboli. Recent data from echocardiography also suggest an enhanced likelihood of embolization from vegetations with *viridans* streptococci. Large emboli also may develop from atrial myxomas, which may be simultaneously infected. Valve replacement should be offered to patients who have had a second major embolus. However, a single embolic event plus echocardiographic evidence of a large (>1.5 to 2.0 cm) vegetation may also be an indication for surgery. Operative intervention based only on vegetation size is controversial. Several recent studies imply that patients with vegetations larger than 1.5 to 2.0 cm carry an excess risk for embolization and that surgery should be strongly considered on this basis alone. This may be especially true for disease on left-sided valves. It should be emphasized, however, that most vegetations are slow to resolve and will still be present at the end of therapy. A recent report demonstrated that echocardiographic persistence at the end of treatment is not an independent predictor of late sequelae.

Recent investigations have assessed the role of cardiac surgery in patients with cerebral embolization or other cerebrovascular complications. An intracerebral event was identified in about 10% of patients with IE, and overall mortality was 11%. An interval of 4 weeks between onset of cerebral complications and surgery is desirable.

Uncommonly, IE recurs following "adequate" antimicrobial therapy. This is usually secondary to localized or metastatic abscess or happens when infection has been associated with a more resistant organism. Consideration for heart surgery should be given if no remedial cause can be located in other areas. TEE and possibly cardiac catheterization should be undertaken to identify occult infectious foci.

### Prosthetic Valve Endocarditis
Prosthetic valve endocarditis (PVE) complicates valve replacement surgery in 1% to 2% of cases. "Early" PVE occurs within the first 60 days, whereas the "late" type occurs

thereafter. The former is associated with more aggressive pathogens and a less favorable prognosis. Pathologically, PVE usually involves infection around the valve ring with extension into adjacent myocardial tissue. This explains the poor results generally noted with medical therapy alone. Fever for more than 10 days following institution of antimicrobials portends extravalvular extension. Table 12-1 lists major reasons for cardiac surgery in PVE. Conditions already outlined for native valve IE also necessitate early operative intervention. These include (a) progressive or severe CHF, (b) recurrent major vessel embolization, (c) failure of appropriate medical therapy, and (d) IE caused by fungi and other resistant pathogens. Virtually all cases of early PVE fulfill these criteria, and surgery should generally be considered. Late PVE is a condition that closely mimics subacute native valve IE. Disease caused by nonstreptococcal organisms is statistically more likely to require valve replacement. A recent 20-year experience with late PVE demonstrated a 52% survivorship at 10 years. However, by the end of the study, only about 25% of patients were alive with the original prosthetic valve. (R.B.B.)

**Bibliography**

Abrams HB, et al. Is there a role for surgery in the acute management of infective endocarditis? A decision analysis and medical claims database approach. *Med Decis Making* 1988;8:165–174.
*Report of a decision analysis to determine the best treatment for patients with left-sided* Staphylococcus aureus *infective endocarditis. Early surgery appeared to be associated with a longer life expectancy. Such data should be substantiated by prospective clinical studies.*

Daniel WG, et al. Improvement in the diagnosis of abscesses associated with endocarditis by transesophageal echocardiography. *N Engl J Med* 1991;324:795–800.
*This large investigation studied almost 120 patients with native or prosthetic valve endocarditis by M-mode, 2-D TTE, and TEE. Forty-six abscesses were identified from surgical or autopsy specimens. The aortic valve was the most common site of infection, and S. aureus was the most common pathogen. Mortality in patients with abscess was higher than in patients without this complication. TEE discovered 40 of 46, whereas TTE found only 13 of these (* p <.001*). It was concluded that TEE is more sensitive and specific for locating abscesses associated with infective endocarditis.*

Dinubile MJ. Surgery in active endocarditis. *Ann Intern Med* 1982;96:650–659.
*This exhaustive review summarizes the indications for surgery in native and prosthetic valve endocarditis. In addition to classic indications, the author summarizes information on the role of echocardiography and vegetation size in determining surgical need and provides tables of major and minor criteria for surgical intervention in active endocarditis.*

Jault F, et al. Active native valve endocarditis: determinant of operative death and late mortality. *Ann Thorac Surg* 1997;63:1737–1741.
*Records of approximately 250 patients who underwent surgery for active native valve IE were reviewed. Involvement of the aortic valve was most commonly noted. Operative mortality was approximately 8%. Risk factors for intraoperative death included advanced age and cardiogenic shock at time of surgery. Duration of antibiotic therapy did not influence surgical outcome. Long-term survival was worst with mitral valve IE and initial neurologic complications.*

Mills SA. Surgical management of infective endocarditis. *Ann Surg* 1982;195:367–383.
*This surgical review points out classic indications for surgical intervention in IE. These include congestive failure resulting from valve disruption, failure of antimicrobials, recurrent emboli, and paravalvular abscess. Major goals of surgery are removal of infected tissue and restoration of valve function.*

Murphy JG, Foster-Smith K. Management of complications of infective endocarditis with emphasis on echocardiographic findings. *Infect Dis Clin North Am* 1993; 7:153–165.
*This review summarizes data concerning the value of echocardiography, especially TEE, in the diagnosis and management of IE. Limitations of TEE are also presented.*

Shively BK, et al. Diagnostic value of transesophageal compared with transthoracic echocardiography in infective endocarditis. *J Am Coll Cardiol* 1991;18:391–397.

*These two modes of echocardiography were employed in 66 patients with suspected IE and compared with a gold standard. TEE was far more sensitive for defining the disease. Neither was associated with false-positive results.*

Steckelberg JM, et al. Emboli in infective endocarditis: the prognostic value of echo-cardiography. *Ann Intern Med* 1991;114:635–640.

*Patients with IE were identified within the first 72 hours of antimicrobial therapy and studied with 2-D echocardiography. First emboli were noted at a rate of 6.2/1,000 patient-days. Rates were similar in those with and without documented vegetations. Streptococcus viridans was associated with higher rates of embolization than S. aureus. Rates of embolization decreased with the length of antimicrobial therapy. Vegetations present by 2-D echocardiography did not appear to have an effect on the likelihood of embolization. S. viridans was associated with higher risks.*

Tornos P, et al. Clinical outcome and long-term prognosis of late prosthetic valve endo-carditis: a 20-year experience. *Clin Infect Dis* 1996;24:381–386.

*The authors describe their experience with 59 patients with late prosthetic valve endocarditis followed for 20 years. Only about 25% remained alive and with their original valve. Mortality with other than streptococcal infection was significantly higher than that noted with streptococcal infection.*

Vuille C, Nidorf M, Picard MH. Natural history of vegetations during successful medical treatment of endocarditis. *Am Heart J* 1994;128:1200–1209.

*Echocardiography was employed to follow the natural history of vegetations during therapy for IE. At the time of termination of therapy, the majority of patients continued to have vegetations that were generally denser that those seen originally. Presence of vegetations was not an independent predictor of adverse outcome.*

## 13. ENDOCARDITIS PROPHYLAXIS

Patients with certain underlying cardiac lesions should receive prophylactic anti-microbials just before undergoing procedures that might cause a bacteremia resulting in infective endocarditis. The subject of endocarditis prevention, however, continues to stir controversy. Although there is agreement on certain aspects of endocarditis prophylaxis, many issues remain unresolved: Which patients should receive prophylaxis? Which therapeutic and diagnostic procedures require prophylaxis? Which antimicrobial regimens are effective for prophylaxis? Are the data derived from the experimental rabbit endocarditis model relevant to prophylaxis in humans? Are bactericidal antimicrobials required for prophylaxis? Is antimicrobial prophylaxis for endocarditis cost effective? Data to answer these and other key questions from controlled clinical studies are unavailable and unlikely to be forthcoming. Thus, the current guidelines for the prophylaxis of endocarditis from the American Heart Association and working party of the British Society for Antimicrobial Chemotherapy are empiric. Adherence to these regimens by practicing dentists is often faulty. In one survey, only 14% of dentists followed the current American Heart Association recommendations for endocarditis prophylaxis.

When bacteria invade the bloodstream, persons who have rheumatic heart disease, congenital heart disease, a prosthetic heart valve, mitral valve prolapse, or other cardiovascular diseases are at risk for the development of infective endocarditis. The mechanism by which endocarditis occurs is still unclear. Organisms may infect a fibrin clot on a previously diseased valve or adhere to a specific receptor site on a valve leaflet. In either case, a key factor in the pathogenesis of infective endocarditis is the occurrence of a transient bacteremia.

Transient bacteremias develop commonly. They may occur spontaneously, as when a person chews food or defecates. They may result from many procedures that traumatize mucous membranes having an indigenous microbial flora, such as a dental extraction or urethral catheterization. Bacteremias following procedures resulting from mucosal trauma are asymptomatic, usually begin about 1 to 5 minutes following the procedure, and generally last for only 15 to 30 minutes. Quantitative blood cultures usually reveal colony counts of fewer than 10 organisms per milliliter of blood. Transient bacteremias are also associated with local infections, such as those resulting from incision and drainage of an abscess or manipulation of the urinary tract in a patient with asymptomatic bacteriuria. The organisms associated with these bacteremias reflect either the normal flora at the manipulated site or the pathogens causing the local infection.

No data accurately define the incidence of infective endocarditis in patients who undergo invasive procedures without antimicrobial prophylaxis. A history of a predisposing event sometimes can be elicited from endocarditis patients. Of patients with nonenterococcal streptococcal endocarditis, 15% to 20% had a preceding dental procedure. In another review, only 3.6% of cases of endocarditis were associated with a dental procedure. A preceding genitourinary tract procedure has been reported in up to 42% of patients with enterococcal endocarditis. Thirty-five percent of patients with staphylococcal endocarditis have had a preceding infection of the skin or soft tissue. Endocarditis often occurs without an obvious predisposing event.

The oropharynx is a frequent portal of entry for organisms into the bloodstream. Blood cultures are positive in 18% to 85% of patients after a dental extraction. The frequency of bacteremia correlates with the severity of gingival infection and the extent of tissue trauma. The organisms isolated reflect the normal mouth flora. *Viridans* streptococci are isolated most frequently, but anaerobic streptococci, coagulase-negative staphylococci, diphtheroids, and *Fusobacterium* also are seen. Strains of *viridans* streptococci account for 50% to 75% of cases of endocarditis and are usually penicillin-sensitive. Streptococci that are relatively resistant to penicillin are found in patients receiving prophylactic penicillin for rheumatic fever and in those given antimicrobial prophylaxis as early as 1 to 2 days before a procedure. Prophylaxis should begin just before a procedure so that serum levels of the antimicrobial are adequate at the time of anticipated bacteremia. Penicillin given just before a dental extraction will decrease the incidence of positive blood cultures after the procedure.

Other dental procedures that may result in a transient bacteremia are periodontal operations, such as gingivectomy, root canal surgery, and dental cleaning. In up to 88% of patients with gum disease, blood cultures are positive, depending on the severity of the disease. The predominant organisms are the same as with dental extraction. Positive blood cultures also are seen after tooth brushing (0 to 26%), the use of oral irrigation devices (7% to 50%) or dental floss (20%), and chewing gum or eating hard candy (0 to 22%). Antimicrobial prophylaxis is impractical for preventing a transient bacteremia secondary to common daily activities. Maintenance of good oral hygiene, however, decreases the amount of gum disease, a key determinant of the frequency of a transient bacteremia following any dental manipulation.

Other procedures involving the oropharynx and respiratory tract may result in bacteremia, including tonsillectomy, nasotracheal intubation, and rigid-tube bronchoscopy. Positive blood cultures, however, rarely are associated with flexible fiberoptic bronchoscopy and lung biopsy.

Diagnostic procedures involving the gastrointestinal tract are another source of transient bacteremias. Positive blood cultures are found in patients undergoing fiberoptic gastrointestinal endoscopy (0 to 10%; 4% overall), rigid sigmoidoscopy (0 to 9.5%; 5% overall), flexible sigmoidoscopy (0%), liver biopsy (3% to 14%), barium enema (11%), and colonoscopy (0 to 27%; 5% overall). Transient bacteremia also occurs in patients having esophageal dilation (mean incidence, 45%), sclerotherapy of esophageal varices (18%), and endoscopic retrograde cholangiopancreatography (6%). The predominant organisms isolated with these procedures are enterococci, a frequent cause of endocarditis, and gram-negative bacilli, organisms rarely involved in native valve endocarditis.

Transient bacteremia and infective endocarditis can occur following urinary tract, obstetric, and gynecologic procedures. The urinary tract is the portal of entry in 20% to 50% of patients with enterococcal endocarditis, whereas 20% of cases caused by this organism are related to obstetric and gynecologic procedures. A transient bacteremia occurs in 8% of patients undergoing urethral catheterization, 24% undergoing urethral dilation, 17% having cystoscopy, and 12% to 31% having transurethral prosthetic resection. The frequency of positive blood cultures increases by several times in patients with infection at the instrumented site, such as a urinary tract infection. Genitourinary tract procedures appear to be the second most common predisposing event.

Transient bacteremia also develops in patients after vaginal delivery, cesarean section, dilation and curettage of the uterus, and insertion or removal of an intrauterine contraceptive device.

Manipulation of an infected focus, such as massage of an infected prostate or incision and drainage of an abscess, is associated with bacteremia and the risk for endocarditis. Transient bacteremia is rare with cardiac catheterization and angiographic procedures. Prevention of endocarditis requires a knowledge of both the events likely to produce bacteremia and the patient with predisposing cardiac lesions. Unfortunately, half of patients with endocarditis have no recognized underlying heart disease, making antimicrobial prophylaxis impossible for this group. Rheumatic valvular disease still remains the most common form of underlying cardiac disease in patients in whom endocarditis develops. The frequency has declined, however, with the decreasing incidence of rheumatic fever. Patients with a bicuspid aortic valve are predisposed to endocarditis, as are patients with calcific or sclerotic changes in the aortic and mitral valves or annulus.

Patients with mitral valve prolapse-click murmur syndrome have been reported to be at increased risk for endocarditis. In a case-control study, the risk for endocarditis in patients with mitral valve prolapse was approximately eight times higher than that for the matched controls. In a study of failures of endocarditis prophylaxis, mitral valve prolapse was the most frequent cardiac abnormality identified, accounting for 33% of cases of endocarditis. One study suggested that the risk for fatal reactions to penicillin far outweighed its benefits in preventing endocarditis in patients with mitral valve prolapse. This is only a theoretical analysis, however, and not a controlled clinical trial. Prophylaxis in all patients with mitral valve prolapse would be difficult because of its high incidence (5% to 6% of the American population). One approach is to prescribe prophylaxis to patients with associated mitral insufficiency, thickened mitral leaflets on the echocardiogram, or men older than 45 years with mitral valve prolapse, but not to those who have only a systolic click and are undergoing procedures associated with endocarditis.

Patients with a previous episode of endocarditis should also receive prophylaxis during predisposing events. Patients with prosthetic or bioprosthetic heart valves are also predisposed. Because infection of a prosthesis is often difficult to eradicate and carries a high mortality, antimicrobial prophylaxis is recommended both for the usual predisposing events and for additional procedures associated with a transient bacteremia but a lower risk for infection, such as upper gastrointestinal endoscopy, barium enema, or colonoscopy.

Only estimates are available for the incidence of endocarditis in susceptible persons after exposure to an event associated with transient bacteremia. The incidence is clearly low, because bacteremias often occur after operative procedures, and resultant endocarditis is relatively rare. Similarly, the effectiveness of antimicrobial prophylaxis for infective endocarditis remains unknown. Because a carefully controlled study with a very large number of patients would be required to answer some of the questions of this issue, animals have been used to study the pathogenesis and efficacy of antimicrobial prophylaxis in infective endocarditis. A major criticism of this model is that a high inoculum of bacteria is used to produce infection, in contrast to the low number of organisms associated with a transient bacteremia.

Antimicrobial prophylaxis is not indicated for patients at risk for endocarditis who are undergoing cardiac catheterization, pacemaker insertion, or peritoneal dialysis. Effective use of prophylactic antimicrobials requires that adequate drug levels be present at the required site at the time of the event posing the risk for transient bacteremia. To accomplish this goal, the antimicrobial drug should be given just before the procedure and continued for 6 to 12 hours. Initiation of an antimicrobial 1 to 2 days before a procedure can result in the replacement of sensitive strains of bacteria by resistant organisms. Selective pressure is also exerted on the local flora, favoring the emergence of resistant strains. Increasing the duration of treatment beyond one dose after the initial loading dose only raises the cost and increases the possibility of an adverse drug reaction. For dental procedures and other procedures involving the airway, the antimicrobial selected should be directed against *viridans* streptococci. Genitourinary manipulation and gastrointestinal, gynecologic, and obstetric procedures require that the antimicrobial prophylaxis be directed against enterococci. Antimicrobials should be adequate for penicillinase-producing staphylococci in a predisposed person undergoing incision and drainage of an abscess. A urine culture should be obtained before a genitourinary procedure, so that any infection can be identified and treated before the instrumentation.

Hematogenous seeding of a prosthetic joint implant is a concern in a patient having a procedure associated with a transient bacteremia as well as for those with an existing infection. No data are available to answer this dilemma, although antimicrobials are frequently administered. Infection of a prosthetic implant has been reported, but the risk appears to be extremely low. Although no medical or legal guidelines exist on this issue, I often recommend antimicrobial prophylaxis, particularly for recently implanted devices, but would not fault a physician for not using it. Whether bactericidal antimicrobials are essential for adequate prophylaxis is unclear. Earlier studies in rabbits favored bactericidal drugs, but recent reports show that bacteriostatic antimicrobials may be sufficient to prevent endocarditis under certain circumstances. Similarly, some strains of *viridans* streptococci are tolerant to penicillin. The relevance of tolerance to successful prophylaxis remains to be determined.

Antimicrobial regimens for prophylaxis are listed in Table 13-1. The recommendations in the United States are derived from the guidelines proposed by advisory

Table 13-1. Endocarditis prophylaxis: dosage for adults

**Dental, oral, and upper respiratory tract procedures**

**Oral**

| | |
|---|---|
| Amoxicillin | 2 g 1 hr before procedure |
| *Penicillin allergy* | |
| Clindamycin | 600 mg 1 hr before procedure |
| OR | |
| Cephalexin* or cefadroxil* | 2 g 1 hr before procedure |
| OR | |
| Azithromycin or clarithromycin | 500 mg 1 hr before procedure |

**Parenteral**\*\*

| | |
|---|---|
| Ampicillin | 2 g IM or IV 30 min before procedure |
| *Penicillin allergy* | |
| Clindamycin | 600 mg IV within 30 min before procedure |
| OR | |
| Cefazolin* | 1 g IM or IV within 30 min before procedure |

**Gastrointestinal, genitourinary, and gynecologic procedures**

**Oral**

| | |
|---|---|
| Amoxicillin | 2 g 1 hr before procedure |

**Parenteral**

| | |
|---|---|
| Ampicillin | 2 g IM or IV within 30 min before procedure |
| plus | |
| Gentamicin | 1.5 mg/kg (120 mg maximum) IM or IV 30 min before procedure |
| *Penicillin allergy* | |
| Vancomycin | 1 g IV infused *slowly over 1 hr* beginning 1 hr before procedure |
| plus | |
| Gentamicin | 1.5 mg/kg (120 mg maximum) IM or IV 30 min before procedure |

*(continued)*

Table 13-1. *Continued*

**Incision and drainage of skin abscesses caused by coagulase-positive staphylococci, not methicillin-resistant**[‡]

**Oral**

| | |
|---|---|
| Dicloxacillin | 500 mg 1 hr before procedure, then 500 mg q6h |

**Parenteral**

| | |
|---|---|
| Nafcillin or oxacillin | 2 g IV 0.5–1 hr before procedure, then 2 grams IV q4h |
| Cefazolin[§] | 1 g IM 1 hr before procedure, then 1 g IV or IM q8h |

***If methicillin-resistant***

| | |
|---|---|
| Vancomycin[‡,§] | 1 g IV over 60 min. Start infusion 1 hr before procedure, then 1 g q12h IV |

---

* Not recommended for patients with history of immediate-type allergy to penicillin.
** Parenteral regimens are recommended for patients with prosthetic or biosynthetic heart valves. Parenteral regimens may be preferred for patients in highest-risk groups, although data to support this practice are not available.
‡ Route and duration of therapy depend on the severity of the infection and on whether the predisposed person is at high risk (e.g., prosthetic heart valve). Results of Gram's stains and cultures should also guide antimicrobial selection.
§ If patient is allergic to penicillin or receiving continuous oral penicillin. Adjust dosage in renal insufficiency for vancomycin and cefazolin.
Modified from Dejani AS, et al. Prevention of bacterial endocarditis. *JAMA* 1997; 277:1794.

committee to the American Heart Association. Amoxicillin has replaced penicillin for prophylaxis in patients undergoing dental or upper respiratory tract surgical procedures, and the dose has decreased from 3 g to 2 g orally. No repeated dose after the procedure is recommended. Patients who have recently received penicillin or who are allergic to it should receive oral clindamycin, azithromycin, clarithromycin, or a cephalosporin for dental procedures. For gastrointestinal, genitourinary, and gynecologic procedures, parenteral ampicillin and gentamicin are recommended. Patients with a penicillin allergy should receive parenteral vancomycin plus gentamicin. Because parenteral regimens are often difficult to use in outpatients, amoxicillin may be substituted in low-risk patients. As the recommendations for endocarditis prophylaxis are empiric, clinical judgment must be carefully exercised in selecting which patients should receive antimicrobial prophylaxis for various procedures that might cause a bacteremia. (N.M.G.)

**Bibliography**

Bayliss R, et al. The bowel, the genitourinary tract, and infective endocarditis. *Br Heart J* 1984;51:339.
  *Patients with underlying cardiac disease should receive an antimicrobial when they undergo genitourinary or alimentary tract surgery or instrumentation.*
Clemens JD, et al. A controlled evaluation of the risk of bacterial endocarditis in persons with mitral valve prolapse. *N Engl J Med* 1982;307:776.
  *Study supports that mitral valve prolapse is a risk factor for bacterial endocarditis.*
Dajani AS, et al. Prevention of bacterial endocarditis. *JAMA* 1997;277:1794.
  *Recommendations for antimicrobial prophylaxis from the American Heart Association are outlined. Prophylaxis should be given to patients with moderate- to high-risk underlying cardiac lesions who are undergoing procedures associated with a high risk for transient bacteremia.*
Devereux RB, et al. Cost effectiveness of infective endocarditis prophylaxis for mitral valve prolapse with or without a mitral regurgitant murmur. *Am J Cardiol* 1994; 74:1024.
  *Administration of amoxicillin to patients undergoing a dental procedure who have mitral valve prolapse and a mitral regurgitant murmur is cost effective.*
Durack DT. Prevention of infective endocarditis. *N Engl J Med* 1995;322:38.
  *Review.*

Durack DT, Bisno AL, Kaplan EL. Apparent failures of endocarditis prophylaxis. Analysis of 52 cases submitted to a national registry. *JAMA* 1983;250:2318.
*Mitral valve prolapse was the most common underlying cardiac lesion. Symptoms began within 5 weeks of the suspected procedure in about 80% of the cases.*

Everett ED, Hirschmann JV. Transient bacteremia and endocarditis prophylaxis. A review. *Medicine (Baltimore)* 1977;56:61.
*Classic comprehensive review cites the frequency of transient bacteremias with various procedures.*

Fitzgerald RH, et al. Antibiotic prophylaxis for dental patients with total joint replacements. *J Am Dent Assoc* 1997;128:109.
*Antibiotic prophylaxis is not indicated for patients undergoing dental procedures who have joint replacements unless there is an increased risk for a hematogenous joint infection. Patients who are at higher risk for infection include those who are immunocompromised, who have undergone implant surgery within the past 2 years or have previously had prosthetic joint infections, and diabetics receiving insulin.*

Garrison PK, Freedman LR. Experimental endocarditis I: staphylococcal endocarditis resulting from placement of a polyethylene catheter in the right side of the heart. *Yale J Biol Med* 1970;42:394.
*Classic article describing the rabbit model used for experimental endocarditis.*

Garrod LP, Waterworth PM. The risks of dental extraction during penicillin treatment. *Br Heart J* 1962;24:39.
*During penicillin treatment, the normal streptococci in the mouth are replaced by penicillin-resistant strains.*

Glauser MP, Francioli P. Successful prophylaxis against experimental streptococcal endocarditis with bacteriostatic antibiotics. *J Infect Dis* 1982;146:806.
*Clindamycin and erythromycin given as single doses were effective in preventing endocarditis.*

Guntheroth WG. How important are dental procedures as a cause of infective endocarditis? *Am J Cardiol* 1984;54:797.
*Dental extractions preceded endocarditis in only 3.6% of cases. Good oral hygiene is the key to preventing endocarditis.*

Hall G, et al. Prophylactic administration of penicillins for endocarditis does not reduce the incidence of postextraction bacteremia. *Clin Infect Dis* 1993;17:188.
*Amoxicillin did not decrease the frequency of transient bacteremia after extraction when compared with placebo. The effect of antibiotics in preventing endocarditis must be based on other mechanisms.*

Hook EW, Kaye D. Prophylaxis of bacterial endocarditis. *J Chronic Dis* 1962;15:635.
*A classic review of the portals of entry of organisms and the risk to the susceptible host.*

Imperiale TF, Horwitz RI. Does prophylaxis prevent postdental infective endocarditis? A controlled evaluation of protective efficacy. *Am J Med* 1990;88:131.
*Antimicrobial prophylaxis was highly effective (91%) in preventing endocarditis.*

Khandheria BK. Prophylaxis or no prophylaxis before transesophageal echocardiography? *J Am Soc Echocardiogr* 1992;5:285.
*Editorial summarizing the frequency of transient bacteremia after common gastrointestinal procedures. Rates are highest with esophageal dilation (45%) and sclerotherapy (18%). Rates are about 5% after transesophageal echocardiography, and it is unclear whether antimicrobial prophylaxis is indicated.*

Kreuzpaintner G, et al. Increased risk of bacterial endocarditis in inflammatory bowel disease. *Am J Med* 1992;92:391.
*Patients with inflammatory bowel disease may be at an increased risk for endocarditis.*

Malinverni R, et al. Antibiotic prophylaxis of experimental endocarditis after dental extractions. *Circulation* 1988;77:182.
*In rats, single-dose amoxicillin or erythromycin given before a dental extraction prevented endocarditis without sterilizing the blood.*

Pelletier LL, Durack DT, Petersdorf RG. Chemotherapy of experimental streptococcal endocarditis IV: further observation of prophylaxis. *J Clin Invest* 1975;56:319.
*Data from the rabbit model are presented for prophylaxis of streptococcal endocarditis.*

Rosen L, et al. Practice parameters for antibiotic prophylaxis—supporting documentation. *Dis Colon Rectum* 1992;35:278.
*Although transient bacteremias occur after lower gastrointestinal endoscopy, the risk for development of endocarditis is low.*
Shorvan PJ, Eykyn SJ, Cotton PB. Gastrointestinal instrumentation, bacteremia, and endocarditis. *Gut* 1983;24:1078.
*A review of gastrointestinal procedures and the risk for endocarditis.*
Taran LM. Rheumatic fever in relation to dental disease. *N Y J Dent* 1944;14:107.
*Risk for development of endocarditis following a dental extraction in children with rheumatic heart disease was 1.1%.*
van der Meer JTM, et al. Efficacy of antibiotic prophylaxis for prevention of native valve endocarditis. *Lancet* 1992;339:135.
*Most cases (87%) of endocarditis were unrelated to any predisposing events.*
van der Meer JTM, et al. Awareness of need and actual use of prophylaxis: lack of patient compliance in the prevention of bacterial endocarditis. *J Antimicrob Chemother* 1992;29:187.
*By history, antimicrobials were given only 22% of the time to patients at risk for endocarditis and undergoing a procedure associated with a bacteremia.*

# IV. GASTROINTESTINAL SYSTEM

## 14. FILLING DEFECTS OF THE LIVER

Filling defects of the liver are defined in this chapter as lesions of sufficient size to be demonstrated by imaging studies, such as standard roentgenograms, computed tomography (CT), radioisotope scanning, or hepatic ultrasonography. Generally, lesions that are 0.5 to 1.0 cm or larger can be documented by newer CT scans with intravenous contrast. Differential diagnosis includes infection, hematoma, neoplasm, and cysts (Table 14-1). Granulomatous processes such as tuberculosis and fungal infection, although capable of involving hepatic parenchyma, are unusual causes of filling defects as defined above.

### Clinical Presentation

Radiographic assessment of the liver is performed for reasons that include (a) hepatomegaly or right upper quadrant (RUQ) tenderness on physical examination, (b) elevation of hepatic enzymes, most notably alkaline phosphatase, (c) jaundice, (d) fever of undetermined origin or other constitutional syndromes, and (e) assessment of metastases in patients with selected known primary malignancies. Clinical presentation is highly variable, depending on the underlying condition. As an example, uncomplicated hepatic cysts may remain asymptomatic and be documented as an incidental finding when roentgenographic studies are performed for other reasons. Alternatively, pyogenic or amebic abscess may present with high-grade constitutional abnormalities including shock. Many patients have subtle complaints of RUQ discomfort and low-grade constitutional abnormalities. Severity and acuteness of presentation may provide useful information about the cause of the process.

### Pyogenic Hepatic Abscess

Hepatic abscess has an incidence of at least 0.016%, is primarily a disease of the elderly, and is felt to be underreported. Recent investigations comparing this disease during two 20-year periods suggest that the incidence is increasing from 13 to 20 cases per 100,000 hospital admissions. Contributory factors include (numbers in parentheses represent percentage of macroscopic abscesses) the following: biliary tract infections (33%), direct extension from contiguous infected foci (25%), bacteremia (10%), blunt trauma to the RUQ (e.g., steering wheel injuries) (15%), and pylephlebitis (e.g., complications of perforated appendix) (6%). Approximately 10% are cryptogenic; this group is becoming more common. Patients with pyogenic hepatic abscess diagnosed within the past 20 years are more likely to have underlying malignancy (typically of the biliary tract or pancreas).

Clinical presentation varies with the predisposing factors. Most cases present subacutely with low-grade constitutional complaints and RUQ discomfort. Fever is the most commonly noted abnormality and is seen in more than 90% of cases. Hepatomegaly is documented in only 50% of patients, and jaundice occurs in approximately 25% of patients. Up to 20% of patients present with pulmonary complaints that include right-sided pleural effusions, elevation of the right hemidiaphragm, or rales on physical examination. Pneumonia may be the initial consideration. Routine laboratory data are often noncontributory. Anemia and leukocytosis are seen in 60% and 70% of cases, respectively. Elevations of the alkaline phosphatase are noted in 75% of patients; hyperbilirubinemia is seen in only 20% to 25%.

Noninvasive imaging techniques are generally employed to assess the patient further. Both RUQ ultrasonography and CT (often with IV contrast) have excellent published results and should be employed preferentially to radioisotope scanning. Neither of the preferred modalities is associated with significant risk for false-negative results. Ultrasound has a reported sensitivity for the diagnosis of pyogenic hepatic abscess of 85% to 95% and has the advantage of providing excellent visualization of the biliary tract (diseases of which may contribute to liver abscess). Additionally, ultrasound may be better at distinguishing solid structures from cysts. CT is more than 95% sensitive for the diagnosis of hepatic abscess and has advantages that include the ability to evaluate selected portions of the liver and discriminate among other abdominal structures,

Table 14-1.  Amebic versus pyogenic hepatic abscess

| Feature | Amebic | Pyogenic |
|---|---|---|
| Male:female ratio | 19:1 | 4:1 |
| Age (median) | 28 y | 44 y |
| Birthplace | Endemic | Any |
| RUQ pain | 59% | 27% |
| Symptoms >14 d | 14% | 37% |
| RUQ tenderness | 67% | 42% |
| Albumin <3.0 g/dL | 16% | 50% |
| Amebic serology (+) | 94% | 6%* |

RUQ, right upper quadrant.
* All had prior amebiasis.
Adapted from Barnes PF, et al. A comparison of amebic and pyogenic abscess of the liver. *Medicine* 1987; 66:472–483.

and usefulness in obese or distended patients. Additionally, patients with multiple pyogenic abscesses may be better diagnosed by CT than by ultrasound. In the absence of pylephlebitis or biliary tract disease, random assessment of the gastrointestinal organs is generally not indicated.

Percutaneous drainage of the filling defect at the time of initial evaluation allows simultaneous diagnosis and therapy. Materials obtained can be sent for Gram's stain, aerobic or anaerobic culture, parasitology, and histopathology. When a filling defect is clinically suspected, percutaneous drainage often can obviate the need for surgical exploration. CT or ultrasonography can then be used to follow clinical response to therapy and ensure resolution of the process.

The bacteriology of pyogenic hepatic abscess is often complex and includes combinations of "gut flora." The role of anaerobes, including *Bacteroides fragilis,* is well defined. These often coexist with enteric gram-negative bacilli, such as *Escherichia coli* or *Klebsiella* species. Trends during the past two decades suggest an increase in hepatic abscesses associated with fungi, streptococci, and *Pseudomonas aeruginosa.* In adults, hepatic abscesses associated with *Actinomycetes* as a single pathogen have recently been reviewed. Most cases presented in typical fashion and had unknown primary sources. Recent reports have also documented the likelihood of metastatic dissemination of *Klebsiella* infection (often causing endophthalmitis) from pyogenic abscess. This has been especially noted in diabetics.

Therapy of pyogenic hepatic abscess consists of long-term parenteral antimicrobials plus drainage. When drainage cannot be performed for technical or medical reasons, certain cases may be managed medically with careful follow-up; however, this should not be considered the standard of care.

Percutaneous catheter drainage is recommended as the drainage procedure of choice. Percutaneous aspiration is generally considered inferior, but comparative studies are needed. Open surgical procedures should be performed when (a) multiple or septated lesions are identified that cannot be drained percutaneously, (b) surgery is indicated to manage the initiating cause of the abscess (e.g., biliary stones), and (c) the patient has failed to respond to percutaneous drainage. Surgical extirpation should also be considered when hydatid disease is in the differential diagnosis. The optimal length of antimicrobial treatment is unknown. Most authorities recommend at least 4 weeks of therapy when drainage has been accomplished, and up to 8 weeks when drainage could not be performed. Agents that include quinolones, metronidazole, and trimethoprim/sulfamethoxazole have excellent bioavailability following oral administration and may be considered in selected cases.

### Amebic Abscess

Amebiasis afflicts up to 10% of the population, is associated with 50 million cases of invasive disease, and may account for as many as 100,000 deaths. Although two species of *Entamoeba* have recently been identified that are morphologically identical, it is only *E. histolytica* that causes invasive disease. Amebic abscess is the most common complication of intestinal amebiasis and can occur many years after exposure in endemic areas. It should be suspected as a cause of intrahepatic filling defects in patients with such an epidemiologic history, and it generally involves the right hepatic lobe. Although many features overlap with those of pyogenic abscess, selected clues summarized in Table 14-1 may occasionally help with differentiation. Geographic areas of risk are Mexico, Central America, and Southeast Asia. Disease is also associated with homosexuality and residence in institutions for the mentally retarded.

Up to 66% of cases present with the acute onset of fever (often with rigors) and abdominal pain with a duration of fewer than 10 days. The others often have complaints for up to 12 weeks. Persons with acute presentations often have high-grade fevers (above 102°F), and abdominal pain is often located in the RUQ. Selected cases may present only as an acute febrile syndrome. Patients with subacute or chronic presentations have lower fevers and more benign presentations. In both groups, pulmonary complaints such as pleurisy and cough may be noted, and the initial consideration may be pneumonia. Only about one third of patients give a history of active diarrhea at any time before clinical presentation. Rarely, initial presentation will be that of rupture—either into the peritoneum, pleural space, or pericardium. Intraabdominal rupture is more likely when abscesses of the left lobe are present.

For patients with acute presentations, laboratory data typically demonstrate leukocytosis with bandemia. WBC counts may be normal in those with more chronic illness. Both groups may become anemic. Approximately 85% of patients have elevations of alkaline phosphatase. This is the most reliable chemical test, and levels are likely to be higher in persons with chronic disease. Hyperbilirubinemia is not commonly noted. Indirect hemagglutination testing is a reliable serologic test for hepatic amebiasis, yielding positive results in at least 85% of patients with extraintestinal disease, and titers often exceed 1:256. It should be performed in all patients with space-occupying lesions when a specific alternative diagnosis cannot be made. Results of serologic testing may be negative early in the course of disease, and a negative result does not preclude this illness in acute cases. However, elevations are almost always noted by 2 weeks into disease and may remain high for many years following successful therapy.

The diagnosis can be suspected by hepatic imaging, but a pathognomonic picture is not seen. Hepatic ultrasound or CT provides highly sensitive results and can be repeated during and after therapy to gauge response. Most authors now feel that the former, because of ease of administration and lower expense, is the study of choice for both diagnosis and follow-up. Satisfactory treatment of amebic abscess can be anticipated to result in return to an echographically normal liver. However, lesion size may actually increase during early therapy, and thus some authorities do not recommend routine radiographic studies if the patient is clinically responding. The time to normalization is 2 to 20 months. Generally, there is no value to gallium or sulfur colloid scans.

Up to 50% of cases demonstrate multiple space-occupying lesions. The most common sites remain the superior or posterior-superior portion of the right lobe. Results of hepatic ultrasonography usually demonstrate round or oval hypoechoic lesions, often containing debris. Fifty percent may appear as cystic lesions, and many that present acutely may appear as either solid or heterogeneous masses. Thus, the ultrasonic presentation, especially in acute cases, is variable.

The average size of abscesses is 7 to 10 cm. Lesions larger than 10 cm can be seen in at least 33% of cases. In acute cases with clinical presentations of fewer than 5 days, however, initial ultrasonographic findings may be falsely negative. The diagnosis should continue to be suspected by the presentation of fever, RUQ discomfort, and elevated alkaline phosphatase in a person with an appropriate epidemiologic history.

The role of percutaneous lesion aspiration for either diagnosis or treatment remains controversial. Surgical intervention is rarely indicated for the uncomplicated case but may be lifesaving if rupture has occurred. Although some recent data suggest that patients with amebic abscess respond more rapidly when aspiration accompanies medication, many patients in whom the diagnosis is secure can be managed without it. Aspiration is indicated if (a) alternative diagnoses are being considered (excluding hydatid disease), (b) lesions are larger than 10 cm, (c) patients fail to respond to standard therapy within approximately 72 hours, or (c) left-sided lesions are at risk for rupture. Material obtained at aspiration should be evaluated for the presence of organisms. Typical fluid does not smell of food and is brownish ("anchovy paste"), often devoid of organisms, and typically without polymorphonuclear leukocytes. Standard cultures (aerobic and anaerobic) and histopathology should be carried out in all cases.

Medical therapy for amebic abscess consists of oral or IV administration of 750 mg of metronidazole three times daily for 5 to 10 days. A regimen of 2.4 g daily by mouth for several days has also been successfully employed. Up to 90% of patients respond clinically within 72 hours. Aspiration of the hepatic lesion should be performed if clinical response is not seen by this time. More toxic regimens that are uncommonly indicated consist of 1 to 1.5 mg of dehydroemetine per kilogram of body weight daily for 5 days plus either diloxanide furoate or paromomycin.

### Echinococcal Cyst (Hydatid Disease)

Echinococcal disease is endemic in areas of southern Europe, the Middle East, and Australia. It represents the larval stage of the canine tapeworm *Echinococcus granulosus*. Cases reported in the United States are primarily imported. Human disease is generally asymptomatic and identified during routine roentgenography for other reasons. Sixty percent to 75% of all cysts occur in the liver. Between 20% and 40% of persons may harbor multiple cysts.

Clinical presentation is often chronic and generally consists of an enlarging space-occupying lesion in the absence of significant constitutional symptomatology. Symptoms are typically vague abdominal pain and pressure. At least one third of patients remain asymptomatic. Complaints are generally not noted until cysts reach 7 cm or more in size; average cyst size at surgery is approximately 11 cm. Hepatic enlargement may be noted, often in association with a palpable mass. Leakage and frank rupture are dreaded complications and can occur spontaneously, after trauma, or at the time of surgical removal. Material is "allergenic," and leakage may be associated with anaphylaxis.

Diagnosis should be suspected in patients with a history of travel to endemic areas. Usual laboratory data are not useful. About 60% of patients will have an elevation of alkaline phosphatase, and 33% may demonstrate eosinophilia. An indirect hemagglutination titer of more than 1:64 is seen in about 50% of cases. CT, ultrasonography, or routine abdominal films often demonstrate single or multiple cystic areas, generally with partial calcification. The presence of intracystic septations associated with partial calcification of the cyst is considered pathognomonic.

Therapy consists of surgical extirpation under carefully controlled conditions to avoid spillage of cyst contents. Percutaneous aspiration is contraindicated because of risk for spillage. Medications are not useful. For the management of cysts when complete excision is not feasible, authorities recommend instillation of cetrimide plus removal of the inner embryonic membranes of the cyst.

### Neoplasm and Other Causes of Hepatic Filling Defects

Benign and malignant neoplasms (both primary and metastatic) often involve the liver. The most common primary neoplasms are hepatocellular carcinoma and cholangiocarcinoma. Primary cancers commonly associated with hepatic metastases include those of the lung, breast, colon, rectum, stomach, and pancreas, and melanoma. One investigation demonstrated that 39% of adults dying with solid tumors had hepatic metastases.

Clinical presentation varies and may overlap that seen with infectious etiologies. Ascites, however, may be seen and is distinctly unusual for infectious causes of hepatic filling defects. Alternatively, patients with pyogenic abscess are more likely to have at least three of the following: leukocytosis, fever, risk factors for pyogenic abscess, shorter clinical course, and normal hepatic size.

CT is considered the best screening test for hepatic metastases. Sensitivity is above 90%, but specificity is low. Lesions larger than 1 cm can be described in this fashion. Hepatic ultrasonography is generally considered the next most important test and (like CT) can distinguish solid from cystic lesions. Up to 90% of these can be discovered with this technique. CT, often with the use of IV contrast, can detect lesions larger than 0.5 cm. Lesions that include cavernous hemangioma, focal fatty deposits, and nodular hyperplasia can often be diagnosed by a characteristic CT scan plus radionucleotide imaging. Both ultrasonography and CT often can discriminate simple cysts and other lesions. Although one or another study can provide clues to etiology, the ultimate diagnosis generally rests on tissue and fluid sampling.

### Summary
Hepatic filling defects are associated with many causes. The clinical presentation is variable, and diagnosis is usually identified by noninvasive radiographic assessment plus sampling of the lesion. Percutaneous evaluation of lesion contents is generally acceptable and well tolerated. However, a consideration for hydatid disease should contraindicate this approach. (R.B.B.)

### Bibliography
Barnes PF, et al. A comparison of amebic and pyogenic abscess of the liver. *Medicine (Baltimore)* 1987;66:472–483.
  *The authors compare the clinical characteristics of 96 patients with amebic abscess with those of 48 patients with pyogenic abscess. Features that included Latin American birthplace, younger age, abdominal pain with RUQ tenderness, symptoms for fewer than 14 days, and selected hepatic enzyme determinations helped predict amebic abscess. Ultrasonographic features of round or oval shape and "hypoechoic appearance with fine, homogeneous, low-level echoes at high gain" were also statistically more common with amebic abscess.*
Cady B. Natural history of primary and secondary tumors of the liver. *Semin Oncol* 1983;10:127–134.
  *This review provides an excellent overview of the likely causes of hepatic neoplasms and their clinical presentation.*
Halvorsen RA Jr, Thompson WM. Imaging primary and metastatic cancer of the liver. *Semin Oncol* 1991;18:111–122.
  *The authors provide an approach to the imaging of hepatic neoplasms. Lesions are placed in several groups according to the presence of characteristic changes by imaging modalities. Unfortunately, most are insufficiently differentiated by imaging alone and require tissue diagnosis.*
Huang CJ, et al. Pyogenic hepatic abscess. Changing trends over 42 years. *Ann Surg* 1996; 223:600–607.
  *The authors assess 233 cases of pyogenic hepatic abscess treated during a 40-year period. They divide patients into two periods: before and after 1972. Differences in bacteriology and treatment were noted. Those cases seen more recently were more likely to be associated with biliary or pancreatic malignancy. Overall mortality decreased from 65% to approximately 30%.*
Klotz SA, Penn RL. Clinical differentiation of abscess from neoplasm in newly diagnosed space-occupying lesions of the liver. *South Med J* 1987;80:1537–1541.
  *The authors recognized the difficulty in differentiating malignant from pyogenic intrahepatic lesions by imaging techniques alone and looked critically at clinical presentations. Patients with pyogenic abscesses had shorter prodromes, risk factors for abscess, fever, leukocytosis, and normal hepatic size. Presence of at least three of these correctly predicted all abscesses.*
Miyamoto MI, Fang FC. Pyogenic liver abscess involving *Actinomyces:* case report and review. *Clin Infect Dis* 1993;16:303–309.
  *The authors report a case of hepatic abscess associated with Actinomyces and review the literature on 35 other cases. Most presented in a subacute fashion and were diagnosed by standard, noninvasive tests. Nonsurgical drainage appears appropriate, and antimicrobial therapy with penicillin or tetracycline resulted in satisfactory outcomes.*
Ravdin JI. Amebiasis. *Clin Infect Dis* 1995;20:1453–1466.
  *The author provides an excellent overview of recent developments in amebiasis. Biology, epidemiology, diagnosis, management, and prevention are explored. Much practical information, obviously provided by a hands-on clinician, is included in this article.*
Rubin RH, Swartz MN, Malt R. Hepatic abscess: changes in clinical, bacteriologic, and therapeutic aspects. *Am J Med* 1974;57:601–610.

*This classic review of the topic summarizes the Massachusetts General Hospital experience with 50 patients during a 12-year period. Most pyogenic abscesses were macroscopic and associated with biliary tract abnormalities. Combinations of enteric flora were most commonly noted. Mortality was greatest in the elderly. Successful treatment required a combination of prolonged antimicrobials and drainage.*

Schaefer JW, Khan Y. Echinococcosis (hydatid disease): lessons from experience with 59 patients. *Rev Infect Dis* 1991;13:243–247.

*This article reports the experience from Saudi Arabia with almost 60 patients who had hydatid disease. Currently, diagnosis can be made by ultrasound or CT presentation. Serologic diagnosis is specific but insensitive. Surgery is the management strategy of choice and should be reserved for symptomatic cases. Outcomes were uniformly satisfactory when surgery was performed electively, but morbidity and mortality were encountered when rupture had occurred.*

Seeto RK, Rockey DC. Pyogenic liver abscess. Changes in etiology, management, and outcome. *Medicine* 1996;75:99–113.

*The authors provide an excellent review of the subject, summarizing information about epidemiology, bacteriology, and management. The central role of CT and ultrasound in both the diagnosis and management of pyogenic hepatic abscess is stressed. The authors feel that drainage rather than aspiration of abscess is the therapy of choice. This therapeutic regimen has cure rates of up to 75%—and up to 90% within the past 5 years.*

Thompson JE Jr, Forlenza S, Verma R. Amebic liver abscess: a therapeutic approach. *Rev Infect Dis* 1985;7:171–179.

*Metronidazole remains the therapy of choice for most amebic abscesses. Failure is occasionally noted and can be anticipated when clinical response is not noted within 72 hours.*

---

## 15. GRANULOMATOUS HEPATITIS

---

Granulomas may be found in the liver of patients with a known systemic disease, such as tuberculosis or sarcoidosis, and in patients who are asymptomatic and whose liver function test findings are abnormal. The term granulomatous hepatitis has been used to describe patients with granulomas in the liver who have abnormal liver function or nonspecific symptoms of fever and malaise.

Recent studies on granulomatous hepatitis appear to show differences in the etiology of this disease in comparison with earlier studies. Guckian and Perry (1965) reviewed 63 cases of granulomatous hepatitis and noted many different causes, including infections (viral, bacterial, fungal, rickettsial), hypersensitivity diseases (drugs and berylliosis), and vascular and connective tissue diseases (Wegener's granulomatosis, rheumatoid arthritis, sarcoidosis). Fifty-three percent of patients had tuberculosis, 12% had sarcoidosis, and 2% had an unknown disease. As might be expected, recent studies show a different distribution of diagnoses, with tuberculosis becoming much less common.

Sartin and Walker (1991) reviewed 88 cases of granulomatous hepatitis from the Mayo Clinic. In 50%, disease was confined to the liver, and a diagnosis of idiopathic granulomatous hepatitis was made. Twenty-two percent of patients had sarcoidosis, and only 3% had tuberculosis. Patients in whom idiopathic disease was diagnosed had a benign course.

Zoutman et al. (1991) reviewed a series of patients with fever of unknown origin who were found to have granulomatous hepatitis on liver biopsy. Of 23 patients, only 26% were given a specific diagnosis, and only two patients had mycobacterial disease. In the remaining 74% of patients, no specific diagnosis was made after 41 months of follow-up. All 17 patients had a benign course and remained well, although seven required long-term prednisone therapy.

Recent reports emphasize the wide differential for granulomatous hepatitis. Infections such as Q fever and Lyme disease may cause granulomatous hepatitis. Lenoir et al. (1988) reported three patients with cat scratch fever. The Warthin-Starry silver stain showed organisms consistent with the cat scratch bacillus. *Bartonella henselae* has been increasingly recognized as a cause of granulomatous hepatitis and splenitis. Granulomatous hepatitis has been reported in association with secondary syphilis. Systemic *Yersinia enterocolitica* infection has caused granulomatous hepatitis with acute necrosis.

Granulomatous hepatitis continues to be reported as a drug effect. Quinidine, diltiazem, hydralazine, methimazole, glyburide, paracetamol, pyrazinamide, and interferon alfa have recently been reported to cause granulomatous hepatitis. Bladder instillation of bacille Calmette-Guérin vaccine for the treatment of bladder carcinoma has also been reported to cause granulomatous hepatitis, both by hematogenous dissemination and as a hypersensitivity reaction. In one study of patients with rheumatoid arthritis receiving gold therapy, gold pigment could be demonstrated in lipogranulomas by radiographic microanalysis.

Mahida et al. (1988) described familial granulomatous hepatitis. Two West Indian parents and three of seven offspring had the disease. No cause or extrinsic etiology could be identified. Granulomatous hepatitis may be a manifestation of lymphoma, although abnormal cells will often be detected with these lesions.

Because of the many etiologies for granulomatous hepatitis, a thorough history and physical examination must direct the workup. Examination of the lung and skin and a search for lymphadenopathy will be particularly important. A detailed history should include all medications and drugs taken by the patient. A history of cough, fever, drenching sweats, and weight loss suggests tuberculosis. Chest roentgenography, determination of serum calcium level, Venereal Disease Research Laboratory (VDRL) test, urine analysis, and tuberculosis skin test will be routinely performed. Liver biopsy material should be cultured for fungi and mycobacteria. Acid-fast, hematoxylin-eosin, and methenamine silver stains should also be performed. Serology for Q fever, brucellosis, syphilis, and hepatitis are recommended. Angiotensin-converting enzyme may be indicated in patients with pulmonary disease in whom sarcoidosis is being considered.

Some patients with miliary tuberculosis may have negative results on stains for acid-fast bacilli. Clinical judgment will be needed to determine when empiric therapy for tuberculosis is indicated. Additional cultures and biopsies of bone marrow, lymph node, or lung lesions may be necessary.

When the suspicion for tuberculosis is low, corticosteroid treatment has proved useful in symptomatic patients with sarcoidosis or idiopathic granulomatous hepatitis. Methotrexate has been reported to be successful therapy in some patients with idiopathic granulomatous hepatitis. (S.L.B.)

## Bibliography

Blest S, Schubert TT. Chronic Epstein-Barr virus infection: a cause of granulomatous hepatitis? *J Clin Gastroenterol* 1989;11:343.
*Granulomatous hepatitis was found in a patient who had IgM antibody to viral capsid antigen.*
Braylan RC, et al. Malignant lymphoma obscured by concomitant epithelioid granulomas. *Cancer* 1977;39:1146.
*Nonnecrotic hepatic granulomas were associated with malignant lymphoma.*
Fitzgerald MX, Fitzgerald O, Towers RP. Granulomatous hepatitis of obscure etiology. *Q J Med* 1971;40:371.
*A discussion of selective aspects of the problem of granulomatous hepatitis, the value of the Kveim test, and the value of therapeutic trials of antituberculosis therapy.*
Guckian JC, Perry JE. Granulomatous hepatitis. An analysis of 63 cases and review of the literature. *Ann Intern Med* 1965;65:1081.
*Excellent classic article and detailed discussion of etiology. Tuberculosis is no longer as common a cause of granulomatous hepatitis.*
Israel HL, Goldstein RA. Hepatic granulomatosis and sarcoidosis. *Ann Intern Med* 1973;79:669.

*Extraabdominal investigation can provide evidence that sarcoidosis is the cause of febrile hepatic granulomatosis. The Kveim reaction has little value in excluding sarcoidosis.*

Knobel B, et al. Pyrazinamide-induced granulomatous hepatitis. *J Clin Gastroenterol* 1997;24:264.
*First documented case of pyrazinamide causing granulomatous hepatitis, with clinical symptoms of hectic fever, chills, and extreme fatigue 4 weeks after pyrazinamide was begun.*

Knox T, et al. Methotrexate treatment of idiopathic granulomatous hepatitis. *Ann Intern Med* 1995;122:592.
*Patients with granulomatous hepatitis for whom no etiologic agent can be found may respond to treatment with methotrexate. Patients who have failed corticosteroid therapy have responded to methotrexate.*

Landas SK, et al. Lipogranulomas and gold in the liver in rheumatoid arthritis. *Am J Surg* 1992;16:171.
*Study of patients with severe rheumatoid arthritis on methotrexate in whom liver biopsy was performed routinely. Patients who had been on gold therapy had lipogranulomas with pigment representing gold deposition.*

Lenoir AA, et al. Granulomatous hepatitis associated with cat scratch disease. *Lancet* 1988;21:1121.
*Describes three patients with granulomatous hepatitis and cat scratch fever. Only one patient had peripheral lymphadenopathy. Results of Warthin-Starry silver stain of the liver were positive.*

Liston TE, Koehler JE. Granulomatous hepatitis and necrotizing splenitis due to *Bartonella henselae* in a patient with cancer. *Clin Infect Dis* 1996;22:951.
*A case report of B. henselae causing granulomatous hepatitis and necrotizing splenitis in an adult cancer patient undergoing chemotherapy. Forty-one cases of Bartonella infection of the liver and spleen are reviewed. Bartonella may cause liver disease in immunocompetent or immunosuppressed patients. Not all patients have contact with dogs or cats.*

Maddrey WC, et al. Sarcoidosis and chronic hepatic disease: a clinical and pathologic study of 20 patients. *Medicine (Baltimore)* 1970;49:375.
*A positive Kveim reaction in patients with sarcoidosis and hepatic granuloma is correlated with the presence of enlarged hilar nodes.*

Mahida Y, et al. Familial granulomatous hepatitis: a hitherto unrecognized entity. *Am J Gastroenterol* 1988;83:42.
*Parents and three offspring had granulomatous hepatitis. Granulomas were also found in muscles, lymph nodes, and pleurae.*

Mathus S, Dooley J, Scheuer PJ. Quinine-induced granulomatous hepatitis and vasculitis. *Br Med J* 1990;300:613.
*Report of quinine as cause of hepatitis and vasculitis. Quinine was also implicated in an earlier report (Br Med J 1983;286:264).*

Mills P, et al. Ultrasound in the diagnosis of granulomatous liver disease. *Clin Radiol* 1990;41:113.
*Patients with granulomatous hepatitis often have suggestive hypoechoic halos on ultrasound.*

Neville E, Piyasena KHG, James DG. Granulomas of the liver. *Postgrad Med J* 1975; 51:361.
*A review of the clinical, biochemical, and immunologic features of diseases that produce hepatic granuloma.*

Port J, Leonidas JC. Granulomatous hepatitis in cat-scratch disease. Ultrasound and CT observations. *Pediatr Radiol* 1991;21:598.
*Case of cat scratch disease and granulomatous hepatitis. Abdominal ultrasound showed multiple well-circumscribed, low-attenuation areas in the liver.*

Rice D, Burdick CO. Granulomatous hepatitis from hydralazine therapy [Letter]. *Arch Intern Med* 1983;143:1077.
*Hydralazine is reported to cause granulomatous hepatitis.*

Sarachek NS, London RL, Matulewica TJ. Diltiazem and granulomatous hepatitis. *Gastroenterology* 1985;88:1260.

*Patient on diltiazem in whom fever and liver function test abnormalities developed had biopsy-proven granulomatous hepatitis.*
Sartin JS, Walker RC. Granulomatous hepatitis: a retrospective review of 88 cases at the Mayo Clinic. *Mayo Clin Proc* 1991;66:914.
*Retrospective review of 88 cases from the Mayo Clinic. Fifty percent of patients had idiopathic hepatitis. Only 3% had tuberculosis.*
Saw D, et al. Granulomatous hepatitis associated with glyburide. *Dig Dis Sci* 1996; 41:322.
*Report of two patients in whom granulomatous hepatitis developed while they were taking glyburide, and review of the literature on the association.*
Scully RE, Galdabini JJ, McNeely BU. Case records of the Massachusetts General Hospital. Case 19-1978. Presentation of a case. *Case Records of the Massachusetts General Hospital* 1978;298:1133.
*Description of a patient with lymphoma who had granulomatous hepatitis.*
Stjernberg U, Silseth C, Ritland S. Granulomatous hepatitis in *Yersinia enterocolitica* infection. *Hepatogastroenterology* 1987;34:56.
*Y. enterocolitica infection was diagnosed by a positive stool culture and serum titer of 1:1280.*
Terplan M. Hepatic granulomas of unknown cause presenting with fever. *Am J Gastroenterol* 1971;55:43.
*Sarcoidosis and tuberculosis were the most frequent causes of hepatic granulomas. A characteristic syndrome appears to accompany nonspecific granuloma.*
Thung SN, et al. Granulomatous hepatitis in Q fever. *Mt Sinai J Med* 1986;53:283.
*Report of Q fever as a cause of granulomatous hepatitis.*
Toft E, Vyberg M, Therkelsen K. Diltiazem-induced granulomatous hepatitis. *Histopathology* 1991;18:474.
*Case report of diltiazem causing granulomatous hepatitis.*
Tucker LE. Tocainide-induced granulomatous hepatitis [Letter]. *JAMA* 1986;27:255.
*Tocainide can be added to the list of cardiac drugs reported to cause granulomatous hepatitis.*
Zoutman DE, Ralph ED, Frei JV. Granulomatous hepatitis and fever of unknown origin. An 11-year experience of 23 cases with 3 years' follow-up. *J Clin Gastroenterol* 1991;13:69.
*Specific diagnosis was made in only 26% of patients with fever of unknown origin and granulomatous hepatitis. Forty-one percent had idiopathic disease. These patients had a benign course, although some required long-term steroid therapy.*

# 16. COMMUNITY-ACQUIRED PERITONITIS

Peritonitis is a commonly encountered illness that occurs in all age groups and is often infectious. Major types of peritonitis discussed in this chapter are spontaneous (primary) bacterial peritonitis (PBP), peritonitis complicating visceral perforation ("secondary" bacterial peritonitis), and that complicating continuous ambulatory peritoneal dialysis (CAPD). An appreciation of the anatomy, pathophysiology, clinical manifestations, and bacteriology of these diseases is important for appropriate management.

## Anatomy and Physiology of the Peritoneal Space

The peritoneum is a closed space with many invaginations and outpockets. In females, the fallopian tubes breach this closure. Upper and lower peritoneal areas are connected by left and right gutters; these are potential conduits for infected material. The most dependent of these areas is the pelvis. Other candidates for accumulation of drainage are the left and right subdiaphragmatic spaces. The lesser sac, one of the largest of the potential spaces, is bounded by the pancreas and stomach and has an opening called the foramen of Winslow. Because of its unique location, it may be spared from general peritoneal infection. Alternatively, it may become infected as an isolated area.

The peritoneal cavity is lined by a single-layered serous membrane that allows rapid bidirectional transfer of materials. Physical forces, including oncotic and hydrostatic pressure, determine flow rate and direction. Antimicrobials such as quinolones, trimethoprim-sulfamethoxazole (TMP-SMX), aminoglycosides, β-lactams, clindamycin, and chloramphenicol penetrate the inflamed peritoneum and can rapidly achieve therapeutic concentrations. Thus, there may be no need for intraperitoneal antimicrobials in the management of some forms of peritonitis. The lymphatics remove proteins and particulate matter. Peritoneal lymphatics interdigitate with those above the diaphragm and allow the rapid dispersal of particulate matter into the pleurae. The diaphragmatic surface is covered with specialized lymphatics bearing stomata of 8 to 12 μm. Bacteria and proteins can be removed through pores of this size.

The peritoneal cavity responds to infection in several ways. Removal of potential pathogens occurs primarily by lymphatics. As an example, at least 50% of an intraperitoneal bacterial challenge is cleared into the bloodstream within 1 hour. Organisms are taken up through peritoneal lining cells, absorbed by lymphatics, and ultimately enter the bloodstream via the thoracic duct. Containment of infection is aided by production of fibrin secondary to inflammation. Normal anatomic barriers such as omentum, abdominal organs, and diaphragm may allow actively infected areas to remain sequestered from the remainder of the peritoneal cavity. Finally, host defenses that include peritoneal macrophages, polymorphonuclear leukocytes, complement, and immunoglobulins can be activated to opsonize, phagocytize, and kill microorganisms.

### Spontaneous (Primary) Bacterial Peritonitis in adults

PBP is that unassociated with a primary intraabdominal source. Adults most often have cirrhosis with ascites as its substrate. In this population, it is a marker of severe liver disease. In-hospital mortality reaches 50%, and rates of relapse of up to 43% at 6 months and 69% at 1 year and 1-year mortality rates of approximately 60% are published. Patients at particular risk are those with ascitic protein concentrations of less than 1 g/dL. Patients with severe liver disease who survive an initial bout of PBP may be candidates for liver transplantation. Symptoms include worsening hepatic failure, abdominal pain or tenderness, and fever. These classic findings may be minimal, however, and the disease occasionally may be diagnosed in the absence of symptoms. Generally, paracentesis should be performed in patients with ascites and any of the classic findings.

PBP most commonly is caused by a single microbe. Identification of multiple enteric bacteria should prompt a search for perforated viscus. *Escherichia coli* (40% to 60%) and streptococci/enterococci (30%) are most often seen. Other enteric gram-negative bacilli, especially *Klebsiella* species, comprise most of the remainder. Anaerobes are rarely identified, probably because of high oxygen tensions in ascitic fluid.

A variant of spontaneous peritonitis, culture-negative neutrocytic ascites, is defined as the combination of ascitic fluid leukocytosis (>500/mm³), no prior antibiotics, and negative cultures. Presentation and natural history are the same as with PBP. The reason for negative cultures involves the immune response of ascitic fluid.

Blood cultures should be performed for patients suspected of having PBP, and individuals should undergo diagnostic paracentesis. The former are positive in about a third of patients. Within ascitic fluid, cell count and differential demonstrate primarily polymorphonuclear leukocytes and cell counts of more than 250 to 500/mm³. Marked peripheral leukocytosis does not affect this. Other parameters that help discriminate between PBP and other ascitic syndromes include an ascitic fluid-serum lactate dehydrogenase ratio above 0.4 and an ascitic fluid-serum glucose ratio below 1.0. Generally, PBP by these criteria has been exudative. Gram's stain typically demonstrates a single morphology (implying a single organism). Paracentesis fluid should be routinely injected into blood culture bottles, and especially the BacT/ALERT system. This results in faster and greater yields than does the use of traditional agar inoculation systems.

Therapy consists of appropriate antimicrobials and supportive care. Choice of agent can be based on Gram's stain. Gram-positive cocci in chains represent streptococci. Two to three million units of aqueous penicillin G IV every 4 hours, plus 5 mg of gentamicin per kilogram IV daily in a single dose provides optimal coverage until identification is completed. *Streptococcus pneumoniae, S. pyogenes,* and most other streptococci can then be treated with penicillin as monotherapy. *Enterococcus faecalis* or *E. faecium* generally requires combination therapy. Unfortunately, some strains of enterococci now produce β-lactamase or may be vancomycin-resistant. Therapy must be individualized based on susceptibilities. Gram-negative bacilli demonstrated on Gram's stain can generally be managed with monotherapy. Options include third-generation cephalosporins, antipseudomonal penicillins, aztreonam, quinolones, TMP-SMX, ticarcillin-clavulanate, piperacillin-tazobactam, or imipenemcilastatin. Choice depends primarily on susceptibility patterns, cost, ease of administration, and patient factors.

Recommendations for empiric therapy if treatment cannot be guided by Gram's stain are generally a third-generation cephalosporin or a β/β-lactamase combination. Aztreonam has been well studied for PBP, and although it works well for illness caused by gram-negative bacilli, gram-positive superinfection has been noted. Thus, its use as empiric monotherapy cannot be supported. For susceptible enteric gram-negative bacilli in patients tolerant of oral therapy, oral quinolones or TMP-SMX could be considered.

Duration of therapy is best guided by the results of a second paracentesis performed 48 hours after initiation of antibiotics. At this time, patients should have ascitic fluid WBC counts of less than $250/mm^3$ and negative cultures. If counts have risen or if cultures remain positive, a ruptured viscus should be considered. For patients with ascitic fluid counts of less than $250/mm^3$ at 48 hours, duration of treatment should be 5 days. Evaluation for ruptured viscus, resistant pathogens, and other reasons for failure should be performed when counts have not fallen at repeated (48-hour) paracentesis.

Primary peritonitis caused by *Mycobacterium tuberculosis* or fungi needs to be considered in patients with negative bacterial cultures and exudative ascites. Tuberculous peritonitis comprises more than 50% of cases of abdominal tuberculosis, is most common in women (71%), and can mimic an acute abdomen, tumor, or cirrhosis. Many of these patients have no evidence of disease elsewhere (46%), and skin tests may be negative (17%). Most cases are associated with exudative ascites and lymphocyte counts above $500/mm^3$. Diagnosis is best made by peritoneal biopsy for smear, culture, and histopathology. Fungal peritonitis is most commonly associated with either *Candida* species or *Cryptococcus neoformans.* The former should be considered in patients with previous intraabdominal surgery and recent broad-spectrum antimicrobial treatment. The latter usually presents a component of disseminated cryptococcosis and is generally diagnosed by aspiration of ascites. Severe underlying hepatic disease is noted, and there may be a history of recent upper gastrointestinal bleeding.

Prevention of PBP should be attempted in all patients who survive an initial bout or who are high risk (variceal bleeding, low ascitic protein concentrations, or prolonged prothrombin times). Oral quinolones and TMP-SMX have been utilized. The latter, at a dose of 1 DS 5 d/wk was associated with a statistically lower likelihood of PBP than placebo, but long-term mortality rates were unchanged. Diuresis to decrease ascitic fluid volume (and therefore raise ascitic fluid protein) is also indicated.

## Secondary Bacterial Peritonitis

Secondary bacterial peritonitis generally results from spillage of the contents of a hollow viscus. Common causes are penetrating trauma, malignancy, diverticular and appendiceal infections, cholecystitis, and pyloric ulcer disease. Consequences depend in part on the bacteriologic composition of the spilled material. Clinical presentation often involves well-defined complexes of symptoms. The elderly and those on high doses of corticosteroids may present in more subtle fashions. In these populations, abdominal pain may be blunted and fever may be lower. As a result, symptoms may last longer before diagnosis, and patients may therefore be sicker on presentation.

### Normal Gastrointestinal Flora

Organisms colonizing the gastrointestinal tract vary qualitatively and quantitatively among different sites (Table 16-1). Such differences have important clinical implications. Polymicrobial contamination with three to five species often follows large-bowel spillage. Anaerobes, including *Bacteroides fragilis,* predominate. *Pseudomonas aeruginosa* may be an important consideration in patients with complicated appendicitis.

Table 16-1. Comparative bacteriology of the intact gastrointestinal tract

| Anatomic area | Enteric gram-negative bacilli | Bacteroides | Streptococci | Other anaerobes |
|---|---|---|---|---|
| Empty stomach | 0.0* | 0.0 | 0.0 | 0.0 |
| Full stomach | 1.5 | 1.5 | 0.0 | 0.0 |
| Gallbladder | 0.0 | 0.0 | 0.0 | 0.0 |
| Jejunum | 1.0 | 1.0 | 2.4–4.2 | 1.0 |
| Distal ileum | 3.3–5.6 | 5.2–5.7 | 2.5–4.9 | 2.5–5.7 |
| Colon | 6.0–7.6 | 8.5–10.0 | 4.0–7.0 | 5.0–10.5 |

* Value is $\log_{10}$ bacteria per milliliter of gastrointestinal contents.

Summarized results from animal and human trials indicate the following: (a) Early mortality from peritonitis approaches 40% and is caused primarily by gram-negative sepsis from *E. coli;* (b) intraabdominal abscesses develop in most survivors with a complex flora that includes *B. fragilis, E. coli,* enterococci, and other anaerobes; (c) the capsule of *B. fragilis* is a virulence factor associated with abscess formation; and (d) there exists a pecking order of antimicrobial agents that vary considerably in their ability to improve survival and decrease abscess formation among survivors and to decrease the number of viable bacteria within experimental abscesses. Conclusions from these studies demonstrate the need for antimicrobials that target both enteric gram-negative and anaerobic (including *B. fragilis*) components of these infections.

In community-acquired peritonitis, the roles of enterococci and *Candida* are controversial. Enterococci are identified in up to 20% of infections, and some recent data identify documentation of enterococcal species as a risk factor for adverse outcome when they are not targeted in therapy. However, there are no data demonstrating enhanced outcomes when enterococcal infection is treated. In general, neither organism needs to be covered empirically unless it is believed to be a predominant pathogen on Gram's stain, associated with positive blood cultures, or noted in pure culture. Vancomycin-resistant enterococci are unlikely to be identified in community-acquired disease. However, both organisms become important considerations following antimicrobial therapy or reoperation for complications.

*Antimicrobials in Secondary Bacterial Peritonitis*
Antibiotics employed in secondary bacterial peritonitis should take into account which pathogens are likely; this is based in part on the initial site of infection. As an example, perforation of a previously healthy stomach is likely to result in either sterile peritonitis or infection associated with low numbers of oropharyngeal flora. Alternatively, peritoneal contamination from the colon will be associated with a complex flora involving enteric bacilli and anaerobes. Numerous antibiotics (when coupled with drainage), administered as monotherapy or in combination, are effective and appropriate for the management of secondary bacterial peritonitis. The author prefers monotherapy when possible, as it is generally easier to manage and may be less expensive. Table 16-2 summarizes some initial treatment regimens. Choice among them requires knowledge of local resistance problems, host factors (allergy, end-organ function), costs, and availability in hospital formularies.

Optimal length of therapy for secondary bacterial peritonitis is unknown. Current data suggest that 5 to 7 days of IV therapy is sufficient for infection associated with recent penetrating trauma or peritonitis in otherwise healthy persons. Complicated peritonitis with residual abscess formation needs longer treatment. Use of oral agents for part of the course may be sufficient in patients with functional gastrointestinal tracts.

*Surgical Management of Secondary Bacterial Peritonitis*
Removal of necrotic tissue, drainage of abscesses, and closure of perforations are major goals of surgery. Penetrating trauma or acute perforation of a viscus requires exploratory laparotomy. Antimicrobials are administered as soon as possible and can often be discontinued by 5 days.

Table 16-2. Antimicrobials useful in
secondary community-acquired bacterial peritonitis

| Antibiotic(s) | Dosage (IV)* |
| --- | --- |
| Ticarcillin-clavulanate | 3.1 g/q6h |
| Cefotetan | 2 g q12h |
| Imipenem/cilastatin | 500 mg q6h |
| Trovafloxacin | 300 mg q24h |
| Piperacillin-tazobactam | 3.375 g q6h |
| Ceftriaxone + metronidazole | 1–2 g q24h + 500 mg q8h |
| Gentamicin + metronidazole** | 5 mg/kg q24h + 500 mg q8h |
| Cefepime + metronidazole | 2 g q12h + 500 q8h |

* Duration of therapy variable, generally 5 to 14 days, use of oral or step-down to oral dependent
on functional gastrointestinal system.
** Regimen popular in parts of Canada, less commonly employed in the United States.

Percutaneous catheter drainage of abscesses should be employed when technically
feasible, but this technique has little value in acute secondary peritonitis. For drainage
of intraabdominal abscesses, success rates in noncomparative studies are more than
85%. Percutaneous drainage should be strongly considered as initial therapy for
patients with approachable intraabdominal abscess and for those who are poor surgical candidates.

### Continuous Ambulatory Peritoneal Dialysis

CAPD-related peritonitis is a significant complicating factor of this procedure and is
noted approximately 1.7 times per patient-year or about every 7 to 10 months. Approximately 60% of patients will have a bout of peritonitis during the first year of CAPD.
Recurrences develop in 20% to 30% of individuals. The relationship between CAPD
peritonitis and mortality is most noted in white, nondiabetic, older patients. Some data
suggest that peritonitis contributes to mortality in about 15% of patients and is most
notable with gram-negative bacilli and fungi. In selected patients on long-term CAPD,
peritonitis does not develop, presuming a role for host defenses or meticulous care. Most
common pathogenetic mechanisms are migration along the dialysis catheter or breaks
in sterile technique during dialysis exchanges. Dialysis fluid inside the peritoneal cavity can support the growth of many pathogens, including most enteric bacilli, *Staphylococcus aureus,* and *P. aeruginosa.* Patients identified as nasal carriers of *S. aureus*
are at higher risk than noncarriers for the development of *S. aureus* peritonitis. Data
also suggest that peritonitis is more likely to develop in patients with enhanced anxiety and decreased quality-of-life scores. The reasons for this are uncertain.

In the context of CAPD, peritonitis can be defined as the presence of turbid dialysate when etiologies other than infection cannot be identified; this condition occurs in
the presence of WBC counts of more than 300/mm³. This definition does not require
the presence of constitutional symptomatology, leukocytosis, abdominal pain, or a
positive Gram's stain or culture. Risk factors include advanced age, use of CAPD
rather than continuous cycling peritoneal dialysis (CCPD), and earlier initiation of
CAPD in the patient's history. The reasons why peritonitis never develops in up to
50% of patients while others have recurrent episodes are uncertain; however, chronic
nasal carriage of *S. aureus* has been identified as a risk factor in some patients with
recurrent infections associated with this organism.

Clinical presentation is generally cloudy peritoneal dialysate. Fever is noted in 33%
of patients, and abdominal pain and tenderness are seen in the majority. Up to one
third of patients will be sick enough to require hospitalization, but therapy is generally rendered in an outpatient setting. It is uncommon for infections to disseminate
beyond the peritoneal cavity.

The bacteriology of peritonitis complicating CAPD is generally monomicrobial. The
presence of polymicrobial infection should prompt an assessment for perforation of a
viscus. *S. aureus* and *Staphylococcus epidermidis* are most commonly implicated and

Table 16-3. Antibiotics for use in peritonitis
complicating continuous ambulatory peritoneal dialysis

| Antibiotic | Route | Dose |
| --- | --- | --- |
| Cefazolin | IP* | 15 mg/kg |
| Ceftazidime | IP | 1 g |
| Cefotaxime | IP | 2 g |
| Aztreonam | IP | 1 g |
| Ciprofloxacin | Oral or IV | 500 mg bid |
| Gentamicin-tobramycin | IP | 0.6 mg/kg |
| Imipenem-cilastatin | IV | 1 g q12h |
| Vancomycin | IP | 15–30 mg/kg q5–7d |
| Metronidazole | Oral or IV | 500 mg tid |

* Intraperitoneal: add dose to one of the daily bags.

are responsible for approximately 50% of infections. Up to 70% of isolates are gram-positive bacteria. *P. aeruginosa* is associated with 5% to 10% of cases but causes significant mortality and morbidity. Miscellaneous organisms, including fungi (mostly *Candida* species) and mycobacteria (not *M. tuberculosis*), and sterile specimens are noted in 10% to 20% of cases. Fungal peritonitis represents 3% to 4% of all cases of peritonitis, is mostly caused by *Candida* species, and is associated with prior use of antibiotics. Removal of catheter, short-term hemodialysis, and catheter replacement at 2 to 8 weeks appears to render satisfactory therapy. Etiology can usually be suspected from Gram's-stained specimens of fluid. This information should be utilized for antibiotic decision making. Culture for aerobic and anaerobic organisms should always be obtained, and special cultures for acid-fast bacilli and fungi should be sought if standard Gram's stain fails to demonstrate bacteria.

The linchpin of management is the administration of appropriate antimicrobials in doses sufficient to exceed the minimum inhibitory concentration for the offending organism at the site of infection for at least part of the dosing interval. Most cases unlikely to be complicated by bacteremia can be managed by intraperitoneal antimicrobials and preservation of the dialysis catheter. *P. aeruginosa* infections are generally managed with two effective agents plus catheter removal.

Table 16-3 summarizes the treatment recommendations for selected antibiotics. Empiric therapy with cefazolin and gentamicin is sensible for patients without positive Gram's stains. Major indications for catheter removal include infection caused by fungi, mycobacteria, *P. aeruginosa*, or *Corynebacteria*. Additional reasons are perforated viscus, relapse of peritonitis, and tunnel infection. Parenteral antimicrobials are initially indicated if bacteremia or sepsis is suspected. Duration of treatment may be 7 to 10 days (gram-positive infection) or 2 to 3 weeks (gram-negative or fungal infection). Amphotericin B in a total dose of up to 500 mg following catheter removal remains the gold standard for susceptible fungal infections.

Prevention of peritonitis in CAPD is difficult and best associated with education and adherence to appropriate techniques. Antibiotic prophylaxis does not work well and is generally not recommended. In patients with *S. aureus* peritonitis, eradication of identified nasal carriage should be attempted with mupirocin. *S. aureus* peritonitis may also be preventable with use of daily mupirocin at the catheter exit site or by use of 600 mg of rifampin for 5 days of every 3 months. (R.B.B.)

### Bibliography
Antillon MR, Runyon BA. Effect of marked peripheral leukocytosis on the leukocyte count in ascites. *Arch Intern Med* 1991;151:509–510.
*This investigation focuses on 29 patients who underwent paracentesis when peripheral leukocyte counts were higher than 20,000/mm³. None had peritonitis as a cause of ascites, and leukocyte counts in ascitic fluid remained low despite the peripheral findings.*
Bhuva M, Ganger D, Jensen D. Spontaneous bacterial peritonitis: an update on evaluation, management, and prevention. *Am J Med* 1994;97;169–175.

*The authors present an excellent overview of spontaneous bacterial peritonitis. Patients with cirrhosis and ascites with fever or abdominal pain should generally undergo paracentesis. Prophylaxis with antibiotics and diuresis may decrease mortality. When possible, drugs without nephotoxic potential should be employed for prophylaxis and treatment.*

Cooper GS, Shlaes DM, Salata RA. Intraabdominal infection: differences in presentation and outcome between younger patients and the elderly. *Clin Infect Dis* 1994; 19:146–148.

*The authors conducted a retrospective study of about 130 eligible patients discharged from a tertiary care center with intraabdominal infections and compared presentation, bacteriology, antibiotic use, and outcomes between younger patients and those over age 65 ("elderly"). Elderly patients had a longer interval until therapy and presented with less obvious symptoms and signs of intraabdominal infection. Bacteriology and use of antibiotics was similar, and mortality rates were not significantly different. However, those over age 65 had prolonged hospitalizations, and normalization of their temperature took longer. Physicians should be aware of the fact that many serious bacterial infections present subtly in the elderly, and a high index of suspicion is warranted.*

Goldie SJ, et al. Fungal peritonitis in a large chronic peritoneal dialysis population: a report of 55 episodes. *Am J Kidney Dis* 1996;28:86–91.

*A retrospective review of records demonstrated that approximately 3% of cases of CAPD-related peritonitis were fungal. Most were caused by* Candida *species. Those with fungal peritonitis had more infections per year and were more likely to have received prior antibiotics. No other risks were identified. Catheter removal and antifungal treatment were mainstays of therapy, and catheter replacement after 2 to 8 weeks of temporary hemodialysis resulted in good salvage.*

Inadomi J, Sonnenberg A. Cost-analysis of prophylactic antibiotics in spontaneous bacterial peritonitis. *Gastroenterology* 1997;113:1289–1294.

*The authors conclude that prophylactic antibiotics are a cost effective strategy for patients with cirrhosis and ascites. Issues addressed include development of PBP, subsequent mortality, and the cost of drugs. Agents primarily assessed were norfloxacin and TMP-SMX. Prophylaxis is cost effective when compared with placebo.*

Jakubowski A, Elwood RK, Enarson DA. Clinical features of abdominal tuberculosis *J. Infect Dis* 1988;158:687–693.

*Eighty-one cases of intraabdominal tuberculosis were reviewed. Most were peritonitis. This was most commonly a disease of women, often not associated with disease elsewhere. More than 80% had positive tuberculin test results. Diagnosis is often difficult, and a long differential diagnosis is considered. Treatment is usually curative.*

Johnson CC, Baldessarre J, Levison ME. Peritonitis: update on pathophysiology, clinical manifestations, and management. *Clin Infect Dis* 1997;24:1035–1047.

*A contemporary review of spontaneous, secondary, and CAPD-associated peritonitis. A good review of issues covered in the title.*

Keane WF, et al. Peritoneal dialysis-related peritonitis treatment recommendations: 1996 update. *Perit Dial Int* 1996;16:557–573.

*The authors provide an exhaustive profile of complications and management strategies of peritoneal dialysis. Antibiotics and dosing regimens are provided, and doses are divided into both continuous and intermittent options. The authors recommend use of a first-generation cephalosporin plus an aminoglycoside as empiric therapy in most instances. They should be praised for recognizing the potential severe problems with vancomycin-resistant enterococci! They also address the general inadvisability of prophylactic antibiotics to prevent peritonitis in this population. An excellent single source of information about the subject.*

McClean KL, Sheehan GJ, Harding GKM. Intraabdominal infection: a review. *Clin Infect Dis* 1994;19:100–116.

*An excellent review of basic pathophysiology, bacteriology, diagnosis, and management of intraabdominal infections. Issues related to imaging are explored, and the authors devote significant space to surgical issues, including type of operation. Controversial issues such as the roles of enterococci and* Candida *species are raised, but no answers are provided. A segment on infections in immunocompromised patients is particularly valuable as an overview of pathogens in difficult hosts.*

Runyon BA, et al. The serum-ascites albumin gradient is superior to the exudate-transudate concept in the differential diagnosis of ascites. *Ann Intern Med* 1992; 117:215–220.
*Although this investigation does not specifically address peritonitis, the article is important because it describes a newer method to evaluate ascites. Assessment of the serum-ascites albumin gradient (high in portal hypertension) may be a better method to manage ascites. Part of the reason for this, the authors claim, is that many cases of bacterial peritonitis may not be associated with "exudative" ascites by classic criteria.*

Silvain C. Can septicemia and ascitic fluid infections in cirrhotic patients be treated by the oral route alone? *Gastroenterol Clin Biol* 1989;13:335–339.
*The investigator utilized oral antimicrobials, primarily quinolones, for the management of primary peritonitis. Outcomes were good.*

Singh N, et al. Trimethoprim-sulfamethoxazole for the prevention of spontaneous bacterial peritonitis in cirrhosis: a randomized trial. *Ann Intern Med* 1995;122:595–598.
*Patients with cirrhosis and ascites, stratified by additional risks, were enrolled in a prospective study to assess whether the use of prophylactic TMP-SMX resulted in fewer cases of PBP. Mean duration of follow-up was 90 days, and PBP or spontaneous bacteremia developed in significantly more patients without antibiotic (27% vs. 3%). Mortality rates were 20% versus 7%. This investigation suggests that antibiotic prophylaxis prevents adverse outcomes in high-risk patients. It should probably be considered a standard of care in this population.*

Wilcox CM, Dismukes WE. Spontaneous bacterial peritonitis. A review of pathogenesis, diagnosis and treatment. *Medicine (Baltimore)* 1987;66:447–456.
*One of the best reviews on all aspects of spontaneous bacterial peritonitis.*

## 17. INFECTIONS OF THE HEPATOBILIARY TRACT

Infections of the hepatobiliary tract hold great potential for mortality and morbidity. Diagnosis may be difficult because of unusual presentations. Patients with advanced HIV and AIDS may present with hepatobiliary disease in which unusual pathogens (many nonbacterial) need to be considered, and for which management may differ significantly from that employed in other cases. Abdominal ultrasonography and computed tomography (CT) have favorably affected both diagnosis and treatment. Invasive radiologic procedures have emerged as an alternative to surgery in many instances.

### Bacteriology of the Biliary Tract

The normal biliary tract is sterile. Approximately 80% of persons with cholelithiasis have biliary tract colonization; pathogenesis is unknown. Common bacteria include *Escherichia coli, Proteus mirabilis, Klebsiella* species, and enterococci and other streptococci. Anaerobes are less common than in other parts of the gastrointestinal tract, although the isolation of *Clostridium perfringens* is well described. *Bacteroides fragilis* may be noted as a colonizer in up to 41% of specimens obtained from elderly persons, but it is rarely pathogenic except in the presence of a stent.

Recent comparative studies demonstrate that the severity of the clinical condition is associated with the intensity of bacterial colonization. Likelihood of biliary colonization is higher when choledochlithiasis is present, and is essentially 100% with acute cholangitis. Age correlates with likely colonization, and in the presence of common duct stones, similar bacteria are recovered from common duct and gallbladder bile.

### Acute Cholecystitis

In the United States, most cases of acute cholecystitis are caused by cystic duct obstruction with subsequent proliferation of colonizing bacteria. Ischemia and tissue necrosis ensue, sometimes resulting in gangrene and perforation. The typical presentation of calculous cholecystitis includes right upper quadrant (RUQ) pain, nausea, and fever. In the elderly, presentation may be subtle, with blunted response to pain and absence of fever. In these situations, the diagnosis must be promptly suspected to avoid perforation, septicemia, and death.

The diagnosis of acute cholecystitis is usually suspected on clinical grounds and should be confirmed radiographically. Ultrasonography of the RUQ is generally considered the procedure of choice and may be able to predict the likelihood of perforation. If this test cannot be obtained for technical reasons, CT provides similar information. Routine blood studies often demonstrate leukocytosis with a left shift, but levels of hepatic enzymes and bilirubin may be normal. Elevation of serum bilirubin above 2 to 3 mg/dL suggests common duct obstruction and possible ascending cholangitis.

Management of acute cholecystitis consists of supportive care, appropriate antimicrobials, and surgery. Although the timing of surgical intervention remains controversial, most authorities recommend prompt cholecystectomy after initial medical stabilization. For patients who are too ill to tolerate major surgery, cholecystostomy may prove lifesaving and may be followed by removal of the gallbladder 4 to 6 weeks later. Patients who fail to stabilize within 24 hours or who demonstrate clinical deterioration should be operated on promptly.

Antimicrobial therapy is guided by the likely causative organisms. Although penetration of antimicrobials into the biliary tract has received attention in the literature, few clinical data confirm the importance of this. Additionally, most agents fail to penetrate the bile in the presence of total biliary tract obstruction. In all cases of acute cholecystitis, high-dose parenteral antimicrobials are initially indicated, as bacteremic disease is not unusual and may be polymicrobial. The regimen should be well tolerated, reasonably safe, and cover most enteric gram-negative bacilli, enterococci, and *C. perfringens*. Coverage for *B. fragilis* is controversial but is reasonable in the elderly. Single agents such as ticarcillin-clavulanate or imipenem-cilastatin are adequate for most cases. Recent investigations employing quinolones as monotherapy (either ofloxacin or ciprofloxacin) have also resulted in satisfactory outcomes. Therapy may be adjusted after the results of cultures become known. Severe sepsis with multiorgan failure or shock, for example, usually indicates a complication (gangrene, perforation) or complete cystic duct impaction.

Acute cholecystitis in the elderly patient is usually associated with higher morbidity and mortality. Up to 40% of the elderly have gangrene, perforation, or empyema at the time of surgical intervention. Fifteen percent have secondary intraabdominal abscesses. The reasons for these age-related differences are not understood. Often, diagnosis is delayed because of more subtle signs of disease. Elderly persons may be afebrile and fail to produce a prompt leukocytosis. Additionally, pain may be poorly localized and vaguely defined. Diagnosis should be suspected in the patient with vague abdominal pain of uncertain origin, and diagnostic studies should be undertaken promptly. Prompt surgical intervention may be necessary in uncertain circumstances.

In 2% to 15% of cases, cholecystitis is acalculous. Severe burns, other critical illnesses, residence within ICUs, and the postoperative state are contributory. Mortality is 30% to 50%, many times higher than that seen in calculous disease. The diagnosis of acalculous cholecystitis is often difficult, in part because of the severity of illness. Many patients cannot be carefully questioned and may be receiving medications that dull response. Fever, leukocytosis, and vague abdominal discomfort may be the sole presentation, and even these may not be simultaneously present. Diagnosis requires a high index of suspicion, and is generally made by RUQ ultrasonography. Laparoscopy can be definitive in selected cases and may obviate the need for formal laparotomy. Alternatively, a recent study employed follow-up sonography 24 hours after a nondiagnostic initial test result. Progressive thickening of the gallbladder wall correlated with acalculous cholecystitis. Therapy usually consists of percutaneous cholecystostomy, which may be curative. Antibiotics are given parenterally and should cover likely enteric flora of an ICU.

Biliary tract candidiasis has been recently reviewed. Approximately 1% of patients undergoing cholecystectomy demonstrate *Candida* as a significant pathogen. Many had uncomplicated cholecystitis. Risk factors include prior use of antimicrobials and corticosteroids. When disease is limited to the gallbladder, cholecystectomy without antifungal therapy is curative in patients who are not neutropenic patients.

*Complications of Acute Cholecystitis*
Gallbladder perforation is seen in 10% to 15% of cases and should be suspected in patients following delays in diagnosis and in men more than 70 years old. Clinical findings include RUQ mass, palpable gallbladder, and peritonitis. Three forms of perforation that occur are (a) free perforation into the peritoneal cavity, (b) rupture with local containment, and (c) rupture into an adjacent viscus. Generalized peritonitis, less common than localized and contained perforation, has the worst prognosis. The clinical presentation is similar to that seen when this disease has other causes, and identification of the gallbladder as the cause of peritonitis is usually made at laparotomy. Perforation with local containment often occurs several days after clinical cholecystitis is evident and usually presents as antimicrobial treatment failure. A palpable mass may become obvious. Rupture into an adjacent viscus, often the stomach, may be at first associated with dramatic clinical improvement. Management of perforation is surgical.

Emphysematous cholecystitis is an uncommon condition diagnosed by the presence of air in either the gallbladder wall or lumen. The clinical presentation is often that of "typical" acute cholecystitis, but with a higher rate of occurrence in male patients and a higher mortality rate (15% vs. 3% to 8%). *C. perfringens* is frequently implicated (45% vs. 10% to 15%). Early surgical intervention is necessary. Empyema of the gallbladder is documented at the time of operation and usually presents in the severely ill patient as RUQ discomfort. At the time of surgery, a pus-filled organ is demonstrated.

## Ascending Cholangitis
Ascending cholangitis results from infection within the common bile duct and is most often caused by an obstructing stone. It may also be noted as an uncommon complication of percutaneous biliary drainage, in the presence of intrahepatic stones, and in cases of AIDS. Fever (92%), chills (65%), and jaundice (67%) are generally observed, whereas RUQ pain (42%) is less commonly noted. Approximately 5% of patients present with septic shock. In the elderly, fever and pain may be subtle. Charcot's intermittent fever is a syndrome of recurrent cholangitis, usually caused by a partially obstructing stone or a series of stones passing through the common duct. In a recent study, it was noted in fewer than 20% of patients with cholangitis.

Laboratory data may demonstrate elevations of both alkaline phosphatase and serum bilirubin. Levels of serum bilirubin above 3 mg/dL are unusual in uncomplicated acute cholecystitis. Leukocytosis is often observed but is nonspecific. Elevation of serum amylase is seen in approximately 40% of cases and does not necessarily imply pancreatitis.

Pathogens include enteric gram-negative bacilli, *Enterococcus faecalis,* and *C. perfringens. B. fragilis* and *Candida albicans* have been rarely noted. Rarely, parasites that include *Ascaris lumbricoides, Clonorchis sinensis,* and *Echinococcus* species have been identified. Ascending cholangitis is the most common cause of polymicrobial bacteremia, and the isolation of multiple pathogens from blood cultures should prompt the clinician to consider the biliary tract as the primary source. Overall, approximately 30% of patients with cholangitis will demonstrate positive blood cultures, and, of these, 25% will be polymicrobial.

Diagnosis can be confirmed by radiographic studies that include ultrasonography and CT. Generally, dilatation of the common duct more than 1.5 cm is noted. Cholangiography, generally by the endoscopic retrograde technique, is indicated in patients requiring urgent biliary decompression and those being prepared for surgery. Antimicrobial therapy is similar to that used for acute cholecystitis. Ticarcillin-clavulanate or imipenem-cilastatin cover most likely pathogens. Recent data demonstrate that parenteral quinolones are also effective. If combinations are to be employed, they should include an agent active against enterococci. Treatment should be continued for 7 to 10 days. Maintenance therapy with low-dose antibiotics has been studied in selected patients with recurrent cholangitis. Quinolones, trimethoprim-sulfamethoxazole, and amoxicillin-clavulanate have been recommended, with suppression continued for 3 to 4 months before reassessment of need. The presence of yeast on Gram's stain (from drainage) as the predominant flora or the heavy growth of *Candida* species on culture merits antifungal therapy. Amphotericin B remains the agent of choice, although newer data suggest a role for IV fluconazole.

Initial stabilization of the patient plus antimicrobials is always indicated. Up to 85% of patients respond favorably to such measures. Urgent drainage is necessary in patients who fail to respond rapidly. For persons who improve, drainage will often be necessary to prevent recurrence. Choice between surgery and endoscopy is dictated by availability and anatomic considerations.

### Biliary Tract Infections in Patients with HIV/AIDS
Recognition of hepatobiliary complications in patients with AIDS dates back to the early 1980s, when patients with biliary tract cryptosporidiosis and obstruction were identified. Although typical bacterial diseases may develop in persons with HIV/AIDS as described above, two syndromes specific to this population are AIDS-related cholangiopathy syndrome and acalculous cholecystitis. However, a recent investigation of patients who underwent cholecystectomy demonstrated that about 25% had cholelithiasis.

Acalculous cholecystitis in this population generally presents with subacute or chronic RUQ pain and fever. Advanced AIDS is usually present. Noninvasive imaging depicts a thickening of the gallbladder wall, but the gallbladder is free of stones. The severity of imaging findings is out of proportion to clinical complaints. Laboratory data demonstrate significant elevations of alkaline phosphatase and absence of leukocytosis. Organisms implicated are usually *Cryptosporidium* or cytomegalovirus (CMV). Other opportunists that have been identified include Microsporidia, *Isospora,* and *Pneumocystis carinii.* Surgery is indicated and alleviates clinical complaints. However, life span is only about 7 months, owing to underlying advanced AIDS.

AIDS-related cholangiopathy is seen in patients with advanced AIDS; the typical CD4 count is less than $100/mm^3$. The presentation is subacute or chronic RUQ pain, but fever, nausea, and vomiting are seen in about 50% of cases. Jaundice is distinctly unusual. Pathogenesis is not known. The diagnosis should be suspected in patients with advanced AIDS and RUQ pain. Ultrasonography or CT are initially indicated and often suggest dilatation of ducts. Endoscopic retrograde cholangiopancreatography is the study of choice. It provides the best definition of ducts and strictures, tissues and materials can be sampled for culture and other microbiologic testing, and therapy with sphincterotomy is possible if indicated. Treatment is geared to relieving obstruction (sphincterotomy or stent placement). Up to 67% of patients will have some measurable relief. Therapy of specific pathogens has been unrewarding. Drugs for CMV have not had a major impact on CMV-related cholangiopathy, and therapy with paromomycin for cryptosporidiosis has also generally been unrewarding.

### Pyogenic Hepatic Abscess
Cases of pyogenic hepatic abscess comprise only 0.016% of hospitalizations. Most cases now occur as a result of common bile duct obstruction. Other causes include (a) perforations of any portion of the gastrointestinal tract, (b) septicemia, (c) blunt trauma, and (d) contiguous spread from adjacent infected foci. However, many cases are cryptogenic. Such abscesses must be differentiated from other space-occupying lesions, including tumors, amebic abscesses, and cysts. Tumors are generally associated with longer prodromes, absence of known risk factors for abscess, and absence of fever and leukocytosis. Amebic abscess should be especially considered in younger patients (often male) with a history of diarrhea who are from underdeveloped countries and in patients with major pleuropulmonary manifestations. Serologic tests for amebiasis are reliable and clinically useful, with results available in only several days. In patients with AIDS, space-occupying lesions may be associated with Kaposi's sarcoma, lymphoma, CMV, and opportunistic fungi and mycobacteria. The opinion of the author is that although in almost 50% of cases a diagnosis is obtained, it is rare to find a treatable etiology.

The clinical presentation of pyogenic hepatic abscess depends on the cause. When it is associated with generalized sepsis, hectic chills and fever may occur along with with RUQ tenderness and hepatomegaly. Localizing findings, however, may be absent. More commonly, hepatic abscess presents as vague RUQ discomfort in the absence of major constitutional complaints. Symptoms may last more than 1 month. Jaundice is unusual except with common duct obstruction. Between 20% and 30% of cases are associated with abnormalities of the right side of the chest, such as atelectasis or elevation of the right hemidiaphragm. Pneumonia may be the first consideration.

Routine hematologic and microbiologic studies are not generally useful except if blood cultures are positive. The most common clue is elevation of serum alkaline phosphatase, which in the proper clinical context suggests infiltrative disease of the liver. The diagnosis can be confirmed by CT or ultrasonography, which usually detects a space-occupying lesion. Results of these procedures are positive in more than 90% of cases, but they may miss lesions smaller than 1 cm in diameter.

Therapy consists of appropriate antimicrobials and drainage. The bacteriology of pyogenic abscess is often polymicrobial and includes enteric gram-negative bacilli, enterococci, and anaerobes (including *B. fragilis*). Septic metastatic complications, often involving the eye or lung, were recently reviewed and found to be associated with *Klebsiella pneumoniae* and underlying diabetes. Liver abscesses complicating bacteremia are often caused by *Streptococcus pyogenes* or *Staphylococcus aureus*.

Antimicrobials should be active against *B. fragilis* and enteric gram-negative bacilli. A potential advantage of clindamycin is its ability to penetrate hepatic tissue in therapeutic levels. No controlled studies have been done comparing various antimicrobial regimens. Therapy should be continued for at least 4 weeks with adequate drainage and for at least 8 weeks if drainage is not performed or is incomplete. Oral therapy has not been well studied. Drainage of all accessible abscesses should now be considered the standard of care. Percutaneous drainage is safe and effective and is generally preferred to surgical intervention when technically feasible. Surgery should be performed to eradicate a feeding focus. (R.B.B.)

## Bibliography

Brandt CP, Priebe PP, Jacobs DG. Value of laparoscopy in trauma ICU patients with suspected acute acalculous cholecystitis. *Surg Endosc* 1994;8:361–364.
*The authors assessed laparoscopic findings in nine patients with suspected acalculous cholecystitis. Diagnosis was essentially 100%. They consider it more accurate than noninvasive studies.*

Csendes A, et al. Simultaneous bacteriologic assessment of bile from gallbladder and common duct in control subjects and patients with gallstones and common duct stones. *Arch Surg* 1996;131:389–394.
*A recent study continues to demonstrate that the normal gallbladder is sterile. The presence of stones increases likelihood of colonization, and in these circumstance gallbladder and common duct bile harbor similar organisms.*

Ducreux M, et al. Diagnosis and prognosis of AIDS-related cholangitis. *AIDS* 1995; 9:875–880.
*Forty-five patients with AIDS-related cholangitis were identified. Several different patterns of disease were demonstrated by endoscopic retrograde cholangiopancreatography, and sphincterotomy was successful in alleviating pain in only about 33%. Survival rates were only 41% (1 year) and 8% (2 years). CMV and* Cryptosporidium *were the most commonly identified organisms.*

Huang CJ, et al. Pyogenic hepatic abscess. Changing trends over 42 years. *Ann Surg* 1996;223:600–607.
*An interesting retrospective study of 223 patients with hepatic abscess seen during a 42-year period. Apparent incidence rose from 13/100,000 hospitalizations (1973) to 20/100,000 hospitalizations (1993). Despite more patients documented with malignancy, mortality decreased substantially, and significantly more patients were treated with percutaneous drainage. This is one of several studies that claim better reduction of mortality with open surgical drainage than with percutaneous approaches.*

Nash JA, Cohen SA. Gallbladder and biliary tract disease in AIDS. *Gastroenterol Clin North Am* 1997;26:323–335.
*The authors review the principles of diagnosis and treatment of biliary tract syndromes unique to AIDS. They stress acalculous cholecystitis and cholangiopathy syndromes, and point out that most cases occur in patients with advanced AIDS, who have limited life spans. Drainage procedures are often indicated, but therapy targeted at offending opportunists is generally unrewarding.*

Sung JJ, et al. Intravenous ciprofloxacin as treatment for patients with acute suppurative cholangitis: a randomized controlled clinical trial. *J Antimicrob Chemother* 1995;35:855–864.

*One of several investigations published during the past several years that indicate the efficacy of fluoroquinolnes as monotherapy for acute bacterial cholangitis. In this study, ciprofloxacin was compared with ceftazidime, ampicillin, and metronidazole. Mortality was less than 5% in each group, and ciprofloxacin as monotherapy was considered equivalent to triple antibiotics.*

van dan Hazel SJ, et al. Role of antibiotics in the treatment and prevention of acute and recurrent cholangitis. *Clin Infect Dis* 1994;19:279–286.

*An excellent review of antibiotic choices and indications for the management of cholangitis. Of particular interest is the information regarding suppressive antibiotics for patients with recurrent disease.*

# V. URINARY TRACT

# 18. URINARY TRACT INFECTIONS: BASIC PRINCIPLES OF THERAPY

Many controversies about the treatment of urinary tract infections remain unresolved. Bacteriuria may be asymptomatic and not require antimicrobial therapy or may be associated with upper or lower tract infection. Although the treatment of cystitis differs significantly from that of pyelonephritis, the physician may not know with certainty where the infection is localized. Despite these controversies and uncertainties, there are several well-documented guidelines for the treatment of urinary tract infection:

1. Patients with upper tract symptoms require 10 days to 2 weeks of antimicrobial therapy.

2. Patients with high fever, chills, and elevated WBC counts require initial IV antimicrobial therapy, guided by urine Gram's stain.

3. Patients with community-acquired upper urinary tract infection who have gram-negative bacilli on urine Gram's stain can be treated with a wide range of antimicrobial agents. Agents such as third-generation cephalosporins, aztreonam, trimethoprim-sulfamethoxazole, and ureidopenicillins are widely recommended. Ampicillin and sulfonamides are not used in this setting because of the increasing resistance of *Escherichia coli*.

4. In patients with hospital-acquired pyelonephritis, a history of recurrent infection, or prior infection with a resistant organism, initial antimicrobial therapy must have an antipseudomonal spectrum. Depending on the institution's antimicrobial resistance profile, agents such as ceftazidime, tobramycin or amikacin, imipenem, ticarcillin-clavulanic acid, or ciprofloxacin may be initiated. When results of antimicrobial susceptibility tests become available, therapy can be revised. If aminoglycoside therapy was begun in an elderly patient or a patient with renal insufficiency, a safer antimicrobial should be chosen once susceptibility results define all options.

5. Bacteria should be cleared from the urine within 24 to 48 hours of therapy. If bacteriuria persists, antimicrobial therapy should be changed based on susceptibility results.

6. Patients who have persistent fever or toxicity despite appropriate antimicrobial therapy should be investigated for perinephric or renal cortical abscess.

7. In patients with uncomplicated upper tract infection, antimicrobial therapy can be switched from IV to oral after a few days of defervescence. The quinolones, particularly ciprofloxacin, have been used extensively in this setting. Selected patients can be treated with oral therapy initially, provided they are not toxic, immunosuppressed, pregnant, or vomiting.

8. Many studies have found that short-course therapy for lower urinary tract infection (3 days or even one dose) is as effective as a 7- to 14-day course. These studies have generally been performed in young women with symptoms of cystitis. Many different oral regimens have been used, including trimethoprim-sulfamethoxazole, norfloxacin, ciprofloxacin, cephalexin, and amoxicillin-clavulanate (Augmentin). Recent reviews have warned that single-drug therapy for cystitis is somewhat less effective than 3-day regimens. Men with cystitis generally receive at least 7 days of antibiotic therapy because of concern for complicating factors, particularly prostatitis.

9. Cystitis in elderly women has not been well studied. Long-term eradication of bacteriuria is less likely to be seen in elderly women, particularly if their functional status is poor. Elderly women with typical symptoms of cystitis should probably be treated for 3 days with a quinolone or trimethoprim-sulfamethoxazole. Relapse after 3 days should be considered evidence for upper tract disease, and treatment guidelines, as previously described, should be followed.

10. Prospective studies have confirmed the value of *in vitro* antimicrobial susceptibility testing. The initial disappearance of bacteriuria is closely correlated with the susceptibility of the microorganism to the concentration of the antimicrobial agent achieved in the urine.

11. The relative importance of antimicrobial concentrations obtained in the serum and urine in the treatment of urinary tract infections remains controversial. When

concomitant bacteremia occurs, blood levels achieve critical importance, and parenteral administration of drugs is required. Urinary tract infections can be cured with drugs that achieve therapeutic concentrations only in the urine. The majority sentiment is that cure of urinary tract infections depends on antimicrobial concentrations in the urine rather than in the serum.

12. Many infectious disease experts prefer to administer a bactericidal drug for urinary tract infections, but there is no documentation that a bactericidal compound has greater efficacy than a bacteriostatic drug. There is no evidence that unselected combinations of multiple antimicrobials given simultaneously produce a higher cure rate than does an effective member of the combination given singly.

13. Drug efficacy can be enhanced by awareness of the fact that the antibacterial activity of many chemotherapeutic agents used in the treatment of urinary tract infections is affected by changes in urinary pH.

   • Alkalinization of urine increases the activity of the aminoglycosides (streptomycin, kanamycin, gentamicin, tobramycin, amikacin), benzylpenicillin, and erythromycin.

   • Acidification of the urine increases the activity of the tetracyclines, nitrofurantoin, and methenamine mandelate.

Controlled studies have demonstrated that efficacy will be enhanced by appropriate modification of urinary pH. (S.L.B.)

### Bibliography

Dembry LM, Andriole VT. Renal and perirenal abscesses. *Infect Dis Clin North Am* 1997;11:663.
   *Renal carbuncles and corticomedullary abscesses usually resolve after 1 week of antibiotic therapy. The patient should then be evaluated by an appropriate imaging technique.*

Fihn SD, et al. Trimethoprim-sulfamethoxazole for acute dysuria in women: a single-dose or 10-day course. A double-blind, randomized trial treatment. *Ann Intern Med* 1985;108:350.
   *A history of urinary tract infection, use of spermicide, and the presence of more than $10^5$ bacteria correlate with failure of the single-treatment regimen.*

File TM Jr, Tan JS. Urinary tract infections in the elderly. *Geriatrics* 1989;44 (Suppl A):15.
   *Describes different approaches to managing urinary tract infection in the elderly.*

Gleckman R, et al. Therapy of symptomatic pyelonephritis in women. *J Urol* 1985; 133:176.
   *Reports that a 10-day course of therapy is adequate for acute pyelonephritis in elderly women.*

Hooton TM, Stamm WE. Diagnosis and treatment of uncomplicated urinary tract infection. *Infect Dis Clin North Am* 1997;11:551.
   *Detailed literature review of treatment for cystitis and uncomplicated pyelonephritis in both men and women.*

Johnson JR, Stamm WE. Diagnosis and treatment of acute urinary tract infections. *Infect Dis Clin North Am* 1987;1:773.
   *Recommends antimicrobial therapy based on changing susceptibility patterns of gram-negative bacilli.*

Naber KG. Use of quinolones in urinary tract infections and prostatitis. *Rev Infect Dis* 1989;11 (Suppl 5):S1321–S1337.
   *Reviews the role of quinolones in complicated and uncomplicated urinary tract infections.*

Norby SR. Short-term treatment of uncomplicated lower urinary tract infections in women. *Rev Infect Dis* 1990;12:458.
   *Reviews of large numbers of patients indicate that short-course therapy for cystitis is not as effective as traditional regimens.*

Philbrick JT, Bracikowski JP. Single-dose antibiotic treatment for uncomplicated urinary tract infections. Less for less? *Arch Intern Med* 1985;145:1672.
   *Single-dose therapy is not recommended for uncomplicated urinary tract infection.*

Raz R, et al. Comparison of single-dose administration and 3-day course of amoxicillin with clavulanic acid for treatment of uncomplicated urinary tract infection in women. *Antimicrob Agents Chemother* 1991;35:1688.
*A 3-day regimen is better than single-dose therapy only in the population with recurrent urinary tract infection.*

Ronald AR, et al. Complicated urinary tract infection. *Infect Dis Clin North Am* 1997;11:583.
*Urinary tract infections may be complicated by structural abnormalities, metabolic abnormalities, immunologic deficiencies, or unusual organisms. Complicated infections usually require longer periods of therapy, although better data are needed to make definitive recommendations.*

Sobel JD, Kaye D. Urinary tract infections. In: Mandell GL, Douglas RG Jr, Bennett JE, eds. *Principles and practice of infectious disease*, 3rd ed. New York: Churchill Livingstone, 1990.
*Expert discussion includes flow diagram of management decisions.*

Stamey TA. Recurrent urinary tract infections in female patients: an overview of management and treatment. *Rev Infect Dis* 1987;9 (Suppl 2):S195.
*Single-dose therapy is not effective in all patients with lower urinary tract infection; a 3-day course gives better overall results.*

Stamm WE, McKevitt M, Counts GW. Acute renal infection in women: treatment with trimethoprim-sulfamethoxazole or ampicillin for 2 or 6 weeks. A randomized trial. *Ann Intern Med* 1987;106:341.
*Supports 2-week course of antimicrobial therapy for uncomplicated pyelonephritis.*

Trienekens TA, et al. Different lengths of treatment with co-trimoxazole for acute uncomplicated urinary tract infections in women. *Br Med J* 1989;299:1319.
*Three days of therapy for cystitis was as effective as 7 days.*

Yoshikawa TT, Nicolle LE, Norman DC. Management of complicated urinary infection in older patients. *J Am Geriatr Soc* 1996;44:1235.
*Describes treatment for recurrent urinary tract infection and catheter-related bacteriuria, including the special considerations in the elderly.*

## 19. CYSTITIS VERSUS PYELONEPHRITIS: LOCALIZING URINARY TRACT INFECTIONS

Antimicrobial therapy will vary depending on whether a urinary tract infection involves the kidney or is confined to the bladder. Hence, the clinician must localize the site of infection as reliably as possible. Many clinical clues are helpful in distinguishing pyelonephritis from cystitis, although none is completely reliable. The symptoms of infection confined to the bladder are dysuria, urgency, and frequency. Symptoms of fever, nausea, rigors, and back pain suggest upper urinary tract infection. On physical examination, suprapubic tenderness occurs in cystitis; costovertebral angle tenderness may be present in pyelonephritis. The peripheral WBC count is normal in bladder infection but is usually elevated in renal infection. In the elderly patient with pyelonephritis, fever and leukocytosis are often absent. Pyuria is almost always present in both upper and lower tract infection. WBC casts occur only in pyelonephritis.

A variety of invasive and noninvasive methods have been employed to distinguish cystitis from pyelonephritis. Two invasive methods, the Stamey test and the Fairley test, are among the most reliable. The Stamey test employs a ureteral catheter to carry out quantitative urine cultures of the bladder. Cultures can be taken from both ureters, and renal infection can be determined to be unilateral or bilateral. The test can even be modified so that percutaneous puncture of the renal pelvis can be performed. The test carries some risk in that patients are instrumented during active infection without antimicrobial therapy. False-positive test results can occur as a consequence of vesicoureteral reflux, especially in children. The Fairley bladder washout test also uses quantitative cultures to localize infection. An indwelling Foley catheter is inserted. Saline solution and an antimicrobial agent are instilled into the bladder. The catheter is clamped for 45 minutes and then rinsed with saline solution periodically in 100-mL samples. The catheter is again clamped and samples are taken at 10, 20, 30, and 60 minutes. In pyelonephritis, infected urine travels from the kidney to the bladder, and a 10% rise in colony count will occur as additional samples are obtained. In cystitis, colony counts remain relatively low because the bladder bacteria have been inhibited by the antimicrobial bladder rinse. This test is very sensitive but is not popular because it requires placing a Foley catheter in an already infected urinary tract.

In 1974, a direct immunofluorescence method for the detection of antibody-coated bacteria (ACB) was reported to differentiate kidney from bladder infection. The test, relatively simple and noninvasive, was based on the premise that bacteria invading kidney parenchyma will stimulate production of specific antibody. This antibody will be present on the bacterial surface and can be detected by a fluorescent antibody against human antibody proteins. Initial studies were very promising, but experience with this test over time uncovered many theoretical and technical problems. The definition of a positive test result has varied among investigators. For example, the percentage of fluorescing organisms for a test result to be considered positive has varied from 1% to 25%. The concentration of the urine evaluated will affect the sensitivity of the test. Cocci can be difficult to distinguish from artifact.

It appears that early in the course of pyelonephritis, the ACB test result may be negative. A direct correlation between a positive ACB test result and duration of upper tract symptoms has been reported in one study. In addition, certain mucoid *Pseudomonas* organisms produce a false-negative test result because they do not bind to specific antibody. An ACB test result can be positive in patients with lower urinary tract infection. Urine can be contaminated with vaginal bacteria that are antibody-coated. Patients with prostatitis or hemorrhagic cystitis are often ACB-positive. Patients with proteinuria, ileal conduit, and bladder tumors also can have false-positive test results.

Excretion of $\beta_2$-microglobulin has also been used as a test for distinguishing upper from lower urinary tract infection. This protein is synthesized by nucleated cells and secreted in serum and other body fluids at a constant daily rate. It passes through glomerular membrane but is almost completely reabsorbed in proximal tubules. When tubular damage is present, as in upper urinary tract infection, urine excretion of $\beta_2$-microglobulin increases. One study showed essentially no overlap in levels of urinary $\beta_2$-microglobulin in 24-hour collection in cystitis versus pyelonephritis. Among patients who have both lower urinary tract infection and tubular renal disease, false-positive tests will certainly occur.

A similar type of test in theory is the urinary lactate dehydrogenase assay. Large quantities of lactate dehydrogenase 4 and 5 are present in the renal medulla and can be detected in urine when the medulla is damaged by pyelonephritis. Considerably more overlap in values has been reported for this test than for urinary microglobulin. A $\beta$-glucuronidase assay is the least discriminating urinary enzyme measurement.

An elevated level of C-reactive protein commonly accompanies acute pyelonephritis. It is rarely elevated in cystitis. However, the test is nonspecific and elevated levels are detectable in many other types of infection.

Maximal urinary concentrating ability has long been considered a useful adjunct in the assessment of urinary tract infection, as upper tract infection can cause loss of concentrating ability. Intrarenal deamino–D–arginine vasopressin has been studied to assess concentrating ability and localize infection in children.

Radiologic methods are rarely used to localize acute urinary tract infection in the United States. Intravenous urograms are used to define structural abnormalities that predispose patients to this infection and to rule out complications such as perinephric abscess. Although signs such as poor concentration of dye and delayed calyceal appearance can suggest upper tract infection, most investigators find the IV pyelogram insensitive and nonspecific for this purpose. Radioisotopic imaging shows some promise in distinguishing upper and lower disease. Schardijn et al. (1984) noted uptake of gallium 67 in all patients with acute pyelonephritis and no uptake in those with lower tract infection. Contrast-enhanced helical computed tomography has also been used in the diagnosis of upper urinary tract infection. The speed of helical scanning allows for better tissue contrast. It has been successful in identifying perinephric fluid collections and small stones and is more sensitive in identifying parenchymal abnormalities.

A practical therapeutic test is highly recommended by most investigators in this field. The cultures of patients with cystitis who are given a short course of oral antimicrobials quickly become negative. Those whose cultures remain positive can then be evaluated further for upper tract infection and treated with more aggressive antimicrobial regimens. (S.L.B.)

### Bibliography

Clark H, Ronald AR, Turck M. Serum antibody response in renal versus bladder bacteriuria. *J Infect Dis* 1971;123:539.
*Determination of hemagglutinating antibody activity is of only limited use in predicting the site of infection in individual patients with bacteriuria.*

Eykyn S, et al. The localization of urinary tract infection by ureteric catheterization. *Invest Urol* 1972;9:271.
*Early study showing that ureteral catheterization will yield infected urine in patients with upper tract infection.*

Fairley KF, et al. Simple test to determine the site of urinary tract infection. *Lancet* 1967;2:427.
*Initial description of the antimicrobial bladder washout method for localizing infection.*

Hooton TM, et al. Localization of urinary tract infection in patients with spinal cord injury. *J Infect Dis* 1984;150:85.
*Investigators localized site of urinary tract infection in asymptomatic bacteriuria patients with spinal cord injury. Study compares bladder washout, ACB, and urinary leukocyte count.*

Hulter HN, et al. Localization of catheter-induced urinary tract infections. Interpretation of bladder washout and ACB tests. *Nephron* 1984;38:48.
*ACB test may not be of value in chronically catheterized patients.*

Kaplan DM, Rosenfield RT, Smith RC. Advances in the imaging of renal infection. Helical CT and modern coordinated imaging. *Infect Dis Clin North Am* 1997;11:681.
*Describes newer imaging techniques in the diagnosis of pyelonephritis, particularly the value of helical computed tomography.*

Komaroff AL. Urinalysis and urine culture in women with dysuria. *Ann Intern Med* 1986;104:212.
*Describes value of urine analysis in assessing type of infection.*

Menon EB, Tan ES. Pyuria: index of infection in patients with spinal cord injuries. *Br J Urol* 1992;69:144.
*Patients with a WBC count of more than 100 per high-power field are more likely to have morbidity from urinary tract infection.*

Montplaisier S, et al. Limitations of the direct immunofluorescence test for antibody-coated bacteria in determining the site of urinary tract infections in children. *Can Med Assoc J* 1981;125:993.
*The ACB test is unreliable in localizing urinary tract infection in children.*

Pappas PG. Laboratory in the diagnosis and management of urinary tract infections. *Med Clin North Am* 1991;75:313.
*A good update on methods to localize urinary tract infection, particularly noninvasive methods, such as the ACB test and $\beta_2$-microglobulin.*

Poirier KP, Jackson GG. Characteristics of leucocytes in urine sediment in pyelonephritis. *Am J Med* 1957;23:579.
*An attempt at a histologic correlation of renal biopsy findings and the detection of glitter cells in the urine by the technique of Sternheimer and Malbin.*

Pollock HM. Laboratory techniques for detection of urinary tract infection and assessment of value. *Am J Med* 1983;75:79.
*Describes laboratory tests used to define urinary tract infection, particularly with respect to specimen collection and localization to upper or lower tract.*

Ronald AR, Boutros P, Mourtada H. Bacteriuria localization and response to single-dose therapy in women. *JAMA* 1976;235:1854.
*Uses single-dose therapy to differentiate upper and lower tract infection.*

Ronald AR, Cutler RE, Turck M. Effect of bacteriuria on renal concentrating mechanisms. *Ann Intern Med* 1969;70:123.
*Provides some evidence that upper tract infection is more likely to cause defect in renal concentrating ability.*

Rumans LW, Vosti KL. The relationship of antibody-coated bacteria to clinical syndromes. As found in unselected populations with bacteriuria. *Arch Intern Med* 1978;138:1077.
*Describes limitations of ACB test in an unselected population with bacteriuria.*

Sanford JP. Urinary tract symptoms and infections. *Annu Rev Med* 1975;26:485.
*Shows that clinical symptoms are often unreliable in distinguishing upper from lower tract infection.*

Schardijn G, Statius van Eps LW, Swaak AJG. Urinary $\beta_2$-microglobulin in upper and lower urinary tract infections. *Lancet* 1979;1:805.
*Urinary microglobulin 24-hour excretion was elevated in all pyelonephritis patients and normal in all patients with lower urinary tract infection.*

Schardijn GH, et al. Comparison of reliability of tests to distinguish upper from lower urinary tract infection. *Br Med J* 1984;289:284.
*Reports excellent results with both $\beta_2$-microglobulin and scintiphotography with gallium 67 in localizing urinary tract infection.*

Seng OB, Kincaid-Smith P. Urine concentration after pitressin administration in upper and lower urinary tract infection. *Med J Aust* 1969;1:982.
*One third of patients with a renal source of infection had a concentrating defect; no patients with bladder infection had a comparable concentrating defect.*

Sheldon CA, Gonzalez R. Differentiation of upper and lower urinary tract infections: how and when? *Med Clin North Am* 1984;68:321.
*Review article on methods to differentiate upper and lower tract infection, including symptomatology, biochemical tests, and radiology.*

Stamm WE. Measurement of pyuria and its relation to bacteriuria. *Am J Med* 1983; 75:53.
*Only 4% to 5% of cases of pyelonephritis do not have pyuria.*

Thomas VL, Forland M, Shelkov A. Antibody-coated bacteria in urinary tract infection. *Kidney Int* 1975;8:520.
*Shows that chronic prostatitis will give a positive ACB test result.*

Thomas V, Shelokov A, Forland M. Antibody-coated bacteria in the urine and the site of urinary tract infection. *N Engl J Med* 1974;290:588.
*Early study suggested that ACB test could distinguish upper from lower urinary tract infection. Later studies showed problems with this test.*

Turck M. Localization of the site of recurrent urinary tract infection in women. *Urol Clin North Am* 1975;2:433.
*A review of the correlation between the indirect techniques of localization and ureteral catheterization in a homogeneous population of women with urinary tract infections but without structural abnormalities.*

Turck M, Ronald AR, Petersdorf RG. Relapse and reinfection in chronic bacteriuria. The correlation between site of infection and pattern of recurrence in chronic bacteriuria. *N Engl J Med* 1968;278:422.
*In women, relapse after antimicrobial therapy suggests upper tract infection.*

## 20. ASYMPTOMATIC BACTERIURIA

How does one approach a patient who has significant bacteriuria but is asymptomatic? Significant bacteriuria is defined as more than $10^5$ bacteria per milliliter of urine obtained by sterile technique on consecutive samples. Patients with significant bacteriuria who have urinary tract symptoms require antimicrobial therapy.

In some patients with asymptomatic bacteriuria, including pregnant women and patients with obstructive uropathy, treatment is recommended. Elderly men and women have a higher incidence of bacteriuria than younger adults, for the following reasons: (a) prostatic hypertrophy in men, (b) loss of bactericidal prostatic secretions in men, (c) perineal soiling in women, (d) bladder dysfunction and genitourinary instrumentation, and (e) loss of hormone-dependent protection against introital colonization in postmenopausal women. The incidence of bacteriuria increases with the degree of debility and institutionalization, from 2% in some ambulatory elderly to 59% in some hospitalized patients.

Because of the high incidence in this setting, the role of antimicrobial therapy has become an area of interest and controversy. In at least two studies, elderly nursing home patients with asymptomatic bacteriuria died earlier than those with sterile urine. Other studies have found no correlation of bacteriuria with longevity. The concern that chronic bacteriuria will cause chronic pyelonephritis is not supported by longitudinal studies. Patients with chronic pyelonephritis have underlying uropathy, hypertension, or diabetes mellitus, but not bacteriuria alone. Progressive abnormalities do not develop on IV pyelogram in patients with asymptomatic bacteriuria. Randomized, controlled trials of antimicrobial therapy for asymptomatic bacteriuria in elderly men and women could demonstrate no effect on mortality. Prospective, randomized studies of therapy for asymptomatic bacteriuria have not benefited elderly men or women, whether bedridden or ambulatory. Recent studies, however, have shown that in patients with asymptomatic bacteriuria studied by a bladder washout technique, localization of bacteria to the kidney is commonly found. Patients with asymptomatic bacteriuria treated with antimicrobials do not maintain urine sterility. Such therapy is associated with side effects, cost, and the development of resistant organisms. Hence, antimicrobials are generally not recommended for asymptomatic bacteriuria in the elderly.

There is no evidence to support the treatment of bacteriuria based on the symptom of foul-smelling urine. The unpleasant odor of urine may be caused by polyamine production of bacteria, but urine may be foul-smelling for other reasons.

Asymptomatic bacteriuria is not in itself an indication for anatomic assessment of the urinary tract. Patients with asymptomatic bacteriuria and obstructive uropathy, as well as patients with asymptomatic bacteriuria, should receive antimicrobial therapy before undergoing genitourinary instrumentation.

In the elderly patient with bacteriuria whose general condition has acutely deteriorated, the term asymptomatic bacteriuria loses its usefulness. Urinary tract infection can present in a more subtle manner in the elderly, and patients with urosepsis may remain afebrile or present only with mental status changes. A patient with a history of bacteriuria who becomes septic will often need to be treated for urosepsis if no definite focus of infection can be found.

Patients who require external condom catheters have a bacteriuria rate of as high as 87%. In patients with long-term Foley catheters, bacteriuria is inevitable.

The pregnant woman with asymptomatic bacteriuria represents a special situation in which benefits of treatment outweigh risks. Reflux and resulting pyelonephritis occur in this group. Preterm delivery and low birth weight appear to be *bona fide* associations with asymptomatic bacteriuria.

The consequences of asymptomatic bacteriuria in patients with diabetes mellitus are not so well defined. The rates of asymptomatic bacteriuria are threefold higher in diabetic women than in nondiabetic women. However, rates for diabetic versus nondiabetic men are similar. In diabetic patients, a 2-week course of antimicrobials is equivalent to a 6-week course for initial eradication of bacteriuria. Reinfection often occurs. The overall benefits of treatment remain unproven.

Screening children for asymptomatic bacteriuria is widely recommended in the hope of preventing pyelonephritis. However, such detection has not been proved to prevent pyelonephritis or renal scarring and is now controversial. (S.L.B.)

**Bibliography**
Abrutyn E, et al. Does asymptomatic bacteriuria predict mortality and does antimicrobial treatment reduce mortality in elderly, ambulatory women? *Ann Intern Med* 1994;120:827.
*No beneficial outcome in the treated group was noted.*

Baldassarre JS, Kaye D. Special problems of urinary tract infection in the elderly. *Med Clin North Am* 1991;75:375.
*Describes rationale for conservative management of asymptomatic bacteriuria.*

Bendall MJ. A review of urinary tract infection in the elderly. *J. Antimicrob Chemother* 1984;13 (Suppl B):69.
*Excellent review of the international literature, particularly with respect to patterns of bacteriuria over time.*

Boscia JA, et al. Epidemiology of bacteriuria in an elderly ambulatory population. *Am J Med* 1986;80:208.
*Different patterns of bacteriuria occur in the elderly. Bacteriuria may be persistent or episodic.*

Dontas AS, et al. Bacteriuria and survival in old age. *N Engl J Med* 1981;304:939.
*In a Greek nursing home, survival is shortened by the presence of asymptomatic bacteriuria.*

Kemper KJ, Avner ED. The case against screening urinalyses for asymptomatic bacteriuria in children. *Am J Dis Child* 1992;146:343.
*Screening children for asymptomatic bacteriuria is considered costly and ineffective in this review.*

Mims AD, et al. Clinically inapparent (asymptomatic) bacteriuria in ambulatory elderly men: epidemiological, clinical and microbiological findings. *J Am Geriatr Soc* 1990;38:1209.
*Of 238 ambulatory elderly men, 29 had asymptomatic bacteriuria. Patients were followed from 1 to 4.5 years. Gram-positive organisms were commonly isolated.*

Mittendorf R, Williams MA, Kass EH. Prevention of preterm delivery and low birth weight associated with asymptomatic bacteriuria. *Clin Infect Dis* 1992;14:927.
*Meta-analysis is used to confirm association of bacteriuria in pregnant women with preterm delivery and low birth weight infants.*

Nicolle LE. Consequences of asymptomatic bacteriuria in the elderly. *Int J Antimicrob Agents* 1994;4:107.
*Foul odor of urine is not an indication for the treatment of bacteriuria.*

Nicolle LE. Asymptomatic bacteriuria in the elderly. *Infect Dis Clin North Am* 1997; 11:647.
*Recent review summarizes outcome data from five of the more recent randomized studies of treatment of asymptomatic bacteriuria. Again, no differences are noted in a comparison of the treatment and nontreatment groups.*

Nicolle LE, Mayhew WJ, Bryan L. Prospective randomized comparison of therapy and no therapy for asymptomatic bacteriuria in institutionalized elderly women. *Am J Med* 1987;83:27.
*A randomized trial of antimicrobial therapy in elderly women with asymptomatic bacteriuria. Despite a lowered prevalence of bacteriuria, no difference in genitourinary morbidity or mortality was found. Antimicrobial therapy was associated with recurrent infection, adverse drug effects, and increasingly resistant organisms.*

Nicolle LE, et al. The association of bacteriuria with resident characteristics and survival in elderly institutionalized men. *Ann Intern Med* 1987;106:682.
*No difference was found in the survival of bacteriuric versus nonbacteriuric elderly men.*

Nicolle LE, et al. Localization of urinary tract infection in elderly, institutionalized women with asymptomatic bacteriuria. *J Infect Dis* 1988;157:65.
*By means of bladder washout technique, it was found that 67% of women with asymptomatic bacteriuria had upper tract infection.*

Ouslander JG, Greengold B, Chen S. External catheter use and urinary tract infections among incontinent male nursing home patients. *J Am Geriatr Soc* 1987;35:1063.
*A high incidence of bacteriuria is reported in patients with external condom catheters.*

Pels RJ, et al. Dipstick urinalysis screening of asymptomatic adults for urinary tract disorders. II. Bacteriuria. *JAMA* 1989;262:1221.
*Recommends that urine culture alone be used to screen pregnant women for bacteriuria. Dipstick screening may be adequate with diabetic patients.*

Ronald AR, Pattullo ALS. The natural history of urinary infection in adults. *Med Clin North Am* 1991;75:299.
*Reviews definitions and data on asymptomatic bacteriuria and renal function.*

U.S. Preventive Services Task Force. Screening for asymptomatic bacteriuria, hematuria and proteinuria. *Am Fam Physician* 1990;42:389.
*Recommends leukocyte esterase and nitrate tests for bacteriuria screening in pregnant women, diabetic patients, and perhaps schoolchildren.*

Zhanel GG, Harding GK, Guay DR. Asymptomatic bacteriuria. Which patients should be treated? *Arch Intern Med* 1990;150:1389.
*An excellent review. The authors recommend that neonates, preschool children, pregnant women, and nonelderly men be treated for asymptomatic bacteriuria.*

Zhanel GG, Harding GK, Nicolle LE. Asymptomatic bacteriuria in patients with diabetes mellitus. *Rev Infect Dis* 1992;13:150.
*Excellent review of the implications of bacteriuria in diabetic patients. A 2-week course of antimicrobials is effective in initial eradication.*

## 21. THE SIGNIFICANCE OF PYURIA

Pyuria is an important laboratory parameter in two different settings:

1. It is extremely important in the assessment of bacterial infection of the urinary tract because it is present in almost all such infections, and its absence must suggest another diagnosis.

2. It is present as a nonspecific reaction to inflammation of the urinary tract. The differential diagnosis for sterile pyuria is therefore a broad one.

Pyuria is often arbitrarily defined as the presence of more than 10 leukocytes per high-power microscopic field from a centrifuged specimen. This method clearly represents only a crude quantitative assessment for several reasons: (a) Initial urine volumes are variable, (b) centrifugation is not standardized with respect to time or speed, (c) the amount of urine placed on a slide is variable, and (d) with no grid for reference, observer bias occurs regarding the area in which cells are to be counted. Several methods for quantifying pyuria are more accurate and useful in clinical studies, though impractical for office evaluation. Measurement of pyuria as the leukocyte excretion rate has been used as a more accurate quantitative method. Hourly rates of leukocyte excretion above 400,000 correlate with symptomatic urinary tract infection. By means of hemocytometer measurement of pyuria, a leukocyte count of more than $10/mm^3$ has been correlated with more than $10^5$ bacteria per colony-forming unit.

More recently, the use of rapid methods to determine pyuria has become widespread. Measurement of leukocyte esterase, an enzyme in neutrophil granules, can be determined within 1 to 2 minutes by using an enzyme-impregnated dipstick. This measurement correlates well with significant pyuria defined as more than 10 WBCs per cubic millimeter of urine. In one study, the test had a 50% positive predictive value for bacterial infection but a negative predictive value of 92%.

Stamm (1983) concluded that accurate estimation of pyuria is important for the following reasons: (a) A leukocyte count of $10/mm^3$ or more occurs in fewer than 1% of asymptomatic, nonbacteriuric patients but in more than 96% of symptomatic patients with significant bacteriuria; (b) most symptomatic women with pyuria but without significant bacteriuria do have urinary tract infection, either with uropathogens at a level below $10^5/mL$ or with *Chlamydia trachomatis;* (c) patients with catheter-associated bacteriuria and pyuria are more likely to have true infection. Several studies in spinal cord-injured patients with indwelling catheters have confirmed that pyuria is a risk factor for increased morbidity secondary to untreated urinary tract infection.

Ouslander et al. (1996) recently studied pyuria among incontinent but otherwise asymptomatic nursing home residents. Pyuria was defined as more than 10 WBCs per high-power field. Forty-five percent of the patients studied had pyuria and 43% had bacteriuria. Of the patients with pyuria, only 56% had bacteriuria. Thirty-one percent of bacteriuric patients did not have pyuria. In the patient population studied, pyuria was common regardless of the presence or absence of bacteriuria.

Any inflammatory reaction in the urinary system can result in sterile pyuria of more than 10 WBCs per cubic millimeter of urine or more than 10 WBCs per high-power microscopic field. (The term sterile pyuria has become a common misnomer; it is used to describe pyuria associated with tuberculosis and other infectious processes in which urine cultures for bacteria are negative.) The differential diagnosis for sterile pyuria includes diseases such as perinephric abscess, urethral syndrome, and chronic prostatitis. Fever in association with sterile pyuria must suggest the possibility of renal tuberculosis.

Fungi such as *Cryptococcus neoformans* and *Coccidioides immitis* may also cause pyuria and renal infection. Sterile pyuria can occur in chronic prostatitis in that bladder urine will usually contain fewer than $10^5$ bacteria per milliliter of urine. Prostatic secretions will have high numbers of the etiologic agent. Renal papillary necrosis should be suspected in patients with sterile pyuria who have diabetes or sickle cell disease, or who are chronic alcoholics. Urethral inflammation may also cause pyuria. Genital herpes can cause dysuria and pyuria. Infection with *C. trachomatis* causes an acute urethral syndrome with dysuria and frequency. Patients with perinephric or renal cortical abscesses may present with signs and symptoms of upper urinary tract infection and pyuria but with negative urine cultures.

Other noninfectious causes of pyuria are uric acid and hypercalcemic nephropathy, lithium and heavy metal toxicity, genitourinary malignancy, sarcoidosis, transplant rejection, interstitial cystitis, and polycystic kidney disease. Pyuria may persist for several months after transurethral prostatectomy. (S.L.B.)

## Bibliography

Christensen WI. Genitourinary tuberculosis. Review of 102 cases. *Medicine (Baltimore)* 1974;53:377.
  *Ninety percent of patients with renal tuberculosis have hematuria or pyuria.*
Cos LR, Cocke TT. Genitourinary tuberculosis revisited. *Urology* 1982;20:111.
  *Reviews clinical and laboratory features of tuberculosis of the genitourinary tract.*
Johnson CC. Definitions, classification, and clinical presentation of urinary tract infection. *Med Clin North Am* 1991;75:241.
  *Good brief descriptions of acute urethral syndrome and perinephric abscess.*
Kenney M, Loechel AB, Lovelock FJ. Urine cultures in tuberculosis. *Am Rev Respir Dis* 1960;82:564.
  *Morning urine specimens are superior to 24-hour collections for isolating Mycobacterium tuberculosis.*
Komaroff AL. Urinalysis and urine culture in women with dysuria. *Ann Intern Med* 1986;104:212.
  *Describes value of urinalysis (including urine culture and WBC in urine) in various disease states.*
Menon EB, Tan ES. Pyuria: index of infection in patients with spinal cord injuries. *Br J Urol* 1992;69:144.
  *Spinal cord patients with indwelling catheters who have more than 100 WBCs per high-power field are more likely to have morbidity from urinary tract infection.*
Murray T, Goldberg M. Analgesic abuse and renal disease. *Annu Rev Med* 1975;26:537.
  *Discusses analgesic nephropathy as a cause of sterile pyuria.*
Norman DC, Yamamura R, Yoshikawa TT. Pyuria: its predictive value of asymptomatic bacteriuria in ambulatory elderly men. *J Urol* 1986;135:520.
  *Pyuria in an elderly, ambulatory population was highly predictive of the presence or absence of significant bacteriuria.*
Ouslander JG, et al. Pyuria among chronically incontinent but otherwise asymptomatic nursing home residents. *J Am Geriatr Soc* 1996;44:420.
  *Prevalence of pyuria and its relationship to bacteriuria was determined. Pyuria was common in patients with and without bacteriuria.*
Pappas PG. Laboratory in the diagnosis and management of urinary tract infections. *Med Clin North Am* 1992;75:313.
  *Describes laboratory methods for defining pyuria.*

Patterson JE, Andriole VT. Renal and perirenal abscesses. *Infect Dis Clin North Am* 1987;1:907.
*Renal abscesses can cause pyuria without positive cultures. Corticomedullary abscesses usually are a complication of reflux or obstruction.*
Pels RJ, et al. Dipstick urinalysis screening of asymptomatic adults for urinary tract disorders. II. Bacteriuria. *JAMA* 1989;262:1221.
*Describes the leukocyte esterase screening test and its correlation with WBCs in urine.*
Petersen EA, et al. Coccidioidouria: clinical significance. *Ann Intern Med* 1976;85:34.
*Discusses infection with C. immitis as a cause of sterile pyuria.*
Pfaller MA, Koontz FP. Laboratory evaluation of leukocyte esterase and nitrite tests for the detection of bacteriuria. *J Clin Microbiol* 1985;21:840.
*Reports a 92% negative predictive value for urinary tract infection when leukocyte esterase screening test is used.*
Randall RE, et al. Cryptococcal pyelonephritis. *N Engl J Med* 1968;279:60.
*Discusses infection with C. neoformans as a cause of sterile pyuria.*
Schaberg DR. Approach to the patient with dysuria or pyuria. In: Kelly WN, ed. *Textbook of internal medicine,* 2nd ed. Philadelphia: JB Lippincott Co, 1992.
*Excellent, succinct discussion of infectious and noninfectious causes of pyuria.*
Stamm WE. Measurement of pyuria and its relation to bacteriuria. *Am J Med* 1983;75 (Suppl): 53.
*Compares methods of measuring urine leukocytes. Excellent summary of the significance of pyuria and its sensitivity and specificity in several clinical contexts.*
Stamm WE, et al. Causes of the acute urethral syndrome in women. *N Engl J Med* 1980;303:409.
*Describes the syndrome of dysuria and pyuria in young women. About a third of the women studied had C. trachomatis infection.*
Teklu B, Ostrow JH. Urinary tuberculosis: a review of 44 cases treated since 1963. *J Urol* 1976;115:507.
*Documents sterile pyuria as a frequent finding in renal tuberculosis.*
Thorley JD, Jones SR, Sanford JP. Perinephric abscess. *Medicine (Baltimore)* 1974;53:441.
*Review of the clinical and radiographic features of perinephric abscess.*

---

## 22. PROSTATITIS

---

Prostatitis is a common but poorly understood inflammatory process in male adults. A recent national survey estimates that almost 2 million visits are made annually in the United States for prostatitis. Eight percent of all urology visits and 1% of all primary care visits are for prostatitis. It is the most common urologic diagnosis in men over 50. The standard classification of prostatitis as acute bacterial and chronic bacterial is now clearly inadequate, as the majority of patients with prostatitis have a chronic condition for which no evidence of infection can be found. The NIH Consensus Conference on Prostatitis divides the disease into six categories. Categories I and II represent the traditional syndromes of acute and chronic bacterial prostatitis. Category III describes a chronic pelvic pain syndrome and is divided into subcategories A and B. Category III A is an inflammatory pelvic pain syndrome evidenced by WBCs in semen, expressed prostatic secretions, or postmassage urine. This category may also be described as a nonbacterial chronic prostatitis. Category III B is a noninflammatory pelvic pain syndrome most consistent with the term prostatodynia. Category IV is asymptomatic prostatitis in which inflammation is noted as part of a work-up for prostatic cancer or infertility.

The clinical diagnosis of acute bacterial prostatitis is usually straightforward. An acute illness develops with chills, fever, and local symptoms of back or perineal pain. Symptoms of frequency and dysuria are also present. Malaise, generalized myalgias, and prostration have been described. On rectal examination, the prostate is tender, swollen, and indurated. Urinary retention resulting from bladder outlet obstruction may be recognized by bladder percussion. Laboratory data will show an elevated peripheral WBC count. A midstream urine sample will usually have WBCs and more than $10^5$ bacteria per milliliter on culture. Macrophages laden with fat droplets may also be seen. In the setting of acute bacterial prostatitis, prostatic massage may lead to bacteremia and is contraindicated.

As in other acute bacterial infections, identification of the etiologic agent is crucial to therapy. Most cases of acute bacterial prostatitis are caused by gram-negative enteric bacilli. *Escherichia coli* causes most community-acquired infections; more resistant gram-negative bacilli, such as *Klebsiella* and *Pseudomonas,* may cause hospital-acquired infection. *Enterococcus faecalis* is the only gram-positive coccus that frequently causes prostatitis. Staphylococci have been reported in some studies. In the antimicrobial era, *Neisseria gonorrhoeae* is only rarely isolated.

These organisms causing acute bacterial prostatitis are also implicated in urinary tract infection. Hypotheses on routes of infection explain this commonality. The several routes of infection in prostatitis are as follows: (a) reflux of infected urine into ejaculatory and prostatic ducts, (b) ascending urethral infection, (c) spread of colonic bacteria through the lymphatic system, and (d) hematogenous spread. Bacterial infections of the prostate are more common in patients with indwelling Foley catheters and condom catheters. Acute prostatitis has occurred in men after transurethral prostatic resection.

Recently, several investigators have described both a systemic and a local immune response in prostatitis. High levels of antigen-specific IgA become detectable immediately on diagnosis. A serum IgG response to specific antigen also occurs and declines slowly over months. Measurement of antigen-specific antibody may also be useful in determining response to therapy.

Patients with acute bacterial prostatitis should have blood cultures and urine Gram's stain and culture before antimicrobial therapy. Gram-positive cocci seen in chains suggest enterococcal infection. Ampicillin plus an aminoglycoside is a regimen of choice. Most patients will have gram-negative bacilli on smear.

Trimethoprim-sulfamethoxazole is commonly used for community-acquired infection, as it provides broad coverage for most gram-negative bacilli. Although only lipid-soluble and basic antimicrobials penetrate the normal prostate gland, diffusion into an acutely inflamed prostate is less of a problem. The severe inflammation of acute prostatitis allows agents that normally diffuse poorly into prostatic secretions to attain therapeutic levels. Quinolones, particularly ciprofloxacin, the monobactam aztreonam, aminoglycosides, and third-generation cephalosporins have all been used successfully. Antimicrobial doses should attain therapeutic levels in the serum. Response is usually dramatic. Analgesia, hydration, bed rest, and stool softener are also recommended.

Complications of acute bacterial prostatitis include septicemia, prostatic abscess, and epididymitis. Chronic prostatitis may occur after infection in some patients. Prostatic abscess results from a mixed gram-negative and anaerobic infection. Treatment of prostatic abscess may require transurethral prostatectomy.

In most patients, chronic bacterial prostatitis presents as recurrent urinary tract infection or bacteriuria. Patients may have dysuria or other voiding symptoms. Chronic pain in the perineum, low back, penis, or scrotum is also described. Chills and fever are not common. Patients may give a prior history of acute bacterial prostatitis. On physical examination, the prostate may be tender, boggy, and indurated, or it may be normal.

The etiologic agents responsible for chronic prostatitis are generally those that cause urinary tract infection. *E. coli* is the most important community-acquired pathogen; more resistant gram-negative bacilli such as *Pseudomonas aeruginosa* are more likely to be hospital-acquired. *E. faecalis* also is responsible for chronic prostatitis, but usually as part of a mixed infection with gram-negative bacilli. Series of patients with *Staphylococcus epidermidis* have been reported. *Mycoplasma hominis* and *Ureaplasma urealyticum* were cultured in 82 of 597 patients in one series. Higher concentrations of these organisms were found in expressed prostatic secretions than in first-voided specimens. *Chlamydia* species have not been as well established as etiologic agents. Granulomatous prostatitis is usually caused by tuberculosis or fungal infection but may occur without a clear-cut etiology.

There is a consensus that the diagnosis of chronic prostatitis is best made by quantitative cultures of concomitantly obtained specimens from urethra, midstream bladder urine, and prostatic secretions. Quantitative cultures of four carefully collected specimens are compared, including first-voided 10 mL (VB1), midstream urine (VB2), prostatic secretions obtained after prostatic massage (expressed prostatic secretions), and first-voided 10 mL after prostatic massage (VB3). In bacterial prostatitis, bacteria in the prostatic specimens (expressed prostatic secretions and VB3) are tenfold higher than in the first two specimens. The test may be simplified by comparing bacterial growth before and after prostatic massage.

The pharmacokinetics of antimicrobials in the prostate is complex. Many antimicrobials with activity against gram-negative bacilli diffuse poorly into prostatic tissue. Trimethoprim-sulfamethoxazole appears to achieve the best prostatic fluid levels. The quinolones also achieve good levels (although many data come from a dog model). In general, antimicrobial bases achieve better levels than acids. To diffuse through the prostate, the antimicrobial must be lipid-soluble and not bound to plasma proteins. Trimethoprim-sulfamethoxazole has been the best-studied antimicrobial for chronic prostatitis. With full-dose therapy for 4 weeks or more, a relapse rate of at least 40% is reported. Some clinicians recommend a more extensive period of therapy, as long as 6 months. Direct injection of antimicrobials into the prostate has been reported to be successful in Belgium, but it is controversial and rarely used in the United States. Extensive studies using quinolones have been undertaken, but criteria for diagnosis and successful therapy vary widely.

When antimicrobial therapy and suppressive therapy fail, transurethral prostatectomy, which has been highly successful in limited studies, may be considered.

It is now commonly accepted that nonbacterial prostatitis, a prostatic inflammatory syndrome in which bacteria are not present, is much more common than chronic bacterial prostatitis. The causes of nonbacterial prostatitis remain elusive. Organisms such as *Mycoplasma, Chlamydia,* and *Trichomonas* may be responsible in some cases, but other, noninfectious etiologies are probably more important. One theory maintains that abnormal voiding results in urinary reflux causing chemical or immunologically mediated reflux. It has also been hypothesized that alcohol, caffeine, and certain foods may induce an inflammatory prostatitis. Recently, the use of alpha blockers for the treatment of chronic prostatitis has been shown to be beneficial for both bacterial and nonbacterial prostatitis. Antibiotics for nonbacterial prostatitis are usually not effective. Transurethral microwave thermal therapy has shown benefit in nonbacterial prostatitis in comparison with sham. Transurethral needle ablation, which heats the prostate, is also being studied.

Prostatodynia or category III B prostatitis causes prostatic symptoms without inflammation or urinary tract infection. Irritative voiding symptoms and prostatic tenderness are common, but prostatic secretions are noninflammatory and not infected. It has been postulated that this syndrome is caused by spasticity of the bladder neck and prostatic urethra. Psychologic factors and stress may also play a role. (S.L.B.)

## Bibliography

Barbalias GA, et al. Alpha-blockers for the treatment of chronic prostatitis in combination with antibiotics. *J Urol* 1998;159:883.
*Alpha blockers were found to be beneficial in bacterial prostatitis, nonbacterial prostatitis, and prostatodynia. Patients with nonbacterial prostatitis did better on alpha blockers than on a combination of antibiotics and alpha blockers.*
Becopoulos T, et al. Acute prostatitis: which antibiotic to use first. *J Chemother* 1990;2:244.
*Describes serum and prostatic tissue concentrations of six antimicrobials administered to 48 patients just before prostatectomy.*
Brunner H, Weidner W, Schiefer H. Studies on the role of *Ureaplasma urealyticum* and *Mycoplasma hominis* in prostatitis. *J Infect Dis* 1983;147:807.
*Provides evidence based on quantitative cultures of expressed prostatic secretions that both* Ureaplasma *and* M. hominis *can cause chronic prostatitis.*

Chodak GW. Prostatitis, epididymitis and balanoposthitis. In: Kass EH, Platt R, eds. *Current therapy in infectious disease*, 3rd ed. Toronto: BC Decker, 1990.
*Outlines a comprehensive treatment approach to acute prostatitis.*

Collins MM, et al. How common is prostatitis? A national survey of physician visits. *J Urol* 1998;159:1224.
*There are more than 2 million office visits annually for prostatitis in the United States. About 1% of all primary care visits are for some syndrome of prostatitis. Fewer than 10% of these cases can be proved to be bacterial.*

Kot T, Pettit-Young N. Acute and chronic bacterial prostatitis: a review of treatment approaches. *Compr Ther* 1990;16:54–59.
*Reviews diagnostic methods and treatment for prostatitis.*

Krieger JN, Egan KJ. Comprehensive evaluation and treatment of 75 men referred to chronic prostatitis clinic. *Urology* 1991;38:11.
*The authors describe their clinical experience with a chronic prostatitis clinic. A comprehensive approach to diagnosis led to specific treatment in 49% of patients.*

Krieger JN, et al. Diagnosing prostatitis: a clinical dilemma. *Patient Care* 1998;2 (Summer Suppl).
*Includes the NIH classification of prostatitis. Summarizes features of the prostatitis syndromes. Describes modification of the four-glass test for diagnosis.*

Lipsky BA. Urinary tract infections in men. Epidemiology, pathophysiology, diagnosis, and treatment. *Ann Intern Med* 1989;110:138.
*Gram-negative bacilli are responsible for 75% of cases of acute bacterial prostatitis.*

Meares EM Jr. Prostatic abscess. *J Urol* 1986;136:1281.
*Editorial summarizes important issues of diagnosis. Transrectal ultrasound and computed tomography are adjunctive diagnostic tools. There is some controversy as to the role of percutaneous aspiration versus transurethral incision.*

Meares EM Jr. Prostatitis. *Med Clin North Am* 1991;75:405.
*Detailed review of types of prostatitis and their diagnosis and treatment. Includes discussion of immune response in bacterial prostatitis. Recommends 30 days of therapy for acute prostatitis.*

Naber KG. Use of quinolones in urinary tract infections and prostatitis. *Rev Infect Dis* 1989;11(Suppl 1321):37.
*Quinolones are shown to achieve good concentrations in prostatic tissue and seminal fluid.*

Naber KG. The role of quinolones in the treatment of chronic bacterial prostatitis. *Infection* 1991;19(Suppl 3):S170.
*A review of 23 studies of the efficacy of quinolones in bacterial prostatitis. Most were not randomized, and many did not include adequate follow-up.*

Neal DE Jr, et al. Experimental prostatitis in nonhuman primates. II. Ascending acute prostatitis. *Prostate* 1990;17:233.
*Summarizes findings on a prostatitis model in primates. Ascending route of infection is documented by serial cultures and histopathology.*

Nickel JC, Costerton JW. Coagulase-negative *Staphylococcus* in chronic prostatitis. *J Urol* 1992;147:398.
*Coagulase-negative staphylococci were cultured from prostatic biopsy specimens and seen on histologic exam.*

Pewitt EB, et al. Urinary tract infections in urology, including acute and chronic prostatitis. *Infect Dis Clin North Am* 1997;11:623.
*Gives brief update of each prostatic syndrome.*

Roberts RO, et al. Prevalence of a physician-assigned diagnosis of prostatitis: the Olmsted County study of urinary symptoms and health status among men. *Urology* 1998;51:578.
*Community-based prevalence of physician-assigned diagnosis of prostatitis is high, similar to that of ischemic heart disease. Men who have a single episode of a prostatitis syndrome had a 20% to 50% chance of a second episode.*

Shortliffe LM, Wehner N. The characterization of bacterial and nonbacterial prostatitis by prostatic immunoglobulins. *Medicine (Baltimore)* 1986;65:399.
*A detailed review of the local and systemic immune response in prostatitis.*

Weidner W, et al. Semen parameters in men with and without proven chronic prostatitis. *Arch Androl* 1991;26:173.
*Compares semen analysis of patients with chronic prostatitis versus controls. An increase in bacteriospermia and an increase in number of leukocytes were present in the chronic group.*
Wolfson JS, Hooper DC. Fluoroquinolone antimicrobial agents. *Clin Microbiol Rev* 1989;2:378.
*Reviews the efficacy of quinolones in prostatitis.*

## 23. COMPLICATED URINARY TRACT INFECTIONS

The term complicated has usually been applied to those urinary tract infections occurring in patients with structural or functional abnormalities of the urinary tract that impede urine flow. The term has also been used to describe urinary tract infections in elderly persons, those with metabolic abnormalities (such as diabetes mellitus and renal impairment), and compromised hosts (persistently neutropenic patients, transplant recipients, patients receiving prednisone to manage a collagen vascular disorder). What these patients share is the tendency to fail to respond to antibiotic therapy.

All patients with complicated urinary tract infections do not require antimicrobial treatment. Drug treatment is not offered to some patients (such as those with spinal cord injury and asymptomatic bacteriuria and elderly patients with asymptomatic bacteriuria) for the following reasons: The natural course of the untreated asymptomatic infection does not appear to represent a threat to life or cause serious morbidity; drug therapy is often unsuccessful and, on occasion, results in superinfection by a drug-resistant pathogen; and drugs not only add to the costs of health care, but also have the potential to produce untoward events.

This chapter focuses on selected disorders that would merit the designation of complicated urinary tract infection: complicated symptomatic pyelonephritis, polycystic kidney disease, infection stone, renal transplantation, spinal cord injury, and emphysematous pyelonephritis. Two additional entities—namely, chronic prostatitis and candiduria—are reviewed in separate chapters.

*Complicated Symptomatic Pyelonephritis*
Complicated (by obstruction, xanthogranuloma, or perinephric abscess) symptomatic pyelonephritis is often manifested by continuous fever and pain despite appropriate antibiotic selection, bacteriuria that persists after drug treatment has commenced, and development of septic shock with or without adult respiratory distress syndrome. These patients are candidates for early drainage of a perinephric abscess, partial nephrectomy for xanthogranuloma, and relief of obstruction. For the patient with symptomatic complicated pyelonephritis, an antibiotic should be prescribed when the disease is first considered and continued for at least 10 to 14 days after the obstruction is relieved or the perinephric abscess is drained.

*Polycystic Kidney Disease*
Polycystic kidney disease is an autosomal dominant hereditary tubular disorder manifested as medullary and cortical cysts accompanied by intervening renal parenchyma that may demonstrate nephrosclerosis or interstitial nephritis. This systemic disease, which affects approximately 500,000 Americans and accounts for approximately 10% of end-stage renal failure, can also be associated with nephrolithiasis, hepatic cysts, hypertension, intracranial aneurysms, mitral valve prolapse, and colonic diverticula. Patients with polycystic renal disease are at risk to experience pain, bleeding, obstruction, and infection as complications of the cysts.

Cyst infections resemble renal parenchymal infections (pyelonephritis) in terms of clinical manifestations and causative organisms (gram-negative aerobic bacilli); however, there are some diagnostic and therapeutic differences. Patients with polycystic kidney disease and uncomplicated pyelonephritis may demonstrate WBC casts, and these patients appear to respond, both clinically and microbiologically, to customary antibiotic treatment. In contrast, patients with infected cysts may not demonstrate bacteriuria, but they are more apt to experience bacteremia, develop a new discrete area of palpable tenderness in the involved polycystic kidney, and be refractory to initial, traditional antibiotic therapy.

Unfortunately, imaging techniques do not reliably identify cysts that are infected. This is a major concern because although infected cysts can occasionally be identified by computed tomography (CT), it becomes necessary, when patients appear to be failing an antibiotic course, to aspirate the infected cyst to identify the causative organism, establish its susceptibility profile, and drain/decompress the infected cyst or perform surgical drainage (partial nephrectomy or total nephrectomy).

A consistent sentiment in the urologic literature, unsupported by clinical investigations but based on measurements of antibiotic concentrations detected in cyst fluid, is that lipophobic antibiotics (including penicillins, cephalosporins, and aminoglycosides) penetrate infected cysts poorly, and that the preferred antimicrobial treatment for the patient with an infected cyst is a lipophilic agent, such as trimethoprim-sulfamethoxazole (TMP-SMX) or a fluoroquinolone.

*Infection Stones*

In selected patients, such as those with continuous or intermittent long-term catheterization to manage a neurogenic bladder, infections stones tend to develop. The stones, consisting of calcium phosphate (apatite) and magnesium ammonium phosphate (struvite), are a threat to life because they are associated with silent obstruction with diminished renal function, xanthogranulomatous pyelonephritis, pyelonephritis, pyonephrosis, renal abscess, perirenal abscess, bacteremia, septic shock, and acute respiratory distress syndrome. Infection stones contain in their interstices urease-producing bacteria, particularly *Proteus mirabilis* and less commonly *Klebsiella pneumoniae* and *Pseudomonas aeruginosa,* and the organisms are protected from host defenses and antibiotics. Such protection explains why infection stones are likely to cause recurrent infections.

Patients who experience acute symptomatic urosepsis are candidates for emergent relief of obstruction, IV administration of an antibiotic, and drainage of perinephric abscess or xanthogranulomatous pyelonephritis. Asymptomatic patients should be considered for stone dissolution with extracorporeal shock wave lithotripsy, percutaneous nephrolithotomy, or a combination of these procedures.

*Renal Transplantation*

When a urinary tract infection is detected within 3 months of a renal transplant, it is most often a pyelonephritis rather than a cystitis, and when treated with the conventional 10 to 14 days of drug, it is frequently associated with relapse. Limited data indicate that these infections respond to a 6-week course of treatment. When urinary tract infections occur more than 3 months after transplantation, a 2-week course of therapy is appropriate. If there is a concern that the disease is pyelonephritis or if the patient experiences a relapse after therapy, the duration of drug treatment should be 6 weeks.

There are, however, important drug interaction risks when immunosuppressive agents are administered to renal transplant recipients, and specific antimicrobial agents are also prescribed. Aminoglycosides, amphotericin B, and TMP-SMX can enhance the nephrotoxicity potential of cyclosporine. Aminoglycosides, amphotericin B, fluconazole, and quinupristin-dalfopristin can lead to tacrolimus-related nephrotoxicity or neurotoxicity by either an additive effect or by reduction of the cytochrome P-450 3A enzymatic metabolism of tacrolimus.

*Spinal Cord Injury*

It has been estimated that approximately 200,000 Americans have sustained severe spinal cord injury. These are usually young men who have experienced a motor vehicle accident, gunshot wound, or fall. Bacteriuria is virtually universal in these patients because of the alterations in the dynamics of voiding, frequent need for catheter drainage of the bladder, concomitant presence of bladder and/or renal calculi, and the use of external collecting devices. Spinal cord-injured patients are at risk for the development of pyelonephritis, septic shock, bacteremia, infection stones, and renal failure.

A consensus has developed that antimicrobial treatment should be offered only to those patients experiencing new signs and symptoms that indicate a symptomatic urinary tract infection. However, because these patients have lost sensation and/or are often catheterized, they do not experience the classic irritative voiding symptoms (frequency, urgency, dysuria), and the clinician must consider what have been referred to as soft or vague symptoms (discomfort over the back or abdomen during urination, onset of incontinence, increased spasticity, sweating, lethargy, cloudy urine with increased odor) in addition to shaking chills and fever. Bacteriuria and pyuria are so universal with these patients that their presence in the symptomatic febrile patient does not establish the diagnosis of a urinary tract infection without the exclusion of alternative infectious (pneumonia, bacteremia, osteomyelitis, infected pressure ulcers) and noninfectious (deep venous thrombosis, pancreatitis, perforated peptic ulcer) conditions.

Symptomatic infection of the urinary tract in the spinal cord-injured patient is most commonly caused by gram-negative bacilli (usually *Escherichia coli, P. aeruginosa, P. mirabilis*), *Enterococcus* species, and *Candida* species. These infections are often polymicrobic. Treatment is initiated with broad coverage, guided by results of urine Gram's stain and culture and blood culture. The duration of therapy has not been established with controlled studies, but 10 to 14 days has been recommended. Recalcitrant infection merits a radiologic assessment (kidneys and urinary bladder with ultrasonography or CT) to detect obstruction and/or abscess. After successful treatment, patients should be considered for urologic consultation to assess the need for cystoscopy and/or urodynamic studies to search for correctable anatomic or functional abnormalities.

*Emphysematous Pyelonephritis*

Emphysematous pyelonephritis is a life-endangering infection characterized by the production of gas within the renal parenchyma and collecting system and/or perirenal tissue. The infection occurs more frequently in elderly female diabetics and on occasion is associated with obstructive uropathy resulting from papillary necrosis or ureteral calculi. This necrotizing disease is usually caused by the traditional gram-negative uropathogens, predominantly *E. coli*. Rarely, multiple organisms can contribute to the infection.

Patients typically present with chills, fever, and lethargy, accompanied by nausea, vomiting, and confusion. Persistent fever in a diabetic patient, despite appropriate antimicrobial treatment, suggests emphysematous pyelonephritis, renal papillary necrosis, intrarenal abscess, or perinephric abscess. A more smoldering form of emphysematous pyelonephritis, caused by *Candida tropicalis,* occurs rarely in diabetics with a history of intravenous drug abuse.

Traditional abdominal x-ray films usually demonstrate the presence of air within the parenchyma of the kidney. CT without contrast offers enhanced diagnostic precision. Retrograde pyelography is performed when there is concern for obstructive uropathy. Blood and urine should be cultured to establish the microbiology and guide antimicrobial treatment.

The initial management consists of infusion of fluids and electrolytes, parenteral administration of an antibiotic, and surgery or CT-guided percutaneous nephrostomy drainage. The antibiotics selected should possess inhibitory activity for Enterobacteriaceae and *P. aeruginosa*. Agents to be considered are ciprofloxacin, ceftazidime, cefepime, imipenem-cilastatin, or merepenem. Surgery has historically consisted of incision/drainage and debridement of necrotic tissue or nephrectomy. Percutaneous image-guided drainage has been successfully performed, resulting in the elimination of the need for surgery and salvage of the kidney.

The quinolones rival TMP-SMX as the preferred medical management for patients with complicated urinary tract infections. The quinolones are available in oral form, have a spectrum of activity that includes most of the gram-negative aerobic bacilli causing urinary tract infection, require infrequent dosing, have an established record of safety and efficacy, and offer appropriate therapy for penicillin-allergic patients. The quinolones have demonstrated therapeutic efficacy in the management of complicated infections caused by bacteria resistant to TMP-SMX and aminoglycosides, and they have also ushered in a new era of oral treatment of *P. aeruginosa*-related urinary tract infections.

There are some concerns with regard to prescribing the new quinolones, however. These are expensive compounds that are not appropriate for pregnant women, and they must be administered in reduced doses to patients with renal failure. The quinolones are not appropriate therapy for patients with infection caused by *Enterococcus* species, and they have the potential to produce hypersensitivity reactions as well as Achilles tendinitis or rupture. In addition, there are potential drug-drug interactions with didanosine (ddi), antacids, sucralfate, multivitamins containing zinc, iron sulfate, and theophylline. Limiting enthusiasm for the new quinolones is the observation that a drug-resistant organism causes a relapse in some patients receiving a quinolone to treat *P. aeruginosa*-related urinary infection, and that superinfection with *Enterococcus* or *Candida* species develops in many recipients of these compounds. (R.A.G.)

## Bibliography

Anderson GA, Degroot D, Lawson RK. Polycystic renal disease. *Urology* 1993; 42:358–364.
*A review of polycystic kidney disease.*

Anderson RU. Treatment of complicated and uncomplicated urinary tract infections. In: Mulholland GS, ed. *Antibiotic therapy in urology*. Philadelphia: Lippincott–Raven Publishers, 1996; 23–27.
*A thorough review of complicated urinary tract infections.*

Cardenas DD, Hooton JM. Urinary tract infection in persons with spinal cord injury. *Arch Phys Med Rehabil* 1995;76:272–280.
*A scholarly review of diagnosis, prophylaxis, and treatment.*

Chapman AB, Thickman D, Gabow PA. Percutaneous cyst puncture in the treatment of cyst infection in autosomal dominant polycystic kidney disease *Am J Kidney Dis* 1990;16:252–255.
*Underscores the value of percutaneous cyst drainage for diagnosis and treatment.*

Gleckman R. Complicated urinary tract infections. *Int J Antimicrob Agents* 1994; 4:125–128.
*A review of classification, disorders, and therapy.*

Montgomerie JZ. Infections in patients with spinal cord injuries. *Clin Infect Dis* 1997;25:1285–1292.
*A contemporary review of infections experienced by patients who have sustained spinal cord injury.*

Nicolle LE. A practical guide to the management of complicated urinary tract infection. *Drugs* 1997;53:538–592.
*A detailed review of the antimicrobial therapy of patients with complicated urinary tract infections.*

Perkash I. Controlling UTI's in patients with spinal cord injuries. *J Crit Illness* 1996; 11:541–548.
*A contemporary discussion of the subject.*

Ronald A, Harding GKM. Complicated urinary tract infections. *Infect Dis Clin North Am* 1997;11:583–591.
*Features a classification, discussion of laboratory diagnosis, and case illustrations.*

Schwab S, Bander SJ, Klahr S. Renal infection in autosomal dominant polycystic kidney disease. *Am J Med* 1987;82:714–718.
*Establishes the principles for antibiotic treatment of the infected renal cyst.*

Yoshikawa TT, Nicolle L, Norman DC. Management of complicated urinary tract infection in older patients. *J Am Geriatr Soc* 1996;44:1235–1241.
*Urinary tract infections in elderly patients are considered "complicated," and this article reviews the epidemiology, diagnosis, and therapeutic approach.*

## 24. CANDIDURIA

Confusion often accompanies a laboratory report indicating the presence of *Candida* or another yeast in the urine (funguria). The vexation that surrounds the detection of funguria is based on the knowledge that the finding may be either inconsequential or of great clinical importance. In fact, a urine culture demonstrating *Candida* can represent contamination, colonization, cystitis, pyelonephritis, or disseminated infection.

Fewer than 5% of all urine cultures will demonstrate the presence of funguria. However, among some groups of patients, funguria is a common finding; for example, candiduria has been detected in up to 25% of hospitalized nursing home residents who have indwelling bladder catheters and are receiving broad-spectrum antimicrobials. The majority of urine isolates are *Candida* species, usually *C. albicans, C. tropicalis, C. parapsilosis,* and on occasion *C. (Torulopsis) glabrata;* the latter microbe is a small, budding yeast that does not form hyphae or pseudohyphae and is capable of producing urinary tract infections in immunocompromised patients. Rarely, *Cryptococcus neoformans, Blastomyces dermatitidis, Histoplasma capsulatum,* or *Coccidioides immitis* will be isolated; the recovery of these fungi from urine always indicates the presence of serious disease, usually disseminated infection.

The first step in evaluation of the patient with a urine culture that reveals funguria is to repeat the test. *Candida* species are common colonizers of the perineum, and they are frequently associated with vulvovaginitis and balanitis, especially in diabetic patients; indeed, a positive finding on urine culture can be the first clue to the presence of diabetes mellitus. In any case, because a urine culture can become contaminated during collection, another sample should be obtained by a clean-catch technique; if necessary, the specimen can be secured by catheterizing the bladder ("straight cath spec"). If the subsequent sample is sterile and pyuria is absent, the initial result can be ignored; if candiduria is repeatedly demonstrated, attempts should be made to determine if the finding represents colonization or infection (i.e., cystitis, pyelonephritis, or disseminated candidiasis).

A simple method to distinguish urinary tract colonization from infection remains to be developed for *Candida* species. In the absence of an indwelling bladder catheter, some experts consider a colony count of greater than 10,000/mL to be important in distinguishing infection from colonization; others believe that any number of *Candida* organisms in a clean-catch urine specimen indicates infection. In the presence of a Foley catheter, large concentrations of yeast are commonly observed, but a role for specific colony counts in differentiating infection from colonization has not been established. Further, the presence or absence of pseudohyphae in the urine sediment is not useful in clarifying the problem. Serologic assays that detect candidal antigens do not yet have the sensitivity or specificity to identify invasive disease reliably.

Insight into the significance of candiduria will usually be gained if the clinician takes into consideration the circumstances in which the finding is made. Colonization of the bladder would be the diagnosis if the patient has risk factors for that problem (indwelling bladder catheter, diabetes mellitus, exposure to broad-spectrum antimicrobials, immunosuppressive therapy, pregnancy) but no symptoms (urgency, frequency, bladder discomfort), signs (suprapubic tenderness), or laboratory evidence (leukocytosis) of infection. Conversely, candidal cystitis would be a likely diagnosis if the patient has risk factors for colonization and clinical or laboratory evidence of locally invasive disease. Cystoscopy in patients with candidal cystitis typically reveals an inflamed mucosa studded with thrushlike plaques.

Candidal infection of the upper urinary tract (renal candidiasis) should be suspected if the patient has risk factors for colonization (indwelling bladder catheter, diabetes mellitus, exposure to broad-spectrum antimicrobials, female sex, immunosuppressive therapy) and symptoms (flank pain, nausea, vomiting), signs (fever, tachycardia, flank tenderness), and laboratory evidence (leukocytosis) of parenchymal disease. It must be emphasized, however, that in some patients, such as debilitated aged persons with diabetes mellitus, the usual clinical manifestations of pyelonephritis can be absent; clues to the presence of renal involvement in such patients include vague constitutional symptoms, a deterioration in kidney function, and persistence of candiduria despite topical antifungal therapy, such as bladder irrigation with amphotericin B. Upper urinary tract infection can be associated with the formation of fungal accretions ("fungus balls"), which can lead to ureteral obstruction and oliguria; thus, the laboratory evaluation may reveal azotemia. In the setting of obstruction by fungus balls, ultrasonography, computed tomography, or IV pyelography may demonstrate the presence of filling defects within the collecting system. Candidal pyelonephritis can also be associated with papillary necrosis. Finally, upper tract infection can lead to fungemia; patients with candidemia arising from the urinary tract usually have anatomic abnormalities causing obstruction and a history of invasive urologic procedures, such as surgery, stent placement, or nephrostomy tube insertion.

Up to 80% of patients with disseminated candidiasis have renal involvement as a complication of the fungemia. Because blood cultures are negative in 40% to 50% of patients with disseminated infection, candiduria can represent a very important clue to the presence of the life-threatening condition. Disseminated candidiasis should be suspected in the patient who has funguria and who has risk factors for blood-borne disease, including malignancy (leukemia, lymphoma), postoperative status, intravascular catheters, immunosuppressive therapy, prior broad-spectrum antimicrobial therapy, and protein-calorie malnutrition. The manifestations of disseminated candidiasis are broad, but most patients exhibit nonspecific symptoms leading to clinical deterioration. The diagnosis should also be considered in hospitalized patients with risk factors for disseminated candidiasis who exhibit enigmatic fever or experience sepsis with sterile blood cultures. Cutaneous lesions (red to pink nodules 0.5 to 1.0 cm in diameter) and retinal abnormalities (iritis, retinal exudates with or without extension into the vitreous) are uncommon but important findings in patients with the problem.

Patients who have candiduria as a consequence of colonization can usually be managed by eliminating the predisposing factor, such as withdrawing systemic antimicrobials, removing indwelling catheters, and treating uncontrolled diabetes mellitus; however, intravesicular or systemic antifungals are occasionally necessary. Symptomatic patients with candidal cystitis may also respond to maneuvers that eliminate risk factors, such as removal of an indwelling bladder catheter; however, if there is no response to removal of the catheter or if the latter is not feasible, antifungal therapy should be given. Fluconazole by mouth (200 mg followed by 100 mg daily for 4 to 7 days) represents one effective therapy. Alternatively, amphotericin B can be administered by continuous infusion through a triple-lumen catheter (25 to 50 mg in 1,000 mL of sterile water infused over 24 hours for 2 to 3 days). In selected circumstances, a single IV dose of amphotericin B (0.3 mg/kg) can be given.

Candidal pyelonephritis can result from ascending infection from the lower urinary tract or from hematogenous seeding in the setting of disseminated disease. Patients with primary renal candidiasis or disseminated infection require systemic antifungal therapy. Amphotericin B and fluconazole represent acceptable agents. The usual dose of amphotericin B is 0.4 to 0.6 mg/kg daily administered intravenously, to a total cumulative dose of 5 to 7 mg/kg; the dose of fluconazole is 400 mg given intravenously for 7 days followed by 400 mg by mouth for an additional 14 days. Of note, although fluconazole is active against the great majority of strains of *C. albicans,* the inhibitory activity of the agent against other candidal species is variable. (A.L.E.)

## Bibliography

Ang BS, et al. Candidemia from a urinary tract source: microbiological aspects and clinical significance. *Clin Infect Dis* 1993;17:662.

*In this retrospective review, the authors present 26 cases of candidemia that originated from the urinary tract. They note that 88% of the patients had structural abnormalities of the urinary tract, which often led to obstruction, and they report that 73% of the patients had undergone an invasive urologic procedure before the fungemia.*

Bross J, et al. Risk factors for nosocomial candidemia: a case-control study in adults without leukemia. *Am J Med* 1989;87:614.

*The administration of two or more antimicrobials or the presence of a central line, bladder catheter, azotemia, diarrhea, or candiduria were among the factors identified as placing nonleukemic adult patients at risk for candidemia.*

Fisher JF, et al. Urinary infections due to *Candida albicans. Rev Infect Dis* 1982; 4:1107.
*This article reviews the epidemiology, pathophysiology, and treatment of the problem and includes an algorithm useful in the management of patients with candiduria.*
Fisher JF, et al. Efficacy of a single intravenous dose of amphotericin B in urinary tract infections caused by *Candida. J Infect Dis* 1987;156:685.
*In this letter describing their experience with four diabetic patients who had chronic candiduria, the authors report that a single IV dose of amphotericin B (0.3 mg/kg) was usually effective in eliminating the fungus.*
Fisher JF, Newman CL, Sobel JD. Yeast in the urine: solutions for a budding problem. *Clin Infect Dis* 1995;20:183.
*Comprehensive review of the problem, with recommendations for therapy.*
Fong IW, Cheng PC, Hinton NA. Fungicidal effect of amphotericin B in urine: *in vitro* study to assess feasibility of bladder washout for localization of site of candiduria. *Antimicrob Agents Chemother* 1991;11:7.
*The authors describe a modified bladder washout technique for distinguishing candidal infection from colonization and for differentiating between invasive disease of the bladder and kidney.*
Frangos DN, Nyberg LM Jr. Genitourinary fungal infections. *South Med J* 1986;79:455.
*The authors review the spectrum of fungi capable of causing invasive disease of the urinary tract.*
Hsu CCS, Ukleja B. Clearance of *Candida* colonizing the urinary bladder by a 2-day amphotericin B irrigation. *Infection* 1990;18:280.
*In this study, 47 of 65 (72%) hospitalized nursing home patients with candiduria had the problem eradicated by a 2-day course of continuous irrigation with amphotericin B (1,000 mL of a 5% dextrose solution containing 50 mg amphotericin B infused during 24 hours).*
Sanford JP. The enigma of candiduria: evolution of bladder irrigation with amphotericin B for management—from anecdote to dogma and a lesson from Machiavelli. *Clin Infect Dis* 1993;16:145.
*The lack of a standard therapeutic approach to the patient with candiduria results from the absence of controlled clinical trials; however, rationales for the usual recommended therapies are presented.*
Trinh T, et al. Continuous versus intermittent bladder irrigation of amphotericin B for the treatment of candiduria. *J Urol* 1995;154:2032.
*In this prospective trial involving 20 patients with candiduria, the authors found that continuous irrigation was superior to intermittent instillation, with cure rates of 80% and 30%, respectively.*
Wise GJ, Silver DA. Fungal infections of the genitourinary system. *J Urol* 1993; 149:1377.
*An in-depth, well-referenced review of a wide range of mycotic infections of the genitourinary tract.*

# VI. GENITAL TRACT

## 25. URETHRAL DISCHARGE

Urethral discharge is the most frequent sexually transmitted disorder occurring in men. In the majority of patients, the discharge has an infectious pathogenesis. If the urethral discharge is not caused by *Neisseria gonorrhoeae,* the patient has nongonococcal urethritis (NGU). These two forms of urethritis, however, are not mutually exclusive, as coinfection with *N. gonorrhoeae* and *Chlamydia* or *Ureaplasma* occurs in 15% to 25% of heterosexual men with urethritis.

NGU is the most common sexually transmitted disease in men and results in about 4 to 6 million visits yearly in the United States. The Centers for Disease Control estimates that there are two and one-half times as many cases of NGU as cases of gonorrhea in men. Whereas the incidence of gonorrhea has declined recently, the proportion of organisms with penicillin resistance is increasing in most areas of the United States. Which type of infection is present depends on the population studied. The highest proportion of NGU cases occurs in college students seen at student health clinics, with rates of 80% to 90% reported. In sexually transmitted disease clinics, cases of gonorrhea appear to be slightly more numerous.

Several organisms are implicated as causes of acute NGU. *Chlamydia trachomatis* is isolated in 30% to 40% of patients with NGU. *Chlamydia* is also recovered from the endocervix of about 70% of women whose partners have chlamydial NGU. A recent study indicated that the frequency of *Chlamydia* infection is decreasing. The organism was found to cause only 15% of cases of urethritis. *Ureaplasma urealyticum* is thought to be responsible for 20% to 25% of cases of NGU. There is a higher incidence of *U. urealyticum* in men having their first episode of NGU. Other, infrequent infectious causes of NGU, which account for 1% to 5% of cases, are *Trichomonas vaginalis,* herpes simplex virus, *Mycoplasma genitalium,* and *Candida.* *M. genitalium* has been found to cause between 12% and 50% of cases of urethritis. The cause of the remaining 20% to 30% of NGU cases is unknown. Thirty to forty percent of patients who do not have intercourse with a new or untreated partner have recurrent urethral discharge within 6 weeks of appropriate therapy for NGU. Most men with recurrent NGU are culture-negative for *Chlamydia* and *Ureaplasma,* and the cause remains unknown. Resistant *Ureaplasma* is implicated as a cause of urethritis that fails to improve following a course of tetracycline. *Chlamydia* appears to be an infrequent cause of persistent or recurrent urethritis. *T. vaginalis* accounts for only a minority of cases of persistent NGU.

Clinically, gonococcal urethritis has an abrupt onset, with an incubation period of 1 to 7 days. The discharge tends to be purulent, and dysuria is a frequently associated syndrome. The clinical picture of NGU is different, with a gradual onset, an incubation period of 10 to 14 days, and mucoid discharge. The symptoms are milder, and patients often wait several days before seeking care. NGU has a tendency to recur, and a prior history of urethritis is common. There is overlap between the symptoms of the two conditions, and a Gram's stain and culture of the discharge are essential for diagnosis. Both *N. gonorrhoeae* and *Chlamydia* can cause asymptomatic urethral infections. About 10% of NGU cases are asymptomatic.

### Diagnosis

When a male patient presents with a discharge or dysuria, or both, the physician should obtain material for Gram's stain and culture by stripping the distal urethra. If no discharge is present or asymptomatic gonorrhea is suspected, a calcium alginate nasopharyngeal swab should be inserted 2 cm into the urethra to obtain a specimen for Gram's stain and culture. Voiding within 2 hours of the examination may interfere with obtaining material for smear. The Gram's-stained specimen shows neutrophils that contain several intracellular gram-negative diplococci in 95% of patients with gonorrhea. The Gram's-stained smear may require a careful search, as the distribution of organisms is uneven. Most neutrophils contain no organisms, and a few cells are loaded with gram-negative diplococci. The hallmark of urethritis is the presence of polymorphonuclear leukocytes (PMNs) on a Gram's-stained smear of urethral discharge. The presence of at least four PMNs per oil-immersion field (1,000×) indicates urethral inflammation.

Patients who are symptomatic but have no evidence of a urethral discharge should have their first 10 mL of urine examined for the presence of PMNs. The urine sample should be centrifuged and the sediment examined for PMNs. Pyuria is defined as the presence of 15 or more PMNs per high-dry field (400×). In some patients with *Chlamydia* isolated, however, urethral Gram's-stained smears and first-voided urine lack enough PMNs to fulfill these criteria for urethral inflammation. In two studies, nearly one third of the patients who had *Chlamydia* isolated did not show evidence of urethral inflammation.

The Gram's stain is also highly sensitive (95%) in the diagnosis of NGU. The smear shows neutrophils without intracellular diplococci; this is confirmed by a culture that is negative for the gonococcus. For many clinicians, the diagnosis of NGU depends on the exclusion of gonococcal infection, as cultures for *Chlamydia* may not be readily available. The swab should be inoculated into an appropriate selective medium (e.g., Thayer-Martin, Martin-Lewis) at room temperature, or inoculated onto a transport system (e.g., Transgrow, Jembec) that yields a carbon dioxide-containing environment. A serologic test for syphilis should always be obtained. In patients with persistent or recurrent NGU, a wet preparation of the urethral discharge may reveal *Trichomonas.*

In addition to the traditional methods of diagnosing gonorrhea by using Gram's stain and culture, rapid diagnostic tests have become commercially available. One test, Gonozyme, is an enzyme immunoassay that can detect gonococcal antigens in urethral, endocervical, and urine specimens. The test requires about 1 hour to perform. For men with a urethral discharge, the immunoassay is essentially equivalent in sensitivity and specificity to the Gram's stain. The Gram's stain, however, is still less expensive and more rapid. For asymptomatic urethral gonorrhea, the Gram's stain has a sensitivity of only 40% in comparison with the culture. In one study of asymptomatic male patients with gonococcal urethritis, the immunoassay for gonococcal antigen had a sensitivity of only 67%. In women with endocervical gonorrhea, the results of the immunoassay were better than those from the Gram's stain (78% vs. 48%). The sensitivity of a single endocervical culture for gonorrhea is about 85%. The immunoassay also appears to be a useful method for the diagnosis of gonorrhea in mailed specimens.

Another rapid test (Gen-Probe PACE 2) utilizes a nonisotopic DNA probe to detect *C. trachomatis* and *N. gonorrhoeae* from the same specimen. The nucleic acid probes are highly specific and can screen large numbers of specimens. The test is expensive and appears to be less sensitive than culture for male urethral specimens. With first-voided urine samples, the leukocyte esterase test can be used to screen for both gonorrhea and NGU. The sensitivity of this nonspecific test is about 80%, and it can be used to identify patients who need further testing.

A number of rapid tests have been developed for diagnosing chlamydial infections. One, a direct immunofluorescent test (Micro Trak), uses a monoclonal antibody conjugated with fluorescein isothiocyanate. The test, which takes about 30 minutes, requires expertise with immunofluorescent microscopy. In one report, the test had a 93% sensitivity and 96% specificity. The other test is an enzyme immunoassay (Chlamydiazyme); it takes 4 hours to perform and has shown a sensitivity of 80% and specificity of 98%. Tests using the polymerase chain reaction (PCR) and ligase chain reaction (LCR) and transcription mediated amplification (TMA) are also available to detect *C. trachomatis.* The cell culture has been the gold standard for diagnosis, and it is too early to determine the role of the various nonculture tests such as PCR, LCR, TMA in the diagnosis of chlamydial infections. The highly sensitive PCR- and LCR-based assays appear to be useful to screen the urine of asymptomatic men. Patients prefer noninvasive tests on urine to the use of urethral swab specimens.

## Treatment

Because 15% to 20% of heterosexual men with gonococcal urethritis have simultaneous chlamydial urethritis, therapy must be directed against both pathogens. Penicillin-resistant and tetracycline-resistant strains of *N. gonorrhoeae* occur frequently, so that penicillin, ampicillin, and tetracycline are no longer recommended. Ceftriaxone administered in a dose of 125 mg intramuscularly is the drug of choice. Ceftriaxone is also likely to be effective against incubating syphilis. A single 400-mg dose of cefixime, administered orally, appears to be as effective as ceftriaxone. Alternatives for penicillin- and cephalosporin-allergic patients with genital or rectal gonorrhea include IM spectin- omycin or an oral quinolone such as ciprofloxacin (500 mg once), ofloxacin (400 mg once), or trovafloxacin (100 mg once). Spectinomycin is not recommended for the treat- ment of pharyngeal gonorrhea, but ceftriaxone and ciprofloxacin appear effective. Men treated with ceftriaxone, cefixime, a single dose of a quinolone, or spectinomycin, which are adequate drugs for gonorrhea, have a persistent mucoid discharge (so-called post- gonococcal urethritis) if *Chlamydia* or *Ureaplasma* infection is also present.

Following treatment of gonorrhea with one of the single-dose regimens, patients should be given a single dose of azithromycin or a 7-day course of doxycycline or tetra- cycline for coexisting chlamydial infection. Azithromycin is preferred because a single dose improves compliance. Erythromycin (1 g/d) may be substituted for tetracycline. Ofloxacin but not ciprofloxacin administered for a 7-day course is another alternative drug for *Chlamydia* infection. *M. genitalium* responds to doxycycline, azithromycin, or erythromycin. A repeated culture is not necessary after treatment unless the patient remains symptomatic or has a recurrence.

Unfortunately, about 33% of patients have persistent or recurrent NGU within 6 weeks of initiation of therapy. The rate of recurrence is the same after 3 weeks of ini- tial therapy as with 1 week. The results of therapy are best if *Chlamydia* is isolated initially, not as good if *Ureaplasma* is present, and poor if neither organism is present initially. Tetracycline-resistant *Chlamydia* is not a problem with recurrent NGU, but resistant *Ureaplasma* has been reported. Erythromycin (2 g/d orally) administered for 7 days is effective against *Chlamydia* and tetracycline-resistant *Ureaplasma*. Trimethoprim-sulfamethoxazole is effective against *Chlamydia* but lacks activity against *Ureaplasma*. Every effort should be made to treat both male and female sex partners of infected patients to prevent reinfection.

Management of recurrent NGU is a difficult problem. The cause is usually unknown. The following must be considered as possible causes of failure to respond or of recur- rence: (a) reinfection, (b) patient noncompliance, (c) mixed infection, (d) *T. vaginalis* urethritis, (e) resistant *Ureaplasma*, (f) herpes simplex virus infection, (g) foreign bod- ies, and (h) trauma (mainly "milking" the urethra). Optimal management is unclear. A urologic evaluation may be beneficial for a minority of patients with unresponsive urethritis. If the patient was compliant with the initial regimen and renewed exposure can be excluded, then metronidazole (2 g orally in a single dose) plus erythromycin (2g/d) for a week is recommended. (N.M.G.)

## Bibliography

Augenbraun MH, Cummings M, McCormack WM. Management of chronic urethral symptoms in men. *Clin Infect Dis* 1992;15:714.
  *Observation is the therapy of choice if known uropathogens are excluded.*
Borchardt KA, Al-Haraci S, Maida N. Prevalence of *Trichomonas vaginalis* in a male sexually transmitted disease clinic population by interview, wet mount microscopy, and the InPouch TV test. *Genitourin Med* 1995;71:405–406.
  *The InPouch TV test was better than the wet preparation to make the diagnosis of tri- chomoniasis and was usually (91%) positive in 24 to 48 hours.*
Bowie WR. Approach to men with urethritis and urologic complications of sexually transmitted diseases. *Med Clin North Am* 1990;74:1543.
  *Review.*
Centers for Disease Control. Recommendations for the prevention and management of *Chlamydia trachomatis* infection. *MMWR Morb Mortal Wkly Rep* 1993;42 (RR11):1.
  *Guidelines.*
Centers for Disease Control and Prevention. 1998 Guidelines for treatment of sexu- ally transmitted diseases. *MMWR Morb Mortal Wkly Rep* 1998;47 (RR1):1.
  *Treatment guidelines.*
Davies PO, Ridgway GL. The role of polymerase chain reaction and ligase chain reac- tion for the detection of *Chlamydia trachomatis*. *Int J STD AIDS* 1997;8:731–738.

*About 60% of men and 75% of women with* Chlamydia *are asymptomatic. These new tests (PCR and LCR) are more sensitive than enzyme-linked immunosorbent assays, but at two to three times the cost.*

Deguchi T, et al. Comparison among performances of a ligase chain reaction-based assay and two enzyme immunoassays in detecting *Chlamydia trachomatis* in urine specimens from men with nongonococcal urethritis. *J Clin Microbiol* 1996;34:1708–1710.
*Use of an LCR assay had a sensitivity of 94%, which was better than the* Chlamydia *culture yield (85%).*

Gordon SM, et al. The emergence of *Neisseria gonorrhoeae* with decreased susceptibility to ciprofloxacin in Cleveland, Ohio: epidemiology and risk factors. *Ann Intern Med* 1996;125:465–470.
*An increase (16%) in ciprofloxacin-resistant* N. gonorrhoeae *was noted.*

Holmes KK, et al. Etiology of nongonococcal urethritis. *N Engl J Med* 1975;292:1199.
*Evidence is given that* Chlamydia *is a frequent cause of NGU.* Chlamydia *organisms were isolated from 42% of patients with NGU and from 7% of controls.*

Hook EW, Holmes KK. Gonococcal infections. *Ann Intern Med* 1985;102:229.
*Classic review.*

Hooton TM, et al. Ciprofloxacin compared with doxycycline for nongonococcal urethritis. *JAMA* 1990;264:1418.
*Ciprofloxacin is effective in treating gonococcal urethritis but not chlamydial urethritis in male patients.*

Hooton TM, et al. Erythromycin for persistent or recurrent nongonococcal urethritis. *Ann Intern Med* 1990;113:21.
*A 3-week course of erythromycin (2 g/d) was more effective than placebo for male patients with persistent or recurrent NGU.*

Horner PJ, et al. Association of *Mycoplasma genitalium* with acute non-gonococcal urethritis. *Lancet* 1993;342:582–585.
*Another cause of NGU.*

Iwen PC, Blair TMH, Woods GL. Comparison of the Gen-Probe PACE 2 system, direct fluorescent antibody and cell culture for detecting *Chlamydia trachomatis* in cervical specimens. *Am J Clin Pathol* 1991;95:578.
*Uses a nonisotopic DNA probe for the direct detection of organisms based on a chemiluminescent detection system.*

Jacobs NF Jr, Arum ES, Kraus SJ. Nongonococcal urethritis: the role of *Chlamydia trachomatis*. *Ann Intern Med* 1977;86:313.
*Classic.* Mycoplasma hominis *does not appear to be major cause of NGU.*

Jacobs NF Jr, Kraus SJ. Gonococcal and nongonococcal urethritis in men: clinical and laboratory differentiation. *Ann Intern Med* 1975;82:7.
*Gram's stain is highly sensitive in the diagnosis of gonococcal urethritis and NGU.*

Jones MF, et al. Detection of *Chlamydia trachomatis* in genital specimens by the Chlamydiazyme test. *J Clin Microbiol* 1984;20:465.
*A 4-hour assay with a sensitivity of 81% and specificity of 98%.*

Judson FN, Ehret JM, Handsfield HH. Comparative study of ceftriaxone and spectinomycin for treatment of pharyngeal and anorectal gonorrhea. *JAMA* 1985;253:1417.
*Ceftriaxone is highly effective for urethral, pharyngeal, and rectal gonococci, including* β- *lactamase-positive strains.*

Martin DH, et al. A controlled trial of a single dose of azithromycin for the treatment of chlamydial urethritis and cervicitis. *N Engl J Med* 1992;327:921.
*A single 1-g dose of azithromycin was highly effective for the treatment of genital chlamydial infections.*

Palmer HM, et al. Detection of *Chlamydia trachomatis* by the polymerase chain reaction in swabs and urine from men with nongonococcal urethritis. *J Clin Pathol* 1991;44:321.
*A PCR for* C. trachomatis *from urethral swabs compared favorably with a direct immunofluorescence test using monoclonal antibodies (Micro Trak).*

Plourde PJ, et al. Single-dose cefixime versus single-dose ceftriaxone in the treatment of antimicrobial-resistant *Neisseria gonorrhoeae* infection. *J Infect Dis* 1992;166:919.
*Cefixime in a dose of 400 mg orally was highly effective (98%) for the treatment of uncomplicated gonococcal urethritis in men and cervicitis.*

Podgore JK, Holmes KK, Alexander ER. Asymptomatic urethral infections due to *Chlamydia trachomatis* in male U.S. military personnel. *J Infect Dis* 1982;146:828.
*Asymptomatic* Chlamydia *infection was noted in 11% of male personnel.*

Schachter J, et al. Noninvasive tests for diagnosis of *Chlamydia trachomatis* infection: application of ligase chain reaction to first-catch urine specimens of women. *J Infect Dis* 1995;172:1411–1414.
*An LCR assay was better than the chlamydial culture in diagnosing infection in women by means of first-voided urine specimens.*

Schwebke JR, et al. Use of a urine enzyme immunoassay as a diagnostic tool for *Chlamydia trachomatis* urethritis in men. *J Clin Microbiol* 1991;20:2446.
*For urine specimens, the enzyme immunoassay (Chlamydiazyme) to detect the presence of chlamydial antigen had a sensitivity of 42% in men with minimal or no symptoms of urethritis. The leukocyte esterase test had a higher sensitivity (88%), but its nonspecificity limits its use as a specific diagnostic test.*

Stamm WE, et al. Antigen detection for the diagnosis of gonorrhea. *J Clin Microbiol* 1984;19:399.
*Sensitivity equal to that of Gram's stain in male patients and significantly better than that of cervical Gram's stain in female patients.*

Stamm WE, et al. Azithromycin for empirical treatment of the nongonococcal urethritis syndrome in men. A randomized double-blind study. *JAMA* 1995;274:545–549.
*Use of a single dose of azithromycin was as effective as 1 week of doxycycline for NGU.*

Stimson JB, et al. Tetracycline-resistant *Ureaplasma urealyticum:* a cause of persistent nongonococcal urethritis. *Ann Intern Med* 1981;94:192.
*A cause of persistent but not recurrent NGU.*

Swartz SL, et al. Diagnosis and etiology of nongonococcal urethritis. *J Infect Dis* 1978;138:445.
*Criteria for the diagnosis of NGU included at least four neutrophils per high-power field in Gram's-stained smears of urethral discharge and a negative culture for N. gonorrhoeae. Gardnerella, group B streptococci, and yeasts were not found as causative organisms of NGU.*

Wong ES, et al. Clinical and microbiological features of persistent or recurrent nongonococcal urethritis in men. *J Infect Dis* 1988;158:1098.
*Ninety percent of patients with urethritis caused by* C. trachomatis *and 70% of cases caused by* U. urealyticum *responded to antimicrobials. When neither organism is involved, more than 50% of cases persist or relapse. The physician should culture or treat for* T. vaginalis *when a second course of antimicrobials fails.*

## 26. SEROLOGIC TESTS FOR SYPHILIS

Most cases of syphilis are diagnosed with a serologic test for syphilis rather than by dark-field microscopic examination of a skin lesion. The causative agent, *Treponema pallidum,* has yet to be grown on artificial culture medium. The dark-field microscopic examination in some cases may not be readily available or is not applicable. It is useful only with moist lesions of primary and secondary syphilis, and the lesions of syphilis may be atypical. Serologic tests for syphilis are invaluable not only for diagnosis but as a measure of response to therapy. Unless the serologic test results are interpreted carefully, however, they can be highly misleading.

Serologic tests for syphilis are of two types: nontreponemal and treponemal. The nontreponemal tests detect an antibody to a cardiolipin-lecithin-cholesterol antigen. The antibodies detected in the nontreponemal tests, called reagins, are immunoglobulins (IgG and IgM). These should not be confused with IgE antibodies, which occur in allergic disorders and are also called reagins. These tests are easy to perform, highly sensitive, and moderately specific. The results are reported as reactive, weakly reactive, and nonreactive, and they are reported quantitatively as the highest dilution of the patient's serum that reacts positively. The test results tend to become negative or at least to demonstrate a drop in titer after treatment. Examples of currently used nontreponemal tests include the Venereal Disease Research Laboratory (VDRL) slide test and various rapid reagin tests, such as the rapid plasma reagin circle card test (RPR-CT). They are used to aid in the diagnosis of symptomatic infections, screen asymptomatic persons, and follow titers in treated cases to determine the effectiveness of therapy. The VDRL slide test and the RPR-CT are the two most frequently used nontreponemal tests. Several tests that link an enzyme-linked immunosorbent assay (ELISA) to a modified version of the VDRL antigen have been developed as nontreponemal screening tests. The ELISA has a sensitivity of 97% but requires equipment, and the patient's serum cannot be quantitated to assess the efficacy of treatment.

Treponemal tests measure specific antitreponemal antibody against treponemal components. These tests are highly sensitive and specific and are the standard laboratory tests that establish the diagnosis of syphilis or confirm the possibility of a false-positive nontreponemal test. The most widely used treponemal tests include the fluorescent treponemal antibody absorption (FTA-ABS) test and the microhemagglutination assay for *T. pallidum* antibodies (MHA-Tp). The hemagglutination test uses antigens of *T. pallidum* adsorbed to erythrocytes. The erythrocytes employed in the various tests differ, but the data fail to show that any one hemagglutination test is superior to another. The most specific test available to diagnose congenital syphilis is the FTA-ABS performed on the purified 19S-IgM fraction of neonatal serum. The test remains investigational and lacks sensitivity. The diagnosis of congenital neurosyphilis is difficult because standard tests are lacking. A potential test uses Western blot analysis to detect IgM antibodies to *T. pallidum* in the cerebrospinal fluid (CSF). New tests need to be compared with the recovery of *T. pallidum* by rabbit inoculation or detection of the organism by the polymerase chain reaction (PCR) technique. Most physicians have been taught that an FTA-ABS test with a positive result usually remains reactive for life, even with adequate therapy, and should not be used to monitor the effectiveness of treatment. Results of a study, however, have demonstrated seroreversal of the treponemal tests after therapy for syphilis in some patients infected with HIV. Another report noted a reversion to seronegativity in the FTA-ABS test of normal hosts in some patients treated for primary syphilis.

The results of the FTA-ABS test depends on the degree of fluorescence and are reported as negative, minimally reactive (1+), and positive (2+ to 4+). This is a qualitative test, and the degree of positivity does not indicate the stage of illness. All patients with an equivocal (formerly designated borderline) FTA-ABS test result should be retested. If the result of the repeated test is again equivocal or negative, syphilis is unlikely. A positive test result indicates past or present infection. A patient with an FTA-ABS test result of 1+ is called a minimal reactor, and this result is considered negative unless the patient has clinical features to suggest syphilis. For patients with an FTA-ABS test result of 1+, the test should be repeated on another specimen. Caution is essential in interpreting the results of any fluorescent test, as laboratory errors may occur. The FTA-ABS test should be performed on serum, and its use on CSF remains controversial. A highly sensitive and specific *T. pallidum* Western blot assay has been developed as a confirmatory test for syphilis, but its place in diagnosis is unknown. The first treponemal test developed was the *T. pallidum* immobilization test (TPI), which is no longer in clinical use. The rabbit intratesticular infectivity test is the oldest and most sensitive test to identify *T. pallidum*. The newest technique is the PCR. The PCR test is used in research settings but could be valuable in the diagnosis of congenital syphilis, neurosyphilis, and early primary syphilis.

In general, treponemal tests are more sensitive than nontreponemal tests. With primary syphilis, nontreponemal tests are positive in 76% of patients, compared with 86% for the FTA-ABS or MHA-Tp test. In secondary syphilis, reactivity is 99% to 100% for both nontreponemal and treponemal tests. In latent and late syphilis, the reactivity of nontreponemal tests is 73%, compared with 96% for treponemal tests. Thus, because the treponemal tests (e.g., the FTA-ABS) are highly sensitive and specific, they are useful in suspected primary or, especially, tertiary syphilis, as the nontreponemal test results are occasionally negative in these patients. An ELISA that measures IgG antibodies against *T. pallidum* is under study for syphilis screening. The test has a sensitivity comparable to that of the RPR-CT but yields fewer false-positives.

Treponemal tests help identify false-positive reactors (positive nontreponemal test and negative treponemal test). The causes of false-positive nontreponemal test results include technical errors, presence of other treponemal diseases such as yaws (not really false-positives), and true, biologically false-positive reactions. Titers in false-positive reactions are usually low (<1:8), and the reactivity is are classified as acute (<6 months of reactivity) or chronic (>6 months). The causes of transiently false-positive nontreponemal test results include a variety of acute viral illnesses, pregnancy (rarely), malaria, and some immunizations. Chronic false-positive reactions may be noted with collagen vascular diseases, drug addiction, advanced age, Hansen's disease, malignancy, thyroiditis, and certain drugs for hypertension. Infrequently (<1% of cases), a test result is false-positive in cases of systemic lupus erythematosus, drug addiction, and pregnancy. A beaded fluorescence pattern (i.e., fluorescence limited to a few portions of the fixed treponeme) is described in patients with systemic lupus erythematosus and a false-positive treponemal test result (the usual pattern being homogeneous fluorescence). A false-positive MHA-Tp test is rarely reported in pregnancy, infectious mononucleosis, and Hansen's disease.

The diagnosis of syphilis in the HIV-infected patient can be a problem. For many patients infected with HIV-1, the serologic tests for syphilis are useful to establish the diagnosis. In selected patients, however, the serologic test results will be negative, and if clinical findings suggest the disease, then dark-field microscopy or a direct fluorescent antibody test for *T. pallidum* (DFA-Tp) should be performed on exudate from a lesion, or a tissue biopsy specimen should be examined with DFA-Tp or a silver stain.

Examination of the CSF is essential for the diagnosis of symptomatic neurosyphilis. The necessity of a lumbar puncture to examine CSF is controversial in regard to immunocompetent patients who are asymptomatic but may have neurosyphilis. Examination of the CSF is essential in an HIV-infected patient with a positive syphilis serology. The gold standard for the laboratory diagnosis of neurosyphilis is the VDRL slide test performed on CSF. The value of tests such as the FTA-ABS or RPR-CT on CSF remains unclear, and therefore they should not be performed on CSF. Unfortunately, results of the CSF VDRL slide test may be negative in 40% to 73% of patients with neurosyphilis. The VDRL cannot be used on CSF to follow response to therapy, as it can on serum. The clinician is usually faced with two situations. First, the physician must determine which serologic test is indicated and what the likely result will be for each patient with suspected syphilis. Second, if the laboratory reports a positive test for syphilis, the physician must decide how to interpret this result and how to manage the patient.

Primary syphilis is a consideration in patients presenting with ulcerative genital or extragenital lesions. Dark-field examination of moist lesions or the DFA-Tp test may be useful in establishing the diagnosis. The DFA-Tp test, which uses a specific fluorescein-labeled antibody against *T. pallidum*, is performed particularly on smears from oral lesions. Nontreponemal test results are positive in 76% of patients, and the FTA-ABS test is positive in 86%. If the initial serologic test result is negative for a patient with a suspected lesion, therapy should be started and the test repeated weekly for 1 month. The clinical manifestations of secondary syphilis are varied, but it is usually suspected on the basis of skin or mucous membrane lesions. Results of the VDRL slide test are positive in all patients at this stage of the illness, usually with high titers (>1:32). A negative test excludes the diagnosis. A prozone reaction may result in a false-negative VDRL test result. In late syphilis, the VDRL slide test is positive in about 70% of patients, and the FTA-ABS test is positive in 96%. Congenital syphilis occasionally can be confirmed by positive findings on dark-field examination. Because the VDRL slide test result may be positive secondary to passive transfer of IgG treponemal antibodies from mother to healthy newborn, presumptive evidence for the diagnosis requires either a significant rise in titer (fourfold) or a stable titer at 3 months of age. Performance of the FTA-ABS test on the purified 19S-IgM fraction of neonatal serum is helpful in the diagnosis of congenital syphilis.

A frequent clinical problem is the management of an asymptomatic patient with an unexpectedly positive nontreponemal test result. The first step is to repeat the test to exclude the possibility of laboratory error. If the repeated test result is positive, a treponemal test is indicated to exclude a false-positive reaction. Then, if the treponemal test result is positive, the clinician should consider the following possibilities: (a) congenital syphilis, (b) treated or untreated acquired syphilis, which can be clarified by the history, and (c) nonvenereal treponemal infection, such as yaws.

Four serologic patterns are observed:

1. Nontreponemal and FTA-ABS tests can be positive with untreated or treated syphilis at any stage, with congenital diseases, or with other spirochetal infections, such as yaws. Clues from the history and physical examination should be helpful.

2. A negative nontreponemal test and a positive FTA-ABS test can indicate adequately treated syphilis, untreated early primary or late infection, Lyme disease, or rarely (<1%) a false-positive FTA-ABS test. Patients with Lyme disease will have a negative VDRL slide test result but may have a positive FTA-ABS test caused by antibody to *Borrelia burgdorferi,* which cross-reacts with *T. pallidum* antigens.

3. A positive nontreponemal test with a negative FTA-ABS test is a false-positive reaction.

4. A negative nontreponemal test and negative FTA-ABS test are seen in incubating syphilis, in the absence of syphilis, and at times in the HIV-infected patient with syphilis. (N.M.G.)

### Bibliography

Catteral RD. Systemic disease and the biological false-positive reaction. *Br J Vener Dis* 1972;48:1.
  *Lists the causes of false-positive reactions.*
Centurion-Lara A, et al. Detection of *Treponema pallidum* by a sensitive reverse transcriptase PCR. *J Clin Microbiol* 1997;35:1348–1352.
  *The PCR is very sensitive and specific and can detect a single organism in clinical samples.*
Dattner B, Thomas EW, DeMello L. Criteria for the management of neurosyphilis. *Am J Med* 1951;10:463.
  *Classic. After appropriate therapy for neurosyphilis, the VDRL slide test may remain reactive for years. CSF cell count and protein should be followed to monitor response.*
Erbelding EJ, et al. Syphilis serology in human immunodeficiency virus infection: evidence for false-negative fluorescent treponemal testing. *J Infect Dis* 1997;176:1397–1400.
  *Some HIV patients with a positive RPR-CT result and a negative FTA-ABS test result, classified as biologic false-positive reactors, may have syphilis based on history and immunoblot testing.*
Fiumara NJ. Biologic false-positive reactions for syphilis: Massachusetts, 1954–1961. *N Engl J Med* 1963;268:402.
  *Classic. Found in 20% of patients and usually with a titer of 1:1 to 1:4.*
Fiumara NJ. Treatment of primary and secondary syphilis: serological response. *JAMA* 1980;243:2500.
  *All patients with primary syphilis had a negative RPR-CT result within 12 months, and all patients with secondary syphilis were negative by 24 months. (See also Guinan ME. Treatment of primary and secondary syphilis: defining failure at 3- and 6-month follow-up. JAMA 1987;257:359. At the 3-month followup visit, cured patients had a fourfold drop in VDRL slide test titer.)*
Flood JM, et al. Neurosyphilis during the AIDS epidemic, San Francisco, 1985–1992. *J Infect Dis* 1998;177:931–940.
  *The median age of patients with neurosyphilis was 39 years, and early symptomatic disease (e.g., acute syphilitic meningitis, uveitis, or meningovascular syphilis) was common.*
Hook EW, Marra CM. Acquired syphilis in adults. *N Engl J Med* 1992;326:1060.
  *Review. Lyme disease may be associated with a positive FTA-ABS test but a negative RPR or VDRL test.*
Hoshmand H, Escobar MR, Kopf SW. Neurosyphilis: a study of 241 patients. *JAMA* 1972;219:726.
  *Nontreponemal tests were reactive in only 48.5% of patients with neurosyphilis when serum was used but in 56.7% when performed on CSF.*

Jaffe HW. The laboratory diagnosis of syphilis. *Ann Intern Med* 1975;83:846.
*Reviews the various serologic tests. The quantitative VDRL slide test on CSF is the serologic test of choice for neurosyphilis.*
Larsen SA, Steiner BM, Rudolph AH. Laboratory diagnosis and interpretation of tests for syphilis [Review]. *Clin Microbiol Rev* 1995;8:1.
*Review of serologic testing.*
Lukehart SA, et al. Invasion of the central nervous system by *Treponema pallidum:* implications for diagnosis and treatment. *Ann Intern Med* 1988;109:855.
*T. pallidum was isolated from the CSF in 30% of patients with untreated primary or secondary syphilis. The CSF should be examined in all patients with syphilis who are positive for HIV.*
Musher DM, Hamill RJ, Baughn RE. Effect of human immunodeficiency virus (HIV) infection on the course of syphilis and on the response to treatment. *Ann Intern Med* 1990;113:872.
*Review of neurosyphilis in HIV-infected patients. The physician should examine the CSF of all HIV-infected patients with a positive serologic test for syphilis.*
Nandwani R, Evans DT. Are you sure it's syphilis? A review of false-positive serology [Review]. *Int J STD AIDS* 1995;6: 241–248.
*Biologic false-positive reactions are classified as acute if they persist for less than 6 months or chronic if they last longer.*
Rawstron SA, et al. Congenital syphilis: detection of *Treponema pallidum* in stillborns. *Clin Infect Dis* 1997;24: 24–27.
*The use of a fluorescent antibody stain against* T. pallidum *was superior to silver staining to identify treponemes in tissue.*
Reeves RR, Pinkofsky HB, Kennedy KK. Unreliability of current screening tests for syphilis in chronic psychiatric patients. *Am J Psychiatry* 1996;153:1487–1488.
*The RPR-CT missed 5% of cases of syphilis in chronic psychiatric patients that were detected by a treponemal test (MHA-Tp).*
Rolfs RT. Treatment of syphilis, 1993. *Clin Infect Dis* 1995;20(Suppl1):S23.
*A comprehensive review of syphilis treatment regimens.*
Rolfs RT, et al. A randomized trial of enhanced therapy for early syphilis in patients with and without human immunodeficiency virus infection. *N Engl J Med* 1997; 337:307–314.
*Current therapy for neurosyphilis with benzathine penicillin is adequate for HIV-positive patients.*
Romanowski B, et al. Serologic response to treatment of infectious syphilis. *Ann Intern Med* 1991;114:1005.
*Seroversion of the RPR occurred in 72% of patients with primary disease by 36 months. Twenty-four percent of patients with an initial episode of primary syphilis will have a negative FTA-ABS test result at 36 months. (See also Lukehart SA. Serologic testing after therapy for syphilis: is there a test for cure?* Ann Intern Med *1991;114:1057.)*
Sanchez PJ, Wendel GD, Norgard MV. IgM antibody to *Treponema pallidum* in cerebrospinal fluid of infants with congenital syphilis. *Am J Dis Child* 1992;146:1171.
*By means of Western blot analysis, the diagnosis of congenital neurosyphilis was supported by detection of IgM antibody to* T. pallidum *in the CSF.*
Scheck DN, Hook EW III. Neurosyphilis [Review]. *Infect Dis Clin North Am* 1994;8:769.
*Only 30% to 70% of patients with central nervous system syphilis have a positive CSF VDRL test result.*
Schroeter AL et al. Treatment for early syphilis and reactivity of serological tests. *JAMA* 1972;221:471.
*A positive treponemal test usually remains so for life, even with adequate therapy.*
Sparling PF. Diagnosis and treatment of syphilis. *N Engl J Med* 1971;284:642.
*Classic. Compares the reactivity of various serologic tests in the different stages of syphilis. The VDRL slide test will usually become negative 6 to 12 months after treatment of primary syphilis or 12 to 24 months after treatment of secondary syphilis.*
Tomberlin MG, et al. Evaluation of neurosyphilis in human immunodeficiency virus-infected individuals. *Clin Infect Dis* 1994;18:288–294.
*The diagnosis of neurosyphilis remains problematic, as the CSF VDRL test is positive in only 9% of cases. A slightly better test is the* T. pallidum *hemagglutination (THPA) index, which measures intrathecal antitreponemal antibody (12.5% positive).*

## 27.  PELVIC INFLAMMATORY DISEASE

Pelvic inflammatory disease (PID) refers to infection of the structures of the upper genital tract, such as the uterus (endometritis), fallopian tubes (salpingitis), and adnexal structures (ovarian abscess); pelvic peritonitis may be present. PID is the most frequently occurring serious infection among sexually active women between the ages of 15 and 24. It is estimated that more than 1 million episodes of PID occur yearly in the United States, resulting in more than 200,000 hospitalizations, more than 100,000 surgical procedures, and about 2.5 million outpatient visits. In recent years, the average cost of hospitalization for PID has increased nearly 150%, and the number of women hospitalized has decreased 25%. Approximately one woman in 50 between the ages of 15 and 24 acquires PID yearly. Most cases (85%) are community-acquired and relate to sexual activity, although the disease can be a complication of a gynecologic surgical procedure, such as a dilation and curettage or induced abortion. PID can develop after the insertion of an intrauterine contraceptive device (IUD), which may cause a cervical infection to spread to the uterus and fallopian tubes.

PID is an ascending infection in which organisms in the vagina and lower cervix spread to the normally sterile endometrial cavity and to the fallopian tubes and adnexal structures. The infecting organisms can be exogenous agents, such as sexually transmitted pathogens, or endogenous agents, such as the normal flora of the vagina or bowel. Acute PID can be either gonococcal or nongonococcal salpingitis, based on the results of endocervical or other cultures, such as that of the peritoneal fluid. When the gonococcus is not isolated, the patient has nongonococcal PID. The frequency of these two diseases varies with the population studied. A high proportion of cases of salpingitis seen at a city hospital are caused by the gonococcus, and a low proportion of gonococcal salpingitis is seen in private practice. The causes of nongonococcal PID include *Chlamydia trachomatis, Mycoplasma hominis,* or a mixture of the aerobic and anaerobic organisms that comprise the normal flora of the lower genital tract.

The frequency of cases caused by the different organisms varies between studies and geographic location. In Sweden, gonococcal disease is infrequent, and *Chlamydia* infection occurs more often. In North America, both *Neisseria gonorrhoeae* and *Chlamydia* are important causes of PID. In some patients, both organisms can be isolated. An endocervical culture yields the gonococcus in 10% to 85% of patients with acute salpingitis. Correlation of an endocervical culture for gonococci with specimens from peritoneal fluid, tubal exudate, or both is variable, with a range of 6% to 70%. In most studies, gonococci are recovered from the peritoneal fluid or fallopian tubes in about 10% to 20% of patients. Whether gonococci are responsible for cases of acute salpingitis when only a cervical culture reveals the organism is unknown. It is hypothesized that gonococci isolated from the endocervix may allow other organisms to ascend to infect the tubes. *Chlamydia* is isolated from both the cervix and fallopian tubes more often than any other organism. *M. hominis* and *Ureaplasma urealyticum* have been isolated from the peritoneal cavity in patients with PID. Gram-negative aerobic bacilli such as *Escherichia coli* and various anaerobes such as peptostreptococci and *Bacteroides* species may also be responsible for cases of PID. *Actinomyces israelii* rarely causes salpingitis in persons who use an IUD. PID caused by anaerobes is usually associated with instrumental trauma of the genital tract rather than sexual intercourse, tends to be more severe, and is often responsible for recurrent rather than first attacks of salpingitis. To date, viruses, except for mumps virus, which can cause oophoritis, have not been implicated as a cause of PID. Many cases of PID are of unknown cause.

Several factors predispose persons to the development of PID. Women who use an IUD have an increased risk compared with those who use other methods of contraception. Most of this risk occurs in the early months after insertion of an IUD and may not be related to sexually transmitted diseases. Women who have multiple sexual partners are also at a higher risk for PID. A single episode of PID increases the risk for a second infection. Thus, 20% of women after one episode of PID have recurrent salpingitis, often within 1 year. Both oral contraceptive agents and condoms appear to protect against PID. Clinical abortion also predisposes to PID, and this complication occurs with a frequency of 0.5%.

PID results from the spread of both exogenous, sexually transmitted organisms and endogenous bacteria in an ascending route to the fallopian tubes. The role of cervical factors (e.g., mucous plug), sexual activity (e.g., frequency and number of partners), sperm, age, and various organisms (e.g., *Trichomonas*) is unknown.

## Diagnosis

The clinical presentation does not distinguish gonococcal from nongonococcal PID; however, certain clues give a hint to the etiologic agent. The patient with gonococcal PID is usually young, febrile, and from a lower socioeconomic group. This is her first episode of PID, and the onset is at the time of or shortly after menses. The patient with chlamydial PID is also young, but she is often afebrile, and the onset is not related to menses. Anaerobic PID, usually seen in an older patient, is often not the first infection and may be associated with an IUD. The patient is sometimes severely ill.

The first problem facing the clinician is to establish the diagnosis and exclude other diseases that may closely mimic this condition, such as acute appendicitis, endometriosis, various types of ovarian cysts or tumors, ectopic pregnancy, urinary tract infection or calculi, and gastrointestinal disease. In one report, the clinical diagnosis of acute salpingitis was confirmed by laparoscopy in only 65% of patients. Of the remaining women, 23% had normal pelvic findings, and in 12% other diagnoses were established.

The diagnosis should be considered in any sexually active woman who presents with lower abdominal pain. Important observations are bilateral lower abdominal pain of less than 3 weeks' duration, purulent vaginal discharge or an endocervical culture of a sexually transmitted pathogen, such as *N. gonorrhoeae,* and tenderness on bimanual pelvic examination. This combination of findings is present in most patients with confirmed PID. The classic findings of pelvic pain, abnormal vaginal discharge, tender adnexa, fever, leukocytosis, and an elevated sedimentation rate are present in only 20% of the patients. Fever (above 38°C) alone is reported in only one third of patients. Salpingitis is usually bilateral, but an 8% incidence of unilateral disease is reported. The presentation spectrum of salpingitis can vary from infection with minimal symptoms to an acute, life-threatening illness.

Right upper quadrant pain suggests the possibility of a concomitant perihepatitis caused by either gonococci or *Chlamydia.* A palpable adnexal swelling can be detected in half of patients with acute salpingitis. Routine laboratory studies such as the erythrocyte sedimentation rate and peripheral WBC count fail to distinguish salpingitis from a lower genital tract infection. The gold standard used to confirm the diagnosis of salpingitis is laparoscopy. A pelvic ultrasound examination can provide guidance in the diagnosis of abscesses, but normal study findings do not exclude the possibility of salpingitis. Serologic tests to detect gonococcal or chlamydial antibodies are not helpful in diagnosis.

When the diagnosis is uncertain, hospitalization is appropriate. Other indications for hospitalization are pregnancy, suspicion of a pelvic abscess, an adolescent patient, severe illness, inability to take oral antimicrobials, failure to respond to outpatient therapy after 72 hours, presence of an IUD, immunodeficient patient, and upper peritoneal signs.

## Treatment

Recommendations to treat PID empirically have been formulated by the Centers for Disease Control. Effective outpatient treatment regimens consist of an initial IM dose of 2 g of cefoxitin, 2 g of cefotetan, or 250 mg of ceftriaxone. Each regimen, except that for ceftriaxone, also includes 1 g of probenecid taken orally. This is followed by a course of 100 mg of doxycycline, taken orally twice a day, for 14 days. Tetracycline may be substituted for doxycycline in 500-mg doses taken orally four times a day for 14 days. The cephalosporins are effective against penicillinase-producing *N. gonorrhoeae.*

Several regimens can be used for hospitalized patients. One effective regimen consists of 2 g of cefoxitin, administered intravenously every 6 hours, or 2 g of cefotetan, given intravenously every 12 hours, plus 100 mg of doxycycline, administered intravenously or orally twice daily. On improvement, patients can be given 100 mg of doxycycline orally twice a day to complete a 14-day course. Alternative regimens for the hospitalized patient consist of clindamycin plus gentamicin, ampicillin-sulbactam plus doxycycline, or ofloxacin plus metronidazole.

Doxycycline or tetracycline should be avoided in pregnancy. If a pregnant woman has PID, an unusual circumstance, cefoxitin or ceftriaxone plus erythromycin or azithromycin should be used. Management of the pregnant woman who is allergic to penicillin is difficult, but spectinomycin plus erythromycin or azithromycin can be used.

Further studies are needed to define optimal treatment regimens. One report showed that cephalosporins, such as cefoxitin alone, resulted in an excellent clinical response but failed to eradicate. *Chlamydia.* Single-drug therapy is inadequate for PID despite an adequate clinical response. Combination therapy directed against *Chlamydia* and the gonococcus is essential for clinical as well as microbiologic cure.

If an IUD is in place, removal should be considered, although controlled studies on this aspect of management have not been performed. All male sexual partners of patients with PID should be tested and treated empirically for *N. gonorrhoeae* and *C. trachomatis,* as a high proportion (58%) of these men will have urethral infection, which is often asymptomatic. Screening of women at risk for chlamydial infection can markedly decrease the frequency of PID. (N.M.G.)

## Bibliography

Aral SO, Mosher WD, Cates W Jr. Self-reported pelvic inflammatory disease in the United States, 1988. *JAMA* 1991;266:2570.
   *A discussion of risk factors associated with PID: age, race, vaginal douching, age at first intercourse, sexually transmitted disease history, and number of lifetime sexual partners.*

Arredondo JL, et al. Oral clindamycin and ciprofloxacin versus intramuscular ceftriaxone and oral doxycycline in the treatment of mild-to-moderate pelvic inflammatory disease in outpatients. *Clin Infect Dis* 1997;24:170–178.
   *Clindamycin plus ciprofloxacin was an effective oral regimen for PID.*

Barbosa C, et al. Pelvic inflammatory disease and human immunodeficiency virus infection. *Obstet Gynecol* 1997;89:65–70.
   *HIV-positive patients who had PID had longer hospital stays and persistent fever compared with HIV-negative patients who had PID.*

Boardman LA, et al. Endovaginal sonography for the diagnosis of upper genital tract infection. *Obstet Gynecol* 1997;90:54–57.
   *A negative vaginal ultrasound examination does not exclude a diagnosis of PID.*

Bowie WR, Jones H. Acute pelvic inflammatory disease in outpatients: association with *Chlamydia trachomatis* and *Neisseria gonorrhoeae. Ann Intern Med* 1981;95:685.
   Chlamydia *was isolated from 22% of patients and* N. gonorrhoeae *from 10%.*

Centers for Disease Control. Pelvic inflammatory disease: guidelines for prevention and management. *MMWR Morb Mortal Wkly Rep* 1991;40(RR5):1.
   *Comprehensive review of diagnosis and management.*

Centers for Disease Control and Prevention. 1998 Guidelines for treatment of sexually transmitted diseases. *MMWR Morb Mortal Wkly Rep* 1998;47(RR1):79–86.
   *Guidelines for management.*

Eschenbach DA, et al. Polymicrobial etiology of acute pelvic inflammatory disease. *N Engl J Med* 1975;293:166.
   *Discusses the two forms of PID: gonococcal and nongonococcal. Anaerobes and aerobic species are important in the latter.*

Falk V. Treatment of acute nontuberculous salpingitis with antibiotics alone and in combination with glucocorticoids. *Acta Obstet Gynecol Scand* 1965;44(Suppl 6):3.
   *Corticosteroids were of no value.*

Hemsell DL, et al. Comparison of three regimens recommended by the Centers for Disease Control and Prevention for the treatment of women hospitalized with acute pelvic inflammatory disease. *Clin Infect Dis* 1994;19:720–727.
   *Three regimens (cefotetan-doxycycline, cefoxitin-doxycycline, clindamycin-gentamicin) were equally effective for hospitalized women with PID.*

Jacobson L, Westrom L. Objectivized diagnosis of acute PID. Diagnostic and prognostic value of routine laparoscopy. *Am J Obstet Gynecol* 1969;105:1088.
*Tumor, acute appendicitis, and ectopic pregnancy can mimic acute PID.*

Kahn JG, et al. Diagnosing pelvic inflammatory disease: a comprehensive analysis and considerations for developing a new model. *JAMA* 1991;266:2594.
*Comprehensive review of diagnostic studies. There is no ideal test for diagnosis of PID.*

Mardh PA. An overview of infectious agents of salpingitis, their biology, and recent advances in methods of detection. *Am J Obstet Gynecol* 1980;138:933.
*A review of infectious causes of salpingitis.*

McCormack WM. Pelvic inflammatory disease. *N Engl J Med* 1994;330:115–119.
*Review. Clinical presentation is often silent or with atypical features. Infertility occurs in about 25% of patients.*

Muller-Schoop JW, et al. *Chlamydia trachomatis* as a possible cause of peritonitis and perihepatitis in young women. *Br Med J* 1978;1:1022.
Chlamydia *infection may mimic the Fitz-Hugh–Curtis syndrome.*

Peterson HB, Galaid EI, Cates W Jr. Pelvic inflammatory disease. *Med Clin North Am* 1990;74:1603.
*Review.*

Rice PA, Schachter J. Pathogenesis of pelvic inflammatory disease. *JAMA* 1991; 266:2587.
*A discussion of the research questions related to pathogenesis of PID.*

Rolfs RT, Galaid EI, Zaidi AA. Pelvic inflammatory disease: trends in hospitalizations and office visits, 1979 through 1988. *Am J Obstet Gynecol* 1992;166:983.
*Hospitalization rates decreased by 36% and were highest for women ages 15 to 29 years.*

Safrin S, et al. Long-term sequelae of acute pelvic inflammatory disease. *Am J Obstet Gynecol* 1992;166:1300.
*In a retrospective study of PID, 24% of patients had pelvic pain for at least 6 months, 43% had a subsequent episode of PID, and 40% were infertile.*

Scholes D, et al. Prevention of pelvic inflammatory disease by screening for cervical chlamydial infection. *N Engl J Med* 1996;334:1362–1366.
*Screening for cervical infection with* Chlamydia *led to a 56% reduction in the incidence of PID.*

Sellors J, et al. The accuracy of clinical findings and laparoscopy in pelvic inflammatory disease. *Am J Obstet Gynecol* 1991;164:113.
*Laparoscopy had a sensitivity of 50% for salpingitis. When findings are negative, the physician should perform endometrial and fimbrial minibiopsy to diagnose PID.*

Soper DE. Pelvic inflammatory disease. *Infect Dis Clin North Am* 1994;8:821–840.
*Review. Patients with atypical PID may lack abdominal pain.*

Swayne LC, Love MB, Karasick SR. Pelvic inflammatory disease: sonographic pathologic correlation. *Radiology* 1984;151:751.
*Abnormal findings could be classified as endometritis, focal mass, or total pelvic distortion.*

Sweet RL, Schachter J, Robbie MO. Failure of β-lactam antibiotics to eradicate *Chlamydia trachomatis* in the endometrium despite apparent clinical cure of acute salpingitis. *JAMA* 1983;250:2641.
*Treatment of acute salpingitis should include an antimicrobial that eradicates* Chlamydia, *such as doxycycline.*

Thompson SE, et al. The microbiology and therapy of acute pelvic inflammatory disease in hospitalized patients. *Am J Obstet Gynecol* 1980;136:179.
N. gonorrhoeae *was isolated from the cervix in 80% of patients and from the peritoneal cavity in 33%.*

Walters MD, Gibbs RS. A randomized comparison of gentamicin-clindamycin and cefoxitin-doxycycline in the treatment of acute pelvic inflammatory disease. *Obstet Gynecol* 1990;75:867.
*The comparison shows similar clinical and microbiologic cure rates in acute PID with both agents.*

Washington AE, et al. Assessing risk for pelvic inflammatory disease and its sequelae. *JAMA* 1991;266:2581.
*A discussion of risk markers, such as socioeconomic status, and risk factors, such as contraceptive practices.*

Wendel GD Jr, et al. A randomized trial of ofloxacin versus cefoxitin and doxycycline in the outpatient treatment of acute salpingitis. *Am J Obstet Gynecol* 1991;164:1390.
*Oral ofloxacin given for 10 days was equal in efficacy to cefoxitin plus doxycycline.*
Zhang J, Thomas AG, Leybovich E. Vaginal douching and adverse health effects: a meta-analysis. *Am J Public Health* 1997;87:1207–1211.
*Frequent vaginal douching is associated with PID.*

---

## 28. THERAPY OF GENITAL HERPES

---

Few other diseases, except AIDS, have attracted such an enormous amount of media attention as genital herpes. The major consequence of genital herpes infection, excluding the emotional toll, is transmission of the virus from mother to infant during birth. Neonatal herpes simplex virus (HSV) infection is a life-threatening illness that occurs in babies up to 4 to 6 weeks of age. If the mother is known to be infected at the time of delivery, transmission of HSV to the newborn can be prevented by delivering the baby by cesarean section. However, neonatal herpes infection develops in most cases because the disease is unsuspected at the time of delivery, as the mother often has no history of genital herpes virus infection. Serial viral cultures are not indicated for most women during late gestation.

It is estimated that 5 to 20 million persons in the United States suffer from recurrent genital HSV infections. Because this is not a reportable disease, nationwide statistics are unavailable. In one study of residents of Rochester, Minnesota, the overall incidence was 50 cases per 100,000 population, with a peak incidence of 128 cases per 100,000. Approximately 20% of the adult population is positive for HSV-2 antibody.

After the first episode of genital herpes infection, the major morbidity of the disease consists of frequent recurrences. One report shows that most patients with symptomatic recurrent genital herpes have five to eight recurrences yearly. The rate of recurrence of genital herpes varies with the HSV type. Only 14% of patients with genital HSV-1 note a recurrence after their first episode, compared with 60% of patients with HSV-2. The recurrence rate is 77% for patients who present with a prior history of genital herpes. Recurrences occur slightly more frequently in men than in women. The median time to the next recurrence is approximately 40 days in patients with recurrent episodes of genital herpes and about 4 months in patients with first episodes.

Few data are available to define the triggering factors responsible for recurrences. One report noted that the recurrence rate diminished with time for some patients, but another shows no difference in recurrence rate between persons who have had the disease for more than 5 years and those who have had the disease for less than 5 years. Most patients cite emotional stress as a triggering factor, and one study noted that recurrence is more frequent 5 to 12 days before menses. Others find no relationship between recurrences and menses or sexual activity. The majority of recurrences result from the endogenous reactivation of latent virus rather than from reinfection.

First episodes of genital herpes can be divided into primary (absence of neutralizing antibody to HSV-1 or HSV-2) and nonprimary initial episodes (serologic evidence of past HSV infection). About 60% of patients who present with a first episode of genital herpes have primary infection with either HSV-1 or HSV-2. Approximately 30% to 70% of patients with a first episode of genital herpes (nonprimary infection) have preexisting antibody to HSV-2, indicating an earlier, asymptomatic infection. Among homosexual men with HSV-2 antibody, 70% denied any history of genital or rectal herpes infection. Eighty-five percent of first-episode genital herpes lesions are produced by HSV-2 and the remainder by HSV-1. The frequency of oral-genital sex may alter these rates. The incubation period for genital herpes is about 6 days (range, 1 to 45 days).

Primary genital herpes is characterized by both systemic and local symptoms. Constitutional complaints, consisting of low-grade fever, headache, malaise, and myalgias, usually subside after 1 week. Local symptoms include pain, itching, dysuria, tender adenopathy, and genital lesions, which are initially single or multiple small vesicles on an erythematous base; these become intensely painful, ulcerative sores. The lesions persist for 2 to 3 weeks and become crusted before healing. The primary infection may also be asymptomatic. The mean duration of viral shedding is about 12 days.

Nonprimary first-episode genital herpes refers to illness in patients with antibody to HSV (Table 28-1). The disease is milder and of shorter duration than primary genital herpes. Systemic symptoms are generally absent. Recurrent genital herpes is a local disease without systemic complaints. Both the severity and duration of the symptoms are significantly less than in primary or nonprimary first-episode disease. Pain in patients with recurrent herpes usually lasts 3 to 4 days, and the lesions resolve in about 1 week.

### Diagnosis

In the United States, HSV is the most frequent infectious cause of genital ulcers. Laboratory confirmation of the diagnosis is usually based on growing the virus in tissue culture. Isolation of the virus generally requires only 1 to 3 days. Multinucleated giant cells are characteristic of herpesvirus, and these cells can be seen by opening a vesicle with a scalpel and taking a scraping from the base of the lesion. The material is smeared on a slide (Tzanck preparation), fixed in alcohol, and stained with either Wright's or Giemsa stain. Vesicles are more likely to be positive on viral culture or Tzanck smear than are crusted ulcer lesions. Results of viral culture for herpes are positive in about 80% of cases, and the positivity rate for the Tzanck smear is 50%. Rapid detection of HSV with immunofluorescent staining or enzyme-linked immunosorbent assay (ELISA) is also available for diagnosis. Viral culture is still the best laboratory confirmation. Serology is generally of minimal value in establishing the diagnosis of genital herpes.

The clinician should be aware that the usual laboratory tests do not reliably distinguish between antibodies to HSV-1 and those to HSV-2. The Western blot assay is capable of separating antibodies to HSV-1 and HSV-2. The methods offered by most commercial laboratories are not reliable to distinguish between HSV-1 antibody and HSV-2 antibody, despite claims to the contrary. The polymerase chain reaction (PCR) is a highly sensitive and specific test for identifying HSV in clinical specimens. This diagnostic approach should be commercially available in the near future. A multiplex PCR assay for the simultaneous detection of *HSV, Treponema pallidum,* and *Haemophilus ducreyi* is under study and appears promising.

### Treatment

Acyclovir has been the drug of choice for genital herpes since 1982 and has a record of efficacy and safety. The drug is now available in generic formulations. Two other drugs available for the treatment of genital herpes include famciclovir and valacyclovir; they offer the advantage of less frequent dosing compared with acyclovir. Topical therapy is of limited value for genital herpes and is not indicated if systemic therapy is administered. Rarely, patients may have an acyclovir-resistant HSV infection, and foscarnet is the drug of choice in this situation. Acyclovir inhibits replication of both HSV-1 and HSV-2. Acyclovir is converted to acyclovir triphosphate, an inhibitor of DNA polymerase, by viral thymidine kinase. The presence of viral thymidine kinase is not necessary for foscarnet activity because this drug does not undergo phosphorylation. Three formulations of acyclovir are available: topical, oral, and IV preparations.

Topical acyclovir is available as a 5% ointment in polyethylene glycol. Topical use usually does not result in serum levels of the drug. Intravaginal use should be avoided.

Table 28-1. Genital herpes

| Type | Antibody present | Patient reports as first episode |
| --- | --- | --- |
| Primary | No | Yes |
| Nonprimary first episode | Yes | Yes |
| Recurrent | Yes | No |

Table 28-2. Genital herpes treatment*

| Use | Acyclovir | Famciclovir | Valacyclovir |
|---|---|---|---|
| Primary genital | 200 mg 5x/d × 10d | 250 mg tid × 5d | 1 g bid × 5d |
| Recurrent | 200 mg 5x/d × 5d | 125 mg bid × 5d | 500 mg bid × 5d |
| Suppression | 400 mg bid | 250 mg bid | 500 mg once daily |

* Nl renal function; creatine clearance ≥ 50 ml/min.

Except for some decrease in viral shedding, topical acyclovir has little therapeutic value in recurrent herpes.

IV acyclovir is effective in the treatment of primary genital herpes. The drug is administered for 5 days as 5 mg/kg of body weight given at 8-hour intervals intravenously over 1 hour. Both systemic and local symptoms resolve more rapidly with IV acyclovir in comparison with placebo. Adverse effects are minimal. Bone marrow depression has not been a problem in normal hosts. Rapid bolus injections should be avoided and adequate hydration maintained. No effect on the recurrence rate is noted. The dosage of the drug should be reduced in patients with renal failure. The IV drug is not indicated for recurrent herpes infections.

Orally administered acyclovir has been found to be effective in treating both primary and recurrent genital herpes. For first-episode genital herpes, the drug is given as 200-mg capsules five times daily or 400 mg three times daily for 10 days; for recurrent disease, it is administered as 200-mg capsules five times daily or 400 mg three times daily for 5 days. The drug is effective in decreasing viral shedding and shortening the healing time. Results are more impressive than expected with primary in comparison with nonprimary first-episode or recurrent disease. Self-initiated therapy is more effective than physician-initiated treatment. There are no significant differences in duration of pain or time to subsequent recurrence between treatment with oral acyclovir and placebo in patients with recurrent genital herpes. Oral acyclovir is well tolerated, and adverse effects are uncommon.

Famciclovir is a prodrug of penciclovir and lacks antiviral activity. The drug is well absorbed (70%) following oral administration and rapidly converted to penciclovir. The intracellular half-life of penciclovir triphosphate ranges from 7 to 20 hours, which permits less frequent dosing in comparison with acyclovir. In patients whose renal function is moderately or severely reduced, dose reduction is recommended. An IV preparation is not available.

Valacyclovir, the L-valine ester of acyclovir, is a prodrug of acyclovir. The drug is rapidly converted to acyclovir following oral absorption. The bioavailability of valacyclovir is about 55%, which is far better than that of acyclovir, which is only 15% to 21%. An IV formulation of valacyclovir is not available. However, the area under the curve (AUC) of oral valacyclovir is similar to that of IV acyclovir.

Table 28-2 lists the doses of acyclovir, famciclovir, and valacyclovir for primary disease, recurrent or episodic disease, and suppression. Except for the cost, long-term suppression of recurrent herpes has been well tolerated. The emergence of resistant strains of HSV has not been a problem. Patients should be given a 1- to 2-month drug holiday each year to assess the recurrence rate.

Condoms appear to decrease the transmission of herpesvirus infection, and their use should be promoted. Intercourse should be avoided during symptomatic episodes of HSV infection. There is also a risk of transmitting herpes when patients are asymptomatic. A vaccine for HSV is under study. A vaccine would be useful for both prevention and treatment. A cure for HSV is still eagerly awaited by millions of genital herpes sufferers. (N.M.G.)

**Bibliography**
Ashley R, et al. Inability of enzyme immunoassays to discriminate between infections with herpes simplex virus types 1 and 2. *Ann Intern Med* 1991;115:520.

*The three licensed enzyme immunoassays provide misleading results in detecting antibodies to HSV-1 and HSV-2 antigens in about 40% of patients.*

Boggess KA, et al. Herpes simplex virus type 2 detection by culture and polymerase chain reaction and relationship to genital symptoms and cervical antibody status during the third trimester of pregnancy. *Am J Obstet Gynecol* 1997;176:443–451.
*PCR was more sensitive than culture for detecting asymptomatic genital HSV.*

Brock BV, et al. Frequency of asymptomatic shedding of herpes simplex virus in women with genital herpes. *JAMA* 1990;263:418.
*Asymptomatic viral shedding occurs commonly and is not related to the menstrual cycle.*

Bryson Y, et al. Risk of acquisition of genital herpes simplex virus type 2 in sex partners of persons with genital herpes: a prospective couple study. *J Infect Dis* 1993; 167:942–946.
*Rate of HSV transmission was about 10% per year. Risk appears to be greater in seronegative women.*

Chuang TY, et al. Incidence and trend of herpes progenitalis: a 15-year population study. *Mayo Clin Proc* 1983;58:436.
*Incidence data.*

Corey L, et al. Genital herpes simplex virus infections: clinical manifestations, course, and complications. *Ann Intern Med* 1983;98:958.
*Review. Twenty-five percent of recurrent episodes were asymptomatic.*

Cowan FM, et al. Relationship between antibodies to herpes simplex virus (HSV) and symptoms of HSV infection. *J Infect Dis* 1996;174:470–475.
*The majority of HSV infections are asymptomatic and unrecognized.*

Evans RM, Brakl MJ, eds. *Genital herpes—a clinician's guide to diagnosis and treatment.* Chicago: American Medical Association, 1997:1–44 (part 1), 1–38 (part 2).
*Review.*

Gold D, Corey L. Acyclovir prophylaxis for herpes simplex virus infection. *Antimicrob Agents Chemother* 1987;31:361.
*Review of prophylaxis. The physician should stop acyclovir after 9 months to see if the recurrence rate warrants continued prophylaxis.*

Guinan ME, Wolinsky SM, Reichman RC. Epidemiology of genital herpes simplex virus infection. *Epidemiol Rev* 1985;7:127.
*Disease may affect 20 million persons in the United States, with fewer than 25% of those infected being symptomatic.*

Johnson RE, et al. A seroepidemiologic survey of the prevalence of herpes simplex virus type 2 infection in the United States. *N Engl J Med* 1989;321:7.
*The prevalence of HSV-2 antibodies was from less than 1% in the group under 15 years old to 20% for those ages 30 to 44 years.*

Koelle DM, et al. Asymptomatic reactivation of herpes simplex virus in women after the first episode of genital herpes. *Ann Intern Med* 1992;116:433.
*Asymptomatic genital shedding occurs more often during the first 3 months after the primary infection than during later periods.*

Koutsky LA, et al. Underdiagnosis of genital herpes by current clinical and viral-isolation procedures. *N Engl J Med* 1992;326:1533.
*The history or clinical examination identified only 39% of women with past or current genital HSV infections. That most cases of genital herpes are unrecognized is a factor in the continued spread of this infection.*

Mertz GJ, et al. Transmission of genital herpes in couples with one symptomatic and one asymptomatic partner: a prospective study. *J Infect Dis* 1988;157:1169.
*Asymptomatic and unrecognized acquisition of HSV-2 infection was common.*

Mertz GJ, et al. Risk factors for the sexual transmission of genital herpes. *Ann Intern Med* 1992;116:197.
*In 69% of patients, transmission occurred from sexual contact during periods of asymptomatic viral shedding. Risk of acquisition of HSV was higher in women than men.*

Mertz GJ, et al. Oral famciclovir for suppression of recurrent genital herpes simplex virus infection in women. A multicenter, double-blind, placebo-controlled trial. *Arch Intern Med* 1997;157:343–349.
*The most effective dose of famciclovir for suppression of recurrent genital HSV was 250 mg twice a day. Emergence of resistant strains to penciclovir was not a problem.*

Molin L, Ruhnek-Forsbeck M, Svennerholm B. One-year acyclovir suppression of frequently recurring genital herpes: a study of efficacy, safety, virus sensitivity and antibody response. *Scand J Infect* 1991;80(Suppl 78):33.
*Four hundred milligrams of oral acyclovir given twice daily for a year was effective in suppressing disease (87%). After stopping the drug, most (69%) patients relapsed.*

Randolph AG, Hartshorn RM, Washington AE. Acyclovir prophylaxis in late pregnancy to prevent neonatal herpes: a cost-effectiveness analysis. *Obstet Gynecol* 1996;88:603–610.
*Based on decision analysis, oral acyclovir prophylaxis in late pregnancy is more cost effective than cesarean section for women with recurrent genital herpes.*

Reeves WC, et al. Risk of recurrence after first episodes of genital herpes. *N Engl J Med* 1981;305:315.
*The recurrence rate is 77% for those with a past history of herpes.*

Reichman RC, et al. Treatment of recurrent genital herpes simplex infections with oral acyclovir. *JAMA* 1984;251:2103.
*Acyclovir is effective in reducing viral shedding and alleviating symptoms.*

Sacks SL, et al. Patient-initiated, twice-daily oral famciclovir for early recurrent genital herpes. A randomized, double-blind multicenter trial. *JAMA* 1996;276;44–49.
*Oral famciclovir (125 mg twice daily for 5 days) was effective for recurrent or episodic genital herpes. The intracellular half-life of penciclovir is 10 to 20 hours, compared with 0.7 hours for acyclovir, permitting dosing twice a day.*

Schmidt OR, Fife KH, Corey L. Reinfection is an uncommon occurrence in patients with symptomatic recurrent genital herpes. *J Infect Dis* 1984;149:645.
*Recurrences result from endogenous reactivation rather than reinfection.*

Scott LL. Perinatal herpes: current status and obstetric management strategies. *Pediatr Infect Dis* 1995;14:827.
*Review. Weekly genital HSV cultures are not indicated. Route of delivery should be based on the presence of identifiable lesions and symptoms.*

Scott LL, et al. Acyclovir suppression to prevent cesarean delivery after first-episode genital herpes. *Obstet Gynecol* 1996;87:69–73.
*Use of acyclovir from 36 weeks of gestation until delivery may have a role in reducing the cesarean section rate.*

Solomon AR, et al. The Tzanck smear in the diagnosis of cutaneous herpes simplex. *JAMA* 1984;251:633.
*This test has a sensitivity of about 50%.*

Spruance SL, et al. A large-scale, placebo-controlled, dose-ranging trial of peroral valacyclovir for episodic treatment of recurrent herpes genitalis. *Arch Intern Med* 1996;156:1729–1735.
*Five hundred milligrams of valacyclovir twice daily for 5 days was effective for recurrent or episodic genital HSV infection. Valacyclovir has the same antiviral activity as acyclovir but superior pharmacokinetics.*

Wald A, et al. Virologic characteristics of subclinical and symptomatic genital herpes infection. *N Engl J Med* 1995;333:770–775.
*Most new HSV infections are acquired from partners with unrecognized or subclinical disease. Subclinical viral shedding of HSV-2 is common.*

Wald A, et al. Suppression of subclinical shedding of herpes simplex virus type 2 with acyclovir. *Ann Intern Med* 1996;124:8–15.
*Acyclovir suppresses shedding of genital HSV.*

Wald A, et al. Frequent genital herpes simplex virus 2 shedding in immunocompetent women. Effect of acyclovir treatment. *J Clin Invest* 1997;99:1092.
*PCR was more sensitive than viral culture in detecting genital HSV-2 shedding, which was noted in 28% of days. Oral acyclovir reduced shedding by 80%.*

Whitley RJ, et al. The natural history of herpes simplex virus infection of mother and newborn. *Pediatrics* 1980;66:489.
*Only 20% of mothers of infants infected with HSV gave a history of recurrent genital herpes infection.*

Whitley RJ, et al. Herpes simplex viruses. *Clin Infect Dis* 1998;26:541–555.
*Review.*

# 29. VAGINITIS

Vaginal discharge is a common gynecologic complaint and accounts for half of patient visits to private gynecologists. Vaginitis, or inflammation of the vagina, is usually associated with an increase in vaginal secretions or discharge. Vaginal discharge may be normal or pathologic. Normal or physiologic vaginal discharge, called leukorrhea, is not associated with vulvar discomfort, is usually nonpruritic, has no offensive odor, contains few white cells, and has normal vaginal flora. The predominant organisms comprising normal vaginal flora are lactobacilli, which are gram-positive rods. Normal vaginal secretions have an acidic pH of about 4.0. Common causes of an increase in physiologic discharge are ovulation, pregnancy, and oral contraceptive use. Discharge may also increase before normal menstruation. An abnormal vaginal discharge usually has an offensive odor, often contains many polymorphonuclear leukocytes, has an abnormal vaginal microflora, and is frequently accompanied by dysuria, dyspareunia, and vulvar itching and soreness.

## Etiology

There are many causes, both infectious and noninfectious, for an abnormal vaginal discharge. Extravaginal disease may mimic vaginal discharge. Dermatologic and psychosomatic disorders may result in vaginal complaints. Rectovaginal or vesicovaginal fistulae may result in the passage of either feces or urine through the vagina. Patients with proctitis may have a discharge that simulates a vaginal discharge. Noninfectious causes of vaginal discharge include chemical irritation or allergy from contraceptive foams or feminine hygiene products, a foreign body such as a forgotten vaginal tampon or device used for masturbation, and atrophic vaginitis. The vaginal mucosa in postmenopausal women may be deficient in estrogen, resulting in a thin, scanty discharge that is sometimes accompanied by vulvar soreness and pruritus. The atrophic vaginal mucosa also may become secondarily infected. Vaginal discharge is sometimes seen with gynecologic neoplasms. The discharge may be scanty and tinged with blood.

The majority of cases of vaginal discharge have an infectious cause, and numerous organisms have been implicated. The three most frequent forms of infectious vaginitis are candidal vaginitis, trichomoniasis, and bacterial vaginosis caused by *Gardnerella vaginalis* and a variety of anaerobes. *Neisseria gonorrhoeae* rarely infects the adult vagina, and the discharge caused by the gonococcus originates in the endocervix. The discharge passes through the introitus and is perceived by the patient as vaginal discharge. Similarly, chlamydial or herpetic cervicitis may be associated with an excessive cervical discharge, which the patient observes as an abnormal vaginal discharge.

The symptoms of vaginitis are vaginal discharge, dysuria, dyspareunia, and foul vaginal odor. Dysuria can indicate infection at a number of different sites: the urethra (acute urethral syndrome), bladder (cystitis), kidneys (pyelonephritis), vulva and vagina (vulvovaginitis), and cervix (cervicitis). A patient may be able to localize the dysuria as either internal (felt inside the body), indicating urinary tract infection, or external (felt over the vaginal labia as urine is passed), suggesting vaginitis. In a large study of women presenting to a primary care clinic with a complaint of dysuria, vaginitis was found far more often than a urinary tract infection (70% vs. 12%). Therefore, women with dysuria should be asked about symptoms of vaginal discharge and vulvar irritation, as well as the presence of internal or external dysuria.

## Candidiasis

The most frequent causes of vaginal infection, depending on the population studied, are vulvovaginal candidiasis and bacterial vaginosis. Most of the fungi isolated from patients with vaginitis are *Candida albicans*. Approximately 10% to 15% of cases are caused by other *Candida* species, such as *Torulopsis glabrata*. Although vaginal candidiasis can be transmitted sexually, sexual acquisition is of limited importance; therefore, there is no need to treat asymptomatic male sexual partners of women with vaginal candidiasis. Moreover, patients can continue intercourse during therapy. Predisposing risk factors for vaginal candidiasis are antimicrobials, pregnancy, oral contraceptives, corticosteroids, exogenous hormones, diabetes mellitus, local allergy to perfumes, HIV, and nylon underwear. The data supporting the importance of some of the risk factors, such as oral contraceptives, remain controversial, and further evidence is needed. Host factors must be involved to explain why some women have infrequent episodes of vaginal candidiasis and others suffer from recurrent infections. Rectal colonization with yeasts is often blamed for recurrent vaginal candidiasis, but in one study the rate of relapse was not related to rectal carriage of *Candida*. The cause of most episodes of recurrent vaginal candidiasis is unknown because the usual predisposing factors are often absent.

As reported for vaginitis of other causes, the clinical features of candidiasis are not distinct enough to permit an accurate etiologic diagnosis. Self-diagnosis is often inaccurate. A curdlike discharge suggests the diagnosis, but a thin discharge occurs as well. The diagnosis can usually be confirmed with a 10% potassium hydroxide preparation or Gram's-stained vaginal smear. Vaginal pH is normal in patients with candidiasis. The diagnosis, however, is not ruled out by a negative result on wet preparation or Gram's-stained smear for yeasts. A culture for *Candida* may be helpful in symptomatic patients when microscopic examination for yeasts is negative. Some 25% to 50% of normal women have yeast as part of their vaginal flora; therefore, for most patients a vaginal culture for *Candida* is not indicated. The diagnosis is made by microscopic examination, and empiric antifungal therapy should be administered.

Various antifungal agents (clotrimazole, miconazole, terconazole, butoconazole, tioconazole, nystatin, ketoconazole, itraconazole, and fluconazole) are used successfully to treat vulvovaginal candidiasis. Cure rates with the different preparations are similar, but duration of therapy varies. Nystatin is administered intravaginally for 14 days, miconazole for 7 days, and clotrimazole for 3 days. Single-dose intravaginal therapy with clotrimazole also yields comparable results. Oral ketoconazole administered for 3 days produces a similar cure rate, but hepatic toxicity has been reported. A single oral dose of 150 mg of fluconazole is effective and convenient. Women with complicated infections are less likely to respond to short-course therapy and require fluconazole for 10 to 14 days. One study shows that even powdered boric acid (600 mg) in gelatin capsules inserted intravaginally produces cure rates better than 90%. Unfortunately, boric acid capsules are not commercially available and must be prepared by a pharmacist or by the patient. Oral ingestion of yogurt containing *Lactobacillus acidophilus* or other *Lactobacillus* preparations may decrease the rate of vaginal candidiasis in comparison with placebo.

Although the various intravaginal preparations can achieve excellent results for an isolated episode of vulvovaginal candidiasis, management of recurrent disease, defined as four or more episodes per year, is a frustrating problem for both patient and clinician. Current therapy has limited value. Use of preparations to decrease *Candida* in the stool and treatment of the male partner do not affect the recurrence rate. In one controlled test, a 2-week course of oral ketoconazole followed by low-dose ketoconazole (100 mg daily) for 6 months was effective in reducing the rates of recurrent disease. After the prophylaxis was discontinued, the recurrence rates were high. Liver function tests should be obtained monthly for patients receiving long-term ketoconazole. Other drugs for recurrent disease after an initial induction regimen has resulted in negative cultures include fluconazole (100 mg a week) and clotrimazole (500-mg vaginal suppositories once weekly). Further studies are needed to help solve the difficult problems of recurrent vaginal candidiasis.

### Trichomoniasis

*Trichomonas vaginalis,* a flagellate protozoan, is a well-recognized and frequent cause of vaginitis. The organism is usually but not invariably transmitted by sexual intercourse. Trichomoniasis facilitates the transmission of HIV. The textbook description of trichomoniasis as vaginitis with frothy discharge and "strawberry appearance" of the cervix is rarely seen. Trichomoniasis, like vaginitis of other causes, cannot be reliably diagnosed by the clinical presentation. Vaginal pH is increased to about 5.0 to 5.5, as in patients with nonspecific vaginitis. In symptomatic patients, a wet mount of vaginal secretions obtained from the posterior vaginal fornix establishes a diagnosis for about 70% of patients. The wet mount is less sensitive in patients with asymptomatic infections. The culture in which modified Diamond's medium is used diagnoses 95% of cases, but this technique requires 2 to 7 days. Another useful diagnostic test, called the InPouch system, consists of two chambers—one for wet preparation and the other for culture. Papanicolaou's smear detects about 70% of infections, depending on the expertise of the cytologist. A test based on monoclonal antibody technology is available for rapid diagnosis; it is a direct immunofluorescence assay having a sensitivity of about 90%. A test in which a DNA probe is used is also available and has a sensitivity of 90%. Secretions for diagnosis should be obtained not from the endocervical canal but from the posterior vaginal fornix.

Both symptomatic and asymptomatic women with trichomoniasis should receive treatment. If trichomoniasis is untreated in pregnancy, there is an increase in premature rupture of the membranes and premature birth. In addition, the regular sexual partners of patients need to be treated to prevent reinfection. A single 2-g dose of metronidazole is highly effective. Male partners can also be treated with a 2-g dose of metronidazole. Alcohol should be avoided for 24 hours after metronidazole is taken. In the first trimester of pregnancy, metronidazole is not recommended, and clotrimazole can be prescribed for intravaginal use, although this drug is less effective than metronidazole. Metronidazole can be used in the last two trimesters of pregnancy without adverse effects. A few patients have intractable trichomoniasis, which usually responds to 2 g of metronidazole taken orally for 7 days. Rarely, IV metronidazole is required to treat this infection when a patient cannot tolerate the oral drug. Paromomycin can be used for the rare patients who fail to respond to metronidazole.

## Bacterial Vaginosis

Bacterial vaginosis, formerly "nonspecific vaginitis," accounts for at least 40% of cases of vaginitis. The origin of the syndrome is polymicrobic; causative organisms include *G. vaginalis* (a small gram-variable coccobacillus) and a variety of anaerobes such as *Bacteroides* species and *Peptococcus* species. A curved, gram-variable to gram-negative anaerobic organism (*Mobiluncus* species) has also been isolated as part of the polymicrobial flora. Confusion has arisen about the taxonomic position of *G. vaginalis*. The former designations were *Haemophilus vaginalis* and *Corynebacterium vaginalis*. Bacterial vaginosis is also associated with a decrease in the lactobacilli that produce hydrogen peroxide.

Features of this diagnosis include a thin, homogeneous vaginal discharge; vaginal pH greater than 4.5; a fishy amine odor after 10% potassium hydroxide is added to a drop of vaginal discharge; vaginal odor resulting from the abnormal amines released; and the presence of clue cells, which are vaginal epithelial cells covered with gram-variable coccobacilli. These cells are noted in 90% of patients with this disease, whereas only 10% of uninfected women have them. A culture for *G. vaginalis* is invariably positive, but 50% of uninfected persons also have this organism as part of the normal vaginal flora. There is little need, therefore, to obtain a culture to confirm the diagnosis. In addition, aerobic lactobacilli and white cells are generally absent from the vaginal smear. A rapid assay to detect proline aminopeptidase activity in vaginal fluid has a sensitivity of 84% and a specificity of 70%. A DNA probe for *G. vaginalis* is available for diagnosis but is expensive.

The mode of disease transmission is not clear, and sexual transmission is unproven. Treatment of the male sexual partner usually is not indicated. Studies of sexual transmission found no beneficial effects on cure rates when partners of women with bacterial vaginosis were treated. However, this issue is still controversial, and partners of women with intractable or recurrent disease should be treated. Studies have reported an increased risk for prematurity linked to chorioamnionitis in women with bacterial vaginosis.

Metronidazole is the drug of choice for this disease. Various treatment schedules may be used, including administering 500 mg orally twice daily for 7 days, or a 2-g single dose. There is no difference in cure rates obtained with a single dose of metronidazole or with a more prolonged course, but the recurrence rate is higher with single-dose therapy. Clindamycin administered in a dosage of 300 mg twice daily for 7 days is also efficacious. Topical intravaginal treatment with 5 g of 2% clindamycin vaginal cream once daily for 3 days, or 5 g of metronidazole vaginal gel twice a day for

5 days, is also effective. Ampicillin cures about one third of patients and is an alternative, especially in pregnancy, without adverse effects. Asymptomatic women from whom clue cells are obtained on a wet mount do not require therapy except in pregnancy and before elective gynecologic surgery. Future studies are needed to define the natural history of asymptomatic disease, identify complications, develop strategies to manage patients with intractable disease, and discover the best screening approaches and treatment in pregnancy. (N.M.G.)

## Bibliography

Ahmed-Jushuf IH, Shahmanesh M, Arya OP. The treatment of bacterial vaginosis with a 3-day course of 2% clindamycin cream: results of a multicentre, double-blind, placebo-controlled trial. *Genitourin Med* 1995;71:254–256.
*Use of 2% clindamycin vaginal cream once nightly for 3 days was effective for bacterial vaginosis.*

Amsel R, et al. Nonspecific vaginitis: diagnostic criteria and microbial and epidemiologic associations. *Am J Med* 1983;74:14.
*Diagnostic criteria for bacterial vaginosis include a vaginal pH greater than 4.5; a fishy odor from the vaginal discharge with the addition of 10% potassium hydroxide; clue cells; and a thin, homogeneous vaginal discharge.*

Brunham RC, et al. Mucopurulent cervicitis—the ignored counterpart in women of urethritis in men. *N Engl J Med* 1984;311:1.
*Illustration of mucopurulent cervicitis caused by* Chlamydia.

DeMeo LR, et al. Evaluation of a deoxyribonucleic acid probe for the detection of *Trichomonas vaginalis* in vaginal secretions. *Am J Obstet Gynecol* 1996;174:1339–1342. *The DNA probe for trichomoniasis had a sensitivity of about 90%.*

Fouts AC, Kraus SJ. *Trichomonas vaginalis:* reevaluation of its clinical presentation and laboratory diagnosis. *J Infect Dis* 1980;141:137.
*A frothy discharge is not pathognomonic for trichomoniasis.*

Geiger AM, Foxman B. Risk factors for vulvovaginal candidiasis: a case-control study among university students. *Epidemiology* 1996;7:182–187.
*Risk factors for vaginal candidiasis included age under 24 years, black race, diagnosis of* Candida *vaginitis in the prior year, and receptive oral sex.*

Greaves WL, et al. Clindamycin versus metronidazole in the treatment of bacterial vaginosis. *Obstet Gynecol* 1988;72:799.
*Oral clindamycin is an alternative drug for bacterial vaginosis.*

Hauth JC, et al. Reduced incidence of preterm delivery with metronidazole and erythromycin in women with bacterial vaginosis. *N Engl J Med* 1995;333:1732–1736.
*In pregnant women with bacterial vaginosis, use of erythromycin plus metronidazole decreased the rates of prematurity.*

Heine RP, et al. Polymerase chain reaction analysis of distal vaginal specimens: a less invasive strategy for detection of *Trichomonas vaginalis. Clin Infect Dis* 1997; 24:985–987.
*Polymerase chain reaction testing had a yield of 92% for trichomoniasis when a swab was inserted about 1 inch into the vagina.*

Hilton E, et al. Ingestion of yogurt containing *Lactobacillus acidophilus* as prophylaxis for candidal vaginitis. *Ann Intern Med* 1992;116:353.
*Daily ingestion for 6 months of 8 oz of yogurt with* Lactobacillus acidophilus *decreased the rate of vaginal candidal colonization and infection. (See also Drutz DJ.* Lactobacillus *prophylaxis for* Candida *vaginitis.* Ann Intern Med *1992;116:419.)*

Joesoef MR, Schmid GP. Bacterial vaginosis: review of treatment options and potential clinical indications for therapy. *Clin Infect Dis* 1995;20 (Suppl 1):S72–S79.
*Oral metronidazole (500 mg twice daily for 7 days) is the drug of choice for bacterial vaginosis.*

Kent HL. Epidemiology of vaginitis. *Am J Obstet Gynecol* 1991;165:1168.
*The incidence of candidal infection has increased during the past decade, with an increased percentage of non-*albicans *candidal strains, such as* C. tropicalis *and* C. glabrata.

Komaroff AL, et al. Management strategies for symptoms of urinary and vaginal infections. *Arch Intern Med* 1978;138:1069.

*Internal dysuria suggests that the patient has a urinary tract infection, and external dysuria favors a diagnosis of vaginitis.*

Krieger JN, et al. Diagnosis of trichomoniasis: comparison of conventional wet-mount examination with cytologic studies, cultures, and monoclonal antibody staining of direct specimens. *JAMA* 1988;259:1223.

*Various methods for the diagnosis of trichomoniasis are compared. The wet-mount examination and Papanicolaou's smear had a sensitivity of about 60%. A false-positive smear was noted in 31% of patients and needs to be confirmed by a wet-mount examination. (See also Lossick JG. The diagnosis of vaginal trichomoniasis. JAMA 1988;259:1230.)*

Lossick JG, Kent HL. Trichomoniasis: trends in diagnosis and management. *Am J Obstet Gynecol* 1991;165:1217.

*Diagnostic methods include saline wet preparation, Papanicolaou's smear, culture, direct immunofluorescence assay, direct enzyme immunoassay, and latex agglutination test. The sensitivities of the saline wet-mount examination and Papanicolaou's smear are about 60%.*

Lugo-Miro VI, Green M, Mazur L. Comparison of different metronidazole therapeutic regimens for bacterial vaginosis: a metaanalysis. *JAMA* 1992;268:92.

*There is no difference between the cure rates of patients with bacterial vaginosis treated with metronidazole as a 2-g single dose, a 2-g single dose given for 2 days, 400 mg three times daily for 5 days, or 500 mg twice daily for 7 days.*

Milne JD, Warnock DW. Effect of simultaneous oral and vaginal treatment on the rate of cure and relapse in vaginal candidiasis. *Br J Vener Dis* 1979;55:362.

*Relapse of vaginal candidiasis was unrelated to rectal carriage of yeast.*

Nyirjesy P, et al. Over-the-counter and alternative medicines in the treatment of chronic vaginal symptoms. *Obstet Gynecol* 1997;90:50–53.

*The most frequent alternative medicines used were* acidophilus *products or yogurt. Most of the yogurt products lack hydrogen peroxide-producing* Lactobacillus *strains that might be of benefit.*

Paterson BA, et al. The tampon test for trichomoniasis: a comparison between conventional methods and a polymerase chain reaction for *Trichomonas vaginalis* in women. *Sex Transm Infect* 1998;74:136–139.

*Polymerase chain reaction testing on a tampon specimen was useful for diagnosis of trichomoniasis.*

Petrin D, et al. Clinical and microbiological aspects of *Trichomonas vaginalis*. *Clin Microbiol Rev* 1998;11:300–317.

*Review. The best diagnostic assay uses the InPouch system, which consists of a two-chambered bag—one for a wet preparation and the other for culture.*

Pheifer TA, et al. Role of *Haemophilus vaginalis* and treatment with metronidazole. *N Engl J Med* 1978;298:1429.

*Metronidazole is highly effective in an oral dose of 500 mg twice daily.*

Reef SE, et al. Treatment options for vulvovaginal candidiasis, 1993. *Clin Infect Dis* 1995;20(Suppl 1):S80–S90.

*Review of therapy for vaginal candidiasis.*

Schaaf VM, Perez-Stable EJ, Borchardt K. The limited value of symptoms and signs in the diagnosis of vaginal infections. *Arch Intern Med* 1990;150:1929.

*An etiology of vaginitis was identified in only half of the patients. Symptoms did not differ for the three diagnoses.*

Schmitt C, Sobel JD, Meriwether C. Bacterial vaginosis: treatment with clindamycin cream versus oral metronidazole. *Obstet Gynecol* 1992;79:1020.

*Cure rate with clindamycin vaginal cream was 72%. No data exist regarding the use of clindamycin cream in pregnancy.*

Sobel JD. Recurrent vulvovaginal candidiasis: a prospective study of the efficacy of maintenance ketoconazole therapy. *N Engl J Med* 1986;315:1455.

*Prophylactic oral ketoconazole (100 mg daily for 6 months) was effective in preventing recurrent vaginal candidiasis. Six months after stopping therapy, half of the patients had recurrence.*

Sobel JD. Pathogenesis and treatment of recurrent vulvovaginal candidiasis. *Clin Infect Dis* 1992;14(Suppl 1):S148.

*Supressing a gastrointestinal focus with nystatin and treating sexual partners does not prevent recurrent vaginal candidiasis.*

Sobel JD. Vaginitis. *N Engl J Med* 1997;337:1896–1903.

*Review.*

Sobel JD, Chaim W. Treatment of *Torulopsis glabrata* vaginitis: retrospective review of boric acid therapy. *Clin Infect Dis* 1997;24:649–652.

*In patients with Torulopsis (Candida) glabrata vaginitis who fail azole therapy, vaginal boric acid may be effective.*

Sobel JD, et al. Single oral dose fluconazole compared with conventional clotrimazole topical therapy of *Candida* vaginitis. *Am J Obstet Gynecol* 1995;172:1263–1268.

*A single oral dose of fluconazole (150 mg) was effective for vaginal candidiasis.*

Sobel JD, et al. Vulvovaginal candidiasis: epidemiologic, diagnostic, and therapeutic considerations. *Am J Obstet Gynecol* 1998;178:203–211.

*Review.*

Spence MR, et al. The minimum single oral metronidazole dose for treating trichomoniasis: a randomized, blinded study. *Obstet Gynecol* 1997;89:699–703.

*The minimum effective dose of metronidazole was 1.5 g.*

Spiegel CA. Bacterial vaginosis. *Clin Microbiol Rev* 1991;4:485.

*Review of diagnosis and treatment.*

Thomason JL, Gelbart SM, Scaglione NJ. Bacterial vaginosis: current review with indications for asymptomatic therapy. *Am J Obstet Gynecol* 1991;165:1210.

*More than 50% of women with bacterial vaginosis are asymptomatic.*

Van Slyke KK, Michel VP, Rein MF. Treatment of vulvovaginal candidiasis with boric acid power. *Am J Obstet Gynecol* 1981;141:145.

*Boric acid powder (600 mg) in a gelatin capsule inserted intravaginally at bedtime had a 91% cure rate.*

Winceslaus SJ, Calver G. Recurrent bacterial vaginosis—an old approach to a new problem. *Internat J STD AIDS* 1996;7:284–287.

*Hydrogen peroxide (3%) used as a single vaginal wash was effective for bacterial vaginosis.*

Wolner-Hanssen P, et al. Clinical manifestations of vaginal trichomoniasis. *JAMA* 1989;261:571.

*Excellent review of the clinical manifestations. Colpitis macularis (strawberry cervix) had a sensitivity of 44% with an odds ratio of 241; a frothy discharge had a sensitivity of 8% with an odds ratio of 21. Overall, the sensitivity of the symptoms and signs of trichomoniasis is low.*

# VII. NERVOUS SYSTEM

## 30. ANALYSIS OF CEREBROSPINAL FLUID

Analysis of cerebrospinal fluid (CSF) is essential in evaluating the patient suspected of having an infection of the central nervous system (CNS), especially acute or chronic meningitis. In addition, analysis of CSF may permit the diagnosis of a noninfectious disease, such as meningeal carcinomatosis. Usually producing much anxiety and potentially causing pain or discomfort, the lumbar puncture requires technical skill and has the potential to lead to life-threatening complications. As a result of the substantial diagnostic value of CSF analysis and the considerable difficulties involved in securing the fluid, anyone contemplating a lumbar puncture must plan the procedure carefully, determining in advance which laboratory studies will be necessary and what volume of CSF will be required for them. Because improper handling of CSF can destroy the usefulness of a specimen, the physician performing the lumbar puncture must ensure that the fluid is processed promptly.

The primary contraindication to lumbar puncture is an increase in intracranial pressure caused by cerebral edema or a mass lesion, such as a brain abscess. A lumbar puncture in a patient with increased intracranial pressure can lead to a continued leak of CSF, precipitating herniation of a temporal lobe over the tentorium cerebelli or of a cerebellar tonsil through the foramen magnum. Obviously, herniation can lead to neurologic deterioration or death. The risk for herniation is low (<2%) in patients with meningitis alone; however, that risk increases substantially (10% to 20%) in patients with mass lesions. Accordingly, patients with papilledema or focal neurologic findings should not undergo a lumbar puncture until the results of computed tomography (CT) or magnetic resonance imaging (MRI) are available. However, antimicrobial therapy must not be delayed in patients with suspected bacterial meningitis, brain abscess with meningitis, or other life-threatening infection while results of CNS radiographic studies are pending. Finally, if possible, a lumbar puncture should be avoided in patients with thrombocytopenia or a coagulopathy until the disorder can be reversed by the transfusion of platelets or clotting factors; patients with hemostatic defects are at risk for development of a hematoma at the site of lumbar puncture, which leads to nerve root or cord compression and permanent neurologic damage. Again, antimicrobials must not be withheld while a clotting defect in a patient with suspected bacterial meningitis is being corrected.

The specific laboratory tests that should be performed on the CSF will depend on a variety of factors, including the following:

1. History of the present illness. Does the history suggest an acute bacterial or viral meningitis, a chronic meningitis syndrome, or an acute encephalitis?
2. Epidemiologic history. Is an underlying disease placing the patient at risk for specific infections, such as syphilitic meningitis (HIV infection) or cryptococcal meningitis (HIV infection, lymphoma, corticosteroid use)?
3. History of prior antimicrobial therapy. Does the patient have a partially treated bacterial meningitis?
4. Availability of laboratory tests. Can the clinical laboratory perform a nucleic acid amplification test for herpes simplex? The importance of defining the most likely etiologic agents has been highlighted by the development of polymerase chain reaction (PCR) assays for the diagnosis of infectious agents not previously detectable in CSF.

When a lumbar puncture is being performed on a patient with a presumptive diagnosis of acute bacterial meningitis, the CSF pressure should be measured and recorded, and the following tests should be carried out on the fluid obtained: RBC and WBC counts, WBC differential analysis, glucose and protein determination, Gram's stain, bacterial cultures, and perhaps an assay to detect bacterial antigens (i.e., latex agglutination test). Depending on the clinical circumstances, other tests may also be appropriate; these include a nontreponemal assay for syphilis [rapid plasma reagin card test (RPR-CT) or Venereal Disease Research Laboratory (VDRL) test], an immunologic assay for cryptococcosis or coccidiodomycosis, smears for acid-fast bacilli, fungal or mycobacterial cultures, and PCR for specific agents not otherwise detectable.

The application of nucleic acid amplification assays to the analysis of CSF is in the process of dramatically enhancing the capacity of clinicians to establish specific etiologic diagnoses rapidly. In many cases, the PCR assays remain investigational; however, once standardized and validated, these tests should become widely available and extremely useful. PCR has already become invaluable for the diagnosis of herpes simplex encephalitis; nucleic acid amplification tests of the CSF are being utilized in clinical investigations to detect a wide variety of viruses (e.g., HIV-1, cytomegalovirus, Epstein-Barr virus, varicella-zoster virus, JC virus, enteroviruses), spirochetes (*Borrelia burgdorferi, Treponema pallidum*), protozoa (*Toxoplasma gondii*) and mycobacteria (*Mycobacterium tuberculosis*)(see Chapter 86, "HIV-1 and Infections of the CNS").

Clear and colorless, normal CSF contains four or fewer WBCs per cubic millimeter, which are characteristically small lymphocytes. The presence of a single neutrophil in the CSF should be considered an insignificant finding if the patient has no signs of meningeal or parameningeal disease and if the glucose and protein levels are normal; higher numbers of neutrophils are abnormal. Turbid fluid implies the presence of 200 WBCs per cubic millimeter, 400 RBCs per cubic millimeter, or $10^5$ bacteria per milliliter; grossly bloody fluid indicates the presence of 6,000 RBCs per cubic millimeter. Grossly bloody CSF that clears as the fluid is collected suggests a traumatic tap; CSF that remains bloody and is xanthochromic indicates a subarachnoid hemorrhage. Of note, xanthochromia may develop in a traumatic tap if there are delays of 1 to 2 hours in processing the specimen. The presence of blood from a traumatic tap can cause confusion in the interpretation of the WBC count. However, the WBC-to-RBC ratios in CSF and in blood should be the same in the setting of a traumatic tap; by extension, if $WBC_{CSF}:RBC_{CSF}/WBC_{blood}:RBC_{blood}$ exceeds 10, the patient very likely has meningitis.

### Bacterial Meningitis

Usually ill for less than 5 days and often symptomatic for only 24 hours, the adult with acute bacterial meningitis classically presents with fever, headache, meningismus, and signs of cerebral dysfunction, such as seizures or a depressed level of consciousness. The CSF in patients with acute bacterial meningitis is characterized by the presence of neutrophils, a depressed glucose, and an elevated protein; the last finding is common but not specific. The total cell counts usually range between 1,000 and 10,000/mm³; about 90% of the cells will be neutrophils. In elderly, alcoholic, or immunosuppressed patients, fewer cells may be present, especially on the initial lumbar puncture. The CSF of patients infected with *Listeria monocytogenes* may contain a relatively large percentage of lymphocytes. Early in the course, the CSF of patients with acute viral meningitis may also contain a preponderance of neutrophils; however, the total WBC count is usually under 1,000/mm³, and the glucose is normal. The presence of eosinophils in the CSF raises the possibility of helminthic infection (angiostrongyloidosis, cysticercosis), neoplastic disease (lymphoma), and rarely tuberculous, syphilitic, rickettsial (Rocky Mountain spotted fever), or fungal (*Coccidioides* infection) meningitis.

The normal CSF glucose concentration is 60% of that in blood, and thus the CSF usually contains about 60 mg/dL. However, a period of 2 to 4 hours is required for an equilibration between CSF and blood glucose levels, and as a result, the CSF concentration may appear to be "normal" in the patient with early bacterial meningitis but a previously elevated blood glucose level. A CSF glucose level of 50% that of the peripheral blood is considered abnormal, and most patients with acute bacterial meningitis will have values below 40 mg/dL. A depressed CSF glucose concentration, also referred to as hypoglycorrhachia, can also be seen in patients with partially treated bacterial meningitis and acute "aseptic" meningitis caused by *T. pallidum, B. burgdorferi,* and some viruses, including mumps virus, the agents of lymphocytic choriomeningitis, and, on rare occasion, herpes simplex virus, varicella-zoster virus, and enteroviruses. Hypoglycorrhachia is a characteristic finding in patients with chronic meningitis syndromes caused by bacteria (*Brucella* species), mycobacteria (*M. tuberculosis*), fungi (*Cryptococcus neoformans, Coccidioides immitis*), spirochetes (*T. pallidum*) and protozoan parasites [*Taenia solium* (cysticercosis)]. Finally, a depressed CSF glucose concentration can also be found in patients with carcinomatous meningitis, CNS sarcoidosis, or subarachnoid hemorrhage.

A Gram's stain must be performed on the CSF of all patients with suspected acute bacterial meningitis; the importance of this simple test is highlighted by the observation that on occasion, the CSF Gram's stain will reveal the presence of bacteria in patients with pneumococcal meningitis who have few inflammatory cells in the fluid. The number of bacteria in the CSF may be low, and thus the Gram's stain of an unconcentrated specimen is not a reliable test. To increase the likelihood of detecting an organism by Gram's stain, the specimen must be concentrated by centrifugation; the microbiology laboratory has protocols to ensure that the sedimentation of the specimen is adequate. If the fluid is processed correctly and the smear is examined carefully, the Gram's stain of the CSF will reveal bacteria in 70% to 80% of patients with untreated meningitis; the sensitivity is reduced by about 20% in patients who have received antimicrobials. The value of the Gram's stain is also influenced by the etiologic agent; for example, the sensitivities of the test in patients infected with *Streptococcus pneumoniae, Haemophilus influenzae, Neisseria meningitidis,* and *L. monocytogenes* are approximately 90%, 85%, 75%, and 50%, respectively.

Several additional tests have been developed to allow rapid and specific diagnoses in patients with acute bacterial meningitis. The most useful and widely employed are assays that detect the presence of capsular polysaccharides of the bacteria commonly associated with the infection, including *S. pneumoniae, H. influenzae,* and *N. meningitidis.* Most hospital laboratories utilize the latex agglutination method. The bacterial antigen tests are rapid and specific, but they are less sensitive than cultures, and thus a negative assay result cannot be interpreted as excluding the presence of infection with one of the microbes noted. Other tests, such as a CSF lactate level, have been used to distinguish bacterial from nonbacterial meningitis; however, they lack the specificity to be employed routinely. Finally, recent observations have indicated that tests that assay for the presence of cytokines, such as tumor necrosis factor, may be reliable in differentiating bacterial from nonbacterial meningitis.

The CSF of patients with partially treated bacterial meningitis is characterized by a neutrophilic pleocytosis, hypoglycorrhachia, and an elevated protein. In many cases, the CSF cultures will be negative, but the immunologic assays for bacterial antigens will remain positive, allowing for a microbiologic diagnosis. These observations again emphasize the folly of withholding antimicrobial therapy in the patient with a presumed bacterial meningitis pending the results of CT or other tests; in short, if CSF is processed properly and if bacterial antigen tests are obtained, the ability to make a specific etiologic diagnosis will not be altered by a few doses of an antimicrobial.

### Acute Nonbacterial Meningitis

The CSF of patients with acute viral ("aseptic") meningitis usually contains fewer than 500 WBCs per cubic millimeter, a normal glucose, and an elevated protein. During the first 48 hours after presentation, the WBC differential can demonstrate a preponderance of neutrophils; however, serial lumbar punctures characteristically demonstrate the rapid conversion to a lymphocytosis. On occasion, viral meningitis may be associated with hypoglycorrhachia; however, the depression in the glucose level is usually mild. Syphilitic meningitis can present as an acute or subacute illness; the CSF usually demonstrates changes suggestive of a viral meningitis, although the glucose will be depressed in about 50% of cases. The diagnosis of syphilitic meningitis can be confirmed by blood and CSF serologies. The CSF abnormalities seen in patients with Lyme disease, which tends to present in subacute manner, are similar to those observed in patients with viral meningitis, although the number of cells tends to be lower (<100 WBCs per cubic millimeter); detection of antibodies to *B. burgdorferi* in the CSF is the usual method of diagnosis. Patients with meningitis caused by *M. tuberculosis* characteristically present with a chronic meningitis syndrome; however, the onset of tuberculous meningitis can be abrupt, and the clinical picture can be that of an acute aseptic meningitis. As noted above, the introduction of nucleic acid amplification assays should substantially enhance the ability of clinicians to diagnose rapidly the conditions traditionally characterized as causes of aseptic meningitis.

A number of noninfectious diseases can present with clinical manifestations and CSF findings suggestive of a viral meningitis; the noninfectious causes of aseptic meningitis include medications [trimethoprim-sulfamethoxazole, nonsteroidal antiinflammatory agents (ibuprofen, sulindac)], malignant diseases (lymphoma, carcinoma), tumors (craniopharyngioma, epidermoid cyst), and miscellaneous conditions, including systemic lupus erythematosus, sarcoidosis, Behçet's disease, and Mollaret's meningitis. Finally, in patients undergoing neurosurgery, especially that involving the posterior fossa, a postoperative aseptic meningitis can develop that is characterized by fever, headache, and neck stiffness. The CSF in the posterior fossa syndrome typically reveals 1,000 to 2,000 WBCs per cubic millimeter with a preponderance of neutrophils, a depressed glucose (<40 mg/dL), and an elevated protein; cultures of the CSF are sterile.

## Chronic Meningitis

The chronic meningitis syndrome is characterized by fever, lethargy, headache, nausea, vomiting, and nuchal rigidity; the patient is usually symptomatic for 1 to 4 weeks before presentation. The CSF typically reveals 100 to 400 WBCs per cubic millimeter with a preponderance of lymphocytes, a depressed glucose concentration, and a moderately or markedly elevated protein level. Patients with a chronic meningitis syndrome should be intensely studied for evidence of treatable infectious diseases, especially tuberculosis, cryptococcosis, coccidioidomycosis, syphilis, Lyme disease, toxoplasmosis, and brucellosis. It is important to emphasize that results of acid-fast stains of the CSF are positive in only 10% to 20% of patients with tuberculous meningitis and that cultures reveal the presence of *M. tuberculosis* in 60% to 80% of cases; to increase the likelihood of a positive result, some authorities recommend that 20 to 40 mL of CSF be submitted for smear and culture. In addition, CSF from patients with suspected tuberculosis but unrevealing smears should be sent to a reference laboratory performing an immunologic or nucleic acid amplification assay for the mycobacterium.

India ink preparations demonstrate *C. neoformans* in about 75% of patients with AIDS and 50% of other patients with meningitis caused by this fungus. Cultures will be positive for *C. neoformans* in 90% of cases, although multiple lumbar punctures may be necessary before the organism is isolated. Fortunately, cryptococcal antigen will be detectable in the CSF in more than 90% of patients, and thus the assay represents the most important test to screen for the presence of the organism. Rarely seen on the smear of CSF, *C. immitis* can be cultured from approximately 50% of patients with coccidioidal meningitis; however, results of the CSF complement fixation test are positive in about 75% to 95% of patients. As is true for patients with tuberculous meningitis, large volumes of CSF may be necessary to permit recovery of these fungi.

Serologic assays in concert with characteristic CSF findings represent the usual method of diagnosing infection caused by *T. pallidum*, *B. burgdorferi*, and *T. gondii;* however, PCR assays have been developed to detect these microbes, and CSF should be forwarded to the appropriate reference laboratory in difficult cases. A number of immunologic assays are being investigated to detect some of the pathogens associated with the chronic meningitis syndrome; for example, assays to detect antigens of *M. tuberculosis* have yielded promising results, with sensitivities of 50% to 80% and specificities greater than 90%. Finally, noninfectious diseases can also produce a chronic meningitis syndrome; these conditions include malignancy (carcinoma, lymphoma, leukemia), sarcoidosis, and vasculitis.

## Other Conditions

Patients with parameningeal infections, such as brain abscesses and epidural abscesses, often have abnormalities of the CSF, including a mixed neutrophilic and lymphocytic pleocytosis, a normal glucose, and an elevated protein. Bacterial antigen test results are negative and cultures are sterile unless the abscess has ruptured into the subarachnoid space. Because of the limited diagnostic utility of the CSF and the risk for herniation, patients suspected of having parameningeal infections should not undergo lumbar punctures. CT or MRI is most useful in confirming the diagnosis in these patients, and aerobic and anaerobic cultures obtained intraoperatively will provide the necessary microbiologic information.

The hallmark manifestations of a viral encephalitis include fever, headache, behavioral changes, speech disturbances, an altered level of consciousness, and perhaps seizures and focal neurologic signs, such as a hemiparesis. Herpes simplex is the most common cause of sporadic, acute encephalitis in the United States. The CSF in patients with herpes encephalitis usually demonstrates 10 to 1,000 WBCs per cubic millimeter (with a lymphocyte predominance), 10 or more RBCs per cubic millimeter, a normal glucose, and an elevated protein; the virus is rarely recoverable from the fluid. The diagnosis of herpes encephalitis is supported by an electroencephalographic, CT, or MRI study demonstrating involvement of the temporal regions of the brain. A definitive diagnosis has traditionally required a brain biopsy; however, PCR to identify viral DNA has been shown to be at least 90% sensitive and specific in patients with herpes encephalitis, and the assay is now widely available. Therapy with acyclovir must be started promptly in the patient suspected of having herpes encephalitis to increase the likelihood of a favorable outcome. (A.L.E.)

## Bibliography

Aharoni A, et al. Postpartum maternal group B meningitis. *Rev Infect Dis* 1990;12:273.
*Group B streptococci represent another bacterial pathogen capable of producing meningitis in fit adults, including postpartum women.*

Ahmed A, et al. Clinical utility of polymerase chain reaction for the diagnosis of enteroviral meningitis in infancy. *J Pediatr* 1997;131:393.
*In this prospective study of 64 infants less than 3 months of age, the authors found that PCR of the CSF was 92% sensitive and 94% specific in establishing a diagnosis of enteroviral meningitis.*

Arditi M, et al. Cerebrospinal fluid cachectin/tumor necrosis factor-$\alpha$ and platelet-activating factor concentrations and severity of bacterial meningitis in children. *J Infect Dis* 1990;162:139.
*In this prospective study, the authors found that CSF levels of tumor necrosis factor and platelet-activating factor in children with bacterial meningitis were correlated with severity of disease. They also noted that the presence of tumor necrosis factor in the CSF reliably distinguishes bacterial from viral meningitis.*

Aurelius E, et al. Rapid diagnosis of herpes simplex encephalitis by nested polymerase chain reaction assay of cerebrospinal fluid. *Lancet* 1991;337:189.
*PCR detected herpes simplex virus in the CSF of 42 of 43 patients with herpes encephalitis confirmed by brain biopsy or intrathecal antibody production, and the assay result was negative in each of the 60 controls who also had a febrile encephalopathy.*

Bailey EM, Domenico P, Cunha BA. Bacterial or viral meningitis? Measuring the CSF lactate can help you know quickly. *Postgrad Med* 1990;88:217.
*These authors conclude that the CSF lactate level represents a useful parameter for differentiating aseptic from bacterial meningitis.*

Berenguer J, et al. Tuberculous meningitis in patients infected with the human immunodeficiency virus. *N Engl J Med* 1992;326:668.
*The authors found that the clinical manifestations and CSF findings in HIV-infected patients with tuberculous meningitis are similar to those of non–HIV-infected patients.*

Berger JR. Neurosyphilis in human immunodeficiency virus type 1-seropositive individuals. A prospective study. *Arch Neurol* 1991;48:700.
*The author concludes that unsuspected neurosyphilis is relatively common in asymptomatic HIV-infected persons, and he recommends that the CSF be evaluated in all HIV-infected patients who have a history of syphilis or serologic evidence of syphilis, regardless of prior antimicrobial therapy.*

Bonadio WA, et al. Distinguishing cerebrospinal fluid abnormalities in children with bacterial meningitis and traumatic lumbar puncture. *J Infect Dis* 1990;162:251.
*The authors provide a rational means of evaluating CSF in children with traumatic lumbar punctures, noting that the diagnosis of bacterial meningitis should rarely be obscured by the presence of blood.*

Chalmers AC, Aprill BS, Shepard H. Cerebrospinal fluid and human immunodeficiency virus. Findings in healthy, asymptomatic seropositive men. *Arch Intern Med* 1990;150:1538.
*The authors detected a lymphocytic pleocytosis (5 to 44 cells per cubic millimeter) or an elevated protein level in the CSF of 48% of the 25 asymptomatic HIV-infected patients studied.*

Coyle PK, Dattwyler R. Spirochetal infection of the central nervous system. *Infect Dis Clin North Am* 1990;4:731.

*The authors review the neurologic manifestations of syphilis and Lyme disease and discuss the role that evaluation of the CSF plays in establishing a diagnosis of these treatable infections.*

Durand ML, et al. Acute bacterial meningitis in adults. A review of 493 episodes. *N Engl J Med* 1993;328:21.

*In this retrospective review of community-acquired and nosocomial bacterial meningitis, the authors found that the initial CSF cell count was below 100/mm³ in about 5% of patients and that the initial CSF glucose level was above 40 mg/dL in about 50% of patients. They also reported that 10% of positive CSF Gram's stains were misinterpreted and that the most common error was the misidentification of Listeria monocytogenes as Streptococcus pneumoniae.*

Girgis N, et al. Tuberculosis meningitis, Abbassia Fever Hospital-Naval Medical Research Unit No. 3, Cairo, Egypt, 1976–1996. *Am J Trop Med Hyg* 1998;58:28.

*In this retrospective review of 875 adult and pediatric patients, the authors make a number of notable observations, including the finding that the mortality and neurologic complication rates were correlated with the duration of symptoms before admission and the neurologic state at presentation. They also conclude that the use of dexamethasone was associated with a significantly reduced case fatality rate.*

Greenlee JE. Approach to diagnosis of meningitis. Cerebrospinal fluid evaluation. *Infect Dis Clin North Am* 1990;4:583.

*A comprehensive review of the use of the CSF in evaluating patients with a variety of infections of the CNS.*

Hansen K, Lebech AM. The clinical and epidemiological profile of Lyme neuroborreliosis in Denmark. A prospective study of 187 patients with *Borrelia burgdorferi*-specific intrathecal antibody production. *Brain* 1992;115:399.

*The authors describe the CSF profiles of patients with second-stage neuroborreliosis, emphasizing the paucity of clinical signs of meningitis despite the presence of substantial inflammatory changes in the fluid.*

Johns DR, Tierney M, Felsenstein D. Alteration in the natural history of neurosyphilis by concurrent infection with the human immunodeficiency virus. *N Engl J Med* 1987;316:1569.

*HIV-infected persons are at risk to experience acute meningitis syphilis following "adequate" treatment for early-stage disease with penicillin benzathine.*

Kuberski T. Eosinophils in the cerebrospinal fluid. *Ann Intern Med* 1979;91:70.

*A review of the many conditions producing eosinophils in the CSF.*

Lopez-Cortes LF, et al. Measurement of levels of tumor necrosis factor-α and interleukin-1β in the CSF of patients with meningitis of different etiologies: utility in differential diagnosis. *Clin Infect Dis* 1993;16:534.

*In this study of 125 patients with meningitis, 20 with other neurologic diseases, and 20 normal controls, the investigators found that elevated levels of tumor necrosis factor-α and interleukin-1β were highly correlated with the presence of bacterial meningitis.*

Marton KI, Gean AD. The spinal tap: a new look at an old test. *Ann Intern Med* 1986;104:840.

*The authors review the indications, risks, and diagnostic utility of a lumbar puncture.*

Mayefsky JH, Roghmann KJ. Determination of leukocytosis in traumatic spinal tap specimens. *Am J Med* 1987;82:1175.

*The authors conclude that the presence of more than 10 times the number of WBCs expected from a traumatic lumbar puncture specimen is a sensitive and specific indicator of meningitis. However, they caution that all clinical and laboratory data available should be considered when decisions are made about initiating antimicrobial therapy in patients with possible bacterial meningitis.*

Mayer SA, et al. Biopsy-proven isolated sarcoid meningitis. *J Neurosurg* 1993;78:994.

*The authors describe a young adult with a chronic, hypoglycorrhachic lymphocytic meningitis resulting from isolated neurosarcoidosis.*

Mouritsen CL, et al. Polymerase chain reaction detection of Lyme disease: correlation with clinical manifestations and serologic responses. *Am J Clin Pathol* 1996;105:647.

*The authors suggest that PCR analysis of the CSF is useful in the diagnosis of neuroborreliosis, especially in the absence of a serologic response.*

Porkert MT, et al. Tuberculous meningitis at a large inner-city medical center. *Am J Med Sci* 1997;313:325.

*In this retrospective review of 34 patients, the authors found that the infection among inner city residents was associated with a mortality rate of 41%, despite the fact that delays in diagnosis did not occur. They also noted that underlying infection with HIV did not substantially alter the clinical presentation or response to therapy.*

Powers WJ. Cerebrospinal fluid lymphocytosis in acute bacterial meningitis. *Am J Med* 1985; 79:216.

*Among 103 patients of all ages with bacterial meningitis, the CSF of 14 had more than 50% lymphocytes, and 13 of these 14 patients had cell counts under $1,000/mm^3$.*

Ragland AS, et al. Eosinophilic pleocytosis in coccidioidal meningitis: frequency and significance. *Am J Med* 1993;95:254.

*In a retrospective review of 27 cases, the authors noted that eight patients had an eosinophilic meningitis, defined as 10 or more eosinophils per cubic millimeter, and that an additional 11 patients had CSF containing a smaller number of eosinophils.*

Ross D, Rosegay H, Pons V. Differentiation of aseptic and bacterial meningitis in postoperative neurosurgical patients. *J Neurosurg* 1988;69:669.

*Based on a retrospective review of cases of postneurosurgical meningitis, the authors found that although the CSF WBC count tends to be higher in patients with bacterial infection, neither that test nor other laboratory parameters are sufficiently sensitive or specific to differentiate pyogenic from aseptic disease. The culture of CSF represented the only reliable method of identifying infected patients.*

Sharma OP, Sharma AM. Sarcoidosis of the nervous system. A clinical approach. *Arch Intern Med* 1991;151:1317.

*A comprehensive review of the clinical and CSF manifestations of neurosarcoidosis.*

Sotelo J, Guerrero V, Rubio F. Neurocysticercosis: a new classification based on active and inactive forms. A study of 753 cases. *Arch Intern Med* 1985;145:442.

*The CSF profile of patients with neurocysticercosis and inflammatory fluid includes eosinophils and, on occasion, hypoglycorrhachia.*

von Herbay A, et al. Whipple's disease: staging and monitoring by cytology and polymerase chain reaction analysis of cerebrospinal fluid. *Gastroenterology* 1997;113:434.

*Based on their experience with 24 patients infected with* Tropheryma whippelli, *the authors conclude that PCR testing of the CSF will prove very useful for the initial staging of Whipple's disease and for monitoring the efficacy of therapy.*

Weber T, et al. Clinical implications of nucleic acid amplification methods for the diagnosis of viral infections of the nervous system. *J Neurovirol* 1996;2:175.

*The authors provide a comprehensive review of the role of PCR techniques in the diagnosis of the various neurologic syndromes caused by herpes simplex virus, cytomegalovirus, varicella-zoster virus, Epstein-Barr virus, human herpesvirus type 6, HIV, enteroviruses, and other viral pathogens.*

Weller PF. Eosinophilic meningitis. *Am J Med* 1993;95:250.

*The author presents an extensive review of the infectious and noninfectious causes of an eosinophilic CSF pleocytosis, emphasizing the fact that parasites represent the most common causes of this finding.*

Yamamoto LJ, et al. Herpes simplex virus type 1 DNA in cerebrospinal fluid of a patient with Mollaret's meningitis. *N Engl J Med* 1991;325:1082.

*At least some cases of Mollaret's meningitis are caused by herpes simplex virus.*

---

## 31. CENTRAL NERVOUS SYSTEM INFECTIONS IN THE COMPROMISED HOST

---

The development of neurologic symptoms and signs in an immunosuppressed patient should alert the clinician to the possibility of an infectious etiology. When persons with AIDS are excluded, organ transplantation patients and persons with an underlying malignancy comprise those at risk for an often life-threatening central nervous system

(CNS) infection. In recent years, the incidence of CNS infection in transplant recipients has diminished because of the use of cyclosporine as the primary immunosuppressive agent. The mortality of CNS infection in immunocompromised hosts, however, ranges from 42% to 77%. Bacteria, fungi, viruses, and protozoa may be involved. Whereas the pneumococcus, meningococcus, or *Haemophilus influenzae* is responsible for 75% of cases of bacterial meningitis in patients with no underlying disease, the causal organisms differ widely in impaired hosts. The common bacterial agents in patients with lymphoma or leukemia are *Listeria monocytogenes,* gram-negative enteric rods, and the pneumococcus.

The predilection for fungal infections with *Cryptococcus, Aspergillus, Mucor,* and *Candida* species has also been emphasized. One study found that one third of patients had meningitis caused by fungi. Unusual organisms such as *Blastoschizomyces capitatus,* a fungus previously known as *Trichosporon,* may cause meningitis in bone marrow transplant recipients. In addition, viral agents such as varicella-zoster virus, herpes simplex virus, papovavirus, and measles virus should be considered, in addition to parasites, especially *Toxoplasma* and *Strongyloides.*

Progressive multifocal leukoencephalopathy, a subacute progressive demyelinating disease, is caused by the JC virus. Patients present with slowly progressive focal defects, which mimic those of a mass lesion. Diagnosis is suggested when magnetic resonance imaging shows a nonenhancing, low-density lesion of the white matter. A brain biopsy is required for definitive diagnosis. In the compromised host, the laboratory must be alerted to the possibility of a common as well as an obscure cause. The differential diagnosis should also include noninfectious problems that may mimic infectious meningitis or a brain abscess, such as carcinomatous or lymphomatous meningitis, cerebral hemorrhage, and adverse reactions to chemotherapeutic agents.

The importance of suspecting an intracranial infection in this group of patients is critical, as the majority of infections are diagnosed only at autopsy and are largely caused by unrecognized fungi. The diagnosis is difficult because the symptoms and signs are often attributed to the patient's underlying disease rather than to a possibly new infectious complication. The clinical features may be subtle, but headache and fever are usually present, even in patients receiving corticosteroids or other immunosuppressive agents. The patient's consciousness will usually be altered at the onset or shortly after admission. Nuchal rigidity is reported in only one third of patients. Seizures may occur, and focal neurologic findings may also be present. One report noted that cerebral metastasis was the most frequent initial diagnosis in patients with CNS infections. Thus, minimal findings of headache and fever in a compromised host should elicit a search to exclude a possible CNS infection.

Cerebrospinal fluid (CSF) analysis is a valuable aid to establishing an etiologic diagnosis. A lumbar puncture should not be performed in patients with a suspected cerebral mass lesion. An elevated pressure, pleocytosis, elevated protein, and low sugar may be found. However, the absence of cells in the CSF does not exclude an infection, and Gram's stain, acid-fast stain, India ink preparation, serologic studies for *Cryptococcus* (latex agglutination test), polymerase chain reaction for suspected pathogen, and appropriate cultures are indicated. A differential cell count showing a predominance of mononuclear cells suggests *Cryptococcus, Listeria, Mycobacterium,* or *Toxoplasma.* An eosinophilic pleocytosis of the CSF rarely occurs and usually indicates a helminthic parasitic infection or lymphoma.

Clues to the specific opportunistic pathogen may be present. *Cryptococcus* has a predilection for patients with lymphomas (impaired cellular immunity). A pulmonary infiltrate, skin lesions, and positive blood or urine cultures are occasionally noted. Other fungi, such as *Aspergillus, Mucor,* and *Candida,* are more difficult to identify, as antemortem cultures will frequently be negative. Fever and a pulmonary infiltrate in a patient with leukemia or a lymphoma unresponsive to broad-spectrum antimicrobial agents suggest a fungal disease. Neurologic involvement usually indicates a disseminated infection.

Of the bacterial opportunists, *Listeria* has a predilection for hosts with impaired T-cell function, such as renal transplant recipients or those with a lymphoma. Whereas most cases of *Listeria* infection are sporadic and the route of infection remains unknown, food-borne outbreaks related to contaminated milk, ice cream, cheese, and coleslaw have been reported. These gram-positive rods may at times appear as gram-positive cocci or be confused with diphtheroids. Patients infected with *Nocardia,* another opportunistic agent, may present with pulmonary, neurologic, and, less often, skin involvement. Gram-negative enteric bacilli may cause hospital-acquired meningitis in patients with acute leukemia and granulocytopenia. Toxoplasmosis is a treatable parasitic infection that presents with any one of three patterns of CNS involvement: (a) diffuse encephalopathy with or without seizures, (b) meningoencephalitis, or (c) single or multiple mass lesions. The diagnosis may be established by noting a fourfold rise in *Toxoplasma* titer on a serologic test, such as the indirect fluorescent antibody titer, or by detecting IgM antibody with an enzyme-linked immunosorbent assay (ELISA). IgM antibody usually disappears in a few months, whereas IgG antibody persists for life. Toxoplasmosis can also be diagnosed with polymerase chain reaction testing of blood or CSF. Finally, a clue to histoplasmosis, coccidioidomycosis, or *Strongyloides* infection may be a history of residence in an endemic area. (N.M.G.)

## Bibiliography

Adair JC, et al. Aseptic meningitis following cardiac transplantation: clinical characteristics and relationship to immunosuppressive regimen. *Neurology* 1991;41:249.
*A neurologic disorder was associated with the use of OKT3 monoclonal antibody. Symptoms resolved within 2 to 5 days of onset without residual defects.*

Armstrong RW, Fung PC. Brainstem encephalitis (rhombencephalitis) due to *Listeria monocytogenes:* case report and review. *Clin Infect Dis* 1993;16:689–702.
*A rare cause of encephalitis in usually normal hosts. Diagnosis was difficult because the blood cultures were positive in only 61% of cases and the CSF in 41%.*

Arnold SJ, et al. Disseminated toxoplasmosis. Unusual presentations in the immunocompromised host. *Arch Pathol Lab Med* 1997;121:869–873.
*In patients with disseminated toxoplasmosis,* Toxoplasma *tachyzoites can be seen by using a Wright's stain on the peripheral blood buffy coat smear.*

Arribas JR, et al. Cytomegalovirus encephalitis. *Ann Intern Med* 1996;125:577–587.
*Diagnosis is usually made by using polymerase chain reaction on CSF, whereas viral cultures are often negative.*

Bayer AS, et al. *Candida* meningitis. Report of seven cases and review of the English literature. *Medicine (Baltimore)* 1976;55:477.
*Meningitis is an infrequent complication of disseminated candidiasis.*

Boes B, et al. Central nervous system aspergillosis. Analysis of 26 patients. *J Neuroimaging* 1994;4:123–129.
*Most cases occurred in the setting of disseminated disease. Amphotericin B was not effective.*

Butler WT, et al. Diagnostic and prognostic value of clinical and laboratory findings in cryptococcal meningitis. *N Engl J Med* 1964;270:59.
*The cell count was abnormal in 97% of patients, protein was elevated in 90%, CSF pressure was increased in 64%, and low sugar was found in 55%.*

Chernik N, Armstrong D, Posner JB. Central nervous system infections in patients with cancer. *Medicine (Baltimore)* 1973;52:563.
*An extensive review. In patients with lymphoma, the three most frequent causes of CNS infection were* Cryptococcus, Listeria, *and pneumococci.*

Chernik NL, Armstrong D, Posner JB. Central nervous system infections in patients with cancer. Changing patterns. *Cancer* 1977;40:268.
*A decline in the incidence of cryptococcal meningitis and an increase in* Listeria *meningitis are reported.*

Choucino C, et al. Nocardial infections in bone marrow transplant recipients. *Clin Infect Dis* 1996;23:1012–1019.
*Soil exposure may be a risk factor. Thirty percent of patients had lesions on computed tomography of the head.*

Denning DW. Diagnosis and management of invasive aspergillosis. In: Remington JS, Swartz MN, eds. *Current clinical topics in infectious diseases.* Boston: Blackwell Science, 19 :277–299.
*In liver transplant recipients,* Aspergillus *is the most common cause of brain abscess, which is usually fatal.*

Denning DW, et al. NIAID Mycoses Study Group multicenter trial of oral itraconazole therapy for invasive aspergillosis. *Am J Med* 1994;97:135–144.
*Itraconazole is an alternative drug for invasive aspergillosis, with a response rate of 39%.*

Deresinski SC, Stevens DA. Coccidioidomycosis in compromised hosts. Experience at Stanford University Hospital. *Medicine (Baltimore)* 1974;54:377.
*Disseminated disease with pulmonary and neurologic involvement can develop in immunosuppressed patients. (See also Meyer RD, et al. An orthotopic heart transplant recipient with subacute meningitis. Rev Infect Dis 1991;13:513.)*

Diamond RD, Bennett JE. Prognostic factors in cryptococcal meningitis. A study of 111 cases. *Ann Intern Med* 1974;80:176.
*A discussion of risk factors associated with the failure of antifungal therapy or relapse. A CSF cryptococcal antigen titer of 1:32 or higher is a poor prognostic sign.*

Drancourt M, et al. Brain abscess due to *Gordona terrae* in an immunocompromised child: case report and review of infections caused by *G. terrae. Clin Infect Dis* 1994;19:258–262.
*A gram-positive coccobacillus is a rare cause of a brain abscess.*

Ellner JJ, Bennett JE. Chronic meningitis. *Medicine (Baltimore)* 1976;55:341.
*The differential diagnosis is reviewed.*

Elmore JG, Horwitz RI, Quagliarello VJ. Acute meningitis with a negative Gram's stain: clinical and management outcomes in 171 episodes. *Am J Med* 1996;100:78–84.
*A cause was identified in only 23% of cases, with transverse myelitis and malignancy being the most frequent.*

Enzmann DR, Brant-Zawadzki M, Britt RH. CT of central nervous system infections in immunocompromised patients. *AJR Am J Roentgenol* 1980;135:263.
*Contrast enhancement may not occur in the compromised host. The etiology could not be predicted by the CT findings.*

Frazier AR, Rosenow EC III, Roberts GD. Nocardiosis. A review of 25 cases occurring during 24 months. *Mayo Clin Proc* 1975;50:657.
*A sputum culture for* Nocardia *may reflect colonization.*

Gantz NM, et al. Listeriosis in immunosuppressed patients. A cluster of eight cases. *Am J Med* 1975;58:637.
*Meningitis may occur with only minimal signs and symptoms.*

Goodman JS, Kaufman L, Koenig G. Diagnosis of cryptococcal meningitis. Value of immunologic detection of cryptococcal antigens. *N Engl J Med* 1971;285:434.
*Results of the latex agglutination test for cryptococcal antigen may be positive in patients with negative India ink preparations.*

Green M, et al. Aspergillosis of the CNS in a pediatric liver transplant recipient: case report and review. *Rev Infect Dis* 1991;13:653.
*An unexplained CNS infarct resulting in a focal seizure may be a clue to* Aspergillus *infection of the CNS in a high-risk patient.*

Greenlee JE. Progressive multifocal leukoencephalopathy. In: Remington JS, Swartz MN, eds. *Current clinical topics in infectious diseases.* Boston: Blackwell Science, 1989:140.
*Magnetic resonance imaging is the diagnostic method of choice and will show areas of increased signal, indicative of demyelination, in the white matter.*

Griffin JW, et al. Lymphomatous leptomeningitis. *Am J Med* 1971;51:200.
*Cytologic study of the CSF may reveal the cause of cranial nerve palsies, headache, and papilledema in a patient with lymphoma.*

Hall WA. Neurosurgical infections in the compromised host. *Neurosurg Clin North Am* 1992;3:435.
*Review.*

Hall WA, et al. Central nervous system infections in heart and heart-lung transplant recipients. *Arch Neurol* 1989;46:173.
*Meningitis was caused by* Listeria *and* Cryptococcus; Aspergillus, Nocardia, *and* Candida *were involved in patients with a brain abscess.*

Heegaard ED, Peterslund NA, Hornsleth A. Parvovirus B19 infection associated with encephalitis in a patient suffering from malignant lymphoma. *Scand J Infect Dis* 1995;27:631–633.
*A rare cause of encephalitis.*

Hooper DC, Pruitt AA, Rubin RH. Central nervous system infection in the chronically immunosuppressed. *Medicine (Baltimore)* 1982;61:166.
*Review. The most common presenting features were fever (78%) and headache (58%). Meningismus was present in only about 25% of patients.*

Jabbour N, et al. Cryptococcal meningitis after liver transplantation. *Transplantation* 1996;61:146–149.
*In liver transplant recipients, headache, fever, and mental status changes occurred most often; meningismus was found in only 30%.*

Louria DB, et al. Listeriosis complicating malignant disease. *Ann Intern Med* 1967;67:261.
*The most common manifestation is bacteremia or meningitis, or both.*

Lukes SA, et al. Bacterial infections of the CNS in neutropenic patients. *Neurology* 1984;34:269.
*Mental status changes (93%) and fever (95%) are common. Seizures were noted in 40% of patients. Platelet transfusions should be given to patients with thrombocytopenia before a lumbar puncture.*

Meyer RD, et al. Aspergillosis complicating neoplastic disease. *Am J Med* 1973;54:6.
*The characteristic clinical features are fever and pulmonary infiltrates, with no response to antimicrobials; CNS findings are usually caused by multiple brain abscesses.*

Murray JF, et al. The changing spectrum of nocardiosis. *Am Rev Respir Dis* 1961;83:315.
*Nocardia is a branching, filamentous, gram-positive, weakly acid-fast organism that causes necrosis and abscess formation but not granulomas.*

Narayan O, et al. Etiology of progressive multifocal leukoencephalopathy. Identification of papovavirus. *N Engl J Med* 1973;289:1278.
*This subacute demyelinating disease occurs in the compromised host, especially in patients with lymphoma.*

Pagano L, et al. Localization of aspergillosis to the central nervous system among patients with acute leukemia: report of 14 cases. *Clin Infect Dis* 1996;23:628–630.
*Primary focus of infection is the lungs. Death occurred usually within 5 days of onset of neurologic symptoms.*

Palmer DL, Harvey RL, Wheeler JK. Diagnostic and therapeutic considerations in *Nocardia asteroides* infection. *Medicine (Baltimore)* 1974;53:391.
*The lungs are the most frequent primary site (in 73%), with the nervous system the most commonly involved secondary site (23%).*

Perfect JR. Fungal meningitis. In: Scheld WM, Whitley RJ, Durack DT, eds. *Infections of the central nervous system.* New York: Lippincott–Raven Publishers, 1997:721–739.
*Review. Fungal meningitis must also be considered in a patient with chronic meningitis.*

Pruitt AA. Central nervous system infections in cancer patients. *Neurol Clin* 1991;9:867.
*Review.*

Rodriguez JC, et al. Evaluation of different techniques in the diagnosis of *Toxoplasma* encephalitis. *J Med Microbiol* 1997;46:597–601.
*Polymerase chain reaction on CSF had a sensitivity of 81% in the diagnosis of Toxoplasma encephalitis in untreated patients and of only 20% in treated patients.*

Ruskin J, Remington JS. Toxoplasmosis in the compromised host. *Ann Intern Med* 1976;84:193.
*A review. Neurologic manifestations predominate in more than half the patients.*

Salaki JS, Louria DB, Chmel H. Fungal and yeast infections of the central nervous system: a clinical review. *Medicine (Baltimore)* 1984;63:108.
*Review.*

Schuchat A, Swaminathan B, Broome CV. Epidemiology of human listeriosis. *Clin Microbiol Rev* 1991;4:169.
*Food-borne sources may be responsible for outbreaks.*

Skogberg K, et al. Clinical presentation and outcome of listeriosis in patients with and without immunosuppressive therapy. *Clin Infect Dis* 1992;14:815.
*Bacteremia and meningitis were the two most common clinical forms of the disease. Mortality was 32% in patients with any underlying illness.*

Stamm AM, et al. Listeriosis in renal transplant recipients: report of an outbreak and review of 102 cases. *Rev Infect Dis* 1982;4:665.
  *Onset often occurs shortly after transplantation.*
Stone MM, et al. Brief report: meningitis due to iatrogenic BCG infection in two immunocompromised children. *N Engl J Med* 1995;333:561–563.
  *A rare cause of meningitis—the accidental intrathecal inoculation of bacillus Calmette-Guérin.*
Strayer DR, Bender RA. Eosinophilic meningitis complicating Hodgkin's disease. *Cancer* 1977;40:406.
  *A case report and differential diagnosis.*
Tabacof J, et al. *Strongyloides* hyperinfection in two patients with lymphoma, purulent meningitis, and sepsis. *Cancer* 1991;68:1821.
  Strongyloides *can be the underlying cause of a gram-negative bacteremia or CNS infection in a patient with lymphoma.*
Thaelkeld SC, Hooper DC. Update on management of patients with *Nocardia* infections. In: Remington JS, Swartz MN, eds. *Current clinical topics in infectious diseases.* Boston: Blackwell Science, 1997:1–23.
  *Review. For disseminated infection, treat for 6 months to 1 year.*
Tunkel AR, Scheld WM. Central nervous system infection in the immunocompromised host. In: Rubin RH, Young S, eds. *Clinical approach to infection in the compromised host,* 3rd ed. New York: Plenum Publishing, 1994:163–210.
  *Comprehensive review.*
Van der Horst CM, et al. Treatment of cryptococcal meningitis associated with the acquired immunodeficiency syndrome. National Institute of Allergy and Infectious Diseases Mycoses Study Group and AIDS Clinical Trials Group. *N Engl J Med* 1997;337:15–21.
  *Use of higher-dose amphotericin B (0.7mg/kg daily) plus flucytosine was associated with an improved outcome compared with lower-dose amphotericin B (0.4mg/kg daily).*
White M, et al. Cryptococcal meningitis: outcome in patients with AIDS and patients with neoplastic disease. *J Infect Dis* 1992;165:960.
  *In this small study, the outcome of cryptococcal meningitis in patients with AIDS was better than in those with underlying neoplastic disease.*
Wilfert CM, et al. Persistent and fatal central nervous system echovirus infections in patients with agammaglobulinemia. *N Engl J Med* 1977;296:1486.
  *Enteroviral infections can be fatal in immunodeficient persons.*
Wilson JP, et al. Nocardial infections in renal transplant recipients. *Medicine (Baltimore)* 1989;68:38.
  *Review. CNS involvement was noted in 16% of patients.*
Winston DJ, Emmanouilides C, Busuttil RW. Infections in liver transplant recipients. *Clin Infect Dis* 1995;21:1077–1091.
  Aspergillus *is the most frequent cause of infection of the central nervous system in liver transplant recipients. Bacterial meningitis is rare, but consider* Listeria.

## 32. NEW ONSET OF FACIAL PARALYSIS

Cranial nerve VII (the facial nerve) is subject to numerous insults that include infection, trauma, and malignancy. Involvement may be unilateral or bilateral, and onset of symptoms is variable. The clinician must be aware of important treatable causes, so that "idiopathic" disease (Bell's palsy) is not overdiagnosed. Anatomic features of the facial nerve with important clinical implications include the fallopian canal and the labyrinthine, geniculate, tympanic, mastoid, and extracranial segments. An understanding of the anatomic relationship between this rather long nerve and the surrounding structures is invaluable for determining likely causes of disease.

Additionally, the facial nerve has three branches (greater superficial petrosal, stapedius, and chorda tympani) with specific functions. An understanding of these functions and the anatomic location of the branches provides clinical information useful in determining the location of lesions and possible etiologies. Idiopathic (Bell's) palsy continues to account for more than 50% of cases of acute facial paralysis, and the most important initial clinical decision is to determine the need for testing beyond the usual care for patients with presumed idiopathic disease. Furthermore, recent data suggest that many cases of acute idiopathic facial nerve paralysis may be associated with herpes simplex virus; this has important implications for management.

## Clinical Evaluation

Facial paralysis is heralded by the inability to move one or both sides of the face. Clinical evaluation must include a complete history and physical examination, with special attention to a comprehensive neurologic examination. Points to be noted on history include rapidity of onset, association with pain, presence of other neurologic and physical complaints, and any recent travel, trauma, vaccinations, or animal exposures. A careful sexual history regarding syphilis and assessment for risk factors for HIV infection is always indicated. Physical examination must be comprehensive and include observations for rash, disease of the head and neck, and neurologic dysfunction. Decisions should be made about the extent of cranial nerve disease, with careful attention to central versus peripheral location of the facial nerve paralysis. The eyes must be carefully examined for corneal ulceration. A decision regarding further testing is based on the likelihood of nonidiopathic disease. Additional studies could include standard blood tests, serologies, computed tomography and magnetic resonance imaging, lumbar puncture, and specific neurologic testing (Schirmer's test, stapedial reflex, taste/salivation, and electric stimulation); however, these are not usually indicated.

## Idiopathic (Bell's) Palsy

Bell's palsy affects 15 to 40 people per 100,000 population, has no predilection for age or race, is a diagnosis of exclusion, and causes more than 50% of cases of acute facial nerve paralysis. There is compelling evidence that many cases are mediated by viral or immunologic mechanisms, and significant attention has been given to the role of herpesvirus. It has been demonstrated that herpes simplex virus is capable of inducing facial paralysis in animals. A recent investigation of 14 patients with Bell's palsy demonstrated that genomes of type 1 herpes simplex virus were detectable in clinical samples of endoneural fluid from cranial nerve VII in 79% of cases, but none of the controls. The authors concluded that herpes simplex virus type 1 was the major etiologic agent for idiopathic facial nerve paralysis. Others have suggested that Bell's palsy be renamed herpetic facial paralysis.

In typical cases, symptoms develop during less than 48 hours, and disease is unilateral. Pain or numbness of the affected area is seen in up to 50% of cases, and approximately 60% of patients note a viral prodrome. Fewer than 15% of patients give a history of recurrence or a family history of similar disease. Up to 13% of patients initially identified with idiopathic facial paralysis will be misdiagnosed. Most common alternatives are tumor, herpes zoster ophthalmicus, and identifiable infection. Physical examination demonstrates evidence of diminished stapedial reflex (90%), and a reddened chorda tympani nerve (40%) is often noted. History and physical examination are otherwise benign. The course of Bell's palsy is self-limited and nonprogressive, with a return of function within 6 weeks in most cases. Occasionally, improvement may take up to 1 year. Atypical Bell's palsy occurs when the clinical course persists for more than 1 year in the absence of other causes. Other causes of acute facial paralysis should be considered when factors other than those already noted are present: (a) positive epidemiologic history (Lyme borreliosis, syphilis, HIV infection), (b) neurologic dysfunction beyond the isolated seventh peripheral cranial nerve, (c) bilateral disease, (d) physical findings outside the nervous system, and (e) failure to improve.

The treatment of idiopathic facial nerve palsy is controversial. Patients need to be reassured about the self-limited nature of the disease and the fact that they have not suffered a "stroke." Eye care may be needed to prevent abrasion or ulceration. Artificial tears and taping of the eye at night can help greatly. The combination of corticosteroids plus acyclovir was recently compared with corticosteroids alone. Patients treated with acyclovir received 400 mg five times daily. Outcome measures were return of volitional muscle motion and prevention of partial nerve degeneration. Patients who received acyclovir improved faster than those who received only corticosteroids, indirectly implying the importance of herpes simplex virus in etiology. Hyperbaric oxygen therapy has recently been studied as another therapy for Bell's palsy. Patients were randomized to either hyperbaric oxygen therapy (two treatments daily, 5 days per week) or prednisone therapy. Patients treated with hyperbaric oxygen therapy had an average time to complete recovery of 22 days, in comparison with 34 days in those treated with corticosteroids. The authors concluded that hyperbaric oxygen therapy is more effective than corticosteroids. Surgical decompression is rarely indicated for idiopathic disease but is indicated for progression associated with neurologic degeneration. This author recommends acyclovir plus prednisone for therapy of acute Bell's palsy. The dose of prednisone is 60 to 80 mg daily for 5 days, with tapering over the next 5 days.

### Acute Facial Paralysis of Other Infectious Causes
Infection accounts for 4% of cases of facial nerve disorders. Table 32-1 depicts possible infectious etiologies. Lyme borreliosis is becoming the most important and treatable cause of acute facial paralysis. In up to 20% of persons, neurologic dysfunction develops following the bite of an infected tick. Facial paralysis, which is often bilateral, develops in at least 10% of persons with Lyme borreliosis. Recent studies of apparent idiopathic acute facial nerve paralysis have demonstrated serologic evidence of Lyme borreliosis in up to 16% of cases. This is more common in children and is more likely to occur during the months when Lyme disease is prevalent. Facial paralysis may be the sole presenting feature and may occur in the absence of a history of erythema migrans or tick bite. However, facial palsy often is noted as a manifestation of early disease, with an average of only 20 days between onset of erythema migrans and neurologic dysfunction.

Lyme disease should be considered in young persons with acute facial paralysis, especially if bilateral or associated with a positive epidemiologic history. Additional features on physical examination include painless facial erythema and swelling preceding paralysis, and associated seventh nerve abnormalities. Serologic confirmation should be sought but results may be negative early in disease or if testing is performed only by enzyme-linked immunosorbent assay (ELISA). The outcome of isolated facial palsy is generally favorable, with better than 95% recovery with or without treatment. Long-term outcome, even in the absence of treatment, remains good. I believe that all suspected cases should be treated with antibiotics. Isolated seventh nerve palsy can be managed with oral doxycycline (100 mg twice daily for at least 21 days). The presence

Table 32-1. Infectious etiologies for acute facial paralysis

| More common | Less common |
| --- | --- |
| Herpes simplex virus | *Mycobacterium leprae* |
| Lyme borreliosis | *Mycobacterium tuberculosis* |
| Epstein-Barr virus | Mucormycosis |
| Varicella-zoster virus | Cat scratch disease |
| Acute otitis media | Malaria |
| Mastoiditis | Enterovirus |
| HIV | Vaccination* |
| Syphilis | Toxins** |
| | *Mycoplasma pneumoniae* |
| | Viral encephalitis |
| | Mumps |

* Viral influenza, poliomyelitis, rabies, tetanus.
** Diphtheria, botulinism.

of other involvement of the central nervous system warrants parenteral treatment with either ceftriaxone (2 g intravenously for 14 days) or aqueous penicillin G (20 million units intravenously for 14 days). There is no identified role for corticosteroids.

Syphilis should be considered in patients with a positive epidemiologic history and in those with either atypical Bell's palsy or associated neurologic dysfunction. Facial nerve palsy is most commonly associated with secondary syphilis but may also be noted in tertiary disease. Presentation may be unilateral or bilateral and is often associated with involvement of other cranial nerves. Aseptic meningitis is often apparent. Diagnosis can be confirmed by serologic testing, and therapy is generally initiated with 2.4 million units of benzathine penicillin units weekly for 3 weeks.

Viral agents other than herpes simplex virus regularly associated with acute facial paralysis include Epstein-Barr virus (EBV) and HIV. Up to 20% of cases of Bell's palsy may actually be associated with EBV on comprehensive testing, and other symptoms of mononucleosis may be lacking. Paralysis may be unilateral or bilateral and may be the presenting symptom. Most commonly, however, other manifestations of EBV infection are apparent. Diagnosis can usually be made by "monospot" testing in early disease, and in about 5% of all cases, more specific EBV serology will be necessary. Therapy is supportive, but the role of specific antiviral agents is being evaluated. Clinical response to supportive care is usually complete, and residua are unusual.

Acute facial paralysis, either unilateral or bilateral, may be a manifestation of acute HIV infection, occurring within 3 months of contraction of the virus. In this regard, it is most often seen as part of an acute mononucleosis-like syndrome. Aseptic meningitis is often noted clinically and on lumbar puncture. A complete epidemiologic history that incorporates questions about HIV risk is mandatory, and diagnosis can be confirmed by HIV testing. In early HIV disease, results of standard ELISA testing may be negative, and follow-up testing is indicated. Treatment is supportive, and the facial palsy usually resolves spontaneously within several weeks.

Varicella-zoster virus has been associated with unilateral acute facial paralysis. Although rare, disease has occurred in the absence of vesiculation. However, most cases are associated with a characteristic rash that may lag behind pain and paralysis by more than 1 week. The most characteristic form of herpes zoster associated with facial palsy, Ramsay Hunt syndrome, is characterized by severe pain about the ear; vesicles on the tympanic membrane, external canal, and external ear; hyperacusis; and vertigo. Sensorineural hearing loss may be noted in up to 40% of cases. Recurrences are more likely to be caused by herpes simplex. Acyclovir is indicated in severe cases and recurrences, and in patients with underlying diseases. The typical dosage is 200 mg 5 times daily for 7 days (herpes simplex) or 800 mg 5 times daily for 7 days (herpes zoster).

Cases of acute unilateral facial paralysis with bacterial causes are uncommon. Most likely are complications of otitis media or mastoiditis; both of these are caused by local compression of the facial nerve. Initial clinical assessment generally demonstrates the underlying cause of the facial paralysis. Otitis media now appears to be less commonly associated with facial palsy than in the pre-antibiotic era. Risk for this complication is higher in adults with otitis media than in children. Remission of facial paralysis is directly related to severity at time of presentation. Therapy is aimed at the underlying disease.

Uncommonly, acute bilateral facial paralysis is associated with botulism or tetanus toxins. Generally, disease will be suspected by the entire clinical syndrome, and response of the paralysis is predicated on overall clinical improvement. Similarly, facial paralysis may occur as an adverse event following vaccination with various agents, including those of poliomyelitis, viral influenza, tetanus, and rabies. Diagnosis is suspected by careful history taking, and improvement is generally noted.

## Acute Facial Paralysis of Noninfectious Causes

Noninfectious causes of acute facial paralysis are summarized in Table 32-2. Congenital, traumatic, malignant, toxic, and metabolic etiologies exist and are usually accompanied by other manifestations of the underlying abnormality. Systemic illnesses that include leukemia, toxicosis, sarcoidosis, and vasculitis may present bilaterally; solid tumors and idiopathic disease are most commonly unilateral.

Table 32-2.  Noninfectious causes of acute facial paralysis

| | |
|---|---|
| Multiple sclerosis | Thalidomide |
| Autoimmune disease | Diabetes mellitus |
| Sarcoidosis | Hyperthyroidism |
| Periarteritis nodosa | Acute porphyria |
| Neoplasia | Congenital/traumatic |
|   Benign parotid lesions |   Basal skull fracture |
|   Cholesteatoma |   Facial fracture |
|   Sarcoma |   Penetrating middle ear injury |
|   Metastatic carcinoma |   Möbius' syndrome |
|   Leukemia |   Barotrauma |
|   Meningioma | |
| Vitamin A deficiency | (Iatrogenic) |
| |   Local anesthesia |
| |   Parotid surgery |
| |   Arterial embolization |

Adapted from May M, Klein SR. Differential diagnosis of facial nerve palsy. *Otolaryngol Clin North Am* 1991; 24:613–645.

**Summary**

The numerous causes of acute facial nerve paralysis include several important infections. Bell's palsy is now most commonly associated with herpes simplex virus and can be successfully treated. Careful history and physical examination are mandatory to identify clues necessary to differentiate it from facial nerve paralysis of other causes. Many laboratory tests are available to help with this decision-making process but should be used judiciously. The most notable infectious etiologies are Lyme borreliosis, HIV infection, syphilis, and mononucleosis. Bacterial etiologies are infrequent, but otitis media may be noted in some cases. (R.B.B.)

**Bibliography**

Adour KK, et al. Bell's palsy treatment with acyclovir and prednisone compared with prednisone alone; a double-blind, randomized, controlled trial. *Ann Otol Rhinol Laryngol* 1996;105:371–378.
*Sophisticated testing was used to compare outcomes in two groups of patients who had Bell's palsy treated with prednisone with or without acyclovir. Those who received acyclovir had a more rapid return of function. The authors conclude that this study provides further indirect evidence of the role of herpes simplex virus as the major cause of idiopathic facial paralysis.*
Ellefsen B, Bonding P. Facial palsy in acute otitis media. *Clin Otolaryngol* 1996; 21:393–395.
*The authors identified 23 patients with facial paralysis associated with acute otitis media. The process was more common in adults, and the frequency appears to have decreased from that of the pre-antibiotic era. Severity of initial presentation correlated with time to resolution.*
Gates GA. Facial paralysis. *Otolaryngol Clin North Am* 1987;20:113–131.
*Excellent discussion of the anatomy and physiology of the facial nerve. Also provides a reasonable approach to the history, physical examination, and laboratory testing useful in differential diagnosis. Includes some information concerning general medical and surgical management considerations.*
Luft BJ, et al. Invasion of the central nervous system by *Borrelia burgdorferi* in acute disseminated infection. *JAMA* 1992;267:1364–1367.
*This study documents early central nervous system invasion by the etiologic agent of Lyme borreliosis in patients with evidence of early infection. Clinical evidence of central nervous system disease was lacking in several patients studied. The article pro-*

*vides food for thought about the potential importance of early parenteral therapy for selected patients.*

May M, Klein SR. Differential diagnosis of facial nerve palsy. *Otolaryngol Clin North Am* 1991;24:613–645.

*Excellent review of the varied causes of facial nerve paralysis that takes into account the large personal experience of one physician. Describes characteristic presentation of typical and atypical idiopathic (Bell's) facial palsy and provides good charts indicating probable causes based on anatomic location of the lesion. Includes 136 references.*

Morgan M, Nathwani D. Facial palsy and infection: the unfolding story. *Clin Infect Dis* 1992;14:263–271.

*Reviews demographics of idiopathic facial paralysis (Bell's palsy) and provides data concerning possible infectious causes of this illness. Includes an excellent section on Lyme borreliosis as a cause of facial palsy and contains 116 references.*

Murakami S, et al. Bell palsy and herpes simplex virus: identification of viral DNA in endoneural fluid and muscle. *Ann Intern Med* 1996;124:63–65.

*The authors studied 14 patients who had presumed idiopathic facial paralysis with comparators that included the presence of Ramsay Hunt syndrome and others. Seventy-nine percent of patients with idiopathic disease were noted to have genomes of herpes simplex virus in endoneural fluid, compared with none of the controls. The authors conclude that most cases of Bell's palsy are caused by herpes simplex virus.*

Racic G, et al. Hyperbaric oxygen as a therapy of Bell's palsy. *Undersea Hyperb Med* 1997;24:35–38.

*The authors conducted a randomized trial of hyperbaric oxygen therapy versus prednisone for Bell's palsy. Neither group received antiviral medication. Long-term outcome, primarily measured as time to complete recovery, was better in those who received hyperbaric oxygen therapy. Given the recent, rather convincing data demonstrating the role of herpes simplex virus and the good outcomes with acyclovir plus prednisone, this modality is unlikely to capture a large following.*

---

## 33. ACUTE INFECTIONS OF THE CENTRAL NERVOUS SYSTEM

---

Infections of the central nervous system (CNS) are associated with mortality and neurologic sequelae. Many are treatable by medical or combined medical and surgical measures. Invasive techniques may also play a diagnostic role. Acute CNS infections can be categorized as meningitis, encephalitis, or mass lesions (Table 33-1). They may differ significantly in clinical presentation, bacteriology, and clinical and laboratory assessment.

### Initial Evaluation

Table 33-2 presents recommendations for the initial evaluation of patients with acute CNS infections. Most patients present with a history of headache and fever. Nausea and vomiting are frequent complaints. The history provides data about the acuteness of presentation, acquisition status (e.g., community or nosocomial), and associated complaints. An epidemiologic history must be obtained, with attention to travel, animal and insect exposures, HIV risks, and recent immunizations. Intrathecal contrast dyes, ibuprofen, and antimicrobials such as trimethoprim-sulfamethoxazole (TMP-SMX) and isoniazid can cause acute meningeal reactions in the absence of infection. Knowledge of underlying illness provides important information about potential pathogens. Alcoholism (*Streptococcus pneumoniae, Listeria monocytogenes*), T cell-mediated immunosuppression such as AIDS (*Toxoplasma gondii, Cryptococcus neoformans*), cerebrospinal fluid (CSF) leaks (*S. pneumoniae*), and trauma (enteric gram-negative bacilli) are examples.

Patients with HIV/AIDS present a special challenge, as the diseases that may manifest as acute CNS infections are diverse and significantly different from those seen in an immunocompetent population. In some instances, an acute CNS presentation is the initial manifestation of AIDS. Table 33-3 presents the most notable acute

Table 33-1.  Acute central nervous system infections

**Meningitis**
Treatable with antiinfectives
  Bacterial
  Granulomatous
  Syphilitic
  Lyme borreliosis
  Other
Nontreatable
  Viral
  Drug-induced
  Other agents (*Leptospira, Mycoplasma*)
  Carcinomatous
**Encephalitis**
Treatable with antiinfectives
  Herpes simplex
  Infective endocarditis, *Naegleria* infection, Rocky Mountain spotted fever, Lyme
    borreliosis
Nontreatable
  Other viral
  Other (postvaccination, toxic-metabolic)
  Reye's syndrome
**Focal lesions**
  Brain abscess
  Subdural or epidural empyema, ruptured brain abscess

CNS diagnoses in patients with AIDS. These have important implications for diagnosis and management. Physical examination provides evidence of focal neurologic abnormalities and non-CNS foci of infection that can act as primary sites for spread. Ear, nose, and throat and cardiopulmonary abnormalities should be sought carefully. Rashes may be manifestations of bacteremia or Rocky Mountain spotted fever.

Routine laboratory data include a CBC, determination of electrolytes, and assessment of renal and hepatic function. Such information may provide evidence for a specific cause of the CNS disease (e.g., Reye's syndrome, leptospirosis, hyponatremia) and baseline values against which to gauge changes resulting from disease or therapy. Blood cultures should be obtained in all patients. Suspected foci should be cultured and roentgenography performed as clinically indicated.

Lumbar puncture (LP) should be performed in most patients unless contraindicated by evidence of substantial elevations of intracerebral pressure. Fluid from an LP should be submitted for Gram's stain and culture (tube 1), glucose and protein analysis (tube 2), and cell count and differential (tube 3). Usually, at least one additional tube should be retained should other tests be needed. These might include Venereal Disease Research Laboratory (VDRL) tests and counterimmunoelectrophoresis (CIE) or latex particle agglutination tests for bacterial antigens, cryptococcal antigen testing, Lyme serology, smears, cultures for mycobacteria and fungi, viral cultures or polymerase chain reaction (PCR) studies, and cytocentrifugation for malignancy. Patients with AIDS may present with a multiplicity of unusual organisms that include *C. neoformans,* HIV, *T. gondii,* and other opportunists. In geographic areas with significant populations of patients with HIV/AIDS, routine CSF testing for cryptococcal antigen and VDRL tests should be performed.

### Meningitis
Typical symptoms of meningitis are fever, headache, nausea and vomiting, and nuchal rigidity. Many patients may not experience all these, especially early in the course of disease. Nuchal rigidity is most often associated with acute bacterial meningitis or tuberculous meningitis. Acute or subacute meningitis present for less than 7 days has

Table 33-2.  Evaluation of acute central nervous system infections

**History**
  Epidemiology (AIDS, travel, animal or insect contacts, immunizations)
  Medications
  Underlying disease (alcohol, immunosuppression)
  Associated complaints
**Physical examination**
  Rash
  Endocarditis, pneumonia
  Focal neurologic abnormalities
  Other focal observations (especially ear, nose, and throat)
**Routine studies**
  Blood cell count with differential, SMA-12, electrolytes
  Urinalysis
  Serology
  **Cultures of blood** and other pertinent sites
  **Lumbar puncture**[a]
  Gram's stain, culture
  Sugar, protein levels
**Other studies as indicated:** VDRL test, fungal and mycobacterial smears and
  cultures, antigen studies (CIE, latex agglutination), Lyme serology (ELISA,
  Western blot)
**Radiography**
  Posterior-anterior and lateral chest x-ray, CT with contrast

SMA, sequential multiple analyzer; VDRL test, Venereal Disease Research Laboratory test; CIE, counterimmunoelectrophoresis; ELISA, enzyme-linked immunosorbent assay; CT, computed tomography.
[a]If mass lesion ruled out.

numerous potential causes, and the prognosis may be improved by prompt diagnosis, particularly if the disease is bacterial. Focal neurologic defects may be noted with "uncomplicated" disease in up to 28% of patients; however, assessment for a mass lesion should be undertaken. The LP may provide specific diagnostic information.

Patients with bacterial meningitis who are not immunosuppressed generally demonstrate CSF leukocytosis. Classic categories for elevations of CSF leukocyte counts are as follows: polymorphonuclear, mixed cellular, and lymphocytic response. Although attempts to classify causes by type of cellular response may be useful, much overlap exists. Additionally, in the granulocytopenic patient, bacterial meningitis may develop with symptoms of fever and obtundation but without significant abnormalities of CSF WBC count. Similarly, in the patient with AIDS and cryptococcal menin-

Table 33-3.  Acute central nervous system infections in patients with AIDS

| Disease | Most common agent | Alternative diagnoses |
|---|---|---|
| Meningitis | *Cryptococcus neoformans* | Tuberculous, HIV (especially acute retroviral syndrome), other granulomatous |
| Encephalitis | *Toxoplasma gondii* | Lymphoma, Kaposi's sarcoma, AIDS dementia syndrome |
| Focal | *T. gondii* | Lymphoma, Kaposi's sarcoma, other granulomatous |

gitis or other opportunistic infections, the WBC response may be small or absent despite the presence of active infection.

*Acute Bacterial Meningitis*
Recent data suggest that acute bacterial meningitis has an annual incidence of about 4/100,000. In cases of community-acquired disease, *Neisseria meningitidis, S. pneumoniae,* and *L. monocytogenes* are most prevalent. Variations among age groups exist, with *N. meningitidis* more common among younger persons and *S. pneumoniae* and *L. monocytogenes* most common among the elderly. Seizures occur in about 10% of cases and are more frequent with pneumococcal meningitis. Mortality rates for bacterial meningitis in adults remain at approximately 20% but rise to at least 40% among those over age 60.

For patients without prior antibiotic therapy, CSF leukocytosis with counts above $1,000/mm^3$ is usual, results of Gram's stains are positive in 50% to 75% of cases, and results of cultures are positive at least about 90% of the time. Prior antibiotics decrease rates of positivity of both Gram's stain and culture. When cell counts are below $500/mm^3$, many patients with bacterial meningitis may demonstrate lymphocytic responses, at least early in the course. Hypoglycorrhachia and elevated protein are anticipated; however, a recent study demonstrated that only 50% of patients had the former. In at least 20% of cases of meningitis caused by *N. meningitidis,* cell counts are below $100/mm^3$. Culture-positive pyogenic meningitis associated with normal LP results has been rarely reported.

When the Gram's stain is negative, CSF antigen-detection tests should be performed. These have the capacity to detect bacterial antigen in the absence of viable organisms. *S. pneumoniae, H. influenzae* type B, most strains of *N. meningitidis,* and group B streptococci may be detected in this manner. False-negative reactions occur, and gram-negative enteric bacilli and *L. monocytogenes* cannot currently be identified in this fashion.

Recently, bacterial meningitis associated with the use of epidural catheters for treatment of pain has been described. Risk for infection is associated with length of surgery for catheter placement and probably with duration of catheter placement. In these circumstances, meningitis may occur in association with other focal infections, including muscle abscess, and therapy includes removal of the catheter, drainage of collections, and administration of appropriate antibiotics. Organisms most commonly encountered are *Staphylococcus aureus,* coagulase-negative staphylococci, and other skin flora.

Gram-negative bacillary meningitis is associated with surgical or nonsurgical trauma and comprises about 5% of all cases of bacterial meningitis. In the absence of such risks, nosocomial fever and mental status changes should not indicate the need for LP. Organisms most commonly implicated are *Escherichia coli* and species of *Klebsiella.* Acute purulent meningitis may be the initial manifestation of acute infective endocarditis. *S. aureus* is often a cause, and septic emboli are usually implicated. Drugs, intrathecal contrast dyes, and exploration of the posterior fossa have also been reported to cause such a response.

Therapy for acute bacterial meningitis requires bactericidal antimicrobials that are effective against the likely pathogens and capable of crossing the inflamed blood–brain barrier. Antibiotics meeting these qualifications include most third-generation cephalosporins, ampicillin, aqueous penicillin G, and TMP-SMX. Chloramphenicol is bactericidal against most strains of *H. influenzae,* meningococci, and some strains of *S. pneumoniae,* but bacteriostatic against *L. monocytogenes* and most enteric gram-negative bacilli.

Changing trends in *S. pneumoniae* resistance have dramatically altered the antibiotic recommendations for empiric treatment of bacterial meningitis. For suspected pneumococcal meningitis, or in the absence of a positive Gram's stain or antigen detection, a third-generation cephalosporin (2 g of cefotaxime every 8 hours, or 2 to 4 g of ceftriaxone every 24 hours) plus vancomycin (1 g given intravenously every 12 hours) is now recommended pending organism identification and susceptibility testing. Aqueous penicillin G (24 million units per day) will treat infections caused by penicillin-sensitive *S. pneumoniae* or *N. meningitidis,* and *L. monocytogenes.* The need to add an aminoglycoside for the latter agent has been poorly substantiated. Four grams of chloramphenicol per day given intravenously is an acceptable alternative in patients with pneumococcal or meningococcal meningitis who cannot tolerate β-lactam antimicrobials.

Third-generation cephalosporins in full parenteral doses for 2 to 3 weeks have revolutionized the therapy of gram-negative bacillary meningitis caused by susceptible pathogens. They are now widely considered to be the drugs of choice for this condition. However, *Enterobacter* organisms often acquire resistance to these agents after only several days, and the agent of choice in this case is probably TMP-SMX (20 mg of TMP equivalent per kilogram per day in two to four divided doses).

The use of ineffective agents or antimicrobials in suboptimal quantities results in higher mortality. Repeated LPs to document the efficacy of treatment are not necessary if the clinical condition is improving.

The length of therapy for bacterial meningitis is controversial. Meningococcal meningitis can usually be managed with 7 days of therapy. Disease caused by *H. influenzae, L. monocytogenes,* and *S. pneumoniae* should be treated for 10 to 14 days. Gram-negative bacillary meningitis usually requires up to 3 weeks of treatment. Outpatient IV antimicrobial therapy can be employed for clinically stable patients to complete the course of treatment.

The efficacy of corticosteroids in adults with meningitis remains unproven. This author would use them in patients with meningococcal disease and shock.

*Aseptic Meningitis: Mixed Cellular Response*

"Aseptic" meningitis usually presents with CSF pleocytosis and 40% to 60% polymorphonuclear leukocytes, and negative results on Gram's stains and routine cultures. CSF glucose is typically normal. The course ranges from acute to chronic. Major differential diagnoses include (a) partially treated bacterial meningitis, (b) parameningeal foci (including emboli from infective endocarditis), (c) syphilitic, Lyme borreliosis, and leptospiral meningitis, and (d) early viral or granulomatous meningitis. Noninfectious conditions include heavy metal encephalopathy, seizures, and carcinomatous meningitis. The clinical approach depends on the status of the patient and pertinent historical and clinical information. If evidence of mass lesions is lacking and the illness is not fulminant, a repeated LP after 6 to 12 hours is indicated. At that time, a change toward either a lymphocytic or polymorphonuclear response may be seen, and CSF glucose may decline. A second LP is especially helpful for patients who may have partially treated bacterial meningitis or viral meningitis. However, some authorities recommend routine treatment of possible bacterial meningitis with subsequent discontinuation of drugs after 48 to 72 hours if assessment is negative.

*Viral and Granulomatous Meningitis: Lymphocytic Response*

A lymphocytic pleocytosis of fewer than 500 cells per cubic millimeter is most commonly seen in viral or granulomatous meningitis. However, some patients with bacterial meningitis may also present with this formula. Granulomatous meningitis (tuberculous, fungal, sarcoid) is often associated with hypoglycorrhachia, which is uncommon in viral meningitis. Tuberculous and fungal meningitis should be considered especially in patients with appropriate epidemiologic histories (including HIV risk factors), evidence of other foci of infection, and hypoglycorrhachia. Cryptococcal antigen tests and smears and cultures for acid-fast bacilli and fungi are indicated. Therapy for tuberculous meningitis may be necessary if other diagnoses cannot be rapidly proved. Intense lymphocytic pleocytosis with cell counts above $5,000/mm^3$ may be seen with lymphocytic choriomeningitis.

Cryptococcal meningitis is the most common type of meningitis in patients with AIDS and is not generally noted with CD4 counts above $100/mm^3$. Presentation is often headache, and initial LP results may demonstrate clear fluid and fewer than 10 cells. In areas endemic for AIDS, cryptococcal antigen testing should be performed routinely on CSF specimens.

**Acute Encephalitis**

Acute encephalitis represents inflammation of brain tissue and may occur concurrently with meningeal irritation ("meningoencephalitis"). Approximately 20,000 cases occur annually in the United States, representing 3.5 to 7.4 cases per 100,000 patient-years, and most are mild. Acute encephalitis is clinically characterized by fever, headache, and altered state of consciousness. Focal neurologic defects, seizures, and autonomic abnormalities may also occur. Herpes simplex encephalitis characteristically is associated with early behavioral disorders because the virus tends to localize in the temporal lobes. Seizures occur early in the course in about half of cases.

In the United States, most encephalitis in non-AIDS patients is viral. Isolated cases are most likely caused by herpes simplex virus or mumps virus but may also be seen with varicella-zoster virus, Epstein-Barr virus (often cerebellar), or rubeola virus. The incidence of herpes simplex is 1/250,000 to 500,000 persons per year, and about 2,000 cases occur annually. It is most common below age 20 or above age 50 and is associated with significant mortality (70%) and neurologic sequelae (almost 100%) if untreated. Thus, it must not be overlooked. When acute encephalitis is encountered with no obvious etiology, empiric therapy for herpes simplex is often warranted. Warm-weather outbreaks are often associated with enteroviruses (coxsackievirus, echovirus, and poliovirus) and togaviruses (equine encephalitis virus).

Nonviral and potentially treatable causes of encephalitis include Rocky Mountain spotted fever, malaria, brucellosis, amebic (*Naegleria*) infection, syphilis, Lyme borreliosis, and toxoplasmosis. The last is an important consideration when encephalitis presents in AIDS patients. Occasionally, chronic meningitides, such as those caused by *Mycobacterium tuberculosis* and *C. neoformans,* may be associated with encephalitis because of hydrocephalus. Measles and rabies vaccines can cause encephalitis. Reye's syndrome, which often follows viral influenza and chickenpox, is a clinical condition that affects children primarily and can cause hepatic dysfunction.

Evaluation of encephalitis requires a comprehensive history, physical examination, and LP. Computed tomography (CT) with contrast or magnetic resonance imaging (MRI) with contrast is generally needed. Initial assessment should rule out treatable diseases, including herpes simplex. With the latter, LP usually reveals an "aseptic" or lymphocytic process with normal or depressed CSF glucose and elevated protein. RBCs in the CSF are often seen. Herpes simplex encephalitis should be suspected if behavioral disorders (often associated with seizures) accompany an episodic illness. The treatment of choice is 10 to 12 mg of acyclovir per kilogram given intravenously every 8 hours for 10 to 14 days.

The approach to diagnosis depends on locally available facilities. MRI defines brain lesions earlier in the course than CT and is preferred. PCR to detect herpes simplex viral DNA in CSF is now known to be highly sensitive and specific and should be considered the strategy of choice when herpes simplex encephalitis is considered. Used in patients with various clinical presentations, it has demonstrated a wider spectrum of disease associated with herpes simplex than originally suspected. Empiric therapy with acyclovir is indicated pending results of this study unless alternative diagnoses have been identified. Table 33-4 depicts other treatable diagnoses to consider.

*T. gondii* is the most common cause of encephalitis in patients with AIDS; such cases most commonly present as mental status changes. The diagnosis is suspected when numerous space-occupying lesions are found in a patient with a CD4 count below 100. Results of tests for serum *Toxoplasma* antibody are positive in more than 95% of cases; thus, a negative test result suggests alternative diagnoses.

## Focal Lesions
Localized CNS infections may present clinically as mass lesions and be confused with tumors or "strokes."

### Brain Abscess
Brain abscess is a focal intracerebral collection of pus that often presents as a mass lesion, with focal neurologic defects related to the area involved. Nonspecific headache is often noted, but fever is variable. Mortality has declined in some series to under 10% as a result of earlier diagnosis. Risk factors for mortality and neurologic sequelae include rapid progression and abnormal mental status on presentation. Suspicion of brain abscess necessitates diagnostic CT or MRI with contrast. LP may be hazardous, especially with lesions that impinge on the ventricles. In some series, 15% to 40% of

Table 33-4. Treatable diseases that mimic herpes simplex encephalitis

---

**Infectious**
  Brain abscess
  Tuberculous meningitis
  Fungal meningitis
  Rocky Mountain spotted fever
  Toxoplasmosis
  Subdural empyema
  Lyme borreliosis
  Syphilitic meningitis
  Leptospirosis
**Noninfectious**
  Central nervous system malignancy
  Systemic lupus erythematosus
  Subdural hematoma

---

Adapted from Whitley RJ. Viral encephalitis. *N Engl J Med* 1990;323:242–250.

patients with brain abscess die within 24 to 48 hours of diagnostic LP. Evidence of infection, especially in the ear, nose, and throat and cardiopulmonary system, should be carefully sought. However, approximately 20% of patients demonstrate no antecedent focus of infection. Only 10% of patients have positive results on blood cultures.

Causative organisms include most commonly oral anaerobes and other oropharyngeal flora. The importance of *S. aureus* is controversial, but abscess associated with staphylococcal bacteremia is regularly encountered. Prior antimicrobial therapy may sterilize lesions. Although there have been reports of successful medical management, most authorities recommend drainage of the lesion(s) unless they are inaccessible. CT-guided drainage is now considered the procedure of choice and can be repeated in cases of re-collection or multiple lesions. Materials should be sent for Gram's stain and culture (aerobic and anaerobic). Length of antibiotic therapy is at least 4 weeks but often should proceed to 6 to 8 weeks; this can be guided by CT response to treatment. Medical therapy alone requires at least 6 to 8 weeks of parenteral treatment. It should be reserved for patients in whom surgery is medically contraindicated or those with numerous or surgically inaccessible lesions. Lesions abutting on ventricles should be drained because of the risk for rupture.

Antimicrobial therapy usually consists of penicillin G (24 million units daily) plus 500 mg of metronidazole three times daily in lieu of chloramphenicol, which had been historically recommended. A third-generation cephalosporin (cefotaxime or ceftriaxone) in full therapeutic doses may be employed instead of penicillin G if considerations include *Haemophilus,* enteric gram-negative bacilli, or HACEK (*Haemophilus, Actinobacillus, Cardiobacterium, Eikenella, Kingella*) organisms. Specific therapy for other pathogens depends on culture and sensitivity results. For clinically stable patients, much of the treatment can be accomplished through outpatient IV antimicrobial therapy.

*Subdural Empyema*
The subdural space lies between the dura mater and arachnoid. Infection usually arises as a complication of sinusitis. Less likely origins include otitis media, or surgical or nonsurgical trauma. A male predominance has been noted; the reason is unknown. The presentation may mimic that of brain abscess, although progression from headache with fever to focal (and often extensive) neurologic defects may be rapid and involve an entire cerebral hemisphere. Seizures are common. Enhanced CT or MRI without LP is indicated, and neurosurgical drainage (generally by burr hole) is mandatory.

Antimicrobial therapy is guided by Gram's stain and culture from drained pus. If the condition is secondary to sinusitis or otitis media, strategies similar to those for brain abscess are reasonable. If it occurs after neurosurgery, coverage of both *S. aureus* and enteric gram-negative bacilli should be initiated. Suitable treatment alternatives include nafcillin-oxacillin or ceftriaxone plus chloramphenicol or metronidazole in full therapeutic doses pending culture results. The length of therapy is at least 1 month, and this can be guided by repeated imaging studies.

*Ruptured Brain Abscess*
Brain abscesses may rupture into the ventricular system, resulting in acute purulent meningitis. The patient is critically ill, and mortality approaches 100%. LP may be necessary in this circumstance because meningitis cannot be ruled out. "Meningitis" associated with focal neurologic lesions should prompt suspicion of this condition. Symptoms are those of acute purulent meningitis. Gram's stain, however, may demonstrate numerous organisms, an unusual observation in other types of meningitis. Therapy consists of high-dose parenteral antimicrobials (based on Gram's stain results), intensive support, and sometimes neurosurgical intervention. (R.B.B.)

## Bibliography

Dill SR, Cobbs CG, McDonald CK. Subdural empyema: analysis of 32 cases and review. *Clin Infect Dis* 1995;20:372–386.
> *The authors categorize cases of subdural empyema as secondary to sinusitis, secondary to trauma, or miscellaneous. Sinusitis was the most common cause and was generally associated with streptococci and anaerobes. Cases resulting from trauma (including neurosurgery) were more likely to harbor gram-negative bacilli or* S. aureus. *Surgical drainage plus at least 1 month of antibiotics is considered appropriate therapy.*

Dominiques RB, et al. Evaluation of the range of clinical presentations of herpes simplex encephalitis by using polymerase chain reaction assay of cerebrospinal fluid samples. *Clin Infect Dis* 1997;25:86–91.
> *Forty-nine patients with various neurologic presentations were studied with PCR for herpes simplex DNA. These studies demonstrate that in patients with more subtle forms of encephalitis, herpes simplex virus may still be the cause. However, temporal lobe localization is often noted.*

Durand ML, et al. Acute bacterial meningitis in adults. *N Engl J Med* 1993;328:21–28.
> *This is a review of almost 500 cases of acute bacterial meningitis seen during a 26-year period at a single tertiary-care hospital.* S. pneumoniae *(37%),* N. meningitidis *(13%), and* L. monocytogenes *(10%) were the most common causes of community-acquired disease. Overall, 40% of cases were nosocomial, and enteric gram-negative bacilli were often noted. Recurrent meningitis was seen in 9% of cases and was often associated with CSF leaks. Advanced age, mental status changes on admission, and seizures within 24 hours of admission were adverse prognostic indicators for patients with community-acquired disease. Mortality for this population was 25%.*

Lakeman FD, Whitley RJ, the National Institute of Allergy and Infectious Diseases Collaborative Antiviral Study Group. Diagnosis of herpes simplex encephalitis: application of polymerase chain reaction to cerebrospinal fluid from brain-biopsied patients and correlation with disease. *J Infect Dis* 1995;171:857–863.
> *This important study documents the role of PCR in identifying herpes simplex viral DNA from CSF. Sensitivity and specificity were 98% and 94%, respectively. Test results were positive in 98% of patients with biopsy-proven herpes simplex encephalitis. The test can be performed on CSF aliquots and obviates the need for brain biopsy in most cases. In cases of encephalitis of undetermined etiology, empiric therapy with acyclovir could be initiated and then discontinued based on the results of this test and clinical response.*

Lebel MH, et al. Dexamethasone therapy for bacterial meningitis. *N Engl J Med* 1988;319:964–971.
> *Although this investigation was carried out in children, it provides insights into the pathophysiology of bacterial meningitis. The authors present compelling data from two prospective, randomized, double-blinded studies that document the efficacy of dexamethasone (in addition to antimicrobial therapy) in preventing sensorineural hearing loss in children with bacterial meningitis. In most cases, disease was caused by* H. influenzae, *and other parameters of response (time to become afebrile and CSF indices) were enhanced in the group that received corticosteroids. The results of this study may not be applicable to adults.*

Mathisen GE, Johnson JP. Brain abscess. *Clin Infect Dis* 1997;25:763–781.
*The authors review recent literature on the pathophysiology, diagnosis, and treatment of brain abscess. Chloramphenicol is less frequently employed, and most cases can now be treated without craniotomy. CT and MRI have revolutionized the diagnosis of this condition, and CT can generally be used to guide percutaneous drainage. Therapy should be continued for 6 to 8 weeks in most instances, and progress can be documented by radiographic follow-up. Currently, the role of oral antibiotics is limited, but outpatient parenteral antibiotic therapy is valuable once stability has been achieved.*

Pegues DA, Carr DB, Hopkins CC. Infectious complications associated with temporary epidural catheters. *Clin Infect Dis* 1994;19:70–72.
*This is one of several articles that deal with the potential for severe infections following the use of catheters for pain control. Risk is related to length of procedure for implantation, and probably to duration of use. Meningitis occurs, often in conjunction with focal muscle or other deep-tissue abscess. Skin flora organisms are most commonly noted, but gram-negative bacilli may also be involved. Therapy consists of drainage, catheter removal, and administration of appropriate antibiotics.*

Powers WJ. Cerebrospinal fluid lymphocytosis in acute bacterial meningitis. *Am J Med* 1985;79:216–220.
*The author reviewed the CSF characteristics of 103 cases of acute bacterial meningitis and noted 14 patients in whom more than 50% lymphocytes / monocytes were noted on CSF cell count. Thirty-two percent of patients with fewer than 1,000 cells per cubic millimeter had lymphocytosis. It was associated with pathogens that included S. pneumoniae, N. meningitidis, and H. influenzae. Most cases were in neonates, but lymphocytosis was observed in all age groups.*

Quagliarello V, Scheld WM. Bacterial meningitis: pathogenesis, pathophysiology, and progress. *N Engl J Med* 1992;327:864–872.
*This comprehensive review of mechanisms of pathogenesis and pathophysiology in bacterial meningitis explores virulence factors of bacteria, immunology of the CNS, features of the blood–brain barrier, and overall host-bacterial interactions. The authors recommend adjunctive corticosteroid therapy for adults (as well as children) with bacterial meningitis that is associated with positive smears on Gram's stain (indicative of high organism load), especially if accompanied by evidence of increased intracranial pressure.*

Seyjdoux Ch, Francioli P. Bacterial brain abscesses: factors influencing mortality and sequelae. *Clin Infect Dis* 1992;15:394–401.
*The authors retrospectively assess 39 patients with confirmed brain abscess in the CT era to document reasons for mortality and neurologic sequelae. All cases were treated within 24 hours of hospitalization. Risk factors for adverse outcome include mental status changes on admission, neurologic abnormalities on admission, and short duration between first symptoms and presentation (rapid progression). Overall, mortality was 13%, and neurologic sequelae were seen in 22% of survivors.*

Talan DA, et al. Role of empiric parenteral antibiotics prior to lumbar puncture in suspected bacterial meningitis: state of the art. *Rev Infect Dis* 1988;10:365–376.
*If LP must be delayed, patients with suspected bacterial meningitis should receive empiric IV antimicrobials. CSF cell count, sugar, and protein determinations are unlikely to be affected, but results of Gram's stain and culture are less likely to be positive. The authors feel that other studies, such as blood cultures or antigen-detection tests, may still allow a bacteriologic diagnosis.*

Tunkel AR, Wispelwey B, Scheld WM. Bacterial meningitis: recent advances in pathophysiology and treatment. *Ann Intern Med* 1990;112:610–623.
*Provides an excellent review of pathophysiologic mechanisms required and responsible for bacterial meningitis. Bacterial virulence factors, the role of the blood–brain barrier, and requirements for antimicrobials used in treatment are reviewed in depth. Several tables are provided with recommendations for antimicrobial use based on patient age and likely pathogens.*

Whitley RJ. Viral encephalitis. *N Engl J Med* 1990;323:242–250.
*This represents a recent and concise overview of encephalitis in the United States. Most cases are viral, with pathogenetic mechanisms that include acute, postinfectious,*

*slow-viral, and chronic degenerative disease. Most infections result from either hematogenous or neuronal spread. Herpes simplex viral encephalitis comprises 10% of all cases and is the most amenable to treatment. An excellent table of diseases mimicking herpes simplex encephalitis is provided.*

Wolff MA, Young CL, Ramphal R. Antibiotic therapy for *Enterobacter* meningitis: a retrospective review of 13 episodes and review of the literature. *Clin Infect Dis* 1993;16:772–777.

*The authors appropriately identify problems with the use of cephalosporins in managing* Enterobacter *meningitis. Treatment with cephalosporins resulted in clinical resistance in 40% of episodes. TMP-SMX, in doses similar to those employed for the management of* Pneumocystis carinii *pneumonia in AIDS patients, appears to be the agent of choice. Mortality with the use of this agent was lower than that seen with cephalosporins.*

---

## 34. CHRONIC MENINGITIS

---

Chronic meningitis is defined as a symptom complex of insidious onset that is characterized by headache, fever, and mental status changes in association with cerebrospinal fluid (CSF) pleocytosis. The CSF protein is usually elevated, and the CSF glucose is often low. This syndrome may be caused by viral, bacterial, fungal, or parasitic agents. Noninfectious causes include malignancy, sarcoidosis, Behçet's syndrome, and vasculitis.

Tuberculosis remains the most common cause of the chronic meningitis syndrome; it is a treatable disease even in the immunosuppressed patient. Hence, the diagnosis must be made and, at times, empiric therapy may be initiated. The diagnosis of tuberculous meningitis continues to be a difficult one. The disease is usually the result of breakdown of a long-standing granuloma. In about half of all patients, this breakdown is associated with some underlying condition, such as sarcoidosis, AIDS, malnutrition, or steroid therapy.

Clinical manifestations of tuberculous meningitis generally are similar to those of other chronic meningitides. A miliary picture on chest x-ray films and inappropriate antidiuretic hormone secretion are the only features useful to distinguish between tuberculous and cryptococcal meningitis. In one study, symptoms of tuberculous meningitis included fever (99°F to 103°F), lethargy, and headache. Duration of symptoms on presentation ranges from 2 days to 6 months. Hospitalization is often precipitated by complaints of headache. Meningeal signs are present in more than half of all cases. Peripheral WBC counts range from low normal to very elevated (>20,000/mm³).

Tuberculous meningitis is often a disease of the inner-city population in the United States. Mortality and morbidity in this group are high. The disease was similar in HIV-positive and HIV-negative patients in two different studies.

Klein et al. reviewed the CSF findings in 21 patients. All but one had a lymphocytic pleocytosis. In 16 of 21, CSF protein levels were above 50 mg/dL; 10 had CSF glucose levels of 40 mg/dL or less. Positivity on acid-fast smear varies dramatically among studies, from a low of 10% to a high of 90%. Prevention of mortality from the disease depends on rapid initiation of therapy; hence, better diagnostic methods are critical.

Several attempts have been made recently to develop rapid, sensitive, specific methods. Ribera et al. have studied the activity of adenosine deaminase in the CSF of patients with tuberculous meningitis. This biologic activity of this enzyme is detected in T lymphocytes, and increased plasma levels of the enzyme have been observed in infectious diseases related to cell-mediated immune response. At levels greater than 9 U/L, the test was found to be sensitive and specific. Levels appeared to correlate with disease activity, and persistently high levels predicted complications. Kadival et al. have used a radioimmunoassay for detecting *Mycobacterium* antigen. Antigen could be detected in 25 of 38 patients with tuberculous meningitis, versus none of 56 patients with nontuberculous meningitis. Assay results become negative after therapy. Krambovitis et al. used a latex agglutination immunoassay, which was also sensitive and specific (one false-positive occurred in a patient with *Haemophilus influenzae meningitis*). Other enzyme-linked immunosorbent assay (ELISA) techniques have also been described. Tuberculostearic acid, a structural component of *Mycobacterium tuberculosis,* can be identified by gas chromatography and was shown to be sensitive and specific in one small study.

The outcome of tuberculous meningitis depends on neurologic status at presentation, time to initiation of therapy, and underlying disease. Three drugs are usually recommended: isoniazid, rifampin, and ethambutol or pyrazinamide. Response occurs after about 1 month, and treatment is continued for 1 year. When empiric therapy is being used, rifampin has broad antimicrobial activity, and clinical response does not necessarily prove tuberculosis as a diagnosis. The use of corticosteroids in tuberculous meningitis remains controversial. Corticosteroids decrease the risk for herniation and may improve the CSF profile; however, survival does not appear to be affected.

The presentation of cryptococcal meningitis is very similar to that of tuberculosis. The disease has become much more common in the AIDS era and may be the first manifestation of AIDS. In addition, lymphoma, systemic lupus erythematosus, sarcoidosis, and renal transplantation are important predisposing conditions. Between 20% and 50% of patients with cryptococcal meningitis have no underlying illness. Cultures of specimens from sputum, bone marrow, or skin lesions may be useful in some patients. Spinal fluid findings, as in tuberculous meningitis, usually show a CSF pleocytosis. An India ink preparation yields positive results in 50% of cases; cryptococcal antigen can be detected in 80% to 90% of cases by a rapid, simple latex fixation test. Computed tomography may be necessary to identify cryptococcomas or to rule out hydrocephalus. The poor prognostic signs in cryptococcal meningitis have been well defined: (a) high opening CSF pressure, (b) low CSF glucose, (c) fewer than 20 WBCs in CSF, (d) high titers of cryptococcal antigen and positive India ink stain, and (e) concomitant disease, such as lymphoma.

Amphotericin is the drug of choice for cryptococcal meningitis. In the absence of bone marrow suppression, flucytosine is usually added. Treatment is generally continued for 4 weeks in patients with mild disease. Those patients with underlying disease, fewer than 10 WBCs in CSF, antigen titer above 1:32, or positive India ink stain should receive 6 weeks of treatment. Flucytosine is generally avoided in the AIDS patient. In some patients refractory to parenteral therapy, intraventricular amphotericin therapy with an Ommaya reservoir has been successful. In AIDS patients, initial treatment is with amphotericin; relapses are prevented with long-term fluconazole therapy. Treatment with fluconazole in acute disease has also been successful.

Coccidioidomycosis is another common cause of chronic meningitis syndrome. A careful travel history may be an important clue to the disease. Residents of southern California, Nevada, Utah, Arizona, New Mexico, Texas, Mexico, and Central America are at risk for the disease by inhaling arthrospores of *Coccidioides immitis.* Visitors to these areas may also contract the disease. Two thirds of patients who contract the disease have no risk factors. However, disseminated disease and meningitis are more likely to develop in blacks, Filipinos, and pregnant women after pulmonary infection. The symptoms of coccidioidomycosis meningitis cannot be distinguished from those of chronic meningitis with other causes, but evaluation for lesions of skin, bone, and lung may provide critical information. CSF parameters are nonspecific. In some patients, a polymorphonuclear leukocyte predominance in CSF may be noted. CSF cultures are often negative.

Culture plates must be handled with care because they are infectious to laboratory personnel. Detection of complement-fixing antibody in the CSF is specific and 75% to 90% sensitive for diagnosis. Systemic and local amphotericin therapy is recommended. IV amphotericin should be continued to a total dose of 3 to 4 g. Most experts recommend an Ommaya reservoir for intraventricular therapy rather than repeated intrathecal injection, which often results in arachnoiditis.

*Blastomyces dermatitidis* can also cause chronic meningitis. Meningitis occurs in about one third of patients with disseminated disease. Diagnosis is usually made by concomitant culture of sputum, skin lesions, bone or joint fluid, and prostatic secretions. The organism is rarely cultured from CSF, and serologic tests are not reliable for extrapulmonary infection.

The presentation of histoplasmosis meningitis is similar to that of *B. dermatitidis* meningitis, and culture of other sites is often required for diagnosis. Half the patients have positive CSF cultures; 90% have CSF antibody. IV amphotericin is recommended for meningitis associated with histoplasmosis or blastomycosis. Intraventricular therapy is used for relapse.

Actinomycosis can be associated with many central nervous system (CNS) lesions, including brain abscess, meningitis, subdural empyema, and epidural abscess. Brain abscesses present with focal neurologic findings, and many patients have evidence of dental infection, mastoiditis, sinusitis, or skin infection. Actinomycosis may involve the meninges alone, producing a basilar meningitis that is indolent and manifested solely by a lymphocytic pleocytosis. In such cases, the disease is frequently misdiagnosed as tuberculous meningitis. *Actinomyces* organisms are fastidious, gram-positive, filamentous bacteria. They often grow slowly and have anaerobic or microaerophilic growth requirements. High-dose penicillin remains the drug of choice.

*Nocardia asteroides* infection may also present as chronic meningitis without brain abscess, but this is unusual. Sulfonamides are the antimicrobials of choice.

Several spirochetes are neurotrophic and can cause a chronic meningitis syndrome. Syphilitic meningitis usually occurs within 2 years of acute infection. Fever is often absent, and headache may be the sole complaint. A CSF pleocytosis with high protein and low sugar may mimic the findings of other chronic meningitides. The diagnosis is suggested by a positive result on treponemal tests and CSF Venereal Disease Research Laboratory (VDRL) tests. Many investigators have reported a change in the clinical spectrum of neurosyphilis recently. Patients may complain of vague chronic symptoms, including headache. They tend not to have classic tertiary signs, such as tabes dorsalis or pupillary changes.

The CNS effects of Lyme disease are receiving increasing attention. *Borrelia burgdorferi* can cause chronic meningitis as a second stage of Lyme disease, months after tick exposure and initial infection. Bell's palsy and radiculopathic syndromes are most common. Meningitis patients present often without fever but with headache, photophobia, and stiff neck, and they may present with long-standing symptoms. A CSF pleocytosis is found. Protein is elevated, and about 15% of patients have low CSF sugar. Results of a CSF VDRL test may be false-positive, but treponemal tests will be negative. Local CSF antibody production occurs, but serologic tests appear to lack sensitivity and specificity. Tests to detect spirochetal DNA in host material may be useful in the future. Recommended treatment includes high-dose penicillin or ceftriaxone.

Other spirochetal diseases, including leptospirosis and relapsing fever, may present with meningitis in addition to other systemic symptoms. These meningitides are usually self-limited.

Other bacteria can cause a chronic meningitis syndrome. Brucellosis usually presents with night sweats, lymphadenopathy, and hepatosplenomegaly. CNS involvement is rare, but when it does occur, a chronic meningitis syndrome is common. Culture from blood or CSF requires special media and longer incubation (2 to 4 weeks). Blood or CSF agglutination titers may be needed for diagnosis. Tetracycline with rifampin or streptomycin is recommended for treatment. *Listeria monocytogenes* and *Neisseria meningitidis* infections, which are more likely to produce an acute meningitis, can also present as a more protracted, insidious disease. An underlying immunodeficiency state may be present in these cases.

Viral infections usually cause meningoencephalitis or aseptic meningitis, with CSF pleocytosis and normal CSF sugar in most cases. Chronic meningitis caused by echovirus or coxsackievirus occurs in patients with agammaglobulinemia or multiple myeloma. HIV infection itself or with concomitant progressive multifocal leukoencephalopathy may cause mental status abnormalities and a chronic CSF pleocytosis.

Noninfectious disease processes may mimic a chronic infectious meningitis syndrome. Metastatic carcinoma from an unsuspected primary carcinoma in the breast or lung can cause a chronic meningitis syndrome, as can lymphoma and melanoma. In many cases, back pain, radicular pain, and cranial nerve abnormalities will also be present. Most patients have a CSF pleocytosis. Cytology is positive for malignant cells in 50% to 80% of patients. CSF lactate dehydrogenase has recently been shown to be a useful test. Findings on computed tomography and magnetic resonance imaging will usually be positive.

Sarcoidosis presents with neurologic findings in 48% of patients. Cranial nerve abnormalities, peripheral neuropathy, and focal cerebral and intraspinal lesions are most common. Aseptic meningitis rarely occurs without other manifestations of sarcoidosis. In one study, CSF pleocytosis was noted in 43% of patients, and hypoglycorrhachia in only 10%. When this disease is suspected, careful examination of optic and other cranial nerves, as well as evaluation of other systems, is crucial. Diagnosis is usually made outside the CNS, such as by biopsy of lymph node, liver, or parotid or other salivary gland. Specific CNS markers for sarcoid have not yet been developed.

Behçet's disease usually is recognized by the triad of oral or genital ulcers, skin lesions, and uveitis. Meningoencephalitis develops in 25% of patients, often in association with flare-up of other symptoms. CSF pleocytosis is present, with elevated protein and normal sugar. (S.L.B.)

### Bibliography

Anderson NE, Willoughby EW. Chronic meningitis without predisposing illness: a review of 83 cases. *Q J Med* 1987;63:283.
*Tuberculosis is still the most common cause of chronic meningitis.*
Bouza E, et al. Coccidioidal meningitis. An analysis of 31 cases and review of the literature. *Medicine (Baltimore)* 1981;3:139.
*Complement-fixing antibody is an important test in coccidioidal meningitis. Intrathecal administration of amphotericin is more effective than IV administration.*
Bouza E, et al. Brucellar meningitis. *Rev Infect Dis* 1987;9:810.
*Review of the neurologic manifestations of systemic brucellosis.*
Bozzette SA, et al. A placebo-controlled trial of maintenance therapy with fluconazole after treatment of cryptococcal meningitis in the acquired immunodeficiency syndrome. *N Engl J Med* 1991;324:580.
*Randomized, controlled trial shows that fluconazole prevents the relapse of cryptococcal meningitis in AIDS patients.*
Buggy BP. *Nocardia asteroides* meningitis without brain abscess. *Rev Infect Dis* 1987; 9:228.
*Case reports of* N. asteroides *meningitis without brain abscess or focal findings.*
Butler WT, et al. Diagnostic and prognostic value of clinical and laboratory findings in cryptococcal meningitis. A follow-up study of 40 patients. *N Engl J Med* 1964;270:59.
*Variability in both clinical symptoms and CSF parameters in patients with cryptococcal meningitis.*
Daniel TM. New approaches to the rapid diagnosis of tuberculous meningitis. *J Infect Dis* 1987;155:599.
*Reviews new developments in the diagnosis of tuberculous meningitis, including biochemical, antigen, and antibody methods.*
Dismukes WE, et al. Treatment of cryptococcal meningitis with combination amphotericin B and flucytosine for 4 as compared with 6 weeks. *N Engl J Med* 1987;317:334.
*Patients with cryptococcal meningitis who have underlying disease should be treated for 6 weeks with amphotericin and flucytosine.*
Dooley DP, et al. Adjunctive corticosteroid therapy for tuberculosis: a critical reappraisal of the literature. *Clin Infect Dis* 1997;25:872.
*Corticosteroids seem to improve neurologic outcomes and decrease mortality.*
Dube MP, Holton PD, Larsen RA. Tuberculous meningitis in patients with and without human immunodeficiency virus infection. *Am J Med* 1992;93:520.
*HIV infection had little impact on the findings and on hospital mortality of patients with tuberculous meningitis. Intracerebral mass lesions were more common in AIDS patients.*
Finkel MF. Lyme disease and its neurologic complications. *Arch Neurol* 1988;45:99.
*Patients with CNS Lyme disease may present with long-standing headache and CSF pleocytosis. CSF IgG and IgM levels should be obtained when CNS Lyme disease is suspected.*
French GL, et al. Diagnosis of tuberculous meningitis by detection of the tuberculostearic acid in cerebrospinal fluid. *Lancet* 1987;1:117.
*Tuberculostearic acid, a structural component of* M. tuberculosis, *can be detected in CSF by gas chromatography.*

Haas EJ, et al. Tuberculous meningitis in an urban general hospital. *Arch Intern Med* 1977;137:1518.
*Acid-fast smears of CSF were positive in only 6 of 19 cases.*

Harvey RI, Chandrasekar PH. Chronic meningitis caused by *Listeria* in a patient infected with human immunodeficiency virus. *J Infect Dis* 1988;157:1091.
L. monocytogenes *may cause a picture of chronic meningitis in the immunosuppressed patient.*

Kadival GV, et al. Radioimmunoassay for detecting *Mycobacterium tuberculosis* antigen in cerebrospinal fluid of patients with tuberculous meningitis. *J Infect Dis* 1987; 155:608.
M. tuberculosis *antigen can be detected in CSF by radioimmunoassay early in the course of disease.*

Kennedy DH, Fallon RJ. Tuberculous meningitis. *JAMA* 1979;241:264.
*Mortality in tuberculous meningitis is strongly associated with delay in diagnosis.*

Klein NC, Damsker B, Hirschman SZ. Mycobacterial meningitis. Retrospective analysis from 1970 to 1983. *Am J Med* 1985;79:29.
*Reviews CNS presentation in 21 patients with mycobacterial meningitis. CSF findings are variable and may include predominance of polymorphonuclear leukocytes, normal protein, and normal sugar.*

Kovacs JA, et al. Cryptococcosis in the acquired immunodeficiency syndrome. *Ann Intern Med* 1985;103:533.
*In AIDS patients with cryptococcal meningitis, CSF WBC count, sugar, and protein were frequently normal. Relapse was very common.*

Krambovitis E, et al. Rapid diagnosis of tuberculous meningitis by latex particle agglutination. *Lancet* 1984;2:1229.
*Results of this test were positive in 17 of 18 patients with tuberculous meningitis. Results in control CSF samples from patients with other meningitides and neurologic diseases were negative in 133 of 134 cases.*

Kravitz GR, et al. Chronic blastomycetic meningitis. *Am J Med* 1981;71:501.
*CSF cultures are rarely positive in blastomycosis meningitis, and serologic tests are not specific.*

Lecour H, Miranda M. Human leptospirosis. A review of 50 cases. *Infection* 1989;17:8.
*Meningitis usually occurs concurrently with other symptoms in leptospirosis.*

Lukehart SA, et al. Invasion of the central nervous system by *Treponema pallidum:* implications for diagnosis and treatment. *Ann Intern Med* 1988;109:855.
*Discusses implications of CNS syphilis in patients with AIDS.*

McKinney RE, Katz SL, Wilfert CM. Chronic enteroviral meningoencephalitis in agammaglobulinemic patients. *Rev Infect Dis* 1987;9:334.
*Echovirus causes a culture-proven chronic meningitis in patients with agammaglobulinemia.*

Meyers BR, Hirschman SZ. Unusual presentations of tuberculous meningitis. *Mt Sinai J Med* 1974;41:407.
*Describes presentation of tuberculous meningitis. Fifty percent of patients have predisposing underlying disease.*

Moosa MY, Coovadia YM. Cryptococcal meningitis in Durban, South Africa: a comparison of clinical features, laboratory findings, and outcome for human immunodefiency virus-positive and -negative patients. *Clin Infect Dis* 1997;24:131.
*Headache, fever, stiff neck, and neurologic findings were more common in HIV-infected patients.*

Ogawa SK, et al. Tuberculous meningitis in an urban medical center. *Medicine (Baltimore)* 1987;66:371.
*Detailed discussion of symptomatology. Fever is almost invariably present in tuberculous meningitis.*

O'Toole RD, et al. Dexamethasone in tuberculous meningitis. *Ann Intern Med* 1969; 70:39.
*Decreased risk of herniation, improved CSF parameters, but no change in mortality is associated with use of steroids in tuberculous meningitis.*

Pachner AR. Spirochetal diseases of the CNS. *Neurol Clin* 1986;4:207.
*Excellent review of CNS syphilis, Lyme disease, leptospirosis, and relapsing fever.*

Polsky B, Depman MR, Gold JWM. Intraventricular therapy of cryptococcal meningitis via a subcutaneous reservoir. *Am J Med* 1986;81:24.
*Retrospective evaluation of intraventricular amphotericin in cryptococcal meningitis. Early intraventricular therapy may be beneficial for those with a poor prognosis.*

Porkert MT, et al. Tuberculous meningitis at a large inner-city medical center. *Am J Med Sci* 1997;13:325.
*Thirty-four patients with tuberculous meningitis were studied at a public hospital in Atlanta. Tuberculous meningitis is a devastating disease in inner-city residents with a delay in diagnosis and has a high mortality rate. Whether or not a patient was HIV-positive did not affect the clinical presentation.*

Reik L. Disorders that mimic CNS infection. *Neurol Clin* 1986;4:223.
*When granulomatous involvement of basal meninges is the predominant pathology, disease will look like tuberculous meningitis.*

Ribera E, et al. Activity of adenosine deaminase in cerebrospinal fluid for the diagnosis and follow-up of tuberculous meningitis in adults. *J Infect Dis* 1987;155:603.
*Adenosine deaminase levels are elevated in the CSF of patients with tuberculous meningitis. The test appears to be both sensitive and specific.*

Richardson EP. Progressive multifocal leukoencephalopathy 30 years later. *N Engl J Med* 1988;318:315.
*Progressive multifocal leukoencephalopathy may occur in as many as 38% of AIDS patients. Article provides a good overview of this disease.*

Rosen MS, Lorber B, Myer AR. Chronic meningococcal meningitis. An association with C5 deficiency. *Arch Intern Med* 1988;148:1441.
*N. meningitidis may cause chronic meningitis in patients with complement deficiency.*

Simon RP. Neurosyphilis. *Arch Neurol* 1985;42:606.
*Describes the many syndromes of neurosyphilis, including CSF parameters.*

Smego RA, Jr. Actinomycosis of the central nervous system. *Rev Infect Dis* 1987;9:855.
*Actinomycosis causes several types of CNS disease, particularly brain abscess. An isolated chronic meningitis picture can occur.*

Southern PM, Sanford JP. Relapsing fever: a clinical and microbiological review. *Medicine (Baltimore)* 1969;48:129.
*Relapsing fever is associated with CNS disease in 8% of tick-borne and 30% of louse-borne infections.*

Steere AC. Lyme disease. *N Engl J Med* 1989;9:593.
*Describes the clinical manifestations of stages 1 through 3 of Lyme disease.*

Steere AC, Pachner AR, Malawista SE. Neurologic abnormalities of Lyme disease: successful treatment with high-dose intravenous penicillin. *Ann Intern Med* 1983;99:767.
*Chronic meningeal symptoms caused by Lyme disease resolve with high-dose penicillin therapy.*

Stern BJ, et al. Sarcoidosis and its neurological manifestations. *Arch Neurol* 1985; 42:909.
*Sarcoidosis presents with neurologic symptoms in 48% of cases. However, an isolated chronic meningitis syndrome is unusual.*

Stern JJ, et al. Oral fluconazole therapy for patients with acquired immunodeficiency syndrome and cryptococcosis: experience with 22 patients. *Am J Med* 1988;85:477.
*Fluconazole was useful in preventing cryptococcal meningitis relapse in AIDS patients.*

Stockstill MT, Kauffman CA. Comparison of cryptococcal and tuberculous meningitis. *Arch Neurol* 1983;40:81.
*The clinical pictures of tuberculous and cryptococcal meningitis are similar. A miliary pattern on chest x-ray films and inappropriate secretion of antidiuretic hormone support a diagnosis of tuberculous meningitis.*

Wasserstrom WR, Glass JP, Posner JB. Diagnosis and treatment of leptomeningeal metastases from solid tumors: experience with 90 patients. *Cancer* 1982;49:759.
*Metastatic carcinoma, particularly from primary carcinoma of lung and breast, can cause chronic meningitis syndrome.*

Wheat J, et al. Cerebrospinal fluid *Histoplasma* antibodies in central nervous system histoplasmosis. *Arch Intern Med* 1985;145:1237.

*CSF antibodies in histoplasmosis meningitis are 90% sensitive. The disease is*
*increasing in HIV-positive patients.*
Yechoor VK, et al. Tuberculosis meningitis among adults with and without HIV infection. Experience in an urban public hospital. *Arch Intern Med* 1996;156:1710.
*Tuberculous meningitis was found to be a relatively common disease in urban non-*
*whites. Underlying HIV disease did not affect clinical or laboratory features of the*
*disease or response to therapy.*

## 35.  GUILLAIN-BARRÉ SYNDROME

Guillain-Barré syndrome (GBS) is an acute demyelinating polyneuropathy. The eponym
comes from a 1916 article by G. Guillain and J. A. Barré, who described a polyneuropathy in association with protein elevation in cerebrospinal fluid (CSF) but no inflammatory cells. Increasing evidence supports the long-standing supposition that GBS is an
autoimmune disease triggered by an infectious or immunologic stimulus. Both plasma
exchange and immunoglobulin therapy have proved to be effective. Acute inflammatory
demyelinating polyneuropathy has been frequently reported as a complication of HIV
disease.
    The clinical features of GBS have been well described; however, the initial presen-
tation may be variable. In general, patients first experience paresthesia and numbness
in the extremities. A symmetric weakness develops over several days, usually in the
lower extremities, making climbing stairs or walking difficult. Weakness characteristically ascends to the trunk and arms. Muscle pain and sciatica are frequent additional
complaints. Weakness may progress for several weeks, affecting respiration, swallowing, eye movements, and autonomic nervous system function. On initial physical examination, symmetric limb weakness and absent deep-tendon reflexes are noted. Loss of
sensation is usually mild despite complaints of paresthesia. Fever is absent.
    Several variations in this clinical picture may be noted. The ascending nature of the
process may not be striking. Miller-Fisher syndrome, which represents about 5% of all
GBS, is characterized by ophthalmoplegia, ataxia, and areflexia. GBS may also present with isolated arm weakness or weakness of the oropharynx, severe ataxia, and
sensory loss or with sudden, complete paralysis.
    As noted, CSF findings confirm the diagnosis. The CSF will show few or no cells
and a protein concentration greater than 0.55 g/L. Protein elevation occurs after
about 1 week of illness. Abnormalities of nerve conduction reflect the demyelination
process. Conduction block in motor nerves and spontaneous discharges in demyeli-
nated sensory nerves make this study both sensitive and specific. Ropper emphasizes
that several findings suggest alternate diagnoses: (a) reflexes that are normal for several days into the illness, (b) marked asymmetry of weakness, (c) fever in the initial
disease presentation, and (d) a CSF protein level above 2.5 g/L. The differential diagnosis depends on the history and physical examination findings but may include
spinal cord compression, transverse myelitis, myasthenia gravis, chronic meningitis,
metabolic myopathies, paraneoplastic neuropathy, poliomyelitis, tick paralysis, botulism, and shellfish poisoning.
    Recent studies suggest a lymphocytic T-cell mechanism for this inflammatory periph-
eral neuropathy. Inflammation is thought to be the result of an aberrant immune
response to myelin antigens. Tumor necrosis factor-α is elevated in many GBS patients
and may contribute to the inflammatory demyelination process. An antibody directed
against myelin might lead to a macrophage response with tumor necrosis factor-α as
the mediating factor in myelin destruction. Serum from patients with GBS causes
demyelination and conduction block in some models. Antineural antibodies have also
been demonstrated. IgM antibody to certain myelin antigens has been shown to correlate with clinical disease.
    The list of infectious organisms that may trigger this process continues to grow. Viral
agents such as herpes simplex virus, Epstein-Barr virus, cytomegalovirus, influenza

virus, measles virus, mumps virus, respiratory syncytial virus, and hepatitis B virus have been implicated. GBS also occurred as a complication of swine flu vaccination in about 500 persons in 1977; however, no other cases of GBS have occurred in subsequent flu vaccination programs. Bacterial pathogens, particularly *Campylobacter, Salmonella,* and *Yersinia* species, appear to cause infections that precipitate GBS. In 1990, Yuki et al. reported that IgM antibody against ganglioside $GM_1$ had been detected in the serum of two patients with GBS following *Campylobacter* infection. This antibody could well be cross-reactive with both the myelin components and the organism itself. In recent years, it has become apparent that *Campylobacter jejuni* is by far the most common agent to precipitate GBS. Thirty percent to 40% of cases are now felt to be caused by preceding *Campylobacter* infection.

The treatment of GBS is supportive and specific. Patients should be hospitalized, at least for observation. GBS is the most common neuromuscular disease requiring respiratory support. Paralysis of the respiratory muscles can occur suddenly without clinical warning. Patients with vital capacities that are declining or below 18 mL/kg should be observed in an ICU setting. Elective intubation for positive-pressure ventilation is recommended at about 15 mL/kg.

Specific treatment for GBS includes plasma exchange or infusion of gamma globulin. Corticosteroids have been used, but randomized controlled trials have not found them to be of benefit.

Plasma exchange has been shown to be beneficial in several randomized trials. The standard regimen appears to be five plasma exchanges (200 to 250 mL/kg in five sessions within 7 to 14 days). Plasma exchange decreased the time until patients could walk unassisted and decreased the need for mechanical ventilation. Benefit was less apparent if exchange was started after 2 weeks of illness. Because immune globulin has been used with beneficial effects in several autoimmune diseases, it was of interest to study its effects in GBS. The Dutch Guillain-Barré Study Group compared IV immune globulin with plasma exchange in 150 GBS patients who were unable to walk but had had the disease for less than 2 weeks. The incidence of improvement was higher in the immune globulin patients (53% vs. 34% in the exchange group) as measured by motor function grading. The median time to improvement by one grade was 41 days in the plasma exchange group and 27 days in the immune globulin group. The immune globulin patients had less need for artificial ventilation.

More recently, the Plasma Exchange/Sandoglobulin Guillain-Barré Syndrome Trial Group completed a randomized trial of plasma exchange versus IV immune globulin versus the combined treatments. The two treatments were equally efficacious, and the combination offered no advantage. Other studies have also concluded the two treatments to be equivalent. The optimal number of plasma exchanges has also been better defined. For mild disease, two plasma exchanges were better than none with respect to time to onset of motor recovery. For moderate disease, four exchanges were better than two. Six exchanges were no better than four, even in severe disease.

GBS has been associated with AIDS and HIV disease. GBS can occur in association with HIV seroconversion or may be a late manifestation of AIDS. As in other patients with GBS, patients with AIDS may report sudden or gradual onset of weakness. It may be particularly difficult in patients with AIDS to distinguish GBS from other causes of peripheral neuropathy. (S.L.B.)

## Bibliography

Allos BM. *Campylobacter jejuni* infection as a cause of Guillain-Barré syndrome. *Infect Dis Clin North Am* 1998;12:173.

*Molecular mimicry between lipopolysaccharide of some* Campylobacter *organisms and ganglioside antigens is the probable explanation for GBS as a sequela of* Campylobacter *infection. In 30% to 40% of cases, GBS is preceded by* C. jejuni *infection.*

Appropriate number of plasma exchanges in Guillain-Barré syndrome. The French Cooperative Group on Plasma Exchange in Guillain-Barré syndrome. *Ann Neurol* 1997;41:298.

*In moderate and severe disease, four plasma exchanges were better than two; six exchanges were no more beneficial than four.*

Berlit P, Rakicky J. The Miller-Fisher syndrome. Review of the literature. *J Clin Neuroophthalmol* 1992;12:57.
*An update on the GBS variant of the Miller-Fisher syndrome, which presents with ataxia, areflexia, and ophthalmoplegia. Prognosis is good, with a mean recovery of 10 weeks.*

Brill V, et al. Pilot trial of immunoglobulin versus plasma exchange in patients with Guillain-Barré. *Neurology* 1996;46:100.
*Results of the two treatments were similar, with no difference in relapse rate.*

Dalakas MC, Pezeshkpour GH. Neuromuscular diseases associated with human immunodeficiency virus infection. *Ann Neurol* 1988;23:S38.
*GBS is one of six subtypes of peripheral neuropathy commonly associated with AIDS. GBS may occur early or late in HIV disease.*

Dyck PJ, Kurtzke JF. Plasmapheresis in Guillain-Barré syndrome. *Neurology* 1985; 35:1105.
*The authors critique the plasmapheresis data of the GBS Study Group (see Guillain-Barré Syndrome Study Group. Plasmapheresis and acute Guillain-Barré syndrome. Neurology 1985;35:1096). The study was not blinded, and 12 patients randomized to plasmapheresis dropped out.*

French Cooperative Study Group on Plasma Exchange in Guillain-Barré Syndrome. Efficiency of plasma exchange in Guillain-Barré syndrome: role of replacement fluids. *Ann Neurol* 1987;22:753.
*The French Cooperative Study found improvement in GBS patients who received plasma exchange. There was no improvement in comparison with controls in an albumin or fresh-frozen plasma group.*

Ginn DR. Guillain-Barré syndrome. An uncommon but severe illness. *Postgrad Med J* 1991;90:145.
*A practical approach to GBS for the practicing physician.*

Guillain-Barré Syndrome Study Group. Plasmapheresis and acute Guillain-Barré syndrome. *Neurology* 1985;35:1096.
*Plasmapheresis was of benefit in GBS patients who received treatment within 7 days.*

Harrison BM, et al. Demyelination induced by serum from patients with Guillain-Barré syndrome. *Ann Neurol* 1984;15:163.
*Serum from 16 patients with GBS caused sciatic nerve conduction block in a rat model. Serum obtained in the recovery phase did not cause block.*

Hartung HP. Immune-mediated demyelination. *Ann Neurol* 1993;33:563.
*Describes the mechanism of the aberrant immune response responsible for GBS. Tumor necrosis factor may contribute to the inflammatory demyelinating process.*

Hughes RA, Rees JH. Clinical and epidemiologic features of Guillain-Barré syndrome. *J Infect Dis* 1997;176(Suppl 2):S92.
*Updates signs and symptoms of the disease and describes worldwide incidence and predisposing factors, emphasizing C. jejuni infection.*

Hund EF, et al. Intensive management and treatment of severe Guillain-Barré syndrome. *Crit Care Med* 1993;21:433.
*Describes the expected complications and treatment of GBS in the ICU. Prevention of thrombosis and pneumonia, psychologic support, and adequate nutrition are all important aspects of management.*

Randomized trial of plasma exchange, intravenous immunoglobulin, and combined treatments in Guillain-Barré syndrome. Plasma Exchange/Sandoglobulin Guillain-Barré syndrome Trial Group. *Lancet* 1997;349:225.
*Plasma exchange and IV globulin were equally effective in the treatment of severe GBS when given during the first 2 weeks after onset of neuropathic symptoms.*

Ropper AH. The Guillain-Barré syndrome. *N Engl J Med* 1992;326:1130.
*Up-to-date comprehensive review that summarizes clinical features, pathophysiology, and results of treatment protocols.*

Ropper AH, Wijdicks EFM, Shahani BT. Electrodiagnostic abnormalities in 113 consecutive patients with Guillain-Barré syndrome. *Arch Neurol* 1990;47:881.
*Describes the types of electrodiagnostic abnormalities found in acute GBS. The types of abnormalities did not generally correlate with prognosis.*

Ropper AH, Wijdicks EFM, Truax BT. *Guillain-Barré syndrome*. Philadelphia: FA Davis Co, 1991.
*Includes detailed clinical descriptions of GBS and its variants.*

Rostami AM. Pathogenesis of immune-mediated neuropathies. *Pediatr Res* 1993;33: S90–S94.
*Review of the pathogenesis of GBS. An animal model of GBS has been induced by immunization with a myelin protein.*

Shearn MA, Shearn L. A personal experience with Guillain-Barré syndrome: are the psychologic needs of patient and family being met? *South Med J* 1986;79:800.
*Describes the personal and psychologic aspects of the disease by means of a patient and family diary.*

Sovilla JY, Regli F, Francioli PB. Guillain-Barré syndrome following *Campylobacter jejuni* enteritis. Report of three cases and review of the literature. *Arch Intern Med* 1988;48:739.
Campylobacter jejuni *is now recognized as a trigger of GBS. Eleven cases are reviewed.*

Tabor E. Guillain-Barré syndrome and other neurologic syndromes in hepatitis A, B, and non-A, non-B. *J Med Virol* 1987;21:207.
*Reviews the association of GBS and viral hepatitis.*

van der Meche FGA, Schmitz PIM, Dutch Guillain-Barré Study Group. A randomized trial comparing intravenous immune globulin and plasma exchange in Guillain-Barré syndrome. *N Engl J Med* 1992;326:1123.
*The Dutch Guillain-Barré Study Group found immune globulin superior to plasma exchange in the treatment of GBS. Patients improved faster on immune globulin and had fewer side effects.*

Winer JB, Hughes RAC, Osmond C. A prospective study of acute idiopathic neuropathy. I. Clinical features and their prognostic value. *J Neurol Neurosurg Psychiatry* 1988;51:605.
*Prospective study gives details of clinical features and prognosis in 100 patients. Age and action potential of abductor pollicis brevis were prognostic factors.*

Yuki N, et al. Acute axonal polyneuropathy associated with anti-GM$_1$ antibodies following *Campylobacter* enteritis. *Neurology* 1990;40:1900.
*Describes two cases of GBS after* Campylobacter *enteritis. In both cases, high titers of IgF antibody against GM ganglioside were demonstrated.*

# VIII. BONES AND JOINTS

# 36. VERTEBRAL OSTEOMYELITIS

Vertebral osteomyelitis is an uncommon but increasingly recognized infection that can be difficult to diagnose and can be complicated by potentially devastating neurologic or vascular catastrophies. It represents 2% to 4% of all cases of osteomyelitis. In adults, hematogenous dissemination is the most common method of spread. Recent data suggest that the risk for vertebral osteomyelitis as a complication of *Staphylococcus aureus* bacteremia is increasing. The reasons for increased recognition of this disease include a higher prevalence of parenteral drug use and nosocomial infection (primarily related to the use of IV catheters), the prevalence of diabetes, an aging population, better imaging techniques, and a greater understanding of this illness.

The disease is more common in adults than in children, and a recent study demonstrated that men were affected in 95% of cases. Most cases occur in persons over the age of 50 years; this may be explained in part by the increased frequency of urinary tract infections in the elderly and the presence of Batson's plexus, a low-pressure, valveless venous plexus that drains the pelvis toward the vertebral column and potentially allows passage of infection into this area. Thus, it differs from other forms of osteomyelitis in that it has a higher male-to-female ratio, occurs in an older population, and is more closely associated with diabetes mellitus. With regard to pyogenic vertebral osteomyelitis, at least 50% of cases involve the lumbar spine (possibly related to the noted anatomic considerations). The thoracic spine (approximately 30% of cases) and cervical spine are involved in decreasing order of frequency. Tuberculous vertebral osteomyelitis most commonly involves the lower thoracic vertebrae (Pott's disease).

## Diagnosis

The clinical presentation is often subtle, and the physician must have a high index of suspicion to make an early diagnosis. Although about 10% of cases present acutely, with positive blood cultures substantiating the diagnosis, subacute or chronic back pain is the most common presentation and is noted in more than 90% of cases. The duration of complaints is frequently longer than 3 months. Unusual clinical presentations may occur as a result of extension into surrounding tissues. Pleural empyema and retropharyngeal abscess have been recently described as initial presentations of pyogenic vertebral osteomyelitis. Neurologic complaints often imply the presence of spinal epidural abscess. IV substance abusers with vertebral osteomyelitis tend to have a more truncated course. Additionally, two cases of gas-forming osteomyelitis caused by enteric gram-negative bacilli have been reported. In both cases, diabetic patients were involved and the course was fulminant. Fever is present in up to 90% of cases but is usually low-grade. Frank rigors are unusual.

Initial assessment must include a careful history to evaluate for a primary focus of infection. Clinical conditions predisposing to vertebral osteomyelitis include a history of IV substance abuse, diabetes mellitus, trauma to the back (including surgery), distant skin or soft-tissue infection, and history of urinary tract infection or instrumentation. In patients currently or recently hospitalized, the IV catheter must be strongly considered. The history should also include an epidemiologic assessment for unusual pathogens, such as *Myobacterium tuberculosis,* fungi, and *Brucella* species. A recent investigation demonstrated that *M. tuberculosis* was the pathogen in approximately 33% of patients with vertebral osteomyelitis, and all came from endemic areas. However, in at least 33% of cases, the predisposing factors for infection will remain undetermined.

The physical examination must include an assessment for localized tenderness over a vertebral body and a search for feeding foci, such as an infected IV line, stigmata of IV substance abuse, and a urinary tract infection. The examination should also assess for neurologic complications.

Initial laboratory data are generally nonspecific. Leukocytosis is seen in fewer than 50% of cases. The erythrocyte sedimentation rate is elevated in more than 80% of cases, but this is a nonspecific finding. However, a decline of this parameter by 33% to 50% during antimicrobial therapy may help to predict cure.

The suspected area should always be assessed radiographically. Plain films may not reveal positive findings for 2 to 8 weeks after clinical presentation, and initial findings are often nonspecific. They may include paravertebral swelling or sclerosis of the vertebral end-plates. However, more advanced cases of vertebral osteomyelitis may involve a disk and adjacent vertebrae. The finding of disk space narrowing with adjacent changes should prompt consideration of this disease. This is in contradistinction to metastatic tumor, which is characteristically confined to the vertebral body and spares the disk. The clinician must have a high index of suspicion when the course of metastatic cancer is other than expected and consider additional diagnoses. Magnetic resonance imaging (MRI) has proved especially useful in this regard. Observations have also been made recently of patients with confirmed vertebral osteomyelitis in the setting of underlying osteoporosis; they presented with localized vertebral disease and resultant collapse mimicking compression fracture, which caused diagnostic delay. Alternatively, findings on routine plain films are usually abnormal when osteomyelitis is of granulomatous origin. This is presumably because of the more indolent nature of the disease and longer time course before clinical presentation.

Gallium, indium [111]In-leukocyte, or technetium bone scanning is more sensitive than standard radiography, and positive results may appear within 7 days. Gallium or [111]In-leukocyte scanning has the capacity to demonstrate complications within adjacent tissues; however, it is not as specific. Computed tomography (CT) and MRI are the best tests for diagnosing vertebral osteomyelitis in a timely fashion, and one or the other should be used early in management. MRI changes suggestive of vertebral osteomyelitis are noted in 90% of patients with symptoms of less than 2 weeks' duration, and in 96% of patients with symptoms lasting beyond 2 weeks.

MRI may prove to be particularly useful in diagnosing vertebral osteomyelitis in the known setting of metastatic tumor to a vertebral body. Changes considered diagnostic of vertebral osteomyelitis include erosion of end-plates and occult paravertebral swelling. Similarly, both MRI and CT can provide timely information concerning complications of the spinal canal or aorta. Thus, in the case of patients with obscure back, chest, or abdominal pain or in the evaluation of fever of unknown origin, CT or MRI can provide invaluable information concerning the diagnosis and potential complications and should be performed early in the evaluation. MRI may also suggest differences between pyogenic and tuberculous osteomyelitis. In the former, fewer vertebral bodies are involved, paravertebral abscesses are smaller, and the magnetic intensity of vertebral bodies is more homogenous. The author recommends initial plain films and then MRI as in the diagnosis of vertebral osteomyelitis. Bone, gallium, and labeled-WBC scans are of limited value.

Once osteomyelitis is suspected, bacteriologic confirmation should be sought. Although blood and urine cultures should be performed, they are unlikely to provide confirmatory data. The best approach is percutaneous bone aspiration of the involved site under CT guidance before the initiation of antimicrobial therapy. This approach may also allow simultaneous drainage of any paravertebral abscesses. Material obtained should be sent for (a) Gram's stain and acid-fast stain; (b) routine (aerobic and anaerobic), mycobacterial, and fungal cultures; and (c) histopathologic analysis. If results of the initial assessment prove negative, routine cultures should be held for several weeks so that pathogens such as *Brucella* species are not overlooked. The yield from percutaneous bone aspiration will decrease if the anterior portion of the bone is involved. In these circumstances, a decision will be needed regarding more aggressive surgery (typically an anterior approach) or empiric therapy.

### Bacteriology

Bacteriology is variable and relates to the underlying cause of disease. A recent investigation demonstrated that the presence of HIV/AIDS did not affect the bacteriology of vertebral osteomyelitis. Most cases involve single isolates. Occasionally, cultures remain sterile, perhaps because of previous antimicrobial therapy. *S. aureus* is the most commonly identified pathogen. Gram-negative enteric bacilli, especially *Escherichia coli* and *Salmonella* species, account for about 30% of cases. The latter are especially noted in patients with sickle cell disease and in those whose illness is complicated by aortic mycotic aneurysm. *Pseudomonas aeruginosa* has been commonly identified in patients whose vertebral osteomyelitis is associated with IV substance abuse. Infections caused by species of *Brucella* should be suspected in persons from selected areas of the world. Tuberculous vertebral osteomyelitis usually involves thoracic or upper lumbar vertebrae and often is associated with evidence of pulmonary tuberculosis. The duration of symptoms is longer in patients with *M. tuberculosis* infection than in those with pyogenic vertebral osteomyelitis. A history of active tuberculosis at other sites should be sought. In some series, it has accounted for almost 40% of cases of vertebral osteomyelitis. *M. tuberculosis* infection should be suspected in patients whose epidemiologic history would suggest exposure to endemic disease. If attempts to identify a bacterial pathogen fail, the search for it should be intensified.

### Treatment
Parenteral antimicrobial therapy active against the offending pathogen is the cornerstone of therapy for uncomplicated pyogenic vertebral osteomyelitis. In most instances, therapy can be withheld until a pathogen is identified. Treatment is usually continued for at least 4 weeks, and the sedimentation rate may be employed to gauge response to therapy. For gram-positive infections, a single β-lactam agent usually suffices. It is important to monitor for adverse reactions, such as interstitial nephritis, toxic hepatitis, or neutropenia or thrombocytopenia, which can occasionally be observed with prolonged β-lactam therapy. Treatment of infections caused by gram-negative bacilli should be guided by susceptibility data. It is the opinion of the author that many cases can be treated with full doses of oral quinolones as monotherapy. Such treatment has been successfully employed with other forms of osteomyelitis. In occasional cases, empiric therapy has been required, as a specific etiologic diagnosis cannot be made. In these instances, the author has had success with a quinolone plus rifampin, given orally for at least 4 weeks. Should tuberculosis also be a consideration, then isoniazid may be added.

Uncomplicated cases of vertebral osteomyelitis are usually managed medically. Surgical or nonsurgical drainage is generally indicated for spinal epidural abscess and other neurologic or vascular complications, or if frank paravertebral abscess is demonstrated by CT. The focal paravertebral collection may be successfully managed with percutaneous drainage.

Immobilization has also generally been recommended; however, this is now generally interpreted to mean modest bed rest early in treatment. Most authorities do not recommend braces or casting for the routine case, although this may occasionally be indicated if spinal instability is noted.

With appropriate diagnosis and treatment, mortality and neurologic sequelae should be modest. Diagnosing this infection remains the major challenge for the clinician, as the presentation may mimic that of numerous other infectious and noninfectious conditions. (R.B.B.)

### Bibliography
Abbey DM, Hosea SW. Diagnosis of vertebral osteomyelitis in a community hospital by using computed tomography. *Arch Intern Med* 1989;149:2029–2035.
   *This report evaluates the radiographic diagnosis of vertebral osteomyelitis in 20 persons with the disease. It points out the failure of routine plain films to document this process and the value of CT in delineating changes consistent with the diagnosis. The most commonly identified abnormality was destruction of the vertebral end-plates. The authors conclude that CT should be performed early in the evaluation of patients who possibly have this disease.*
An HS, et al. Differentiation between spinal tumors and infections with magnetic resonance imaging. *Spine* 1991;16(Suppl 8):S334–S338.
   *The authors studied 30 patients with proven spinal tumors or infections. MRI correctly diagnosed 29 of 30 processes. Involvement of disk spaces was seen only with infectious processes, as was involvement of contiguous vertebrae. The authors believe MRI to be the best imaging modality to differentiate infection from tumor.*
Arnold PM, et al. Surgical management of nontuberculous thoracic and lumbar vertebral osteomyelitis: report of 33 cases. *Surg Neurol* 1997;47:551–561.
   *Indications for surgery were either neurologic deficit or failure of antibiotic therapy. Long-term outcomes following surgery were good.*

Carragee EJ. The clinical use of magnetic resonance imaging in pyogenic vertebral osteomyelitis. *Spine* 1997;22:780–785.

*One hundred three cases of vertebral osteomyelitis were reviewed by the author. Within the first 2 weeks of symptoms, MRI findings were either positive or suggestive of the diagnosis in about 90% of cases. After 2 weeks, this rate rose to about 96%. The author feels that MRI is valuable for the initial diagnosis of vertebral osteomyelitis. However, its role in follow-up is uncertain, as the MRI often demonstrates worsening disease while clinical improvement has been noted.*

McHenry MC, et al. Vertebral osteomyelitis presenting as spinal compression fracture. Six patients with underlying osteoporosis. *Arch Intern Med* 1988;148:417.

*The authors identified six patients with underlying osteoporosis complicated by pyogenic vertebral osteomyelitis (one patient was infected with* Nocardia asteroides*). All demonstrated infection of a single vertebra, which initially was felt to represent compression fracture rather than infection. In the experience of the authors, this clinical presentation represented 10% to 15% of cases of vertebral osteomyelitis and 2% to 3% of cases of presumed compression fracture. The presentation was associated with significant sequelae because of long delays in diagnosis. The presence of elevated sedimentation rate, fever, severe pain, or discomfort that does not improve with standard treatment should make the clinician suspect the presence of infection.*

McHenry MC, et al. Vertebral osteomyelitis and aortic lesions: case report and review. *Rev Infect Dis* 1991;13:1184–1194.

*This report summarizes data on 70 patients whose vertebral osteomyelitis was complicated by involvement of the aorta. Mortality was more than 70%. Infected aneurysms were most commonly noted, and pathogens included an extended list of enteric gram-negative bacilli (including* Salmonella *species), gram-positive cocci, and mycobacteria. The best outcomes were noted with a combination of targeted antimicrobial therapy plus aortic resection.*

Patzakis MJ, et al. Analysis of 61 cases of vertebral osteomyelitis. *Clin Orthop* 1991; 264:178–183.

*The authors compared diagnostic imaging techniques in 61 patients with confirmed vertebral osteomyelitis and conclude that MRI is the most sensitive technique for making the diagnosis. Further prospective studies are necessary before their recommendation of MRI as a front-line study for this disease can be totally accepted.*

Perronne C, et al. Pyogenic and tuberculous spondylodiskitis (vertebral osteomyelitis) in 80 adult patients. *Clin Infect Dis* 1994;19:746–750.

*This retrospective study demonstrated that almost 40% of patients had tuberculous disease, based primarily on the population that was studied. This points out the need for a careful epidemiologic history. Cases of both tuberculosis and* Staphylococcus *infection were associated with histories of prior active infection, which could help the clinician in making the diagnosis. In this investigation, more than 50% of patients with pyogenic disease had positive blood cultures, and about 75% had positive bone aspirate cultures.*

Sapico FL, Montgomerie JZ. Pyogenic vertebral osteomyelitis: report of nine cases and review of the literature. *Rev Infect Dis* 1979;5:754–776.

*An excellent review of the subject that evaluates 318 cases. Elderly men and diabetic patients were particularly predisposed, and the most commonly identified predisposing focus was the urinary tract. Parenteral antimicrobials for more than 4 weeks plus bed rest were the major therapeutic modalities. Treatment of lesser duration increased failure rates. Failure of the sedimentation rate to decline by at least one third was an adverse prognostic indicator.*

Sapico RL, Montgomerie JZ. Vertebral osteomyelitis. *Infect Dis Clin North Am* 1990; 4:539–550.

*The authors review data on the diagnosis, bacteriology, and management of vertebral osteomyelitis. They rightfully conclude that diagnosis may be subtle, and all attempts should be made to isolate a pathogen rather than treat empirically.*

Torda AJ, Gottleib T, Bradbury R. Pyogenic vertebral osteomyelitis: analysis of 20 cases and review. *Clin Infect Dis* 1995;20:320–328.

*In this investigation, most patients were elderly and only 30% presented with fever. Nosocomial infection, often associated with IV cannula use and methiciliin-resistant* S. aureus, *was common. MRI or CT was the most useful radiographic modality.*

## 37. INFECTIONS OF PROSTHETIC JOINTS

Total hip and knee replacements are frequent orthopedic procedures, with about 450,000 arthroplasties performed each year in the United States. Infection is the most dreaded complication of joint replacement operations. For most series, the overall infection rate after total hip replacement is 0.5% to 2.0%. The rate of infection after knee replacement is higher, 0.6% to 3.9%. The rate of infection is still higher for certain types of prostheses, such as a metal-hinged knee (11%). Infection is more likely to develop following total joint arthroplasty in patients with rheumatoid arthritis or who have had prior surgery than in those who have underlying osteoarthritis or are undergoing a primary operation. Although the overall infection rate after hip replacement is low (approximately 1%), more than 1,000 infected patients are seen annually in the United States.

Prosthetic joint infections can be classified as early (within the first 3 months after replacement), delayed (within the first 2 years), and late (after 2 years). In the early category, most of the infections occur within the first month after operation. The majority (67%) of prosthetic infections are detected within the first 2 years after replacement, and about one third of patients present with late infections after 2 years. Under-reporting of late infections may occur; moreover, the potential for late infections persists indefinitely. Infections that develop within the first 2 years are largely the result of contamination of the prosthetic joint or wound at the time of replacement or of other nosocomial events, such as undetected line-related bacteremias. Infections that occur after 2 years are the result of hematogenous seeding from an infected focus, such as a distant cellulitis, a urinary tract infection, or a transient bacteremia related to a minor dental or surgical procedure. Late infections can also develop from very low-grade infections initiated at the time of replacement or during the perioperative period. The proportion of late infections attributed to a hematogenous source compared with that of infections from other sources is debatable.

Early prosthetic joint infections often result from the contiguous spread of bacteria from a local wound infection to the prosthesis. The patient may have an obviously infected wound early in the postoperative period. Whether the infection is superficial and does not involve the prosthesis or is deep and does affect the joint replacement is often unclear. Surgical exploration of the wound may be required to establish the correct diagnosis. The patient may also have a painful hematoma that proves to be infected after it is aspirated. Frequently, joint pain is the prominent symptom, and the wound may appear entirely normal (no warmth, erythema, tenderness, or inflammation) or only slightly inflamed. Pain usually occurs with active and passive motion of the affected joint. Another clue to deep infection is persistent wound drainage. Fever is usually present.

The clinical presentation of delayed infection is more insidious, key findings being pain on bearing weight and on motion of the joint. Clues that usually indicate infection, such as inflammation, drainage, and fever, are often absent. Late infection is usually characterized by the acute onset of joint pain and fever after a long asymptomatic period following the initial surgery. The history may reveal an earlier distant focus of infection that may have been untreated. The diagnosis of an infected joint is frequently difficult to make and may be established only at reoperation. Pain, usually constant, is the hallmark of joint infection. The pain caused by mechanical loosening of the prosthesis is generally related to motion and weight bearing and is not present at rest.

A number of laboratory studies are used to support the clinical diagnosis of an infected prosthetic joint: WBC count, erythrocyte sedimentation rate (ESR), plain radiographs, sinogram, arthrogram, joint aspiration, technetium bone scan, and gallium and indium 111 scans. The WBC count in patients with infection is variable. An elevated ESR (>20 mm/h) suggests infection if no other explanation for the increase, such as underlying rheumatoid arthritis, can be found. A normal ESR makes infection unlikely (3% to 11% of cases) but does not exclude it entirely. The ESR usually falls to 20 mm/h at 6 months after an uncomplicated joint replacement. Serial plain radiographs are helpful in assessing the presence of infection. Deep infections may produce radiolucencies at the prosthesis-cement-bone interface. These changes of bone resorption may also result from mechanical loosening of the prosthesis. Arthrography and sinography may also provide useful information to establish the diagnosis of infection.

Aspiration of the joint is the most reliable test to diagnose infection. Fluoroscopy ensures proper placement of the needle. A Gram's stain should be performed, and the aspirate should also be cultured aerobically and anaerobically, as well as fungi and mycobacteria in selected cases. Positive results on technetium bone, gallium, and indium 111 scans suggest infection; however, with mechanical loosening of the prosthesis, results of the gallium scan are normal, and the technetium bone scan result is abnormal.

Another approach to differentiate infection from mechanical loosening of the prosthesis is to obtain five biopsy samples for culture. Bacterial growth in one or two cultures indicates contamination, and growth in all five samples suggests infection. Growth in both solid and broth media indicates infection; growth only in broth medium indicates contamination.

Staphylococci are the most common cause of prosthetic joint infections, accounting for at least 30% to 40% of all infections. Previous studies showed that *Staphylococcus aureus* is the leading cause of infection in the early, delayed, and late-onset periods. In one report, however, *Staphylococcus epidermidis* was shown to cause 40% of the infections and *S. aureus* only 19%. In another report, staphylococci accounted for almost half of the infections, evenly divided between *S. aureus* and *S. epidermidis*. *S. epidermidis* infection usually appears as an indolent infection, causing minimal symptoms and signs. The symptoms and signs of *S. aureus* infection can vary from fulminant sepsis to an indolent infection. Because *S. epidermidis* is also a frequent cause of contamination of culture specimens, more than one isolate is needed to confirm this as the etiologic agent.

After staphylococci, gram-negative bacilli, such as *Escherichia coli, Proteus* species, *Enterobacter* species, and *Pseudomonas aeruqinosa,* account for 20% to 30% of infections. Gram-negative bacilli are more common in the early-onset period than in late-onset infections. Genitourinary and gastrointestinal tract procedures or infections are associated with gram-negative prosthetic infections. Other organisms that are implicated less often include streptococci of different groups, anaerobic streptococci, *Propionibacterium acnes,* and, rarely, fungi or mycobacteria. Anaerobes account for about 16% of cases, and in about 10% of patients, all cultures are negative despite clinical evidence of infection. Cultures can be negative because of prior administration of antimicrobials and, occasionally, inadequate bacteriologic techniques. Polymicrobial infections can also occur.

A number of studies address the problems of treating prosthetic joint infections. If the patient has an early-onset infection, the prosthesis can be left in place if during surgical procedures there is no evidence of loosening of the device. Adequate debridement should be performed, and appropriate antimicrobials, depending on the results of culture and sensitivity testing, must be given parenterally for 6 weeks. Most studies report better results with gram-positive than with gram-negative bacilli.

A loose hip prosthesis can be replaced with a new one even when infection is present. This procedure is limited to gram-positive infections, and a favorable outcome is reported in up to 85% of selected patients. Appropriate antimicrobials should then be continued for 6 weeks. Some authorities favor surgical debridement of the wound, removal of the prosthesis, a subsequent 6-week course of parenteral antimicrobials, and then reimplantation of another joint. If reimplantation is not possible, an excision arthroplasty and prolonged antimicrobial suppression can be attempted. In delayed infections, salvage of the prosthetic hip is rare, and the prosthesis should be removed at the time of the debridement. An attempt can be made to save the hip prosthesis in patients with acute hematogenous joint infection. Some patients (30%) can be cured with debridement and prolonged parenteral antimicrobials. In the majority of these patients, however, either removal and a reimplantation procedure or an excision arthroplasty is required.

The management of prosthetic knee infections is similar to that of hip infections. If the prosthesis is not loose and the etiologic agent is a gram-positive organism, then debridement and parenteral antimicrobials may be adequate. More often, however, the prosthesis must be removed.

Administering antimicrobials to prevent late-onset joint infection in patients who undergo procedures involving dental or genitourinary tract manipulation, which causes a transient bacteremia, is controversial. Most late-onset infections in patients with rheumatoid arthritis result from hematogenous seeding of a joint from established distant foci of infection. Examples of these infections are skin abscesses and urinary tract infections. Prompt treatment of these infections with appropriate antimicrobials prevents hematogenous seeding and subsequent joint infection. The risk for hematogenous seeding of a prosthetic joint from a transient bacteremia, such as that caused by a dental cleaning, appears to be extremely low. In one report, the risk associated with dental procedures was 0.05%, so low that the cost to prevent a single case of joint infection would be high. Legal issues must also be considered in such situations. Because most late-onset infections result from established infections, patients should be treated promptly when infections are present.

An advisory committee of the American Dental Association and American Academy of Orthopaedic Surgeons has formulated guidelines to determine the need for antibiotic prophylaxis to prevent hematogenous prosthetic joint infections in patients undergoing a procedure such as a dental extraction. The panel of experts has suggested that antibiotics are not necessary for patients undergoing a dental procedure if they have a pin, plate, or screw, or for most patients with a total joint replacement. Patients who are at increased risk for hematogenous joint infection and who should receive antibiotic prophylaxis include those who are immunosuppressed (e.g., rheumatoid arthritis or systemic lupus erythematosus), have had a joint replacement within the previous 2 years, have had previous prosthetic joint infections, or have diabetes and are receiving insulin. These patients should receive a single dose of amoxicillin, or a cephalosporin such as cephalexin or cefazolin, or clindamycin if they are penicillin-allergic. In addition to antibiotic prophylaxis to prevent hematogenous seeding of a prosethetic joint, maintenance of good oral health is critical. (N.M.G.)

## Bibliography

Ainscow DAP, Denham RA. The risk of hematogenous infection in total joint replacement. *J Bone Joint Surg Br* 1984;66:580.
*Patients with rheumatoid arthritis are at increased risk for development of hematogenous infection of a prosthetic joint.*

Anonymous. Advisory statement. Antibiotic prophylaxis for dental patients with total joint replacements. American Dental Association; American Academy of Orthopaedic Surgeons. *J Am Dent Assoc* 1997;128:1004–1008.
*Antibiotic prophylaxis is not indicated for patients with pins, plates, and screws or for most patients with total joint replacements who are undergoing a dental procedure, such as an extraction.*

Booth RE Jr, Lotke PA. The results of spacer block technique in revision of infected total knee arthroplasty. *Clin Orthop* 1989;248:57.
*Describes use of a tobramycin-impregnated polymethylmethacrylate spacer block to treat infection locally during the exchange interval.*

Bose WJ, et al. Long-term outcome of 42 knees with chronic infection after total knee arthroplasty. *Clin Orthop* 1995;319:285–296.
*Overall success rate was 74%. Use of a two-stage reimplantation procedure was most effective.*

Brandt CM, et al. *Staphylococcus aureus* prosthetic joint infection treated with debridement and prosthesis retention. *Clin Infect Dis* 1997;24:914–919.
*Debridement of an infected prosthetic joint without replacement has a high failure rate (69%).*

Brause BD. Infected orthopedic prostheses. In: Bisno AL, Waldvogel FA, eds. *Infections associated with indwelling medical devices*. Washington, DC: American Society for Microbiology, 1989.
*Review.*

Cherney DL, Amstutz HC. Total hip replacement in the previously septic hip. *J Bone Joint Surg Am* 1983;65:1256.
*The success rate was better for gram-positive prosthetic infections.*

Deacon JM, et al. Prophylactic use of antibiotics for procedures after total joint replacement. *J Bone Joint Surg Am* 1996;78-A:1755–1770.
*Prophylactic antibiotics are usually not indicated in patients with a prosthetic joint who are undergoing a procedure associated with transient bacteremia.*
Fitzgerald RH, et al. Deep wound sepsis following total hip arthroplasty. *J Bone Joint Surg Am* 1977;59:847.
*Hip infections were classified as acute fulminant infection (occurring within the initial 3 months), delayed sepsis (occurring in the initial 26 months), and late hematogenous infection.*
Forster IW, Crawford R. Sedimentation rate in infected and uninfected total hip arthroplasty. *Clin Orthop* 1982;168:48.
*An elevated sedimentation rate suggests infection rather than aseptic loosening of the prosthesis.*
Gillespie WJ. Infection in total joint replacement. *Infect Dis Clin North Am* 1990; 4:465.
*Review.*
Gillespie WJ. Prevention and management of infection after total joint replacement. *Clin Infect Dis* 1997;25:1310–1317.
*Review of management.*
Goksan SB, Freeman MAR. One-stage reimplantation for infected total knee arthroplasty. *J Bone Joint Surg Br* 1992; 74-B:78.
*In a small series of infected knee prostheses caused by gram-positive organisms, a one-stage exchange procedure was effective in eradicating the infection.*
Goldman RT, Scuderi GR, Insall JN. Two-stage reimplantation for infected total knee replacement. *Clin Orthop* 1996;331:118–124.
*Infected prosthetic knees responded (77%) to an approach with three phases: (a) removal of the prosthesis and debridement, (b) 6 weeks of antibiotics, and (c) reimplantation with a new knee.*
Green SA, Ripley MJ. Chronic osteomyelitis in pin tracks. *J Bone Joint Surg Am* 1984; 66:1092.
*Management reviewed.*
Inman RD, et al. Clinical and microbial features of prosthetic joint infection. *Am J Med* 1984;77:47.
*Presenting symptoms included pain (95%), fever (43%), swelling (38%), and drainage (32%).*
Kamme C, Linderg L. Aerobic and anaerobic bacteria in deep infections after total hip arthroplasty. *Clin Orthop* 1981;154:201.
*A normal sedimentation rate does not exclude infection.*
Lachiewicz PF, Rogers GD, Thomason HC. Aspiration of the hip joint before revision total hip arthroplasty. Clinical and laboratory factors influencing attainment of a positive culture. *J Bone Joint Surg Am* 1996;78-A;749–754.
*In patients with a high sedimentation rate (mean of 80 mm/h), aspiration of the hip joint was helpful in predicting infection (sensitivity of 92%).*
McDonald DJ, Fitzgerald RH Jr, Ilstrup DM. Two-stage reconstruction of a total hip arthroplasty because of infection. *J Bone Joint Surg Am* 1989;71-A:828.
*The rate of recurrence was lower for patients who had a reimplantation more than 1 year after the resection arthroplasty. For gram-negative bacilli and enterococci, antimicrobial therapy should be given for at least 28 days.*
Mont MA, et al. Multiple irrigation, debridement, and retention of components in infected total knee arthroplasty. *J Arthroplasty* 1997;12:426–433.
*In patients with an infected knee prosthesis less than 30 days after surgery and no radiographic signs of osteitis or a loose prosthesis, debridement and antibiotics produced a high cure rate (83%).*
O'Neill DA, Harris WH. Failed total hip replacement: assessment by plain radiographs, arthrograms, and aspiration of the hip joint. *J Bone Joint Surg Am* 1984; 66:540.
*Aspiration of the hip joint is useful to diagnose infection.*
Oyen W, et al. Diagnosis of bone, joint, and joint prosthesis infections with In-111-labeled nonspecific human immunoglobulin G scintigraphy. *Radiology* 1992;182:195.

*Use of IgG labeled with indium 111 was valuable in the diagnosis of infections involving prosthetic hips and knees.*

Pagnano MW, Trousdale RT, Hanssen AD. Outcome after reinfection following reimplantation hip arthroplasty. *Clin Orthop* 1997;338:192–204.

*Patients in whom infection develops after reimplantation of a new prosthesis are candidates for an attempt at a third prosthesis in which a two-stage approach is used (success rate of 27%).*

Pellegrini VD, Jr. Management of the patient with an infected knee arthroplasty. *Instr Course Lect* 1997;46:215–219.

*Review. Factors that predispose patients to infection include use of steroids, rheumatoid disease, prior knee surgery, and the presence of open skin lesions on the affected leg.*

Powers KA, et al. Prosthetic joint infections in the elderly. *Am J Med* 1990;88:5–9N, 1990.

*In the elderly, only 61% of prosthetic joint infections responded with removal of the device; none resolved without removal of the prosthesis.*

Rand JA, Brown ML. The value of indium 111 leukocyte scanning in the evaluation of painful or infected total knee arthroplasties. *Clin Orthop* 1990;259:179.

*Indium 111 had a sensitivity of 83% and a specificity of 85% in the diagnosis of infected prosthetic knees.*

Rushton N, et al. The value of technetium and gallium scanning in assessing pain after total hip replacement. *J Bone Joint Surg Br* 1982;64:313.

*Suggests the use of both technetium bone and gallium scans to diagnose prosthetic joint infection.*

Salvati EA, et al. Infection rates after 3,175 total hip and knee replacements performed with and without a horizontal unidirectional filtered air-flow system. *J Bone Joint Surg Am* 1982;64:525.

*Infection rates were 0.9% after total hip replacement and 3.9% after total knee replacement.*

Schmalzried TP, et al. Etiology of deep sepsis in total hip arthroplasty. *Clin Orthop* 1992;280:200.

*The incidence of infection after a total hip arthroplasty is 1.5%. The major source for late infections is the genitourinary tract.*

Tsukayama DT, Estrada R, Gustilo RB. Infection after total hip arthroplasty. *J Bone Joint Surg Am* 1996;78:512–523.

*Infections were classified into four groups—positive intraoperative culture (at least two specimens positive), early postoperative infection (within 1 month of surgery), late chronic infection, and hematogenous infection (documented or suspected bacteremia). Aerobic gram-positive cocci were isolated in 74%, gram-negative bacilli in 14%, and anaerobes in 8% of cases.*

Wilde AH, Ruth JT. Two-stage reimplantation in infected total knee arthroplasty. *Clin Orthop* 1988;236:23.

*When a two-stage reimplantation with an antimicrobial-impregnated cement spacer was used in the treatment of infected knee prostheses, the cure rate was 90%.*

Wilson MG, Kelley K, Thornhill TS. Infection as a complication of total knee-replacement arthroplasty. *J Bone Joint Surg Am* 1990;72:878–883.

*Infection occurred in 1.6% of patients after knee replacement arthroplasty. Risk factors associated with infection included underlying rheumatoid arthritis, presence of skin ulcers, and prior surgery.*

Wininger DA, Fass RJ. Antibiotic-impregnated cement and beads for orthopedic infections. *Antimicrob Agents Chemother* 1996;40:2275–2279.

*Review. (see also Duncan CP, Masri BA. The role of antibiotic-loaded cement in the treatment of infection after hip replacement. Instr Course Lect 1995;46:305–313).*

Zimmerli W, et al. Role of rifampin for treatment of orthopedic implant-related staphylococcal infections: a randomized controlled trial. Foreign-Body Infection (FBI) Study Group. *JAMA* 1998;279:1537–1541.

*In selected patients with staphylococcal infections, rifampin plus ciprofloxacin for 3 to 6 months after an initial debridement was effective without removal of the implant.*

## 38. FEVER AND JOINT PAIN

Joint effusion is a common problem and a diagnostic challenge because septic arthritis is a medical emergency. Failure to establish an early diagnosis and administer appropriate therapy may lead to loss of joint function or death. The differential diagnosis in a patient with one or more warm, swollen joints is extensive and includes both infectious and noninfectious causes. Bacteria (including mycobacteria), viruses, and fungi are all among the infectious causes.

Bacterial arthritis can be classified as gonococcal or nongonococcal. The frequency distribution of organisms depends on differences in the population studied, such as location (city hospital vs. suburban community hospital), patient age, and the presence of an underlying illness. At one city hospital, approximately 60% of the patients with septic arthritis had gonococcal infection. This finding contrasts with the distribution in a community hospital, where nongonococcal disease predominates. In recent years, there appears to have been a decrease in the incidence of gonococcal arthritis. Of the nongonococcal causes, *Staphylococcus aureus* is seen most often and accounts for 30% to 50% of cases. This is followed by various species of streptococci (25%), including groups A, B, and G. Gram-negative bacilli have emerged as an important cause (20%) and are responsible for disease particularly in IV drug users and immunosuppressed patients. *Pseudomonas aeruginosa* tends to affect drug users and often attacks the sternoclavicular joint. *Streptococcus pneumoniae* is an infrequent cause of septic arthritis and accounts for 5% of cases. Pneumococcal arthritis usually results from bacteremic seeding of a joint in a patient with pneumococcal pneumonia. *Haemophilus influenzae* was formerly a common cause of septic arthritis in infants and young children but only infrequently produces disease in adults (<1%).

A number of viruses are associated with arthritis, the most frequent causes being hepatitis B virus, hepatitis C virus, rubella virus, mumps virus, parvovirus B19, HIV, and arbovirus. A painful, subacute, oligoarthritic syndrome involving the knees and ankles has been described in patients with AIDS. The pathogenesis is unknown. Other musculoskeletal disorders that have been reported in association with HIV infection include Reiter's syndrome, psoriatic arthritis, and avascular necrosis of bone.

Fungal and tuberculous causes of joint pain are rarer. Lyme disease, rheumatic fever, subacute bacterial endocarditis, Whipple's disease, and *Yersinia enterocolitica* infection are other infectious causes. Lyme disease is possible in a patient with a sudden onset of monoarthritis or oligoarthritis. Joint pains are usually preceded by the characteristic skin lesion, erythema chronicum migrans, in 60% to 70% of patients. The interval between appearance of the skin lesion and start of the joint symptoms is approximately 4 weeks, with a range of 0.6 to 24 weeks. The knee is the joint most often affected, followed by the shoulder. The arthritis usually lasts 1 week, but attacks recur frequently. A chronic arthritis, usually of the knees, is reported in 10% of patients. Serologic testing is an invaluable aid in the diagnosis, as most patients will have an increased IgG antibody titer to *Borrelia burgdorferi*. The synovial fluid is inflamed, with a median WBC count of 25,000/mm$^3$. Most of the cells are polymorphonuclear leukocytes. Oral doxycycline or amoxicillin and probenecid for 1 month are recommended for Lyme arthritis. Two grams of ceftriaxone per day given intravenously or high-dose penicillin administered intravenously for 2 to 3 weeks is also effective. Intraarticular steroid injections should be avoided because they may increase the risk for antimicrobial failure.

Joint pain of noninfectious causes, such as the inflammatory diseases (gout, pseudogout, rheumatoid arthritis, Reiter's syndrome, psoriatic arthritis, collagen diseases), and the arthritis of ulcerative colitis, or regional enteritis, can mimic septic arthritis. Hemarthrosis, secondary to hemophilia or other hemorrhage disorders, and trauma, such as an auto accident, should also be considered.

Organisms reach the synovium and joint space by one of three routes: direct introduction, extension from a contiguous focus, or hematogenous spread. Direct involvement can occur after trauma, surgery, or, rarely, the intraarticular injection of steroids. Spread from an overlying cellulitis or from an adjacent osteomyelitis is an example of a contiguous focus as the source. Hematogenous seeding of the synovium occurs most often. With a hematogenous origin, an extraarticular focus may be present. For example, a patient with pneumococcal arthritis may have pneumonia, or the organism may be found in the cervix or pharynx of a woman with disseminated gonococcal arthritis. A careful search for a bacterial source is often rewarding.

Factors that predispose the host to septic arthritis include damaged joints from prior rheumatoid arthritis, diabetes mellitus, cirrhosis, neoplasms, immunosuppressive therapy, and extraarticular foci of infection. The factors that permit an organism such as the gonococcus to infect a joint space during dissemination are unknown. The joint symptoms in patients with gonococcal disease often appear as a result of immune system processes.

Clinically, the onset of bacterial arthritis is usually abrupt. The symptoms include chills, fever, and monoarthritis with warmth, redness, swelling, and tenderness. Polyarthritis occurs in about 10% of patients. Any joint can be affected, but the large joints are the main targets, especially the knees, ankles, and wrists. The sternoclavicular joint may be infected in IV drug users or as a rare complication of subclavian venous catheterization, and the hip or sacroiliac joints can become infected in patients with inflammatory bowel disease; however, these joints are less commonly involved. The presentation can be cryptic in patients with rheumatoid arthritis and in infants, who may show only irritability and immobility. Patients with bacterial arthritis of the hip may have only knee pain.

The gonococcus is a common cause of septic arthritis in adults. Two forms are known, although overlap can occur. The disease usually occurs in young, healthy women, and it typically begins during the menses, pregnancy, or early postpartum period. An asymptomatic genital, pharyngeal, or rectal infection is the usual source. In one form, symptoms are chills, fever, migratory polyarthritis, and characteristic skin lesions. Tenosynovitis may occur and strongly suggests a gonococcal origin. Blood cultures are positive in 20% of patients, but little synovial fluid is present, and the results of a joint culture are often negative. Monoarthritis occurs in the other form, and the gonococcus is usually isolated from the joint fluid.

Synovial fluid analysis is the critical test for establishing the cause of an arthritis. Typical results of this analysis of a pyogenic joint infection are a WBC count of 50,000 to 100,000/mm$^3$ with 90% neutrophils, a poor mucin clot, and a sugar concentration at least 50 mg/dL below that of the blood sugar; occasionally, the joint fluid WBC count may be as low as 10,000/mm$^3$. A Gram's stain of a sediment is necessary for a diagnosis. The use of polymerase chain reaction may yield a diagnosis. Blood cultures, Gram's stains, and cultures for the gonococcus or meningococcus from other sites of infection, particularly the throat, cervix, rectum, and skin pustules, may be helpful. Synovial fluid should be plated on blood and chocolate agar and immediately incubated in 10% carbon dioxide for both aerobes and anaerobes. Thayer-Martin medium is not used, as it inhibits bacteria other than the gonococcus. Acid-fast stains, synovial biopsy, and cultures are performed if mycobacteria and fungi are suspected. Results of joint roentgenography are negative in septic arthritis unless an associated osteomyelitis is present.

Treatment consists of drainage and administration of antimicrobials directed toward the specific organism. The initial antimicrobial therapy should be guided by the patient's age and underlying disease, as well as the results of the synovial fluid Gram's stain. Needle aspirations must be repeated whenever the effusions reaccumulate to prevent cartilage destruction by leukocytic enzymes and debris. Open drainage is indicated for all hip joint infections, often for the shoulder joint, and when closed drainage does not permit adequate removal of the fluid because of adhesions and loculation. Arthroscopic techniques may be used for debridement as an alternative to the open arthrotomy. Intraarticular antimicrobial injections are unnecessary and may result in chemical synovitis.

The effectiveness of therapy can be judged by the clinical response and serial synovial fluid analyses. Physical therapy is instituted to maintain joint function. The joint fluid should become sterile after a few days, the WBC count should decrease progressively, and the sugar concentration should rise. The outcome depends on the duration of symptoms before treatment, the infecting organism, and the nature of the patient's underlying illness. The prognosis is poor in patients whose symptoms have been present for more than 5 days before initiation of antimicrobial therapy and in those with infections caused by gram-negative bacilli or staphylococci. Rapid improvement without sequelae can be expected in patients with gonococcal arthritis after 24 to 48 hours of therapy. Any warm, swollen joint should be considered infected until proved otherwise, and it should be treated as a medical emergency to avoid complications. (N.M.G.)

## Bibliography

Aglas F, et al. Sternoclavicular septic arthritis: a rare but serious complication of subclavian venous catheterization. *Clin Rheumatol* 1994;13:507–512.
*A bone scan is useful to diagnose sternoclavicular septic arthritis.*

Amirault JD. Septic arthritis in the elderly. *Clin Orthop* 1990;215:241.
*Most patients were afebrile and had a normal WBC count.*

Bayer AS, et al. Gram-negative bacillary septic arthritis: clinical, radiographic, therapeutic, and prognostic features. *Semin Arthritis Rheum* 1977;7:123.
*Sternoclavicular joint involvement in heroin addicts was caused by* P. aeruginosa.

Black J, et al. Oral antimicrobial therapy for adults with osteomyelitis or septic arthritis. *J Infect Dis* 1987;155:968.
*A small series reporting the successful use of oral antimicrobials to treat osteomyelitis or septic arthritis in adults while monitoring trough serum bactericidal titers.*

Borenstein DG, Simon GL. *Haemophilus influenzae* septic arthritis in adults: a report of four cases and a review of the literature. *Medicine (Baltimore)* 1986;65:191.
*Although uncommon, septic arthritis is suspect in an immunocompromised host with an extraarticular focus of* H. influenzae *infection.*

Bronze MS, Whitby S, Schaberg DR. Group G streptococcal arthritis: case report and review of the literature. *Am J Med Sci* 1997;313:239–243.
*A rare cause of septic arthritis.*

Cimmino MA. Recognition and management of bacterial arthritis. *Drugs* 1997;54:50–60.
*Review. Septic arthritis is caused by hematogenous seeding of a joint or by direct extension from a contiguous focus of infection.*

Ellis LC, et al. Joint infections due to *Listeria monocytogenes:* case report and review. *Clin Infect Dis* 1995;20:1548–1550.
*A rare cause of septic arthritis, usually seen in renal transplant recipients or patients with rheumatoid arthritis.*

Fitzgerald RH Jr, et al. Anaerobic septic arthritis. *Clin Orthop* 1982;164:141.
*Although rare, most cases occur as a complication of surgery or following trauma.*

Gardner GC, Weisman MH. Pyarthrosis in patients with rheumatoid arthritis: a report of 13 cases and a review of the literature from the past 40 years. *Am J Med* 1990;88:503.
S. aureus *is the most common infecting organism, and the skin is often the source.*

Garrido G, et al. A review of peripheral tuberculous arthritis. *Semin Arthritis Rheum* 1988;18:142.
*Review.*

Goldenberg DL. Infectious arthritis complicating rheumatoid arthritis and other chronic rheumatic disorders. *Arthritis Rheum* 1989;32:496.
*Diagnosis is often delayed. Twenty percent of patients had polyarticular septic arthritis.*

Goldenberg DL. Bacterial arthritis. *Curr Opin Rheumatol* 1995;7:310–314.
*Polymerase chain reaction may be useful in the diagnosis of culture-negative cases.*

Goldenberg DL, Reed JI. Bacterial arthritis. *N Engl J Med* 1985;312:764.
*Review.*

Hansen BL, Andersen K. Fungal arthritis. A review. *Scand J Rheumatol* 1995;24:248–250.
Candida *is the most frequent fungal cause of septic arthritis.*

Hirsch R, et al. Human immunodeficiency virus-associated atypical mycobacterial skeletal infections. *Semin Arthritis Rheum* 1996;25:347–356.
*Consider atypical mycobacteria in HIV patients with septic arthritis and a CD4 cell count below* $100/mm^3$.

Hollander JL. Examination of synovial fluid as a diagnostic aid in arthritis. *Med Clin North Am* 1966;50:1281.
*A discussion of synovial fluid analysis.*

Kauffman CA, Watanakunakorn C, Phair JP. Pneumococcal arthritis. *J Rheumatol* 1976;3:409.
*Associated with endocarditis and / or meningitis in almost half of cases.*

Kay BR. Rheumatic manifestations of infection with human immunodeficiency virus (HIV). *Ann Intern Med* 1989;111:158.
*The foot and ankle are the most common sites of involvement.*

Krey PR, Bailen DA. Synovial fluid leukocytosis: a study of extremes. *Am J Med* 1979;67:436.
*Search for crystals in synovial fluid with high as well as low cell counts.*

Laster AJ, Michels ML. Group B streptococcal arthritis in adults. *Am J Med* 1984; 76:910.
*A rare cause of septic arthritis.*

Lawson JP, Rahn DW. Lyme disease and radiologic findings in Lyme arthritis. *AJR Am J Roentgenol* 1992;158:1065.
*Joint effusion involving the knee is the most common radiologic manifestation of Lyme arthritis.*

Li F, et al. Molecular detection of bacterial DNA in venereal-associated arthritis. *Arthritis Rheum* 1996;39:950–958.
*Polymerase chain reaction is useful to detect* Neisseria gonorrhoeae, Chlamydia *species, and* Ureaplasma *species from synovial fluid.*

Mader JT, Mohan D, Calhoun J. A practical guide to the diagnosis and management of bone and joint infections. *Drugs* 1997;54:253–264.
*Review.*

McCutchan HJ, Fisher RC. Synovial leukocytosis in infectious arthritis. *Clin Orthop* 1990;257:226.
*Synovial leukocytosis may be less severe than expected in the compromised host.*

Nelson JD. Antibiotic concentrations in septic joint effusions. *N Engl J Med* 1971; 284:349.
*The penicillins and cephalothin penetrate into joint fluid.*

O'Brien JP, Goldenberg DL, Rice PA. Disseminated gonococcal infection: a prospective analysis of 49 patients and a review of pathophysiology and immune mechanisms. *Medicine (Baltimore)* 1983;62:395.
*More than 60% of patients had tenosynovitis and more than 70% had skin lesions.*
N. gonorrhoeae *was isolated in half of the joint effusions.*

Parisien JS, Shaffer B. Arthroscopic management of pyarthrosis. *Clin Orthop* 1992; 275:243.
*Describes the use of arthroscopic techniques to drain infected joints.*

Phillips PE. Viral arthritis. *Curr Opin Rheumatol* 1997;9:337–344.
*Update on viruses, particularly parvovirus B19, rubella virus, and hepatitis viruses B and C as causes of acute arthritis.*

Pinals RS. Polyarthritis and fever. *N Engl J Med* 1994;330:769.
*An approach to the differential diagnosis.*

Pioro MH, Mandell BF. Septic arthritis. *Rheum Dis Clin North Am* 1997;23:239–258.
*Review. Septic arthritis is a medical emergency.*

Rahman MU, Shenberger KN, Schumacher HR Jr. Initially unrecognized calcium pyrophosphate dihydrate deposition disease as a cause of fever. *Am J Med* 1990; 89:115.
*Pseudogout can mimic septic arthritis when fever is present.*

Rahn DW, Malawista SE. Lyme disease: recommendations for diagnosis and treatment. *Ann Intern Med* 1991;114:472.
*Reviews diagnostic methods and therapy.*

Rompalo AM, et al. The acute arthritis-dermatitis syndrome: the changing importance of *Neisseria gonorrhoeae* and *Neisseria meningitidis*. *Arch Intern Med* 1987;147:281.
*Consider* N. meningitidis *as well as* N. gonorrhoeae *as a cause of the acute arthritis-dermatitis syndrome. A decrease in the incidence of disseminated gonococcal infection was noted.*

Rynes RI, et al. Acquired immunodeficiency syndrome-associated arthritis. *Am J Med* 1988;84:810.
*The synovial fluid is noninflammatory.*

Sack K. Monoarthritis: differential diagnosis. *Am J Med* 1997;102:30S–34S.
*Review. Acute monoarthritis should be regarded as infectious until an arthrocentesis excludes the diagnosis.*

Sapico FL, Liquete JA, Sarma RJ. Bone and joint infections in patients with infective endocarditis: review of a 4-year experience. *Clin Infect Dis* 1996;22:783–787.
*About half (44%) of the patients with endocarditis will have musculoskeletal complaints.*

Smith JW, Piercy EA. Infectious arthritis. *Clin Infect Dis* 1995;20:225–231.
*The knee is the most frequently affected joint, and in 10% of patients, multiple joints are involved.*

Solomon G, Brancato L, Winchester RW. An approach to the human immunodeficiency virus-positive patient with a spondyloarthropathic disease. *Rheum Dis Clin North Am* 1991;17:43.
*A discussion of the musculoskeletal syndromes associated with HIV infection.*

Sonnen GM, Henry NK. Pediatric bone and joint infections. Diagnosis and antimicrobial management. *Pediatr Clin North Am* 1996;43:933–947.
*Review.*

Steere AC. Diagnosis and treatment of Lyme arthritis. *Med Clin North Am* 1997;81:179–194.
*Lyme arthritis usually involves the knee and responds to a 2-month course of oral doxycycline or amoxicillin.*

Steere AC, Schoen RT, Taylor E. The clinical evolution of Lyme arthritis. *Ann Intern Med* 1987;107:725.
*In approximately 10% of patients with untreated Lyme arthritis, chronic synovitis develops later in the illness.*

Steere AC, et al. Erythema chronicum migrans and Lyme arthritis. The enlarging clinical spectrum. *Ann Intern Med* 1977;86:685.
*Onset is usually in the summer, with the characteristic skin lesion.*

Syrogiannopoulos GA, Nelson JD. Duration of antimicrobial therapy for acute suppurative osteoarticular infections. *Lancet* 1988;1:37.
*In children, a shorter duration of therapy is often effective.*

Taillandier J, et al. *Aspergillus* osteomyelitis after heart-lung transplantation. *J Heart Lung Transplant* 1997;16:436–438.
*A rare complication of solid-organ transplantation.*

Tesh RB. Arthritides caused by mosquito-borne viruses. *Annu Rev Med* 1982;33:31.
*Symptoms consist of fever, arthralgias, and rash with a 2- to 10-day incubation period.*

Vincent GM, Amirault JD. Septic arthritis in the elderly. *Clin Orthop* 1990;215:241.
*Most patients were afebrile and had a normal WBC count.*

Vyskocil JJ, et al. Pyogenic infection of the sacroiliac joint: case reports and review of the literature. *Medicine (Baltimore)* 1991;70:188.
*Pyogenic sacroiliitis is usually unilateral, and diagnosis depends on fine-needle aspiration of the joint under fluoroscopic guidance or during open biopsy.*

Wise CM, et al. Gonococcal arthritis in an era of increasing penicillin resistance. Presentations and outcomes in 41 recent cases (1985–1991). *Arch Intern Med* 1994;154:2690–2695.
*The clinical features are unchanged in recent years, and ceftriaxone is the drug of choice.*

Zimmermann B 3rd, Mikolich DJ, Lally EV. Septic sacroilitis. *Semin Arthritis Rheum* 1996;26:592–604.
*Magnetic resonance imaging is useful to diagnose septic sacroiliac joint arthritis.*

# IX.  SKIN AND SOFT TISSUE

# 39. INFECTIOUS DISEASE INDICATIONS FOR HYPERBARIC OXYGEN THERAPY

In hyperbaric oxygen (HBO) therapy, patients are entirely enclosed within a pressure vessel so that they breathe $O_2$ at a pressure greater than that at sea level, which is 1 atmosphere absolute (1 ATA). In practice, patients are placed entirely within a chamber (either monoplace or multiplace) and breathe 100% $O_2$ under pressures of at least 1.4 ATA and generally 2.0 to 3.0 ATA (equivalent to pressure at 33 to 66 ft below sea level). Published data suggest that about 30% of cases treated with HBO in the United States have an infectious disease indication. The therapeutic efficacy of $O_2$ is related both to the enhanced concentrations available to tissues (with resultant positive effects on parts of the immune system and wound healing, and deleterious effects on some bacteria) and to the salutary effects exerted by increased pressures on bubble size. These are in part explained by the Laws of Dalton, Henry, and Boyle.

Dalton's Law demonstrates that the total pressure of a gas mixture is the sum of the pressures exerted by the individual components. At 1 ATA, the partial pressure of oxygen (comprising approximately 21% of air, which has a total pressure of 760 mm Hg) is about 160 mm Hg. At 3 ATA, the partial pressure of $O_2$ in compressed air would be 480 mm Hg, whereas in a 100% $O_2$ environment, the partial pressure of $O_2$ rises to approximately 2,280 mm Hg. Boyle's Law relates pressure to volume at a constant temperature. As pressure increases, volume inversely decreases. Henry's Law relates the pressure of a gas to the amount that is contained in solution. Tripling the pressure on a gas triples the amount that is driven into solution.

Reimbursement issues have had an important effect on the progress of HBO therapy. Although the direct costs of HBO therapy are high (typically at least $300 per treatment, with many chronic indications requiring 20 to 40 treatments), evolving data suggest that HBO therapy may be cost effective when compared with prolonged hospitalization and additional surgery.

## Delivery of Hyperbaric Oxygen Therapy

HBO therapy can be delivered in either a monoplace or multiplace setting. In all situations, the patient is completely contained within the chamber and breathes 100% $O_2$. The monoplace chamber allows one person to receive therapy. Such a chamber generally resembles a Plexiglas tube that is continuously flooded with $O_2$ under pressures of up to 3 ATA. This is sufficient to treat virtually all clinical conditions. Major advantages of a monoplace chamber include decreased expense and space needs. Disadvantages include decreased patient accessibility and an increased risk for chamber fire because the entire internal environment is 100% $O_2$. Multiplace chambers can be custom-designed to fit the needs of an individual institution and can accommodate many persons. They allow room for an inside "tender" who has ready access to patients and can perform procedures as indicated. An additional benefit is that the chamber can be pressurized to 6 ATA, a historical advantage in the management of selected diving accidents. The multiplace chamber is flooded with air under pressure while the patient breathes 100% $O_2$ through a close-fitting plastic helmet. The cost of such a chamber may be millions of dollars, and substantial space is required. Additionally, tenders are at risk for nitrogen saturation illness (the "bends") because they breathe air under pressure, as do scuba divers.

## Adverse Effects and Risks of Hyperbaric Oxygen Therapy

Adverse effects from HBO therapy are rare, the most common being auditory barotrauma. A recently reported series demonstrated that only 0.37% of patients had to have a treatment curtailed because of this condition, and all ultimately resumed treatment. Similar problems with barotrauma can occur to the sinuses (sinus squeeze) or dentition. Pulmonary barotrauma can result in pneumothorax. Patients with advanced chronic obstructive pulmonary disease, especially in the setting of known bullae, need to consider the risks and benefits of HBO therapy very carefully.

The likelihood of oxygen toxicity, generally manifested as central nervous system agitation (including seizures), is directly related to the length of time spent within a 100% $O_2$ environment and to the degree of pressure in atmospheres. The likelihood is approximately 0.0009%. Fever, prior seizure history, and selected medications can increase the risk for seizures. Risk can be decreased by careful patient assessment and use of air breaks.

### Rationale for Hyperbaric Oxygen Therapy in Infectious Disease

HBO therapy augments the medical and surgical management of selected infectious diseases, as summarized in Table 39-1. The ability of anaerobic bacteria, including *Peptostreptococcus, Peptococcus, Clostridium,* and *Bacteroides* species, to tolerate environmental $O_2$ is variable. HBO can be associated with either bactericidal or bacteriostatic activity against many of these organisms. The explanation for this is the lack of selected enzymes, such as peroxidases, that serve a protective function against oxygen radicals.

Toxins, such as the alpha toxin produced by *Clostridium perfringens,* are associated with much of the toxicity and mortality caused by this species. The high $O_2$ tensions provided by HBO are capable of terminating toxin production and inactivating circulating toxin.

Many killing functions of polymorphonuclear leukocytes are oxygen-dependent. As an example, oxidative burst becomes negligible under anaerobic conditions, and killing of many bacteria declines. This appears to be especially true for *Staphylococcus aureus.*

Oxygen concentration can have an important impact on the efficacy of antibiotics. Products that include aminoglycosides, quinolones, and trimethoprim-sulfamethoxazole are far less active in an anaerobic environment. Alternatively, enhanced $O_2$ may augment the effects of tobramycin, trimethoprim-sulfamethoxazole, and nitrofurantoin.

The pharmacokinetic parameters of antibiotics given in an HBO environment have been poorly assessed. A recent investigation of gentamicin demonstrated no difference in pharmacokinetics between an HBO and normal environment.

### Infectious Disease Indications for Hyperbaric Oxygen Therapy

*Clostridial Myonecrosis*

Clostridial myonecrosis (gas gangrene) is caused by selected species of *Clostridium. C. perfringens* infection accounts for at least 80% of cases in most series. These organisms are generally considered to be anaerobic but are quite aerotolerant and can survive in $O_2$ pressures as high as 70 mm Hg. Gas gangrene is one of several distinct syndromes associated with clostridial infection, and it is the most severe and life-threatening. It often follows penetrating traumatic injury, often to an extremity. The injury is frequently accidental and may be clinically of little significance, but it invariably involves muscle. Pathogenesis requires both the introduction of an appropriate clostridial species and a decreased oxidation-reduction potential locally within the wound. The full-blown acute clinical syndrome is characterized by local pain, major constitutional symptomatology, and the finding on clinical examination of blue-brown discoloration of the involved skin part, often associated with formation of bullae. The diagnosis can be confirmed by discovery of the organism in representative clinical specimens. Pathologically, this infection is caused by local invasion of muscle, with

Table 39-1. Approved indications for hyperbaric oxygen therapy

| | |
|---|---|
| Air embolism | Clostridial gas gangrene |
| Decompression sickness | Refractory osteomyelitis |
| Osteoradionecrosis | Necrotizing soft-tissue infections |
| Carbon monoxide poisoning | Refractory mycoses |
| Thermal burns | Chronic nonhealing wounds |
| Crush injuries | Graft/flap preparation |
| Exceptional blood loss anemia | Cyanide poisoning |

resultant release of major toxins from vegetative *C. perfringens*. The alpha toxin (lecithinase C) has been demonstrated to be a significant hemolysin and is considered to be a major component of the disease process. Hemolysis can be rapid and complete, and much of the symptomatology is a consequence of this. Thus, gas gangrene is primarily a disease of toxin production rather than one of fulminating infection with a highly virulent organism.

HBO therapy should always be considered adjunctive to surgical debridement of devitalized tissue, clinical support of the patient, and appropriate antibiotic therapy. Postponement of either surgical debridement or initiation of antibiotic therapy to transport a patient long distances to a hyperbaric facility is generally ill-advised. Antimicrobials active against *Clostridium* species include penicillin G, clindamycin, chloramphenicol, metronidazole, and selected cephalosporins, such as cefoxitin, cefotetan, and (usually) cefazolin. Penicillin G remains the agent of choice. Surgical excision of devitalized muscle is of paramount importance. However, delineation of dead from dying tissue is difficult, and preservation of viable tissue is essential.

Although recent experimental data have called into question the value of HBO, most publications suggest strongly that HBO is well established as a modality of care. Major effects of HBO, when administered in conjunction with surgery and antibiotics, include delineation of viable from dead tissue, decrease in extent of amputation required in patients with clostridial myonecrosis of an extremity, and general clinical improvement. HBO may decrease mortality from more than 50% to less than 20% and reduce the need for amputation from 50% to less than 20%. When HBO is used within 24 hours of diagnosis, disease-specific mortality may be as low as 5%. The scientific rationale for these observations has been substantiated by animal data that demonstrate the ability of HBO to decrease production of alpha toxin and aid in the killing of *C. perfringens*. Concentrations of $O_2$ of at least 40 mm Hg are needed to arrest clostridial growth, whereas concentrations of at least 80 mm Hg are needed to stop synthesis of alpha toxin.

HBO therapy should be employed early and often in the management of clostridial gas gangrene. If feasible, initial treatment should be performed preoperatively. Thereafter, therapy should be continued two to three times daily for several days. All treatments should be performed at 3.0 ATA for 90 minutes, and treatments can generally be discontinued at 5 to 7 days.

*Necrotizing Soft-tissue Infections*

Necrotizing soft-tissue infections exist in the literature under the rubric of Fournier's gangrene, anaerobic cellulitis, necrotizing fasciitis, and Meleney's synergistic gangrene, among others. Despite the variations in terminology, they share the capacity to cause rapid and serious damage to subcutaneous tissues. Bacteriologically, many are associated with infections involving polymicrobial flora. This often includes both anaerobes (*Bacteroides* and *Peptostreptococcus* species) and aerobes (*Escherichia coli, Klebsiella* species, *Enterococcus* species, among others). Pathogenesis often involves breaches of normal mucocutaneous barriers (e.g., by trauma or tumor) such as can occur in diverticulitis, appendicitis with perforation, penetrating trauma of the abdomen (with involvement of the large intestine), many infections of the female genital tract, and infected decubitus and diabetic ulcers. Selected necrotizing soft-tissue infections may be caused by a single aerobic species, such as *Streptococcus pyogenes* ("flesh-eating" bacteria), and in these situations the value of HBO remains controversial.

Clinically, redness, heat, and tenderness of involved skin are usually seen early in the course, but the disease is often more severe that that generally noted with uncomplicated cellulitis. Bullae and crepitus are important guides to a more complicated process. Progression is often noted despite administration of appropriate antibiotics, and the patient remains ill. The diagnosis can often be confirmed by aspiration of bullae for Gram's stain and culture or by frozen section of involved fascia.

Therapy consists of surgical debridement and antibiotics. Debridement must remove all devitalized tissue, and often the surgeon must operate on multiple occasions ("second look") to ensure the adequacy of debridement.

The use of HBO for anaerobic soft-tissue infections should always be considered adjunctive to adequate surgical debridement and appropriate systemic antibiotic ther-

208    IX.  Skin and Soft Tissue

apy. It should be considered in those cases likely to be associated with mortality or significant morbidity from surgery. The rationale for HBO includes reversal of hypoxia, enhancement of WBC function, aid in delineating viable from dead tissue, and direct toxic effect on selected bacteria. The usual treatment is 2.5 ATA for 90 minutes one to two times daily for several days. For necrotizing infections other than clostridial gas gangrene, HBO generally begins after initial surgical debridement.

*Refractory Bacterial Osteomyelitis*
Osteomyelitis is said to be refractory when it has not responded to standard therapy with appropriate systemic antibiotics and surgical debridement. Most cases are associated with bone infection under contiguous soft-tissue foci of infection and may be complicated by compromised vascularity. The latter often results in hypoxic tissue, often below 23 mm Hg $O_2$, a number too low for effective healing. HBO therapy at $\geq 2$ ATA can raise $O_2$ tensions to levels above 45 mm Hg $O_2$ and has been noted to result in effective healing. The reasons for this include enhancement of both polymorphonuclear leukocyte function and selected antibiotic activity. Although clinical data are limited and a true placebo-controlled, double-blinded study has yet to be conducted, at least one completed study documents a success rate greater than 80%.

*Problem Wound Healing*
Problem wounds are those that fail to heal after intense medical and/or surgical therapy. In general, they have existed for at least 4 weeks with therapy or 8 weeks with or without treatment. Although not inevitably associated with infection, many are associated with bacterial colonization and can be managed with antibiotics. Infectious disease specialists are often consulted in this regard. The evaluation of problem wounds requires a multidisciplinary approach, and testing to assess arterial and venous patency, the presence of infection, and local $O_2$ tensions may be required.

HBO therapy has been successfully employed in the management of problem wounds, and its use is based on sound logic. Infection and hypoxia are two major reasons for problem wounds. Enhanced oxygenation augments fibroblast proliferation, angiogenesis, and collagen formation. Effects on infection have been previously discussed.

*Hyperbaric Oxygen Therapy for Other Infectious Diseases*
HBO therapy has been successfully utilized for numerous other infections. As an example, recent data suggest that HBO may successfully impact on survivorship from rhinocerebral mucormycosis. Malignant otitis externa may also benefit from HBO therapy employed as an adjunct to antipseudomonal antibiotics and surgery.

### Bibliography
Davis JC, et al. Adjuvant hyperbaric oxygen in malignant external otitis. *Arch Otolaryngol Head Neck Surg* 1992;118:89–93.
  *Sixteen patients with malignant external otitis were treated with HBO. Approximately 40% were considered to have advanced disease that had failed combined medical and surgical treatments. All patients improved with adjuvant HBO and were free of relapse at reassessment at least 1 year later. The authors conclude that HBO should be utilized in either advanced or recurrent cases.*
Gütter MF, et al. Adjunctive hyperbaric oxygen therapy in the treatment of rhinocerebral mucormycosis. *Infect Med* 1996;13:130–136.
  *Four patients with extensive rhinocerebral mucormycosis are presented. All failed to improve until HBO was added to a surgical and antifungal regime. The rationale for use of HBO was that the necrotic (anaerobic) environment caused by the infection and its complications made it difficult for antifungals to be effective. Furthermore, the disfiguring surgery necessary for cure may be limited by timely use of HBO.*
Merritt GJ, Slade JB. Influence of hyperbaric oxygen on the pharmacokinetics of single-dose gentamicin in healthy volunteers. *Pharmacotherapy* 1993;13:382–385.
  *Gentamicin was administered to five healthy men in a randomized crossover study. No effect of HBO on the pharmacokinetics of gentamicin was demonstrated. Because so few data are available on the pharmacokinetics of antibiotics in the HBO environment, the authors caution about the use of narrow-spectrum antibiotics in HBO, by which their effects could be altered.*

Park MK, et al. Oxygen tensions and infections: modulation of microbial growth, activity of antimicrobial agents, and immunologic reponses. *Clin Infect Dis* 1992;14: 720–740.

*An extensive review of the role played by oxygen in infection and its impact on antimicrobial activity. Many activities of WBCs and antibiotics are enhanced in a hyperoxic environment. However, prolonged periods of enhanced oxygen tensions may diminish oxidative burst and impair activities mediated by T cells.*

Stevens DI, et al. Evaluation of therapy with hyperbaric oxygen for experimental infection with *Clostridium perfringens*. *Clin Infect Dis* 1993;17:231–237.

*A model that assessed the efficacy of various antibiotic regimens with HBO for experimental clostridial myonecrosis was developed. HBO appeared to be additive to selected antibiotic regimens only when the inoculum size was larger than $10^9$ organisms.*

Tibbles PM, Edelsberg JS. Hyperbaric oxygen therapy. *N Engl J Med* 1996;334: 1642–1648.

*A major recent review article that emphasizes the approved uses for HBO as well as the proposed mechanisms by which HBO works. A table provides useful information concerning available controlled studies of HBO.*

---

## 40. LYME DISEASE—A DIAGNOSTIC CHALLENGE

---

Lyme disease is a multisystem disease with protean manifestations. The illness was brought to attention in 1977 when it was thought that the "juvenile rheumatoid arthritis" of a group of children in Lyme, Connecticut, had an infectious cause. Subsequent studies identified *Ixodes* ticks as vectors of the disease, and in 1982, a spirochete, now called *Borrelia burgdorferi*, was isolated from *Ixodes scapularis* (formerly *Ixodes dammini*). Features of the illness were recognized in Europe early in this century.

Lyme disease is the most commonly reported tick-borne disease in the United States. Cases have occurred in all states except Alaska, Arizona, Colorado, Montana, Nebraska, and New Mexico, although the disease is regional, with more than 90% of cases reported from the northeastern states, Maryland, Wisconsin, Missouri, and California. The disorder has also been noted in Europe, China, Japan, Australia, and the former Soviet Union. Cases have been reported worldwide except in the Antarctic.

Although the disorder is not rare, confusion exists for most clinicians regarding the diagnosis. For every case of Lyme disease that is diagnosed, it is estimated that 50 to 100 serologic tests for Lyme disease are performed. A number of factors have contributed to the diagnostic dilemma for clinicians and confusion for patients. First, unlike most bacterial infections, Lyme disease is not diagnosed by isolation of the etiologic agent or demonstration of the antigen or organism by special stains in tissue. Second, the clinical features are protean and may mimic those of several other diseases. The pathognomonic skin lesion, erythema migrans, which develops at the site of the tick bite, is absent in one third of patients. Third, confusion exists regarding the interpretation of a positive or negative result of the serologic test for Lyme disease antibody. Clinicians believe that a positive Lyme disease test result alone confirms the diagnosis. A positive Lyme serology may be a false-positive because of cross-reacting antibodies; alternatively, it may indicate past infection with *B. burgdorferi* or suggest active infection. Elevated antibody titers may persist for years with or without therapy and do not indicate the presence of an active infection that requires antimicrobial therapy. A false-negative serologic test result may be seen early in the illness because the antibody response may not appear until 3 to 6 weeks after the tick bite. Antimicrobial therapy can also diminish the antibody response, resulting in a false-negative serologic test result. Finally, confusion exists regarding how to manage a patient who reports a tick bite and is concerned about the development of Lyme disease.

Lyme disease can be classified into early and late infection. Early infection can be further subdivided into localized infection (stage 1) or disseminated infection (stage 2). Erythema migrans is the hallmark of early localized disease. The rash usually occurs 3 to 32 days (median, 7 days) after the initial tick bite. The rash is described as an annular, expanding, erythematous lesion with central clearing that is at least 5 cm in diameter. The center of the lesion may become vesicular and necrotic or remain erythematous. Secondary annular skin lesions occur in half the patients. These lesions resemble those of erythema migrans. The skin lesions usually fade within 3 to 4 weeks, even if untreated. Fever and minor constitutional symptoms, such as malaise and fatigue or regional lymphadenopathy, may accompany the classic skin rash. It is extremely difficult to diagnose Lyme disease in a patient with flulike symptoms alone without a rash because the serology is usually negative at this time.

Manifestations of early disseminated disease may involve the nervous, cardiovascular, or musculoskeletal system. The spectrum of neurologic disease includes lymphocytic meningitis; cranial neuritis, such as Bell's palsy; radiculoneuropathy; or, rarely, encephalomyelitis. Bell's palsy is the most common cranial neuropathy. Headache, paresthesia, and a mild stiff neck alone are not accepted as criteria for the diagnosis of neurologic disease. Symptoms of musculoskeletal involvement can include migratory arthralgias, muscle and bone pain, and transient arthritis affecting the large joints, such as the knees. The arthritis usually begins 6 months after onset. Cardiac manifestations begin about 2 to 6 weeks after onset and include atrioventricular block and, less often, myocarditis or pericarditis. Syncope caused by cardiac conduction abnormality may be the presenting complaint. Late or persistent infection is manifested as a chronic arthritis, lasting a year or more, involving the knees; neurologic disorders, such as an encephalomyelitis; and a localized cutaneous disorder, acrodermatitis chronica atrophicans. Ocular abnormalities may occur as part of early disseminated disease.

Because it is difficult to culture the spirochete from most patients with Lyme disease, the diagnosis must rely heavily on the clinical presentation and epidemiologic clues. The diagnosis is often a challenge because laboratory support depends on detection of an immune response to the organism, which has the limitations already noted. Current methods of testing use mainly an enzyme-linked immunosorbent assay (ELISA) and Western blot (immunoblot) test. Specific IgM antibodies against the organism appear about 1 month after the onset, peak at 2 months, and then decline. Specific IgG antibodies are detectable in the second month and may remain elevated for life. Antibody levels decline with treatment but usually persist indefinitely. Antibody levels should not be monitored to indicate success or failure of therapy. Similarly, the presence of antibodies may indicate a previous infection, with the patient's acute symptoms having another cause. Serologic testing is not helpful to diagnose recurrent disease.

Immunoblot testing (Western blot) can support the diagnosis of Lyme disease, but a negative test result does not exclude the disorder. In early disease, an antibody response to a flagellar protein (flagellin) and to a fragment of this protein, designated as 41G, develops in some patients. In late disease, the antibody response is directed to outer-surface proteins A and B in addition to the flagellar proteins. Again, cross-reacting antibodies directed against other spirochetes can confuse the picture, and the clinician should discuss with the laboratory personnel the criteria used to classify a Western blot test as positive. Some laboratories require the presence of four or five bands on the Western blot to consider the result positive. Serologic tests for Lyme disease can easily be misinterpreted. A two-step approach is advised. The first step is to perform an ELISA or indirect immunofluorescence test. A positive or equivocal result should be followed by a Western blot assay. This second test is supplemental rather than confirmatory because of suboptimal specificity. A negative test result does not exclude the diagnosis, and another sample should be obtained 1 month later.

In addition to antibody responses to infection, specific cellular immune responses occur. In a group of seronegative patients with Lyme disease, a T-cell proliferative assay may be useful to demonstrate exposure to *B. burgdorferi*. However, this test is still confined to research purposes, and the results must be interpreted with caution. Other laboratory methods, such as antigen detection and the polymerase chain reaction (PCR), are still experimental. In one report in which material obtained by 2-mm skin biopsy was used, the sensitivity of the PCR was about 60%. These new methods may prove to be invaluable considering the limitations of making the diagnosis by means of the various antibody tests.

The topic of Lyme disease has generated numerous questions from both clinicians and patients:

1. *How long must a tick be attached to transmit the disease?* In experimental studies, it is unlikely for ticks attached for less than 48 hours to transmit disease. It is important to prevent tick bites by using appropriate insect repellents and protective clothing. Ticks should be removed with a forceps.

2. *How would you interpret a positive ELISA or a positive immunoblot test?* A positive test result indicates possible exposure to *B. burgdorferi* but does not confirm active infection. The diagnosis of Lyme disease is a clinical one supported by laboratory studies.

3. *Does a negative serologic test result for Lyme disease exclude the diagnosis?* No. False-negative results occur mainly during the first several weeks of the illness. Late infection is usually associated with a positive serologic test result. Rarely, patients will have a negative serologic test for Lyme antibody with late infection and have a positive T-cell response to *B. burgdorferi*. The specificity of this test is unclear, and it is not recommended for diagnosis at present.

4. *What are the causes of a false-positive serologic test result for Lyme antibody?* Causes of a false-positive Lyme serology include systemic lupus erythematosus, rheumatoid arthritis, Rocky Mountain spotted fever, infectious mononucleosis, and various spirochetal diseases, such as syphilis, relapsing fever, and periodontal disease. Patients with Lyme disease will have a negative result on a nontreponemal test for syphilis, such as the Venereal Disease Research Laboratory (VDRL) test or rapid plasma reagin circle card test (RPR-CT), and may have a false-positive result on the fluorescent treponemal antibody absorption test (FTA-ABS) test. Another problem that should always be considered is the patient with an asymptomatic *B. burgdorferi* infection and a positive Lyme serologic test. In this situation, the patient's symptoms may be falsely attributed to Lyme disease because of the positive antibody test result, and the correct diagnosis is missed.

5. *Does Lyme disease cause chronic fatigue syndrome?* The diagnosis of chronic fatigue syndrome depends on excluding other diseases. The diagnosis of Lyme disease should not be searched for as a cause of fatigue unless a patient has epidemiologic evidence to suggest infection with *B. burgdorferi,* plus other clinical manifestations of Lyme disease. Rarely, fibromyalgia may develop in patients with treated Lyme disease. In patients with fibromyalgia triggered by prior Lyme disease, there is no evidence that antimicrobial therapy alters the course of the illness.

6. *Is there a role for prolonged antimicrobial therapy in a patient with Lyme disease?* Although the optimal therapy for Lyme disease is unknown, it appears that antimicrobials usually should be administered for 3 weeks to eradicate the organism. There is no evidence that antimicrobial therapy for longer than 30 days, even for patients with Lyme arthritis, provides any advantage. After therapy is started, patient symptoms may worsen because of a Jarisch-Herxheimer reaction. Oral therapy should be adequate for most infections, and IV therapy should be reserved for patients with well-documented chronic disease, such as Lyme arthritis, or disseminated disease with major organ involvement, such as Lyme carditis or Lyme meningitis.

7. *How should you manage someone in an endemic area who is asymptomatic and has a positive Lyme serology?* In endemic areas, rates of Lyme seropositivity may be as high as 22.5%. No data are available to indicate whether late complications of Lyme disease will develop in patients who are asymptomatic. The role of antimicrobials in this setting is unclear.

8. *What is the role for prophylactic antimicrobials to prevent Lyme disease after the bite of a deer tick?* The risk for acquiring Lyme disease, even in an endemic area, after a deer tick bite is low. Therefore, prophylactic antimicrobials are not usually indicated. One exception might be a pregnant patient, but this issue has not been studied.

9. *Is there a risk for transmitting* B. burgdorferi *infection to the fetus during pregnancy?* Although there is a potential for maternal-to-fetal transmission of *B. burgdorferi* during pregnancy, the risk appears to be extremely low. There is no need to screen for Lyme antibodies in asymptomatic women during pregnancy. However, suspected or documented cases of Lyme disease should be treated during pregnancy. Controlled studies are needed to assess the risk to the fetus associated with maternal Lyme disease.

10. *After a patient with Lyme disease is treated, should antibody titers be monitored to assess cure?* Antimicrobial therapy usually causes a decline in antibody levels against *B. burgdorferi.* However, the patient usually remains seropositive indefinitely, and repeated serologic testing is not indicated.

Despite a tremendous increase in our understanding of Lyme disease, controversies and confusion still exist regarding this illness. It is hoped that better answers to many questions concerning Lyme disease will be forthcoming. (N.M.G.)

## Bibliography

Agger W, et al. Lyme disease: clinical features, classification, and epidemiology in the upper Midwest. *Medicine (Baltimore)* 1991;70:83.
*Half of the early cases and about 10% of the late cases recalled a tick bite. In the Midwest, onset of early disease occurred mainly from June through November.*
Bakken LL, et al. Performance of 45 laboratories participating in a proficiency testing program for Lyme disease serology. *JAMA* 1992;268:891.
*A false-positive rate of 2% to 27% was noted. Interlaboratory results were highly variable.*
Committee on Infectious Diseases. Treatment of Lyme borreliosis. *Pediatrics* 1991; 88:176.
*Guidelines for diagnosis and treatment from the American Academy of Pediatrics (see also Canadian Pediatric Society. How to diagnose and treat Lyme disease in children.* Can Med Assoc J *1992;147:169).*
Corpuz M, et al. Problems in the use of serologic tests for the diagnosis of Lyme disease. *Arch Intern Med* 1991;151:1837.
*A marked variability was noted in the results of serologic testing between different laboratories, with sensitivities ranging from 13% to 73%.*
Cox J, Krajden M. Cardiovascular manifestations of Lyme disease. *Am Heart J* 1991; 122:1449.
*Atrioventricular block usually resolves within 6 weeks with antimicrobial therapy.*
Coyle PK. *Borrelia burgdorferi* infection: clinical diagnostic techniques. *Immunol Invest* 1997;26:117–128.
*Use a two-test approach for serologic diagnosis. If results of the enzyme immunoassay are positive, then obtain a Western immunoblot. (Order immunoglobulin M immunoblot if the illness has been present less than 1 month; otherwise obtain an immunoglobulin G immunoblot.)*
Dattwyler RJ, et al. Seronegative Lyme disease: dissociation of specific T- and B-lymphocyte responses to *Borrelia burgdorferi. N Engl J Med* 1988;319:1441.
*A test that measures T-cell blastogenic response to* B. burgdorferi *may be helpful in the diagnosis of the rare patient with clinical evidence of chronic Lyme disease and a negative serology.*
Dinerman H, Steere AC. Lyme disease associated with fibromyalgia. *Ann Intern Med* 1992;117:281.
*Fibromyalgia may develop in treated patients with Lyme disease; antimicrobials are not indicated for these patients.*
Dressler F, et al. Western blotting in the serodiagnosis of Lyme disease. *J Infect Dis* 1993;167:392.
*With the Western blot test, the sensitivity varied between 32% and 83%, and the specificity was 95% to 100%.*
Dressler F, Yoshinari NH, Steere AC. The T-cell proliferative assay in the diagnosis of Lyme disease. *Ann Intern Med* 1991;115:533.
*A test measuring the T-cell proliferative response to* B. burgdorferi *antigens had a sensitivity of 45% and specificity of 95% in a small group of patients with late Lyme disease.*
Dumler JS. Is human granulocytic ehrlichiosis a new Lyme disease? Review and comparison of clinical, laboratory, epidemiological, and some biological features. *Clin Infect Dis* 1997;25(Suppl 1):S43–S47.
*Although ehrlichiosis and Lyme disease are both transmitted by deer ticks (*Ixodes scapularis*), leukopenia, thrombocytopenia, and abnormal hepatic transaminases occur with the former and are usually absent in Lyme disease.*

Feder HM Jr, Whitaker DL. Misdiagnosis of erythema migrans. *Am J Med* 1995;99: 412–419.
*A typical lesion of erythema migrans is annular, erythematous, and at least 5 cm in diameter, and it begins to develop 3 to 30 days after a tick bite.*

Fikrig E, et al. Serologic diagnosis of Lyme disease using recombinant outer surface proteins A and B and flagellin. *J Infect Dis* 1992;165:1127.
*Measurement of antibodies to outer-surface proteins A and B, flagellin, and region of flagellin (41G) from B. burgdorferi with an immunoblot and ELISA was useful in the serodiagnosis of Lyme disease.*

Fix AD, Strickland GT, Grant J. Tick bites and Lyme disease in an endemic setting. *JAMA* 1998;279:206–210.
*Overuse of serologic testing and prophylactic antibiotic therapy.*

Gerber MA, Shapiro ED. Diagnosis of Lyme disease in children. *J Pediatr* 1992;121: 157.
*A skin lesion that appears immediately after a tick bite, resolves within 1 to 2 days without appropriate antimicrobial therapy, and is less than 5 cm is unlikely to be erythema migrans.*

Golightly MC. Lyme borreliosis: laboratory considerations. *Semin Neurol* 1997;17: 11–17.
*Diagnosis should be based on the history and clinical findings, with the laboratory providing supporting evidence.*

Keller TL, Halperin JJ, Whitman M. PCR detection of *Borrelia burgdorferi* DNA in cerebrospinal fluid of Lyme neuroborreliosis patients. *Neurology* 1992;42:32.
*PCR on cerebrospinal fluid is a useful method to detect B. burgdorferi. This test appears to be an alternative to the measurement of intrathecal production of specific Lyme antibody.*

Kuiper H, et al. Absence of Lyme borreliosis among patients with presumed Bell's palsy. *Arch Neurol* 1992;49:940.
*Lyme disease was identified in 6% of patients with peripheral facial palsy, compared with a rate of 4.5% in controls. Screening for Lyme disease is not indicated in this setting unless other evidence suggests the diagnosis.*

Lawson JP, Rahn DW. Lyme disease and radiologic findings in Lyme arthritis. *AJR Am J Roentgenol* 1992;58:1065.
*The most frequent abnormality is a joint effusion involving the knee. Loss of cartilage occurs in about 25% of patients with chronic Lyme arthritis.*

Luft BJ, et al. Invasion of the central nervous system by *Borrelia burgdorferi* in acute disseminated infection. *JAMA* 1992;267:1364.
*In a small study, B. burgdorferi was identified in the cerebrospinal fluid of 67% of patients with early disseminated disease when a PCR assay was used.*

Luger SW, Krauss E. Serologic tests for Lyme disease: interlaboratory variability. *Arch Intern Med* 1990;150:761.
*Serologic testing should not be the sole criterion used to make the diagnosis of Lyme disease because of wide variability in the test results among laboratories.*

Malane MS, et al. Diagnosis of Lyme disease based on dermatologic manifestations. *Ann Intern Med* 1991;114:490.
*A review of the cutaneous lesions. Erythema migrans occurs in about 75% of patients with Lyme disease.*

Nadelman RB, et al. Comparison of cefuroxime axetil and doxycycline in the treatment of early Lyme disease. *Ann Intern Med* 1992;117:273.
*A 20-day course of cefuroxime axetil (500 mg twice daily) or doxycycline (100 mg three times daily) was effective in patients with early Lyme disease.*

Nocton JJ, Steere AC. Lyme disease. *Adv Intern Med* 1995;40:69–115.
*Review.*

Pachner AR, Ricalton NS. Western blotting in evaluating Lyme seropositivity and the utility of a gel densitometric approach. *Neurology* 1992;42:2185.
*Use of a quantitative Western blot test was helpful in establishing the diagnosis. Patients with secondary syphilis had positive results on immunoblots.*

Rahn DW. Lyme disease: clinical manifestations, diagnosis, and treatment. *Semin Arthritis Rheum* 1991;20:201.
*Review.*

Rahn DW, Malawista SE. Lyme disease: recommendations for diagnosis and treatment. *Ann Intern Med* 1991;114:472.
*A review of the national surveillance case definition for diagnosis and treatment guidelines.*
Reid MC, et al. The consequences of overdiagnosis and overtreatment of Lyme disease: an observational study. *Ann Intern Med* 1998; 128:354–362.
*Of a group of referred patients with presumptive Lyme disease, only 21% met criteria for active Lyme disease. Most positive results on serologic tests for Lyme disease are false-positives.*
Schwartz I, et al. Diagnosis of early Lyme disease by polymerase chain reaction amplification and culture of skin biopsies from erythema migrans lesions. *J Clin Microbiol* 1992;30:3082.
*The sensitivity of PCR for the detection of* B. burgdorferi *in skin biopsy specimens was about 60%. The yield was similar when culture was used.*
Shapiro ED, et al. A controlled trial of antimicrobial prophylaxis for Lyme disease after deer tick bites. *N Engl J Med* 1992;327:1769.
*In an endemic area, prophylactic amoxicillin is not indicated to prevent Lyme disease after a deer tick bite.*
Sigal LH. Summary of the first 100 patients seen at a Lyme disease referral center. *Am J Med* 1990;88:577.
*Lyme disease was diagnosed in only 37% of patients referred for evaluation. Fibromyalgia was common.*
Steere AC. Lyme disease. *N Engl J Med* 1989;321:586.
*Review.*
Steere AC. Musculoskeletal manifestations of Lyme disease. *Am J Med* 1995;98(Suppl 4A);44S–51S.
*Lyme arthritis usually responds to a 1-month course of antibiotics—doxycycline, amoxicillin, or ceftriaxone (see also Steere AC. Diagnosis and treatment of Lyme arthritis. Med Clin North Am 1997;81:179–194).*
Steere AC, Schoen RT, Taylor E. The clinical evolution of Lyme arthritis. *Ann Intern Med* 1987;107:725.
*The spectrum of disease in untreated patients with Lyme arthritis includes intermittent episodes of arthritis (64%), arthralgias alone (23%), and chronic arthritis (14%).*
Steere AC, et al. The early clinical manifestations of Lyme disease. *Ann Intern Med* 1983;99:76.
*Erythema migrans is illustrated. Multiple annular secondary skin lesions developed in half the patients.*
Steere AC, et al. Treatment of the early manifestations of Lyme disease. *Ann Intern Med* 1983;99:22.
*Erythema migrans responded to antimicrobial therapy in 5 days with and in 10 days without treatment. Major late complications did not occur in patients who were treated with tetracycline.*
Steere AC, et al. Evaluation of the intrathecal antibody response to *Borrelia burgdorferi* as a diagnostic test for Lyme neuroborreliosis. *J Infect Dis* 1990;161:1203.
*Measurement of intrathecal antibody production, most commonly IgA, was useful in the diagnosis of Lyme neuroborreliosis. A negative study result, particularly in patients with peripheral nervous system involvement, does not exclude the diagnosis.*
Treatment of Lyme disease. *Med Lett Drugs Ther* 1997;39:47–48.
*For erythema migrans, doxycyline, amoxicillin, or cefuroxime axetil is recommended.*
Tugwell P, et al. Laboratory evaluation in the diagnosis of Lyme disease. *Ann Intern Med* 1997;127:1109–1123.
*Although Lyme disease is the most common tick-borne disease in North America, laboratory testing is indicated only if the pretest probability is .20 or higher (see also American College of Physicians. Guidelines for laboratory evaluation in the diagnosis of Lyme disease. Ann Intern Med 1997;127:1106–1108).*
Warshafsky S, et al. Efficacy of antibiotic prophylaxis for prevention of Lyme disease. *J Gen Intern Med* 1996;11:329–333.
*A metaanalysis of clinical trials failed to establish the efficacy of antibiotics as prophylaxis for tick bites.*

Wormser GP. Treatment and prevention of Lyme disease, with emphasis on antimicrobial therapy for neuroborreliosis and vaccination. *Semin Neurol* 1997;17:45–52.
*Ceftriaxone is the drug of choice for neuroborreliosis.*

Wormser GP, et al. Use of a novel technique of cutaneous lavage for diagnosis of Lyme
disease associated with erythema migrans. *JAMA* 1992;268:1311.
*Culture of material obtained by a 2-mm skin biopsy and fluid from a technique called
cutaneous needle lavage yielded* B. burgdorferi. *Skin biopsy culture was more sensitive than lavage culture (74% vs. 40%).*

---

## 41. CELLULITIS AND OTHER SKIN AND SOFT-TISSUE INFECTIONS

---

### Cellulitis

Erysipelas remains a common cause of cellulitis. A sharply demarcated, advancing,
and palpable border suggests this infection. The etiologic agent is almost always group
A β-hemolytic streptococci. *Staphylococcus aureus* can rarely cause the same clinical
picture. However, the lesions of *S. aureus* cellulitis usually have less distinct borders
and may be associated with bullae, pustules, or other primary localized areas of infection. Other hemolytic streptococci, such as groups C and G, may also cause cellulitis,
often in patients with underlying malignancy.

An erysipeloid cellulitis, particularly around the fingers or on the hand, has been
associated with the occupations of fishermen, butchers, and other persons handling
raw fish and poultry. The organism causing this cellulitis is *Erysipelothrix rhusiopathiae.* The cellulitis often has a violet hue. There is local tenderness but little systemic reaction. Penicillin G is the antimicrobial of choice. More recently, cellulitis
caused by a fish pathogen, *Streptococcus iniae,* has been described in association with
an outbreak in Canada. All the patients had handled live or freshly killed fish.

Cellulitis caused by Enterobacteriaceae can occur in association with trauma and
diabetes or after surgery. *Escherichia coli* and *Klebsiella* species can cause a gas-forming gangrene that must be distinguished from purely anaerobic soft-tissue infection.
Necrotizing fasciitis is a potentially life-threatening infection because of the virulence
of the causative organism and the depth of involvement to the fascia. Bacteremia is
common, and mortality from the disease is high. Toxic strains of hemolytic streptococci have made the disease more common. Necrotizing fasciitis requires rapid diagnosis and early antibiotic therapy and surgical intervention. Although definitive
diagnosis is difficult, clues to deeper infection include bullae formation, anesthesia
over the infected area, dusky discoloration, and failure to respond to antibiotics. Deep-
tissue infection may be the result of mixed anaerobic and gram-negative infection.
Fournier's gangrene of the scrotum may often be caused by anaerobic streptococci and
gram-negative bacilli. This infection presents as scrotal swelling and pain with rapidly
advancing necrosis of soft tissue. Pain and systemic toxicity are associated.

Breast cellulitis has recently been reported as a complication of breast-conservation
therapy. More than 80% of patients had radiologically demonstrated fluid collections
at the site of lumpectomy. Episodes of cellulitis developed, on average, 4.9 months
after the end of radiotherapy for stage I or II breast carcinoma.

*Pseudomonas aeruginosa* folliculitis has been recently described, almost exclusively
in association with the use of hot tubs and whirlpools. Papules or nodules that are red
or violaceous appear on the abdomen or trunk. The neck and face are usually spared.
Patients may have low-grade fever but do not become bacteremic or systemically ill.
Avoidance of the source of infection is usually sufficient therapy because the rash is
self-limited.

*Vibrio vulnificus* has caused a spectrum of skin infections in saltwater wounds.
Immunocompromised patients and patients with liver disease are prone to life-
threatening infection. A cellulitis may be acquired from the exposure of abraded skin

to seawater. Bites, fishing injuries, or puncture by a fin or spine may be the predisposing event. Cellulitis, bullous disease, necrotizing fasciitis, and myositis have all been well described.

*V. vulnificus* bacteremia may develop in immunocompromised patients after ingestion of shellfish. Metastatic skin lesions, particularly vesicles and bullae, may be associated with this bacteremia. Antimicrobial therapy (tetracyclines and aminoglycosides have been most commonly used), blood pressure support, and often wound debridement are required because the disease is rapidly progressive.

### Animal Bites

Animal bites are a common cause of soft-tissue infection, with more than a half million bites, mostly from dogs and cats, occurring in the United States each year. Several factors are important in developing a diagnostic and therapeutic plan: the animal involved, severity and location of the wound, circumstances of the attack, and interval between injury and presentation. A plan for treatment must include (a) local care, with thorough cleaning of the wound with soap and water and adequate irrigation; (b) tetanus prophylaxis; (c) rabies prophylaxis, depending on the animal involved and the epidemiology of rabies in the specific locale; and (d) antimicrobials. Prophylactic antimicrobial therapy is controversial; however, routine prophylaxis for dog bites is becoming increasingly recommended. Patients with deep wounds or wounds of the face and patients with wounds who are immunocompromised or have liver disease probably should receive prophylaxis (prospective studies are lacking). The antimicrobial of choice is controversial. A broad-spectrum agent such as amoxicillin-clavulanate is often recommended.

Treatment of animal bite soft-tissue infection should be directed against the etiologic agent. *Pasteurella multocida,* the most common organism in dog and cat bites, is a small, gram-negative rod (appearing much like *Haemophilus* species organisms on Gram's stain). Penicillin is the drug of choice; tetracycline is an effective alternative.

Dysgonic fermenter 2 (DF-2), now called *Capnocytophaga canimorsus,* recently has been recognized to cause soft-tissue infection and overwhelming sepsis after dog bites. The disease has also occurred after cat bite. Patients with cirrhosis and splenectomized patients are at high risk for septic shock and disseminated intravascular coagulation. Penicillin in high doses is the drug of choice. *Bacteroides* and *Prevotella* species are commonly isolated from bite wounds and are now better characterized.

### Lyme Disease

The variable cutaneous manifestations of Lyme borreliosis are important to review in the context of the differential diagnosis of skin infection. Erythema migrans is an erythematous lesion occurring at the site of tick bite and borrelial inoculation. It is an annular lesion that shows centrifugal spread. Borrelial lymphocytoma has been described as a blue-red nodular lesion. A dense lymphocytic infiltration is seen histologically. The ear and breast may be sites of predilection for this lesion. Multiple erythema migrans lesions suggest disseminated disease. Acrodermatitis chronica atrophicans is a chronic skin lesion that starts as a localized inflammatory process but is followed by an atrophic phase. Sclerotic skin lesions may also develop secondary to Lyme disease. Different species of *Borrelia* tend to cause different types of skin lesions. For example, *Borrelia afzelii* is the predominant etiologic agent in acrodermatitis chronica atrophicans.

### Herpes Zoster

Herpes zoster, or shingles, is caused by reactivation of latent varicella-zoster virus in the dorsal root ganglia. Clinical diagnosis is usually not difficult; the patient presents with a painful vesicular rash in a dermatomal distribution. Herpes simplex can rarely present in a dermatomal distribution, and herpes zoster can disseminate and resemble primary varicella. The vesicular lesions of all three diseases appear the same histologically, with multinucleated giant cells and intranuclear inclusions.

Antiviral therapy has a well-established role in patients with herpes zoster. For both localized and disseminated disease, acyclovir has been shown to improve the rate of viral clearing and provide faster relief of pain. Acyclovir prevents dissemination of virus in immunosuppressed patients. IV acyclovir was shown to be more effective than vidarabine in preventing disseminated disease. Acyclovir has been used to decrease the incidence of zoster after bone marrow transplantation.

In the normal host with localized disease, the role of acyclovir is not completely defined. IV acyclovir improves healing and decreases the duration of acute pain. This effect is modest; the incidence of long-standing herpetic neuralgias is not affected by antiviral therapy. When started within 2 days of the onset of rash, acyclovir reduces the incidence of formation of new lesions.

Herpes zoster ophthalmicus, because of its high rate of ocular complications and vision loss, requires antiviral therapy. Although a positive effect with oral therapy has been reported, most experts recommend IV acyclovir for zoster ophthalmicus.

### Decubitus Ulcers

With the aging of the population in the United States, decubitus ulcers have become an increasingly common soft-tissue infection. Five percent of the 23.5 million Americans over age 65 live in nursing homes. In this institutional setting, decubitus ulcers are prevalent in 6% to 35% of patients. The pathogenesis of decubitus ulcers has been well defined. Sustained pressure is the principal predisposing factor. Shearing forces, such as occur when a patient is raised up in bed, also contribute to the process. Moisture secondary to incontinence, perspiration, and drainage from a wound infection may also be contributing factors. Malnutrition, as reflected by serum albumin levels, is an important predictor of the development of a pressure ulcer. Altered states of consciousness, diabetes mellitus and neuropathy, and sensory deficits also contribute indirectly to the process.

Clinical assessment of a pressure ulcer will include examination to determine the degree of hyperemia (blanching or nonblanching), the presence or absence of blistering or eschar formation, and the depth of tissue ulceration. The base of an ulcer should be carefully palpated to determine whether it extends to muscle or bone. Any spreading edge of erythema should be marked and carefully followed.

The microbiologic assessment of a pressure ulcer is difficult. Superficial swab cultures do not correlate with organisms grown from bone biopsy specimens when osteomyelitis has developed by contiguous spread. There are usually fewer species present in the deeper tissues than superficially. When bacterial cultures are obtained by reliable methods, such as needle aspiration, a combination of anaerobic and aerobic bacteria is isolated. The most common aerobic isolates are *E. coli, Proteus mirabilis,* enterococci, and *Pseudomonas* species. Common anaerobic organisms include *Peptostreptococcus, Bacteroides fragilis,* and *Clostridium perfringens.* When patients become septic from decubitus ulcers, anaerobes, particularly *B. fragilis,* are most commonly isolated. In addition to sepsis, other complications of decubitus ulcers include contiguous osteomyelitis, pyarthrosis, and rarely tetanus. Table 41-1 summarizes the basic principles for management of decubitus ulcers.

As with other infectious disease, prevention is the most important weapon in the fight against decubitus ulcers. A good prevention program first identifies patients at

Table 41-1. Principles of management for decubitus ulcers

1. Improvement of general medical conditions, including better nutrition, oxygenation, and tissue perfusion; control of diabetes.
2. Local care of ulcer, which includes careful wound cleansing and debridement. Use of enzymatic preparations that liquefy necrotic tissue without damaging granulation appears promising. Keeping pressure off the involved area is critically important.
3. Treatment of complications. Empiric broad-spectrum antimicrobial therapy to cover both anaerobes and gram-negative bacilli in the septic patient. Osteo myelitis requires prolonged therapy directed against the specific organism.
4. Surgical treatment, including excision of necrotic tissue and establishment of drainage.

greatest risk. Vigilance and meticulous attention to early blanching hyperemia are critical. Frequent turning and cleanliness of sheets are the basis of prevention. Patients should be lifted and not dragged across sheets. Activity and good nutrition should be maximized. (S.L.B.)

## Bibliography

Alexander CJ, et al. Characterization of saccharolytic *Bacteroides* and *Prevotella* isolates from infected dog and cat bite wounds in humans. *J Clin Microbiol* 1997; 35:406.
  *Many species of* Bacteroides *and* Prevotella *can be isolated from human bites. Clinical laboratories need to be aware of these species.*

Asbrink E. Cutaneous manifestations of Lyme borreliosis. Clinical definitions and differential diagnoses. *Scand J Infect Dis* 1991;77(Suppl):44.
  *Cutaneous manifestations of Lyme borreliosis as described during the Fourth International Conference on Lyme Disease.*

Auerbach PS. Natural microbiologic hazards of the aquatic environment. *Clin Dermatol* 1987;5:52.
  *Describes risk for* Erysipelothrix *infection in fish handlers.*

Balfour HH, et al. Acyclovir halts progression of herpes zoster in immunocompromised patients. *N Engl J Med* 1983;308:1448.
  *In immunocompromised patients, IV acyclovir decreased the progression of disease and incidence of dissemination.*

Brenner DJ, et al. *Capnocytophaga canimorsus* sp. nov. (formerly CDC group DF-2), a cause of septicemia following dog bite, and *C. cynodegmi* sp. nov., a cause of localized wound infection following dog bite. *J Clin Microbiol* 1989;27:231.
  Capnocytophaga *may cause sepsis after dog bite, particularly in the splenectomized or cirrhotic patient.*

Burdge DR, Chow AW. The pressure ulcer. In: Verghese A, Berk SL, eds. *Infections in nursing homes and long-term care facilities.* Basel: Karger, 1990.
  *Detailed discussion of pathogenesis.*

Chuang YC, et al. *Vibrio vulnificus* infection in Taiwan: report of 28 cases and review of clinical manifestations and treatment. *Clin Infect Dis* 1992;15:271.
  *Summary of 28 episodes of* V. vulnificus *infection. Twenty-three of 27 patients had skin involvement.*

Clayton MD, et al. Causes, presentation and survival of 57 patients with necrotizing fasciitis of the male genitalia. *Surg Gynecol Obstet* 1990;170:49.
  *Clinical description of Fournier's fasciitis. Infection was caused by both anaerobes and gram-negative bacilli.*

Cobo M. Reduction of the ocular complications of herpes zoster ophthalmicus by oral acyclovir. *Am J Med* 1988;85:90.
  *Oral therapy prevented complications. However, evidence for continued viral replication was of concern. Most experts recommend IV acyclovir for zoster ophthalmicus.*

Goldstein EJ. Management of human and animal bite wounds. *J Am Acad Dermatol* 1989;21:1275.
  *The spectrum of organisms in animal bites is wide, and broad-spectrum antimicrobial therapy is recommended.*

Gustafson TL. *Pseudomonas* folliculitis: an outbreak and review. *Rev Infect Dis* 1983;3:1.
  *Clinical description of hot-tub folliculitis.*

Huff JC, et al. Therapy of herpes zoster with oral acyclovir. *Am J Med* 1988;85:84.
  *Normal hosts treated with oral acyclovir reported less acute pain than the placebo group.*

Kertesz DK, Chow AW. Infected pressure and diabetic ulcers. *Clin Geriatr Med* 1992; 8:835.
  *Review of decubitus ulcers, including physiology, staging, diagnosis, and treatment. Emphasizes the team approach to prevention.*

Koenig KL, Mueller J, Rose T. *Vibrio vulnificus.* Hazard on the half shell. *West J Med* 1991;144:400.
  *Describes clinical syndromes and predisposing factors for* V. vulnificus *skin infection.*

Merz KR, et al. Breast cellulitis following breast conservation therapy: a novel complication of medical progress. *Clin Infect Dis* 1998;26:481.
*Cellulitis, which is sometimes recurrent, is now more commonly seen after breast-sparing surgery, often after radiation therapy. Most episodes occur less than 3 months after treatment.*

Ohlenbusch A, et al. Etiology of the acrodermatitis chronica atrophicans lesion in Lyme disease. *J Infect Dis* 1996;174:421.
*B. afzelii is associated with acrodermatitis chronica atrophicans—skin lesions that persist over atrophied skin.*

Parenti DM, Snydman DR. *Capnocytophaga* species: infections in non-immunocompromised and immunocompromised hosts. *J Infect Dis* 1985;151:140.
*Describes* Capnocytophaga *as a cause of traumatic hand wounds.*

Pers C, et al. *Capnocytophaga canimorsus* septicemia in Denmark, 1982–1995: review of 39 cases. *Clin Infect Dis* 1996;23:71.
*Disseminated disease occurred in alcoholics and splenectomized patients. Twelve of 39 patients died. Disseminated intravascular coagulation was a common complication.*

Shepp DH, Dandliker PS, Myers JD. Treatment of varicella-zoster virus infection in severely immunocompromised patients. *N Engl J Med* 1986;314:208.
*Acyclovir was more effective than vidarabine in preventing progression of zoster in compromised patients.*

Stone DR, Gorbach SL. Necrotizing fasciitis. The changing spectrum. *Dermatol Clin* 1997;15:213.
*Describes the clinical picture and management of this infectious disease emergency. There is an increasing incidence of toxic shock strains of streptococci.*

Weber DJ, Hansen AR. Infections resulting from animal bites. *Infect Dis Clin North Am* 1991;5:663.
*Review of epidemiology and treatment of animal bites, including infections with* Pasteurella multocida *and* C. canimorsus.

Weinstein MR, et al. Invasive infections due to a fish pathogen, *Streptococcus iniae*. *N Engl J Med* 1997;337:589.
*Describes nine patients with invasive skin infections caused by this organism after they handled fresh fish.*

Weiss HB, Friedman DI, Coben JH. Incidence of dog-bite injuries treated in the emergency departments. *JAMA* 1998;278:51.
*There are 12.9 dog-bite injuries per 10,000 population. Most occur in children ages 5 to 9 years.*

Wood MJ, et al. Efficacy of oral acyclovir treatment of acute herpes zoster. *Am J Med* 1988;85:79.
*Eight hundred milligrams of oral acyclovir given five times per day for 7 days (within 48 hours of rash onset) reduced formation of new lesions and reduced acute pain. No benefit was shown in reduction of postherpetic neuralgia.*

# X. BACTEREMIA

## 42. GRAM-NEGATIVE BACTEREMIA AND THE SEPSIS CASCADE

### Gram-negative Bacteremia

More than 300,000 episodes of gram-negative bacteremia occur yearly in the United States, and the incidence of the problem has increased, especially among persons age 65 years and older. Despite the availability of potent antimicrobial drugs and sophisticated life-support facilities, 20% to 25% of all patients with this condition succumb, and approximately 50% of bacteremic patients who also experience severe sepsis expire; among geriatric patients with gram-negative bacteremia in whom severe sepsis and the adult respiratory distress syndrome (ARDS) develop, the mortality rate can approach 90%. Finally, although this chapter focuses on gram-negative bacteremia, it must be emphasized that contemporary studies of blood-borne infection have shown that the prevalence of bacteremia (and the associated sepsis) caused by gram-positive microbes, such as staphylococci and enterococci, is increasing; indeed, in some recent surveys of bacteremia, the frequency of blood-borne infections due to gram-positive microbes has exceeded that of disease caused by gram-negative organisms.

The urinary tract is the most common source of both community-acquired and nosocomial gram-negative bacteremia. Bacteremia frequently complicates bladder catheterization or surgical manipulation. Gram-negative bacteria can also invade the bloodstream following infection of the lungs (pneumonia), hepatobiliary system (cholecystitis, cholangitis), abdominal cavity (abscess, perforated viscus, peritonitis), skin (decubitus ulcer, surgical wounds, burns), and female reproductive organs (pelvic abscess). In hospitalized patients, bacteremia can result from infected intravascular catheters—both peripheral and central lines. Infected pacemaker wires and endovascular prostheses (cardiac valves, arterial grafts) are uncommon causes of gram-negative bacteremia that are very difficult to cure. On occasion, diagnostic procedures, such as upper gastrointestinal endoscopy, can produce life-threatening hematogenous infection. In some patients, especially those with granulocytopenia, bacteremia can occur in the absence of an apparent focus of infection; in that circumstance, the lower gastrointestinal tract is the source of the problem.

The risk for a gram-negative bacteremia appears to be greatest in patients of advanced age who are hospitalized for long periods of time, who have received prior antimicrobial therapy, and who have serious underlying diseases, such as neoplasms, renal failure, cirrhosis, diabetes mellitus, congestive heart failure, and skin lesions (burns, decubitus ulcers). The incidence of bacteremia has been noted to be up to fourfold greater in geriatric patients than in younger adults; however, underlying diseases and other factors beyond advanced age play substantial roles in placing a geriatric patient at risk. Medical interventions that disrupt host defenses, such as catheterization of the urinary tract, corticosteroid administration, and surgical procedures, clearly increase the likelihood of bacteremia. Nevertheless, granulocytopenia (cell counts of <1,000/mm$^3$) is the most important factor predisposing the host to gram-negative bacteremia. The risk for bacteremia increases with the magnitude and duration of the neutropenia; for example, infection will occur within 3 weeks in 50% of patients with granulocyte counts below 1,000/mm$^3$ and in 100% of those with counts below 100/mm$^3$.

The organisms most frequently isolated from patients with community-acquired gram-negative bacteremia are *Escherichia coli, Klebsiella pneumoniae, Proteus mirabilis, Haemophilus influenzae,* and *Bacteroides* species; those recovered from patients with hospital-acquired infection include *E. coli, Klebsiella* species, *Enterobacter* species, *Serratia* species, and *Pseudomonas aeruginosa.*

### Clinical Manifestations

Because they are varied and not unique to the disorder, the clinical manifestations of gram-negative bacteremia are similar to those caused by other infectious agents, including gram-positive bacteria and fungi. Moreover, spiking fevers and severe constitutional symptoms can be prominent in certain viral illnesses (e.g., acute Epstein-Barr viral disease) and in a number of noninfectious illnesses, such as drug toxicity (e.g., methyldopa) and connective tissue disorders (e.g., Still's disease). Nevertheless,

223

the possibility of gram-negative bacteremia must be considered in the patient with fever and rigors who has a known or suspected localized infection, such as cholecystitis or pyelonephritis, that is typically caused by gram-negative bacilli. Blood-borne infection should also be suspected in febrile patients who are elderly or granulocytopenic or who have intravascular or urinary tract catheters. With advanced age, uremia, corticosteroid use, or severe debilitation, the magnitude of the fever may be blunted; therefore, subtle or unexplained changes in the patient's clinical status can be important clues to the presence of infection. Among the isolated observations that can indicate gram-negative bacteremia are hypothermia, hypotension, tachypnea, a change in mental status, the adult respiratory distress syndrome (ARDS), acute pulmonary edema, oliguria, leukopenia, thrombocytopenia, hyperbilirubinemia, disseminated intravascular coagulation (DIC), hypoglycemia, metabolic acidosis, and respiratory alkalosis. On occasion, the presence of bacteremia will be suggested by the appearance of ecthyma gangrenosum, bullous lesions, or petechiae.

*Evaluation*
The initial evaluation of the patient with suspected gram-negative bacteremia is directed at confirming the diagnosis and identifying the source of infection. Blood cultures are mandatory in patients with presumed bacteremia. Samples for three aerobic and anaerobic blood cultures should be obtained during a 15- to 30-minute period; that number of cultures will detect organisms in more than 95% of untreated bacteremic patients. The isolation of a bacterium from the blood and the results of antimicrobial susceptibility testing will ensure that appropriate drug therapy is administered. Blood cultures may also reveal the presence of a bacterium other than that suggested by the Gram's stain of sputum, urine, wound drainage, or other clinical material. Finally, the identification of an organism in the blood can provide insight into the source of the bacteremia in patients with occult infection. For example, the isolation of a *Klebsiella* species from an elderly patient with normal chest radiographic findings and a negative urine culture would suggest an intraabdominal infection (cholecystitis, perforated viscus); the recovery of a *Haemophilus* species from a young adult without radiographic evidence of respiratory tract infection may indicate infective endocarditis; the presence of *Burkholderia* (*Pseudomonas*) *cepacia* or other unusual microbes in the blood of a hospitalized patient raises the possibility of contaminated IV equipment or solutions; and the finding of *Salmonella choleraesuis* in the blood of a geriatric patient with atherosclerotic cardiovascular disease brings into focus the possibility of an infected aneurysm.

To identify the source of the bacteremia, clues must be detected in the history and physical examination that might indicate the presence of a localized infection, such as pyelonephritis, cholecystitis, or pelvic abscess. In granulocytopenic patients, the significance of modest complaints, such as perirectal discomfort, must not be overlooked, and the importance of subtle physical findings, such as erythema and tenderness, must not be underestimated. In general, the preliminary laboratory evaluation will be guided by the results of the history and examination. In aged, debilitated, or granulocytopenic patients, a Gram's stain and culture of secretions (sputum), excretions (urine), and body fluids (pleural or peritoneal specimens) should be considered, even in the absence of suggestive historical data or physical examination findings. Biopsy specimens of cutaneous lesions may need to be obtained for Gram's stain, culture, and histologic assessment.

*Treatment*
Antimicrobials remain the cornerstone of therapy for patients with suspected or confirmed gram-negative bacteremia. In general, the initial selection is guided by epidemiologic considerations (e.g., community-acquired vs. nosocomial infection), by the results of the history and physical examination, and by the findings on the Gram's stain of clinical material. Obviously, because the clinical manifestations of disease caused by gram-positive bacteria can be similar to those caused by gram-negative microbes, because gram-positive microbes play some role in all the common infectious syndromes (e.g., pneumonia, cholecystitis), and because gram-positive bacteremia can lead to severe sepsis and death, all empiric regimens must contain an agent with activ-

ity against pertinent gram-positive bacteria. Examples of empiric therapy include the following:

1. For the patient with community-acquired biliary tract infection, ampicillin-sulbactam, with or without an aminoglycoside; clindamycin plus gentamicin, aztreonam, or a fluoroquinolone (e.g., ciprofloxacin), with or without ampicillin; cefoxitin or cefotetan, with or without ampicillin; or a third-generation cephalosporin plus flagyl, with or without ampicillin.
2. For the patient with community-acquired pyelonephritis, an aminoglycoside; a fluoroquinolone (e.g., ciprofloxacin); aztreonam; or a third-generation cephalosporin.
3. For the patient with an ICU-acquired pneumonia, an aminoglycoside plus a third-generation cephalosporin (e.g., ceftazidime), an antipseudomonal penicillin (e.g., ticarcillin), or aztreonam; or imipenem or meropenem alone. If methicillin-resistant *Staphylococcus aureus* is prevalent in the ICU, add vancomycin.
4. For the granulocytopenic patient admitted from home with fever, ceftazidime or imipenem, with or without an aminoglycoside; or an antipseudomonal penicillin (e.g., ticarcillin) plus an aminoglycoside. In the setting of hypotension, frank infection at a central venous catheter site, or a history of colonization or infection with methicillin-resistant *S. aureus,* add vancomycin.

To reiterate, because the clinical manifestations of gram-negative and gram-positive sepsis are indistinguishable, the seriously ill patient who has no obvious focus of infection and who requires empiric therapy should be given agents that have activity against gram-negative bacilli and *S. aureus* and, perhaps, streptococci, such as *Streptococcus pneumoniae* and *Enterococcus faecalis*. Finally, among patients with suspected hospital-acquired gram-negative bacteremia, the empiric choice of aminoglycoside or third-generation cephalosporin should be guided by a knowledge of the organisms usually recovered in the institution and their susceptibility patterns.

The importance of appropriate antimicrobial therapy in the management of the patient with gram-negative bacteremia cannot be overemphasized. Prompt treatment with adequate doses of at least one drug to which the offending pathogen is susceptible *in vitro* reduces the frequency with which shock complicates the bacteremia and increases the likelihood of a successful outcome. Thus, care must be given to the initial selection of drugs for the patient who requires empiric treatment.

Regardless of which empiric regimen is selected for the patient with presumed gram-negative bacteremia, therapy should be adjusted once a pathogen is isolated and the results of antimicrobial susceptibility testing are available. In general, broad-spectrum empiric therapy should be replaced by more focused treatment, and drugs that are less toxic should replace antimicrobials with the potential for serious side effects.

The optimal antimicrobial therapy for gram-negative bacteremia is not known. Some enthusiasm for the use of combinations of antimicrobials remains. Selected combinations of these agents can exert synergistic killing activity against many aerobic gram-negative bacilli, and in a few clinical circumstances, combination therapy with synergistic agents is more efficacious than other regimens. However, it is frequently not possible to predict which combination of drugs will act synergistically, and the *in vitro* studies necessary to confirm synergy are difficult to perform in most clinical microbiology laboratories. The use of combination therapy increases the risk for an untoward drug reaction and enhances the possibility of superinfection. In general, the combination of an aminoglycoside plus a β-lactam agent [i.e., antipseudomonal penicillin, third-generation cephalosporin, or monobactam (aztreonam)] will usually result in the synergistic killing of most aerobic gram-negative bacilli. A regimen of aminoglycoside plus β-lactam should be considered for patients who are infected with gram-negative bacilli and who have granulocytopenia, an endovascular focus of sepsis (i.e., endocarditis), or a pneumonia caused by *P. aeruginosa, Enterobacter* species, *Serratia* species, or another organism that is difficult to eradicate.

*Supportive Measures*
Supportive measures are essential for patients with gram-negative bacteremia. Fluids should be administered to optimize the cardiac output and ensure adequate tissue per-

fusion. Hyperglycemia, hypoxemia, acid-base disturbances, and electrolyte abnormalities should be quickly identified and promptly treated. Surgical interventions should be vigorously pursued, and abscesses should be drained, visceral obstructions relieved, and necrotic tissue debrided. Percutaneous drainage procedures guided by computed tomography, such as cholecystostomy and nephrostomy, should be considered in patients who may be too unstable for a definitive surgical intervention. The patient must be monitored closely for complications of the bacteremia, including ARDS, renal failure, gastrointestinal bleeding, and DIC. Blood cultures should be repeated in patients with persistent fever or other evidence of ongoing bacteremia. The persistence of bacteremia may indicate an undrained abscess, an obstruction within the biliary or urinary tract, inappropriate antimicrobial therapy, or an endovascular focus of infection, such as a septic thrombophlebitis or mycotic aneurysm.

## Sepsis Cascade

*Definitions*

The magnitude of the problem of sepsis and related syndromes is enormous; 400,000 to 500,000 episodes of sepsis occur annually in the United States, and the condition is associated with a case-fatality rate of 30% to 40%. To facilitate the study of this prevalent and serious condition, attempts have been made to provide more helpful clinical classifications of the infection-related syndromes that can evolve as a consequence of gram-negative or gram-positive bacteremia, or occasionally fungemia.

Sepsis is currently defined as the presence of the systemic inflammatory response syndrome (SIRS) when it is attributable to a documented infectious disease. The essential features of SIRS include fever (>38°C) or hypothermia (<36°C), tachypnea (>20/min), and tachycardia (>90/min); obviously, SIRS can occur in the absence of an infectious illness, and the condition can be precipitated by pancreatitis, trauma, and burns. Severe sepsis is the presence of sepsis plus evidence of hypotension or hypoperfusion leading to organ dysfunction (e.g., altered mental status, hypoxia, oliguria, increased plasma lactate). Septic shock is severe sepsis plus hypotension and organ dysfunction refractory to fluid resuscitation. These distinctions are useful because data have shown that even if it is precipitated by infection, the sepsis cascade can become self-perpetuating; indeed, by the time that sepsis becomes clinically manifest, the triggering infection may not be apparent. As a result, in the setting of sepsis, severe sepsis, or septic shock, therapies beyond antimicrobials are necessary to increase the likelihood of survival.

Septic shock occurs in 25% to 40% of patients with gram-negative bacteremia, usually within the first 12 hours of infection. Factors that predispose to shock are advanced age, a history of prior therapy with antimicrobials or immunosuppressive agents (corticosteroids, antimetabolites, cytotoxic drugs), and the presence of diabetes mellitus, congestive heart failure, azotemia, or a rapidly fatal illness. The risk for shock does not seem to be influenced by the magnitude of the bacteremia, species of the bacterium, or presence of detectable quantities of endotoxin.

*Pathophysiology*

Derived from the cell wall of gram-negative bacteria, endotoxin contains lipopolysaccharide (LPS), outer-membrane structures, and capsular polysaccharides. LPS consists of a core polysaccharide, O (somatic) antigen side chains, and lipid A. LPS plays the central role in precipitating the sepsis cascade; for example, many of the manifestations of sepsis can be induced in laboratory animals by the administration of cell wall fragments, LPS, or lipid A. Of note, the components of gram-positive bacteria that can precipitate sepsis include cell wall constituents (e.g., peptidoglycan) and extracellular products, such as the superantigens, pyrogenic exotoxin A (elaborated by *Streptococcus pyogenes*), and toxic shock toxin 1 (produced by *S. aureus*).

Substantial insight into the molecular mechanisms through which endotoxin or LPS precipitates the sepsis cascade has been gained, and new observations concerning mediators of the syndrome and their interactions are being published regularly. In general, once in the circulation, LPS binds to LPS-binding protein (LBP), and the LPS-LBP complex attaches to specific receptors on monocytes and macrophages, stimulating the release of a large number of biologically active molecules. The endogenous mediators induced by LPS-LBP include tumor necrosis factor (TNF), interleukin-1, -2, and -6

(IL-1, IL-2, IL-6), and platelet-activating factor; TNF and IL-1 represent the most important proinflammatory cyokines released in response to LPS. The endogenous mediators in turn activate a variety of cellular and humoral inflammatory systems, including T lymphocytes, neutrophils, platelets, endothelial cells, and the coagulation and complement cascades. Furthermore, endotoxin and the inflammatory mediators increase the expression of nitric oxide synthetase found in vascular smooth muscle; that enzyme in turn results in an overproduction of nitric oxide, a potent vasodilator recently implicated in the pathogensesis of septic shock. The activation of these inflammatory systems leads to DIC, ARDS, and circulatory collapse. With insight into the pathogenesis of septic shock, researchers have attempted to alter the course of the condition by blocking the effects of mediators. Unfortunately, controlled clinical trials have failed to demonstrate a benefit of monoclonal or polyclonal antibodies to endotoxin, monoclonal antibodies to TNF, or antagonists to platelet-activating factor and the IL-1 receptor.

*Management*

The biologic effects of the potent endogenous mediators result in increased cellular metabolism and therefore increased oxygen requirements. They also produce an increase in capillary permeability, a peripheral vasodilation, a fall in systemic vascular resistance, and a global depression of myocardial contractility. These cardiovascular changes contribute to septic shock. By extension, the goals of therapy of septic shock include a restoration of adequate tissue perfusion and oxygen delivery. The rapid administration of large volumes of fluid is essential. Although the roles of crystalloids versus colloids (e.g., hydroxyethyl starch solutions) remain controversial, the importance of monitoring the progress of fluid administration with a pulmonary artery (Swan-Ganz) catheter is widely accepted. These catheters allow measurements of wedged pulmonary artery pressures and so permit an accurate assessment of left ventricular filling pressures. In general, a wedged pulmonary artery pressure of 12 to 14 mm Hg should be maintained, although higher levels may be required in some patients. An improved mental status, a urine output of 40 to 50 mL/h, and a decline in serum lactate concentration are indicative of a favorable response.

Vasoactive drugs must be administered if volume expansion does not result in a prompt clinical improvement, including a rise in systolic blood pressure to about 100 mm Hg. The adrenergic agent of choice, dopamine, produces a variety of dose-dependent effects on the cardiovascular system. At low doses (2 to 5 g/kg per minute), dopamine raises the heart rate and enhances cardiac contractility, resulting in increases in stroke volume and cardiac index; it also augments renal blood flow and the glomerular filtration rate. At higher doses, dopamine produces generalized vasoconstriction. If hypotension persists despite administration of high doses of dopamine (20 to 25 g/mL), treatment with norepinephrine should be initiated. The roles of other agents, including the combination of dobutamine and norepinephrine, vasopressin, and nitric oxide synthetase inhibitors, remain under study.

To ensure the delivery of sufficient oxygen to tissues, a hemoglobin saturation approaching 100% is essential. To achieve an arterial hemoglobulin saturation of greater than 90%, the arterial oxygen tension must be maintained above 60 mm Hg. Accordingly, endotracheal intubation and mechanical ventilation are usually indicated in patients in whom respiratory insufficiency, progressive hypoxemia, and an arterial oxygen tension of less than 50 mm Hg develop. The addition of positive end-expiratory pressure is often required to maintain an arterial oxygen tension of 60 to 70 mm Hg without increasing the fraction of inspired oxygen to above 50%.

A variety of additional therapeutic interventions are often required to address the multiple manifestations of septic shock: insulin for hyperglycemia; glucose for hypoglycemia; platelet and red blood transfusions for thrombocytopenia with active bleeding; fresh-frozen plasma, platelets, and RBC transfusions for DIC with active bleeding; nasogastric lavage, histamine$_2$-receptor antagonists and RBC transfusions for upper gastrointestinal bleeding; and glucocorticoids for acute adrenal insufficiency, an overlooked condition in this setting that can lead to refractory hypotension. (A.L.E.)

**Bibliography**

The ACCP/SCCM Consensus Conference Committee. Definitions for sepsis and organ failure and guidelines for the use of innovative therapies in sepsis. *Chest* 1992; 101:1644.

*Clinical definitions for systemic inflammatory response syndrome, sepsis, severe sepsis, septic shock, multiple organ dysfunction syndrome, and related entities are provided.*

Aube H, Milan C, Blettery B. Risk factors for septic shock in the early management of bacteremia. *Am J Med* 1992;93:283.
*Multivariate statistical analysis identified the following risk factors for septic shock: male sex and age over 75 years, elevated serum creatinine, abnormal prothrombin time, and interstitial pattern on chest radiograph.*

Baxter F. Septic shock. *Can J Anaesth* 1997;44:59.
*A contemporary overview of the pathogenesis and management of the problem.*

Bisbe J, et al. *Pseudomonas aeruginosa* bacteremia: univariate and multivariate analysis of factors influencing prognosis in 133 episodes. *Rev Infect Dis* 1988;10:629.
*Among the factors predicting a poor outcome in patients with this infection were a granulocyte count of less than $500/mm^3$, inappropriate antimicrobial therapy, and the development of septic shock.*

Bone RC, Grodzin CJ, Balk RA. Sepsis: a new hypothesis for pathogenesis of the disease process. *Chest* 1997;112:235.
*The failure of antiinflammatory cytokines to control the production and effects of TNF and the other proinflammatory cytokines contributes to SIRS.*

Gribes AR, Smit AJ. Use of dopamine in the ICU. Hope, hype, belief and facts. *Clin Exp Hypertens* 1997;19:191.
*After critically reviewing the data concerning the benefits of dopamine in patients with septic shock, the authors suggest that the widespread use of dopamine remains unsupported by scientific findings and that alternate interventions be used to restore blood pressure.*

Jaber BL, Pereira BJ. Extracorporeal adsorbent-based strategies in sepsis. *Am J Kidney Dis* 1997;30:(5 Suppl 4):S44.
*Review of data from preliminary observations on the benefit of blood purification methods in which extracorporeal adsorbent techniques are used, and discussion of the potential role of this therapy in managing patients with sepsis.*

Kilbourn RG, Szabo C, Traber DL. Beneficial versus detrimental effects of nitric oxide synthetase inhibitors in circulatory shock: lessons learned from experimental and clinical studies. *Shock* 1997;7:235.
*An excellent overview of nitric oxide and its role in physiologic and pathologic vasodilation.*

Kreger BE, et al. Gram-negative bacteremia. III. Reassessment of etiology, epidemiology and ecology in 612 patients. *Am J Med* 1980;68:332.
*Outstanding clinical review.*

Kreger BE, Craven DE, McCabe WR. Gram-negative bacteremia. IV. Re-evaluation of clinical features and treatment in 612 patients. *Am J Med* 1980;68:344.
*Outstanding clinical review.*

Leibovici L, et al. Predictive index for optimizing empiric treatment of gram-negative bacteremia. *J Infect Dis* 1991;163:193.
*Among the factors predicting isolation of an antimicrobial-resistant gram-negative bacterium from blood were hospital acquisition of the infection, prior antimicrobial therapy, endotracheal intubation, and thermal trauma as the reason for hospitalization.*

Lorente JA, et al. Time course of hemostatic abnormalities in sepsis and its relation to outcome. *Chest* 1993;103:1536.
*The authors present a detailed analysis of the coagulation and fibrinolytic abnormalities detected in 48 patients with septic shock.*

Martin MA, Silverman HJ. Gram-negative sepsis and the adult respiratory distress syndrome. *Clin Rev Respir Dis* 1992;14:1213.
*A contemporary review of the pathogenesis and prognosis of ARDS.*

Miller PJ, Wenzel RP. Etiologic organisms as independent predictors of death and morbidity associated with bloodstream infections. *J Infect Dis* 1987;156:471.
*Among patients with hospital-acquired blood-borne infection, the risk for hypotension, oliguria, respiratory failure, or mortality can be correlated with specific microbes; for example, bacteremia caused by* P. aeruginosa *often predicts death.*

Moreau R, et al. Septic shock in patients with cirrhosis: hemodynamic and metabolic characteristics and intensive care outcome. *Crit Care Med* 1992;20:746.
*In cirrhotic patients, septic shock is often associated with hypothermia and a marked lactic acidemia; the condition carries a 100% mortality rate for patients admitted to the ICU.*
Nys M, et al. Sequential anti-core glycolipid immunoglobulin antibody activities in patients with and without septic shock and their relation to outcome. *Ann Surg* 1993;217:300.
*The authors monitored endogenous levels of anti-LPS antibody levels in septic surgical patients, and they found that the absence of anti-core glycolipid IgM antibodies was correlated with the evolution of septic shock and that the presence of high or rising IgG antibody levels was associated with a better outcome.*
Redl-Wenzl EM, et al. The effects of norepinephrine on hemodynamics and renal function in severe septic shock states. *Intensive Care Med* 1993;19:151.
*In a prospective study of 56 patients with septic shock and hypotension refractory to fluids, dopamine, and dobutamine, the authors found that the administration of norepinephrine was associated with increases in mean arterial pressure, systemic vascular resistance, stroke volume, and glomerular filtration rate; the drug had no deleterious effect on cardiac index, oxygen delivery, or oxygen consumption.*
Reuben AG, et al. Polymicrobial bacteremia: clinical and microbiologic patterns. *Rev Infect Dis* 1989;2:161.
*The finding of an aerobic gram-negative bacillus and* S. aureus *in the blood indicates a cutaneous focus of infection; the recovery of a gram-negative bacillus and* Streptococcus faecalis *correlates with an intraabdominal source.*
Reynolds KL, Brenner ER. Analysis of 1,186 episodes of gram-negative bacteremia in non-university hospitals: the effects of antimicrobial therapy. *Rev Infect Dis* 1983; 5:629.
*The use of inappropriate antimicrobial therapy was associated with a mortality rate of 45%; the administration of appropriate antimicrobials resulted in a case fatality rate of 28%.*
Sprung CL, et al. Impact of encephalopathy on mortality in the sepsis syndrome. *Crit Care Med* 1990;18:801.
*Among patients with the sepsis syndrome, hypothermia, hypotension, thrombocytopenia, the absence of shaking chills, and an altered mental status independently predict an increased mortality rate.*
Tuchschmidt J, et al. Elevation of cardiac output and oxygen delivery improves outcome in septic shock. *Chest* 1992;102:216.
*Interventions that augmented cardiac output reduced the mortality rate from 74% to 40%.*

## 43. METHICILLIN-RESISTANT *STAPHYLOCOCCUS AUREUS*

Following its introduction into clinical practice in the 1940s, penicillin became the treatment of choice for infections caused by *Staphylococcus aureus;* however, penicillin-resistant strains of *S. aureus* rapidly emerged. The problem of resistant staphylococci appeared to have been eliminated with the development of the semisynthetic penicillins, such as methicillin and oxacillin, in the early 1960s. However, in 1961, strains of *S. aureus* resistant to the semisynthetic penicillins were isolated in England, and within 10 years, outbreaks of hospital-associated infections became common throughout Europe.

Before 1976, only sporadic outbreaks of nosocomial infection with methicillin-resistant *S. aureus* (MRSA) were reported in the United States. Since that time, hospital-acquired disease caused by MRSA has reached epidemic proportions. Although the initial outbreaks were confined to university medical centers, by 1979, more than 30% of community hospitals had patients with MRSA bacteremia, and by 1989, more than

90% of all acute-care hospitals reported having patients infected with this microbe. The fact that few antimicrobials are available to treat infected patients and the observation that the organism can be difficult to eliminate from an institution contribute to the concern about MRSA as a nosocomial pathogen. That concern has been dramatically accentuated since strains with reduced susceptibililty to vancomycin have been isolated in Japan and the United States.

The resistance of *S. aureus* to penicillin is mediated by a β-lactamase, which is an enzyme usually produced under the control of extrachromosomal DNA (plasmid). The β-lactamase is capable of hydrolyzing the β-lactam ring and thus chemically inactivating penicillin. In contrast, resistance to methicillin and related drugs is chromosomally linked, and it does not involve the inactivation of the antimicrobial. Rather, methicillin-resistant staphylococci express a penicillin-binding protein that possesses a greatly reduced affinity for β-lactam antimicrobials, including the semisynthetic penicillins; this protein is referred to as penicillin-binding protein 2a. The phenotypic expression of this intrinsic resistance can be modified by a number of factors; for example, raising the pH of the culture media or lowering the incubation temperature below 35°C increases the expression of methicillin resistance. The heterogeneity in the phenotypic expression of resistance is clinically relevant; if an intrinsically resistant strain is incubated at 37°C, only 1 in $10^5$ or $10^6$ bacteria will express resistance, and the isolate may be incorrectly characterized as methicillin-susceptible. Of note, MRSA often contains plasmids that convey resistance to other antimicrobials. Finally, methicillin-resistant strains possess all the virulence factors found in methicillin-susceptible staphylococci, and so the organism is capable of producing life-threatening disease in humans.

### Epidemiology

MRSA is usually introduced into a hospital by patients who are transferred from other institutions, especially nursing homes, in which the organisms are endemic. Physicians have also been implicated as the source of interhospital spread. On occasion, spouses of patients have been found to be reservoirs of MRSA. Once introduced into a hospital, MRSA can disseminate rapidly and colonize patients and personnel, who then serve as sources of continued transmission. Diseases of the skin, including decubitus ulcers, burns, surgical wounds, and chronic dermatitis, increase the probability of colonization. In addition, colonization of the anterior nares of patients and hospital employees can occur and contribute to the spread of MRSA.

The risk for development of infection with MRSA is increased among colonized patients who are aged and debilitated, who have received prior antimicrobial therapy, who reside in ICUs, who undergo chronic hemodialysis, or who are hospitalized for prolonged periods of time. Resistant staphylococci can produce a number of potentially life-threatening diseases, including endocarditis, pneumonia, bacteremia, osteomyelitis, and septic thrombophlebitis. Because of the prevalence of serious underlying illnesses among patients infected with MRSA, case-fatality rates are high; among patients with bronchopneumonia, for example, mortality rates above 50% have been reported.

### Treatment

The management of patients with infections caused by MRSA remains problematic, in part because of the limited number of useful antimicrobials. These organisms are invariably resistant to all penicillins. Some strains are susceptible *in vitro* to the cephalosporins; however, clinical experience indicates that patients infected with MRSA and treated with cephalosporins respond poorly, and MRSA must be considered resistant to this class of antimicrobials. Virtually all strains of MRSA exhibit susceptibility to vancomycin, and clinical studies have confirmed that vancomycin is an effective drug in the management of patients with serious infections. Vancomycin is the treatment of choice for patients with potentially life-threatening disease caused by MRSA, but it is not an ideal agent; some strains of MRSA are only inhibited by the drug, not killed, and treatment failures can occur in patients infected with these tolerant strains. Some strains of *S. aureus* resistant to the β-lactam antimicrobials are sensitive to trimethoprim-sulfamethoxazole, and the drug can be employed to treat patients infected with MRSA. Ciprofloxacin has also been used on occasion with success. The glycopeptide teicoplanin, which is not yet available in the United States, also appears to have excellent activity against MRSA, and the drug has been used with success abroad. Of note, patients cured of MRSA infection often remain colonized by the pathogen.

Vancomycin is usually administered at a dosage of 1 g every 12 hours, although alternate dosing regimens are under investigation. Because the drug is excreted by the kidneys, dosage adjustments are mandatory in patients with renal dysfunction. Serum levels should be monitored, and peak concentrations of 30 to 40 g/mL and trough levels of 5 to 10 g/mL should be maintained. Vancomycin alone rarely produces nephrotoxicity; however, the potential for renal injury is substantially augmented in patients also receiving aminoglycosides. In general, renal function should be assessed two to three times weekly, and the use of other nephrotoxic drugs should be avoided. Vancomycin has been reported to cause hearing loss, although this complication is very rare. Finally, antimicrobial antagonism can occur when a second drug is combined with vancomycin; therefore, in most circumstances, vancomycin should be used alone. If the patient fails to respond to therapy with vancomycin, the addition of rifampin or an aminoglycoside should be considered; in general, the combination of vancomycin with rifampin or an aminoglycoside will produce synergistic killing.

## Infection Control

To control the spread of MRSA within a hospital, patients known to be infected with the organism should be isolated or perhaps cohorted with other infected patients. Stringent adherence to the isolation techniques is mandatory, and scrupulous attention must be paid to hand washing and the use of gloves, gowns, and masks, as required by the type of isolation implemented. Patients who are colonized and require prolonged hospitalization should be cohorted with other carriers; the specific isolation precautions necessary should be determined by the infection control officer on a case-by-case basis. Carriers of MRSA should be discharged as soon as possible; many adult patients discharged to home will eliminate the bacterium within a month.

If standard infection control measures fail to arrest an outbreak of MRSA disease, surveillance cultures should be obtained to identify colonized patients who may be the source of continuous person-to-person transmission. Physicians, nursing personnel, and other persons in contact with patients who are infected or colonized with MRSA should be screened for carriage by culturing the anterior nares and cutaneous lesions, including furuncles, carbuncles, and areas of paronychia and chronic dermatitis. If the survey of personnel fails to detect MRSA carriage but the outbreak continues, additional cultures of the health care workers' nares, throat, hands, axillae, rectums, and inguinal regions should be considered; environmental cultures will also be required in selected circumstances. Hospital personnel colonized with MRSA should be removed from direct patient contact. Occasionally, ICUs must be closed to new admissions to control an outbreak of infection.

In the setting of outbreaks of infection, the use of antimicrobials in the management of patients and health care workers who are carriers of MRSA in concert with other infection control measures has proved effective in controlling the epidemics. In particular, studies have shown that treatment of carriers is frequently associated with eradication of colonizing MRSA and control of epidemics. Thus, antimicrobials should be employed if an outbreak of MRSA disease is not terminated by alternate infection control procedures.

Data from a number of studies have shown that topical 2% mupirocin applied to the anterior nares two to three times daily for 5 to 7 days represents a highly effective means of eliminating the nasal carrier state. Most experts recommend the concurrent use of rifampin (600 mg daily for 5 days) and trimethoprim-sulfamethoxazole (1 DS tablet for 5 to 10 days). Because of a number of unique properties, rifampin is effective in treating the carrier state; it is active against most strains of MRSA, appears in high concentrations in external secretions, and achieves high levels within phagocytic cells, where it kills sequestered organisms. Resistance to rifampin can develop rapidly; thus, the agent should never be use alone to treat staphylococcal carriers. Minocycline (100 mg twice daily) together with mupirocin and rifampin has also been highly effective in eradicating the nasal carrier state. Of note, although these antibiotic regimens have produced nasal clearance rates approaching 100%, antimicrobial combinatiions have been found to be only 60% to 80% effective in eradicating MRSA from extranasal sites, such as surgical wounds or decubitus ulcers.

Most carriers of MRSA will be cleared of the organism with one of the outlined protocols; however, patients with MRSA at sites that contain copious secretions, such as decubitus ulcers and tracheostomy wounds, often fail treatment. Further, the use of topical or systemic antimicrobials in the setting of foreign bodies, such as nasogastric or percutaneous gastrostomy tubes, will usually be unsuccessful in eliminating colonization, and the intervention may lead to the development of drug resistance. Finally, after the completion of a course of antimicrobials directed at the carrier state, follow-up cultures are necessary to ensure that the methicillin-resistant staphylococci have been eradicated from colonized patients and health care workers. (A.L.E.)

### Bibliography

Bradley SF, et al. Methicillin-resistant *Staphylococcus aureus:* colonization and infection in a long-term care facility. *Ann Intern Med* 1991;115:417.
  *Even in a chronic care facility with endemic MRSA, in 65% of the residents colonization never developed, and only 3% of the colonized patients experienced an infection.*

Brumfitt W, Hamilton-Miller J. Methicillin-resistant *Staphylococcus aureus. N Engl J Med* 1989;320:1188.
  *A comprehensive, well-referenced review of the topic.*

Centers for Disease Control. Update: *Staphylococcus aureus* with reduced susceptibility to vanomycin—1997. *MMWR Morb Mortal Wkly Rep* 1997;46:765.
  *In 1997, the first U.S. isolate of S. aureus intermittently susceptibe to vancomycin (minimum inhibitory concentration, 8 μg/mL) was isolated in Michigan.*

Cohen SH, Morita MM, Bradford M. A 7-year experience with methicillin-resistant *Staphylococcus aureus. Am J Med* 1991;91 (Suppl 3B):233S.
  *The authors detail a comprehensive infection control program that has been effective in restricting the spread of MRSA in a university hospital setting.*

Darouiche R, et al. Eradication of colonization by methicillin-resistant *Staphylococcus aureus* by using oral minocycline-rifampin and topical mupirocin. *Antimicrob Agents Chemother* 1991;35:1612.
  *By using a combination of systemic (minocycline and rifampin) and topical (mupirocin) antimicrobial therapy, the authors eradicated MRSA colonization from 91% of the patients and 95% of the sites.*

Doebbeling BN, et al. Elimination of *Staphylococcus aureus* nasal carriage in health care workers: analysis of six clinical trials with calcium mupirocin ointment. *Clin Infect Dis* 1993;17:466.
  *After analyzing the data from double-blinded studies performed at six institutions that involved 339 health care workers with stable nasal carriage of S. aureus, the authors concluded that calcium mupirocin ointment administered intranasally for 5 days was safe and effective in eliminating the organism.*

Fung-Tomac J, et al. Emergence of homogeneously methicillin-resistant *Staphylococcus aureus. J Clin Microbiol* 1991;29:2880.
  *In a study of 47 clinical isolates, the authors note that 100% of the strains recovered before 1987 were inhibited in vitro by ciprofloxacin but that only 60% of the strains obtained after 1987 were susceptible to the drug.*

Haley RW, et al. The emergence of methicillin-resistant *Staphylococcus aureus* infections in United States hospitals. *Ann Intern Med* 1982;97:297.
  *Describes the onset of the problem of MRSA in U.S. hospitals and implicates "the house staff-patient transfer circuit" as contributing to the interhospital spread of the microbe.*

Harbarth S, et al. Impact of methicillin resistance on the outcome of patients with bacteremia caused by *Staphylococcus aureus. Arch Intern Med* 1998;158:182.
  *In a retrospective study of almost 200 patients with staphylococcal bacteremia, the authors concluded that methicillin resistance alone exerted no significant impact on mortality rates.*

Hershow RC, Khayr WF, Smith NL. A comparison of clinical virulence of nosocomially acquired methicillin-resistant and methicillin-susceptible *Staphylococcus aureus* in a university hospital. *Infect Control Hosp Epidemiol* 1992;13:587.
*Patients infected with methicillin-susceptible and methicillin-resistant strains have similar demographic features, underlying diseases, clinical presentations, and outcomes.*

Hicks NR, Moore EP, Williams EW. Carriage and community treatment of methicillin-resistant *Staphylococcus aureus:* what happens to colonized patients after discharge? *J Hosp Infect* 1991;19:17.
*The majority of infants and mothers colonized with MRSA at discharge had persistent carriage after 4 weeks; the most common site of colonization was the perineum in mothers and the throat in infants.*

Hsu CC. Serial survey of methicillin-resistant *Staphylococcus aureus* nasal carriage among residents in a nursing home. *Infect Control Hosp Epidemiol* 1991;12:416.
*In this prospective study of nursing home patients, the authors found that MRSA colonization was present in 70% to 80% of the residents who were bedridden or had decubitus ulcers or foreign bodies, and that the presence of the organism within the facility was perpetuated by persistently or intermittently colonized residents.*

Kauffman CA, et al. Attempts to eradicate methicillin-resistant *Staphylococcus aureus* from a long-term care facility with the use of mupirocin ointment. *Am J Med* 1993;94:371.
*Although mupirocin ointment was effective in eliminating MRSA from the nares and wounds of colonized patients in a long-term care institution, recurrence rates were high and long-term use selected for resistant strains; these observations led the authors to conclude that mupirocin should be utilized only in the setting of an outbreak of infection with MRSA.*

Kitagawa Y, et al. Rapid diagnosis of methicillin-resistant *Staphylococcus aureus* by nested polymerase chain reaction. *Ann Surg* 1996;224:665.
*The use of polymerase chain reaction to detect the gene that codes for methicillin resistance represents a potential technique for the rapid determination of resistance.*

Levine DP, Fromm BS, Reddy BR. Slow response to vancomycin or vancomycin plus rifampin in methicillin-resistant *Staphylococcus aureus* endocarditis. *Ann Intern Med* 1991;115:674.
*In this randomized study of 42 consecutive patients with MRSA endocarditis, therapy with vancomycin alone or vancomycin plus rifampin was equally effective.*

Muder RR, et al. Methicillin-resistant staphylococcal colonization and infection in a long-term facility. *Ann Intern Med* 1991;114:107.
*In this prospective cohort study, the investigators noted that staphylococcal infection was almost four times more likely to develop in patients colonized with methicillin-susceptible strains.*

Mulhausen PL, et al. Contrasting methicillin-resistant *Staphylococcus aureus* colonization in Veterans Affairs and community nursing homes. *Am J Med* 1996;100:24.
*In this prospective survey of more than 200 nursing home patients, the authors found that the prevalence of colonization was about 30% in Veterans Affairs nursing homes and 10% in community facilities.*

Mulligan ME, et al. Methicillin-resistant *Staphylococcus aureus:* a consensus review of the microbiology, pathogenesis, and epidemiology with implications for prevention and treatment. *Am J Med* 1993;94:313.
*Superb review that contains recommendations for the eradication of the carrier state and guidelines for infection control in a variety of settings.*

Panlilio AL, et al. Methicillin-resistant *Staphylococcus aureus* in U.S. hospitals, 1975–1991. *Infect Control Hosp Epidemiol* 1992;13:582.
*In a retrospective review of susceptibility data from 66,132 hospital isolates of S. aureus, the authors found that the percentage of strains resistant to methicillin had risen from 2.4% in 1975 to 29% in 1991; for hospitals with 500 beds or more, 38.3% of the isolates in 1991 were methicillin-resistant.*

Piercy EA, et al. Ciprofloxacin for methicillin-resistant *Staphylococcus aureus* infections. *Antimicrob Agents Chemother* 1989;33:128.
*The use of ciprofloxacin in the therapy of infections with MRSA can produce clinical cures; however, ciprofloxacin-resistant strains can emerge during therapy.*

Sheretz RJ, et al. A cloud adult: the *Staphylococcus aureus*-virus interaction revisited. *Ann Intern Med* 1996;124:539.
  *The importance of the colonized anterior nares as a potential reservoir for epidemics of MRSA infection is highlighted by this report.*
Tokue Y, et al. Comparison of a polymerase chain reaction assay with a conventional microbiologic method for detection of methicillin-resistant *Staphylococcus aureus*. *Antimicrob Agents Chemother* 1992;36:6.
  *The polymerase chain reaction assay was found to be a sensitive method for the detection of MRSA.*

## 44. COAGULASE-NEGATIVE STAPHYLOCOCCI

A report from the microbiology laboratory that a blood culture is positive for gram-positive cocci in grapelike clusters suggests that the organism most likely is *Staphylococcus aureus* or *Staphylococcus epidermidis*. Rarely, the organism will be identified as a *Micrococcus* or a *Peptococcus* (an anaerobic gram-positive coccus) species. Staphylococci are catalase-positive organisms that belong to the family Micrococcaceae. The staphylococci that produce coagulase are *S. aureus,* and those that are coagulase-negative are designated as coagulase-negative staphylococci or *Staphylococcus* not *aureus.* There are multiple species of coagulase-negative staphylococci, but *S. epidermidis* is the most common. Another pathogenic coagulase-negative staphylococcal organism is *S. saprophyticus,* a well-recognized cause of urinary tract infections, especially in women. Resistance to novobiocin is the characteristic used most often to distinguish *S. saprophyticus* from other species of coagulase-negative staphylococci. All the factors that determine the virulence of *S. epidermidis* are unknown. The organism can adhere to and proliferate on prosthetic devices. Coagulase-negative staphylococci produce a slime-like substance that covers the organism but is not a true capsule. This substance interferes with phagocytosis.

Most (85%) coagulase-negative staphylococci isolated from a blood culture are contaminants, as the organisms colonize human skin and mucosal surfaces. In the other 15% of cases, the organisms are considered pathogens, especially in patients with indwelling medical devices such as prosthetic valves, central venous catheters, central nervous system shunts, vascular grafts, and pacemakers. *S. epidermidis* can also cause bacteremia in neutropenic patients with malignancy, neonatal bacteremia in low-birth-weight infants, and native valve endocarditis. To be able to interpret the meaning of a positive blood culture for a gram-positive coccus in clusters, the clinician must ask the following questions:

1. *How many blood cultures are positive?* A single positive culture suggests contamination unless the patient has an indwelling prosthetic device; if that is the case, repeated blood cultures are indicated, depending on the clinical situation. Obtaining a single set of blood cultures in an adult with a prosthetic device poses a dilemma for the clinician if the culture becomes positive. To avoid this problem, three sets of blood cultures should be obtained in the setting of suspected infection in a patient with an indwelling medical device.

2. *What if there are multiple positive blood cultures?* The finding of multiple positive blood cultures for coagulase-negative staphylococci suggests true invasive disease. The clinician should compare the antibiograms of the staphylococci isolated from the different blood culture bottles to determine if they are the same or different strains. The advantage of using the antimicrobial susceptibility test results to compare the strains is that the antibiograms are readily available. However, the technique is limited by the resistance of most nosocomial staphylococci to multiple antimicrobials, and the resistance may be unstable. Other methods of epidemiologic analysis are phage typing, biotyping, plasmid profile analysis, and restriction endonuclease analysis. The various techniques used to determine strain uniqueness are costly and may not be

readily available, so that it is imperative to obtain blood cultures with the utmost care to avoid contamination.

3. *Does the patient have a persistent bacteremia?* Persistent recovery of a unique organism from the blood is powerful evidence that the coagulase-negative staphylococcal organism is a real pathogen and not a contaminant.

4. *Were the positive blood cultures obtained in a patient with intravascular lines?* Intravascular lines are often the source of S. epidermidis and should be inspected, removed, and cultured. If there is no obvious primary focus such as an IV line and the patient has persistent bacteremia, infective endocarditis must be suspected.

5. *Does the patient have cardiac valve involvement?* Two-dimensional or transesophageal echocardiography may be of value in documenting a vegetation on a cardiac valve, which supports the diagnosis of infective endocarditis.

If the interpretation of the blood culture reports supports the diagnosis of a real bacteremia rather than contamination, therapy should be selected based on the results of antimicrobial susceptibility testing. Several caveats must be considered when therapy is selected for a coagulase-negative staphylococcal infection.

1. If the organism is β-lactamase-negative, penicillin can be used. However, this rarely occurs.

2. If the organism is β-lactamase-positive and susceptible to methicillin, nafcillin can be selected. However, these organisms can be heteroresistant—that is, a culture can comprise two populations, one susceptible to methicillin and the other resistant. This resistance can be overlooked unless testing is performed with a large inoculum on salt-containing media and the culture is incubated at 30°C to 35°C. Unfortunately, methicillin resistance can be seen in as many as 40% to 80% of strains, depending on the hospital.

3. If an organism is resistant to methicillin, it must be assumed that it is resistant to all the cephalosporins, even if it is found to be susceptible by testing.

4. Vancomycin susceptibility testing is reliable.

5. Prospective studies to determine the optimal therapy of S. epidermidis native valve infection are lacking. Retrospective studies favor the use of a β-lactam antimicrobial (e.g., nafcillin or oxacillin), or vancomycin plus gentamicin. The dosage of gentamicin is that used for synergy (1 mg/kg every 8 hours) in a patient with normal renal function. The duration of gentamicin administration varied between 3 and 42 days in different studies. Rifampin can be substituted for gentamicin and given with nafcillin or vancomycin for the duration of therapy (4 weeks). I favor using gentamicin only for the initial 5 days, unless the patient is doing poorly, and then using a single drug for the remainder of the therapy.

6. If the patient has a prosthetic device and an infection caused by a methicillin-susceptible S. epidermidis, then nafcillin or oxacillin plus rifampin should be selected for a 6-week course. Antimicrobial susceptibility testing of the S. epidermidis must be appropriate to detect the presence of heteroresistance. If the organism is susceptible to gentamicin, administer gentamicin in doses to achieve a peak serum concentration of 3 g/mL. Gentamicin should be given only for the initial 2 weeks of therapy. In patients with infection caused by a methicillin-resistant S. epidermidis, use vancomycin plus rifampin along with gentamicin for the first 2 weeks, then continue vancomycin plus rifampin for the remaining 4 weeks of therapy. The role of teicoplanin, a glycopeptide antimicrobial, and quinupristin-dalfopristin in patients unable to tolerate vancomycin remains to be determined.

7. The mortality rate for native valve S. epidermidis endocarditis ranges from 13% to 36%.

8. The mortality rate for S. epidermidis prosthetic valve endocarditis is about 20%. However, a cure rate of 80% usually requires a combination of surgery plus 6 weeks of antimicrobial therapy. (N.M.G.)

## Bibliography

Arber N, et al. Native valve *Staphylococcus epidermidis* endocarditis: report of seven cases and review of the literature. *Am J Med* 1991;90:758.

*In this small series, the authors describe a disease with an indolent course and few complications.*

Boyce JM, et al. A common-source outbreak of *Staphylococcus epidermidis* infections among patients undergoing cardiac surgery. *J Infect Dis* 1990;161:493.
*The hands of a cardiac surgeon were identified as the source of infection. The authors used plasmid profiles and restriction endonuclease digest analysis to determine that the strains were identical.*

Calderwood SB, et al. Risk factors for the development of prosthetic valve endocarditis. *Circulation* 1985;72:31.
*The risk for prosthetic valve endocarditis was 3.1% at 12 months and 5.7% at 60 months.*

Caputo GM, et al. Native valve endocarditis due to coagulase-negative staphylococci. *Am J Med* 1987;83:619.
*Although the presentation is usually subacute, complications such as arterial emboli, conduction system abnormalities, congestive heart failure, myocardial abscesses, and valve leaflet disruption occur frequently.*

Garcia R, Raad I. *In vitro* study of the potential role of quinupristin-dalfopristin in the treatment of catheter-related staphylococcal infections. *Eur J Clin Microbiol Infect Dis* 1996;15:933–936.
*Quinupristin-dalfopristin is an alternative drug to vancomycin for catheter-related staphylococcal infections.*

Hedin G. A comparison of methods to determine whether clinical isolates of *Staphylococus epidermidis* from the same patient are related. *J Hosp Infect* 1996;34:31–42.
*Biotyping and antibiotic resistance testing were helpful in determining whether the strains isolated were causing infection or were contaminants.*

Herwaldt LA, et al. The positive predictive value of isolating coagulase-negative staphylococci from blood cultures. *Clin Infect Dis* 1996;22:14–20.
*Twenty-six percent of coagulase-negative staphylococci isolated represented infections. Clues to infection-associated isolates included identification of the species as* S. epidermidis, *in one of five biotypes, and demonstration of resistance to at least five antibiotics.*

Karchmer AW. Staphylococcal endocarditis: laboratory and clinical basis for antibiotic therapy. *Am J Med* 1985;78(Suppl 6B):116.
*Outline of guidelines for therapy.*

Karchmer AW, Archer GL, Dismukes WE. *Staphylococcus epidermidis* causing prosthetic valve endocarditis: microbiologic and clinical observations as guides to therapy. *Ann Intern Med* 1983;98:447.
*Surgery is indicated for patients on appropriate therapy who have persistent fever for more than 9 days or evidence of prosthetic valve dysfunction.*

Kloos WE, Bannerman TL. Update on clinical significance of coagulase-negative staphylococci. *Clin Microbiol Rev* 1994;7:117.
*Review.*

Lowy FD, Hammer SM. *Staphylococcus epidermidis* infections. *Ann Intern Med* 1983;99:834.
S. epidermidis *is an important cause of infection in patients with a prosthetic valve, prosthetic hip, central nervous system shunt, vascular graft, or peritoneal dialysis catheter.*

Martin MA, Pfaller MA, Wenzel RP. Coagulase-negative staphylococcal bacteremia: mortality and hospital stay. *Ann Intern Med* 1989;110:9.
*The leading cause of nosocomial bacteremia, associated with an 8.5-day increase in length of stay.*

Patrick CC. Coagulase-negative staphylococci: pathogens with increasing clinical significance. *J Pediatr* 1990;116:497.
*Review.*

Rupp ME. Coagulase-negative staphylococcal infections: an update regarding recognition and management. In: Remington JS, Swartz MN, eds. *Current Clinical Topics in Infectious Diseases*. Clin Boston: Blackwell Science, 1997;17:51–87.
*Review.*

Rupp ME, Archer GL. Coagulase-negative staphylococci: pathogens associated with medical progress. *Clin Infect Dis* 1994;19:231–245.
*Review. Most infections are nosocomial and involve indwelling foreign devices.*
Tenover FC, Arbeit RD, Goering RV. How to select and interpret molecular strain typing methods for epidemiological studies of bacterial infections: a review for health care epidemiologists. *Infect Control Hosp Epidemiol* 1997;18:426–439.
*A review of strain typing methods. For coagulase-negative staphylococci, pulse-field gel electrophoresis is preferred.*
Whitener C, et al. Endocarditis due to coagulase-negative staphylococci. *Infect Dis Clin North Am* 1993;7:81.
*Review. Cure of prosthetic valve endocarditis usually requires a combination of antimicrobials plus surgery.*
Winston DJ, et al. Coagulase-negative staphylococcal bacteremia in patients receiving immunosuppressive therapy. *Arch Intern Med* 1983;143:32.
*An important pathogen in the patient with granulocytopenia and an IV catheter.*

# 45. VANCOMYCIN-RESISTANT ENTEROCOCCI

Vancomycin, a glycopeptide, was discovered in the mid-1950s. The drug inhibits peptidoglycan synthesis. Vancomycin has been the mainstay of therapy for infection with gram-positive organisms, including methicillin-resistant *Staphylococcus aureus,* coagulase-negative staphylococci, penicillin-resistant *Streptococcus pneumoniae,* and enterococci. The two most important enterococcal species are *Enterococcus faecalis* and *Enterococcus faecium,* with the former accounting for 80% of clinical isolates. Among vancomycin-resistant enterococci (VRE), 90% of the isolates are *E. faecium.*

In the late 1980s, the first clinical isolate of VRE was identified first in Europe and then in the United States. From 1989 through 1993, the percentage of nosocomial VRE isolates reported to the surveillance system of the Centers for Disease Control increased from 0.3% to 7.9%. In patients in ICUs, the increase in VRE was more dramatic, with almost 14% of isolates being resistant. Rates of resistance of enterococci to vancomycin in the non-ICU setting have increased and are now similar to rates in the ICU. Most hospitals in the United States have encountered at least one strain of VRE. VRE in the community has not been a problem in the United States, but the risk exists for transmission of strains of VRE from colonized patients after they leave the hospital.

Resistance of vancomycin can be classified as three phenotypes. Strains with van A resistance show a high level of resistance to vancomycin [minimum inhibitory concentrations (MICs) ≥64 µg/mL] and resistance to another glycopeptide, teicoplanin (MICs ≥16 µg/mL). Van A resistance occurs in both *E. faecalis* and *E. faecium.* Isolates with van B resistance are resistant to vancomycin (MICs from 4 µg/mL to 1,000 µg/mL or higher) but remain susceptible to teicoplanin. Strains with van C resistance have a low level of resistance to vancomycin (MICs of 4 to 32 µg/mL) and are susceptible to teicoplanin. Van C resistance occurs in all isolates of *Enterococcus gallinarum,* an organism found in stool that does not appear to cause disease. VRE would not be such a serious problem if it were not for the fact that VRE are also resistant to ampicillin, oxacillin, cephalosporins, aminoglycosides, sulfa-trimethoprim, clindamycin, and the fluoroquinolones.

Enterococci, which are gram-positive cocci, are part of the normal gastrointestinal flora, and they are also found in small numbers in the mouth, vaginal secretions, and perineal skin. Enterococci rank second or third in frequency as causes of nosocomial infections in the United States. The sources of enterococci, which can either infect or colonize patients, are the patient's own normal flora (endogenous) and the hands of hospital personnel (exogenous). Enterococci have also been isolated in the hospital environment from bed rails, blood pressure cuffs, electronic thermometers, telephone handsets, and the surfaces of stethoscopes. Cultures of the surface environment yielded

Table 45-1. Precautions to prevent patient-to-patient transmission
of vancomycin-resistant enterococci

1. Place VRE-infected or VRE-colonized patient in a private room, or cohort two
   patients with VRE in the same room.
2. Wear gloves when entering the room. Change gloves after contact with stool,
   which may contain high colony counts of VRE.
3. Wear a gown if there will be contact with the patient or environment.
4. Remove gloves and gown before leaving room and wash hands with antiseptic soap.
5. Designate equipment such as the stethoscope, blood pressure cuff, or thermometer to a single patient with VRE or a cohort of VRE patients.
6. Continue VRE isolation until three stool or other cultures obtained at weekly
   intervals are negative.
7. Establish a system to identify patients with VRE so that they can be placed in
   isolation on readmission to the hospital.

VRE, vancomycin-resistant enterococci. Modified from Centers for Disease Control and Prevention. Recommendations for preventing the spread of vancomycin resistance: recommendations of
the Hospital Infection Control Practices Advisory Committee (HICPAC). *MMWR Morb Mortal
Wkly Rep 1995;44(RR12):7–9.*

VRE in 7% to 46% of samples. Use of the usual disinfectants should be adequate to
eradicate VRE from environmental surfaces. However, one report found that 8% of cultures after terminal cleaning still showed VRE.

Risk factors for acquiring VRE include serious underlying illness, advanced age,
immunosuppression, ICU residence, prior surgery, renal insufficiency, long hospital
stay (7 days or more), presence of a urinary or vascular catheter, and use of antibiotics,
especially third-generation cephalosporins, vancomycin, and drugs for anaerobes.
Once colonized with VRE, patients may remain so for years. When patients are not
taking antibiotics, VRE counts in the stool may decrease, resulting in false-negative
stool cultures for VRE. Cultures may again become positive when the patient is again
given an antibiotic.

Once a patient is identified as being either colonized or infected with VRE, contact
precautions as recommended by the Hospital Infection Control Practices Advisory
Committee (HICPAC) are instituted (Table 45-1).

Prudent use of vancomycin has been reported to decrease the risk for colonization and infection with VRE. Hospitals should adopt the guidelines recommended by
HICPAC, which list the situations in which vancomycin use is appropriate and those
in which its use should be discouraged (Tables 45-2 and 45-3). In addition to the prudent use of vancomycin and institution of barrier precautions, a decreased use of cefotaxime, ceftazidime, and clindamycin was noted in one report to result in a marked
decrease (from 47% to 15%) in stools positive for VRE. Contamination of the environ-

Table 45-2. Indications for vancomycin treatment

1. Treatment of infections caused by MRSA, *Staphylococcus epidermidis* and enterococci in a penicillin-allergic patient.
2. Treatment of infections caused by gram-positive organisms in patients with a
   life-threatening penicillin allergy.
3. Treatment of antibiotic-associated colitis when metronidazole fails.
4. Prophylaxis for endocarditis in patients at high risk for infection.
5. Surgical prophylaxis in patients with a history of life-threatening penicillin allergy.

MRSA, methicillin-resistant *Staphylococcus aureus.* Modified from Centers for Disease Control
and Prevention. Recommendations for preventing the spread of vancomycin resistance: recommendations of the Hospital Infection Control Practices Advisory Committee (HICPAC). *MMWR
Morb Mortal Wkly Rep 1995;44(RR12):3–4.*

Table 45-3.  Situations in which the use of vancomycin should be discouraged

1. Surgical prophylaxis other than in a patient with life-threatening allergy to β-lactam antibiotics.
2. Empiric antimicrobial therapy for a febrile neutropenic patient, unless there is strong evidence that the patient has an infection caused by a gram-positive microorganism.
3. Treatment of a single blood culture positive for coagulase-negative *Staphylococcus,* if other blood cultures drawn in the same time frame are negative.
4. Selective decontamination of the digestive tract.
5. Eradication of MRSA colonization.
6. Routine prophylaxis for patients on continuous ambulatory peritoneal dialysis or hemodialysis.
7. As a vancomycin solution for topical application or irrigation.
8. Initial treatment of *Clostridium difficile* colitis.

MRSA, methicillin-resistant *Staphylococcus aureus.* Modified from Centers for Disease Control and Prevention. Recommendations for preventing the spread of vancomycin resistance: recommendations of the Hospital Infection Control Practices Advisory Committee (HICPAC). *MMWR Morb Mortal Wkly Rep* 1995;44(RR12):4.

ment and equipment for patient care with VRE is a problem, especially when patients have diarrhea. Because many patients may have both VRE and *Clostridium difficile,* measures to reduce the incidence of *C. difficile* may decrease the environmental contamination with VRE.

Treatment of infections caused by VRE remains a major problem. Chloramphenicol shows activity *in vitro* against many strains and has been used with modest success. Oral chloramphenicol is not available; the drug must be given intravenously. Treatment with high doses of ampicillin-sulbactam (30 g/d) has also had some success. Also effective has been surgical debridement with drainage of an abscess, and removal of a Foley catheter or IV catheter without any specific antibiotic treatment. Dalfopristin-quinupristin, a streptogramin antibiotic, may be effective against some strains of *E. faecium,* but not *E. faecalis.* Experimental agents, which include linezolid and the ketolides as well as a semisynthetic glycopeptide designated as LY333328, may have a role in the management of VRE. (NMG)

## Bibliography

Anderson RL, et al. Susceptibility of vancomycin-resistant enterococci to environmental disinfectants. *Infect Control Hosp Epidemiol* 1997;18:195–199.
*No special disinfectants or procedures are needed to eradicate VRE from environmental surfaces.*
Beezhold DW, et al. Skin colonization with vancomycin-resistant enterococci among hospitalized patients with bacteremia. *Clin Infect Dis* 1997;24:704–706.
*Skin colonization (inguinal area and or antecubital fossa) was common (86%) among patients with bacteremia and may be the source of catheter-related sepsis.*
Bonilla HF, et al. Colonization with vancomycin-resistant *Enterococcus faecium:* comparison of a long-term-care unit with an acute-care hospital. *Infect Control Hosp Epidemiol* 1997;18:333–339.
*VRE was found frequently (13% to 41%) on the hands of health care workers.*
Boyce JM. Vancomycin-resistant enterococcus. Detection, epidemiology, and control measures. *Infect Dis Clin North Am* 1997;11:367–384.
*Review.*
Centers for Disease Control and Prevention. Recommendations for preventing the spread of vancomycin resistance: recommendations of the Hospital Infection Control Practices Advisory Committee (HICPAC). *MMWR Morb Mortal Wkly Rep* 1995; 44 (RR12):1–13.
*Control of VRE will require (a) appropriate use of vancomycin, (b) staff education regarding VRE, (c) detection of VRE, and (d) implementation of infection control measures.*

Edmond MB, et al. Vancomycin-resistant enterococcal bacteremia: natural history and attributable mortality. *Clin Infect Dis* 1996;23:1234–1239.
*The mortality rate for patients with VRE bacteremia was 67%, which was twice that for matched controls.*

Eliopoulos GM. Vancomycin-resistant enterococci. Mechanism and clinical relevance. *Infect Dis Clin North Am* 1997;11:851–865.
*Review.*

Evans ME, Kortas KJ. Vancomycin use in a university medical center: comparison with Hospital Infection Control Practices Advisory Committee guidelines. *Infect Control Hosp Epidemiol* 1996;17:356–359.
*Only 35% of the vancomycin orders were consistent with HICPAC guidelines.*

Joshi N, Milfred D, Caputo G. Vancomycin-resistant enterococci: a review. *Infect Dis Clin Pract* 1996;5:528–537.
*Review. Risk factors for VRE infection include advanced age; severe underlying illness; immunosuppression; ICU residence; surgery; antibiotic exposure, especially with vancomycin and third-generation cephalosporins; and use of invasive devices.*

Lai KK. Treatment of vancomycin-resistant *Enterococcus faecium* infections. *Arch Intern Med* 1996;156:2579–2584.
*Removal of the IV catheter or Foley catheter and surgical debridement without antibiotics were effective in eradicating VRE.*

Lai KK, et al. The epidemiology of fecal carriage of vancomycin-resistant enterococci. *Infect Control Hosp Epidemiol* 1997;18:762–765.
*VRE carriage is often prolonged (19 to 303 days).*

Montecalvo MA, et al. Natural history of colonization with vancomycin-resistant *Enterococcus faecium*. *Infect Control Hosp Epidemiol* 1995;16:680–685.
*The rate of VRE colonization was 10 times the rate of infection among oncology patients and often persists for a year.*

Montecalvo MA, et al. Bloodstream infections with vancomycin-resistant enterococci. *Arch Intern Med* 1996;156:1458–1462.
*VRE bacteremia often persists in the immunocompromised patient.*

Noskin GA, et al. Recovery of vancomycin-resistant enterococci on fingertips and environmental surfaces. *Infect Control Hosp Epidemiol* 1995;16:577–581.
*Enterococcus faecalis survived for 5 days and* Enterococcus faecium *for 7 days on countertops.*

Porwancher R, et al. Epidemiological study of hospital-acquired infection with vancomycin-resistant *Enterococcus faecium:* possible transmission by an electronic ear probe thermometer. *Infect Control Hosp Epidemiol* 1997;18:1771–1773.
*VRE transmitted by an electronic ear probe.*

Quale J, et al. Manipulation of a hospital antimicrobial formulary to control an outbreak of vancomycin-resistant enterococci. *Clin Infect Dis* 1996;23:1020–1025.
*Decreased use of cefotaxime, ceftazidime, and clindamycin was associated with a decrease in stool colonization with VRE.*

Rafferty ME, et al. Vancomycin-resistant enterococci in stool specimens submitted for *Clostridium difficile* cytotoxin assay. *Infect Control Hosp Epidemiol* 1997;18:342–344.
*Seventeen percent of stools submitted for* C. difficile *testing were positive for VRE.*

Saurina G, Landman D, Quale JM. Activity of disinfectants against vancomycin-resistant *Enterococcus faecium*. *Infect Control Hosp Epidemiol* 1997;18:345–347.
*Except for 3% hydrogen peroxide, phenolic and quaternary ammonium compounds were effective in eradicating VRE after a 10-minute exposure.*

Slaughter S, et al. A comparison of the effect of universal use of gloves and gowns with that of glove use alone on acquisition of vancomycin-resistant enterococci in a medical intensive care unit. *Ann Intern Med* 1996;125:448–456.
*Use of gloves and gowns was no better than gloves alone in preventing rectal colonization by VRE.*

Stroud L, et al. Risk factors for mortality associated with enterococcal bloodstream infections. *Infect Control Hosp Epidemiol* 1996;17:576–580.
*The mortality rate was 69% for patients with VRE bacteremia. The high mortality caused by bacteremia occurred in a cohort of severely ill patients.*

Tornieporth NG, et al. Risk factors associated with vancomycin-resistant *Enterococcus faecium* infection or colonization in 145 matched case patients and control patients. *Clin Infect Dis* 1996;23:767–772.
*Prolonged hospitalization (≥ 7 days), intrahospital transfers, and use of vancomycin or third-generation cephalosporins were associated with an increased risk for VRE infection or colonization.*
Tucci V, Haran MA, Isenberg HD. Epidemiology and control of vancomycin-resistant enterococci in an adult and children's hospital. *Am J Infect Control* 1997;25:371–376.
*The majority (83%) of cases of VRE were nosocomial.*
Weber DJ, Rutala WA. Role of environmental contamination in the transmission of vancomycin-resistant enterococci. *Infect Control Hosp Epidemiol* 1997;18:306–309.
*Environmental contamination in patients with VRE ranges from 7% to 46%.*

# XI. FEVER

## 46. THE FEBRILE PATIENT WITHOUT AN OBVIOUS SOURCE OF INFECTION

Infection represents only one of several important groups of illnesses that can initially manifest with fever. Other examples include connective tissue disease, malignancy, and myocardial or pulmonary infarction. Certain medications may also be associated with fever. In addition to the broad differential diagnosis it entails, fever may be further confounded because it is sometimes absent in persons with significant infection. This consideration is especially important in elderly patients and those who are immunosuppressed. Moreover, neither the degree of fever nor the fever curve correlates with etiology or severity of disease. Finally, in numerous important infections, the source may not initially be obvious.

The likelihood that the acute onset of fever is caused by bacterial infection is statistically associated with advanced age, presence of indwelling urinary catheters, residence in a nursing home, and leukocytosis. Examples of diseases in which acute onset of fever may be unaccompanied by focal complaints or significant physical findings are given in Table 46-1. Identification of the source of acute fever may be complicated in circumstances in which the history and physical examination are difficult to obtain (e.g., elderly persons, severely debilitated or noncompliant patients, those with overwhelming illness or language barriers). Thus, the clinician must have a sound understanding of the potential causes of fever as well as a studied approach to the patient who presents with this complaint.

### Etiology

The history and physical examination provide important initial clues on which to base management decisions. The history must be comprehensive and include questions concerning travel, pet exposures, similar illness in family members and colleagues, medications (prescribed, over-the-counter, and illicit), and duration of fever. The travel history may be the initial important clue toward consideration of diseases such as malaria, yellow fever, and dengue. If a patient has returned with fever from a malarious area, malaria should be considered until the diagnosis has been excluded. A history of animal and bird exposure may expand the differential diagnosis to include ornithosis, infection with *Pasteurella multocida,* plague, hantavirus infection, or tularemia.

In general, fevers of longer duration may be evaluated in a more relaxed fashion. Special attention should be paid to a review of systems because subtle complaints may be uncovered that will help target the physical examination and provide clues to management. The clinician should also assess patient age, length of illness, any underlying diseases, and gross severity. Information concerning immunosuppression

Table 46-1. Common acute febrile diseases that may be nonfocal

| All hosts | Elderly/debilitated hosts |
| --- | --- |
| Viral influenza | Pneumonia |
| Malaria | Genitourinary infection |
| Primary bacteremia (meningococcemia, *Staphylococcus aureus* infection, typhoid fever) *Capnocytophaga* (DF-1) infection | Cholecystitis/cholangitis |
| Rocky mountain spotted fever | Myocardial/pulmonary infarction |
| Occult abscess | Apathetic hyperthyroidism |
| Hypoadrenalism | Drug fever (β-lactams, sulfonamides, procainamide, hydralazine) |
| | Cerebrovascular accident |

should be elicited because selected processes may predispose to potentially life-threatening infections. Examples are splenectomy, neutropenia, infection with HIV, hypogammaglobulinemia, and intake of medications (e.g., corticosteroids) that may alter cell-mediated immunity.

In patients with HIV/AIDS, fever almost always accompanies the acute retroviral syndrome, and otherwise is generally noted as a component of opportunistic disease. In last-stage AIDS, fever may be the manifestation of disseminated infection with *Mycobacterium avium* complex. It is also noted as an adverse effect of certain drugs (e.g., trimethoprim-sulfamethoxazole) and may accompany lymphoma, tuberculosis, or pneumonia caused by *Pneumocystis carinii.*

The presence of foreign bodies, such as joint implants and prosthetic heart valves, should also be noted. A history of rigors is generally sought but does not provide information beyond the fact that the temperature became rapidly elevated; it does not imply a specific etiology.

The physical examination must be comprehensive. Vital signs provide an important initial clue to the severity of illness and may help with the decision of whether to hospitalize. In general, the degree of fever does not correlate with etiology. Nevertheless, fevers above 103°F generally are of more concern and often point to infection. Recent data suggest that for some infections, such as shigellosis, the degree of temperature elevation may correlate with the severity of illness. Adults with fevers above 105.6°F should be hospitalized for fever reduction; temperatures at this level may cause tissue damage. Contrary to the classic dictum, many patients with temperatures at this level have treatable bacterial disease and should be treated empirically with antimicrobials.

Hypothermia is associated with impending sepsis, hypothyroidism, environmental exposure, and diabetes mellitus with autonomic instability. In the hypothermia associated with infection, the systemic vascular resistance is likely to be statistically lower and the cardiac index higher than in the noninfectious conditions already listed.

The respiratory rate is an often overlooked sign. Elderly patients with rates above 25/min often have lower-respiratory infection, even in the absence of initial physical findings. In the setting of community-acquired pneumonia, rates above 30/min are associated with increased mortality. Low or unstable blood pressure may suggest impending septic shock and is an important reason for hospitalization. An elevated pulse is anticipated with temperature elevation. Physiologic elevation is 10 to 15 beats/min per degree rise in temperature.

Temperature-pulse dissociation is associated with beta blockade and intrinsic coronary disease. Infectious causes include viral influenza, Legionnaires' disease, yellow fever, typhoid fever (or less commonly other gram-negative bacteremias), and other viral syndromes. Rash should be sought in all body areas; even if it is subtle, it can provide useful information both etiologically and diagnostically. Careful attention must be paid to physical examination of the mouth, sinuses, and rectum.

### Management

Initial decision making focuses on requirements for hospitalization, empiric or targeted antimicrobial therapy, route of administration if a need for antimicrobials has been determined, and further testing. Hospitalization is indicated primarily for persons who are clinically unstable or believed to be at risk for rapid deterioration. The criteria are best determined for patients with community-acquired pneumonia. Recent studies in patients seen in emergency departments demonstrate that advanced age and leukocytosis (>15,000/mm$^3$) correlate with serious disease and can help determine the need for hospitalization. Other reasons must be individualized; they can include the need for IV antimicrobials or other fluids, rapid evaluation likely to require sophisticated testing, and intense monitoring. Other potential reasons for hospitalization, such as lack of compliance, unfavorable home environment, and uncertain diagnosis, are less likely to be allowable under current reimbursement guidelines. In general, the acutely febrile elderly patient, especially if the fever is associated with underlying disease, is more likely to be infected and to require hospitalization. Similarly, the person with known major alterations of immunity should be hospitalized if significant infection cannot be rapidly ruled out. On the other hand, the younger, fit person is more likely to be treatable as an outpatient.

Table 46-2.  Acute febrile conditions often warranting empiric antimicrobial treatment

| |
| --- |
| Fever >105.6°F |
| Immunosuppression<br>  Neutropenia/granulocytopenia<br>  Asplenia<br>  Hypogammaglobulinemia<br>  Cirrhosis |
| Fever in an elderly patient |
| Unstable vital signs |
| Presence of prosthetic device or foreign body |
| Epidemiologic evidence suggestive of infection<br>  Recent bite<br>  Recent travel |

Management of the febrile patient without an obvious focus of infection will vary depending on the need for hospitalization. Basic laboratory data should be obtained from the hospitalized patient, including CBC count, urinalysis, and (generally) several sets of blood cultures. Decisions regarding other tests (e.g., chest x-ray films, further blood tests, and cultures from sites other than blood) will depend on clinical presentation and subtle clues obtained from the history and physical examination. The urgency of testing depends on the clinical status. Generally, acutely febrile patients, especially those who have high-grade fevers or are unstable, require more intensive evaluation. If hospitalization is not felt to be warranted, testing is generally more limited and based on symptoms and signs.

Antimicrobial needs are determined by the likelihood of treatable infection. Table 46-2 depicts conditions that usually warrant empiric antimicrobial therapy. This management strategy should be reserved for inpatients believed to have either a high probability of treatable infection or of significant adverse outcome if untreated. Antimicrobials should always be initiated after cultures have been obtained from appropriate sites, and the need should be reassessed after several days when more information is returned from the laboratory and clinical response has been evaluated. The choice of empiric antimicrobials is based on presumed site of infection and likely microbe(s) from that site. As an example, *Pseudomonas aeruginosa* is an unlikely pathogen in most patients with community-acquired infection. For most hospitalized patients requiring antimicrobials, therapy is initiated parenterally to ensure uniform absorption and attain high systemic levels quickly.

In febrile patients not sufficiently ill to be hospitalized, especially those with a subacute or chronic onset, antimicrobials should not be overused. Overuse of oral antibiotics for viral infections has been identified as a major problem in the United States, and one that may be associated with emerging antibiotic resistance of common bacteria. Persons with neither focal abnormalities nor significant underlying disease may often be observed. However, all patients should be followed regularly for changes in clinical status that either point to improvement or a more focused process.

The need for further testing is based on the presence of ongoing fever. Although no clear guidelines can be presented, blood tests that determine the CBC count (with differential), liver function, sedimentation rate, antinuclear antibody, and renal function are often warranted. Early in the evaluation, posteroanterior and lateral chest x-ray images should be obtained. The need for other blood, radiographic, microbiologic, and invasive tests for tissue must be individualized. (R.B.B.)

**Bibliography**
Gallagher EJ, Brooks F, Gennis P. Identification of serious illness in febrile adults. *Am J Emerg Med* 1994;12:129–133.
  *The authors conducted a prospective observational study within a cohort of approximately 600 adults who presented to an emergency department with fever above*

*100°F. Serious disease was defined as (a) associated with bacteremia or (b) fatal. Twelve percent of febrile patients met the criteria for serious illness. By regression analysis, only advanced age (50 years or more) and leukocytosis (>15,000/mm³) were associated with serious disease. The authors concluded that approximately one third of adults exhibiting both these parameters will be seriously ill. However, the absence of the two parameters does not preclude serious disease as defined.*

Leibovici L, Cohen O, Wysenbeek AJ. Occult bacterial infection in adults with unexplained fever. *Arch Intern Med* 1990;150:1270–1272.

*This investigation of more than 100 patients admitted to a hospital with unexplained fever depicted a strategy to determine the likelihood of bacterial infection. Patients who were of advanced age, had indwelling urinary catheters, resided in nursing homes, or had elevated WBC counts were more likely to harbor bacterial infection.*

Mackowiak PA, et al. Concepts of fever: recent advances and lingering dogma. *Clin Infect Dis* 1997;25:119–138.

*This round-table discussion on a variety of issues related to fever covers pathogenesis, fever patterns, and fever in the HIV/AIDS population. The authors describe situations likely to be associated with fever and discuss selected tests of value. Fever is most commonly noted during the acute retroviral (mononucleosis-like) syndrome and accompanies many opportunistic processes. Fever is unlikely to resolve spontaneously in advanced disease.*

McFadden JP, et al. Raised respiratory rate in elderly patients: a valuable physical sign. *Br Med J* 1982;284:626–627.

*A normal respiratory rate in elderly patients was 16 to 25/min. Higher rates were noted in those with acute lower respiratory infection. The observation of an increased rate preceded diagnosis. An elevated respiratory rate was not seen in other infections.*

Pinson AG, et al. Fever in the clinical diagnosis of acute pyelonephritis. *Am J Emerg Med* 1997;15:148–151.

*Adult women who had pyuria with or without fever were studied as two groups to determine the presence of acute pyelonephritis. They were further stratified by need for hospitalization. Among both the hospitalized women and those treated as outpatients, the absence of fever predicted alternative diagnoses that included pelvic inflammatory disease and cholecystitis. The authors conclude that fever is associated with pyelonephritis in patients with pyuria.*

Sioson PB, Brown RB. Hyperpyrexia in a large community hospital: etiologies, features, and outcomes. *South Med J* 1993;86:773–776.

*Within a defined population of 39 patients with fever above 105.6°F, potentially treatable bacterial infections were commonly noted. This finding differs from observations reported in earlier literature and has important implications for management. The authors feel that most patients with hyperpyrexia warrant empiric antibiotic therapy pending results of cultures and other assessments for treatable infection.*

---

## 47. FEVER AND PROSTHETIC HEART VALVES

Fever occurring in a patient with a prosthetic heart valve may signal infective endocarditis or numerous other conditions. It is estimated that an infection will develop in 1% to 4% of patients with prosthetic devices during the life span of the device.

In diagnosis, it is helpful to note how long after the operation the fever developed. Any major surgical procedure can be associated with a low-grade fever (100°F or 37.8°C) for a few days. Possibilities during the initial 24-hour period include a transfusion reaction, atelectasis, aspiration pneumonia, or wound infection, especially with group A hemolytic streptococci or *Clostridium* species. Fever developing after the first 24 hours may be caused by an anesthetic. Fever with lymphadenopathy and atypical lymphocytes, called the postperfusion syndrome, usually occurs 2 to 4 weeks after surgery. It is caused by the transfusion of fresh blood with cytomegalovirus or Epstein-Barr virus. Hepatitis C and, rarely, malaria may develop after blood transfusions.

Other infectious complications to consider are phlebitis related to numerous IV lines, infusion of contaminated fluids, drug fever, abscesses secondary to IM injections, bacterial pneumonia, pulmonary infarction, urinary tract infection, wound infection, deep-vein thrombophlebitis, sternal osteomyelitis, and mediastinitis. A syndrome of unknown etiology, the postcardiotomy syndrome, occurs 10 days to 3 months after surgery and is characterized by fever, chest pain, and often a pericardial friction rub. Reactivation of rheumatic fever also may be responsible for fever.

It is important to obtain blood cultures from patients with fever and a prosthetic heart valve. Infective endocarditis occurring within 60 days after valve insertion is called early endocarditis; infection after that time is called late endocarditis. Some authors consider endocarditis as early if it occurs within the first 12 months of surgery and late if it is seen after a year. The source of organisms responsible for early-onset infections may be contamination of the prosthetic valve or bloodstream at the time of operation or an infectious complication developing during the postoperative period, such as a sternal wound infection, pneumonia, or an infected IV line. The same organism can often be isolated from a peripheral site (a wound), sputum, or the blood. The prosthetic valve, like any other foreign body, is at high risk for becoming infected as a consequence of bacteremia. Late-onset infections may be caused by a transient bacteremia associated with either a dental, skin, or genitourinary tract procedure or an infection. Other organisms responsible for late-onset infections may be acquired at the time of operation and have a long incubation period.

The organisms causing prosthetic valve infections differ from those producing classic endocarditis. Certain bacteria, such as diphtheroids and, especially, coagulase-negative staphylococci, usually considered blood culture contaminants, account for about one third of all infections in these patients. Of the early-onset cases, half are caused by *Staphylococcus aureus* or *Staphylococcus epidermidis,* 20% are caused by gram-negative bacilli, and 10% are produced by fungi such as *Candida* or, rarely, *Aspergillus*. The major causative organisms of late-onset infections are streptococci (36%), staphylococci (38%), gram-negative bacilli (10%), and other pathogens (10%). However, any organism can infect a prosthetic valve, and when blood cultures are positive for unusual pathogens or so-called nonpathogens, these should not be dismissed as contaminants. Approximately 5% to 10% of patients have culture-negative endocarditis.

The clinical features of early-onset infections are often dominated by other, concomitant infectious complications, such as pneumonia, wound infection, suppurative phlebitis, or urinary tract infection. Symptoms and signs include fever (90% to 100%), new insufficiency murmurs (60%), splenomegaly (20%), and shock (33%). The presence of petechiae, hematuria, or anemia is difficult to interpret during the early postoperative period, as these conditions may relate to the operation. A more fulminant clinical course often occurs in patients with early-onset prosthetic valve endocarditis (PVE). The manifestations of late-onset infection caused by streptococci are similar to those in patients without a prosthetic heart valve. Fever, a new aortic or mitral insufficiency murmur, splenomegaly, anemia, and peripheral stigmata such as petechiae and splinter hemorrhages are often present in late-onset infections.

Sustained bacteremia is characteristic of endocarditis, and blood cultures are positive in 95% of patients with prosthetic valve infections. Blood cultures may be negative in patients with *Candida* or *Aspergillus* endocarditis. Emboli occluding major arteries are common in fungal endocarditis. Culture and histologic examination of the clot may be useful for establishing the cause. Fastidious microorganisms such as members of the HACEK group (*Haemophilus, Actinobacillus, Cardiobacterium, Eikenella, Kingella*) and *Legionella* should be considered. Noninvasive cardiac procedures such as transesophageal echocardiography, cinefluoroscopy, and electrocardiography may be helpful. Cardiac cinefluoroscopy, although used less often now than in the past, may show an abnormal rocking motion of the prosthesis. A new murmur of aortic insufficiency or large vegetations on a valve may be detected on an echocardiogram. Selective cardiac catheterization with quantitative blood cultures may be useful for determining the site of infection if the patient has more than one prosthetic valve.

A diagnostic dilemma occurs in the interpretation of positive blood cultures during the postoperative period. Although the presence of a sustained bacteremia may indicate bacterial endocarditis, it is important not to assume that the positive blood cultures confirm the diagnosis of endocarditis. Other criteria that help to establish the diagnosis are the presence of a new or changing heart murmur or of embolic phenomena, and the absence of an extracardiac source for the bacteremia. However, no criterion will absolutely distinguish bacterial endocarditis from a sustained bacteremia without endocarditis. If the blood cultures are positive during this period, remove the IV and arterial lines, drain any focus of pus, and begin antimicrobials. If during the next 2 to 3 weeks no new murmur develops, the peripheral stigmata of endocarditis are absent, and the repeated blood cultures are sterile, discontinue therapy. If a new murmur develops, peripheral manifestations of endocarditis appear, or the blood cultures remain positive after the source has been eliminated, continue therapy for 4 to 6 weeks.

A bactericidal antimicrobial given in high doses parenterally is the cornerstone of therapy for prosthetic valve infections. Peak serum bactericidal levels should be present at a dilution of at least 1:8. Commonly accepted indications for surgery along with high-dose antimicrobial agents include a significant valvular leak or congestive heart failure, or both; persistent or recurrent bacteremia after 1 to 2 weeks of optimal treatment; multiple peripheral emboli; new-onset conduction abnormalities; and endocarditis caused by fungi. Recurrent emboli are a controversial indication for surgery. Surgery combined with antimicrobials may be indicated for infections caused by *S. aureus* and *S. epidermidis,* as well as for early-onset prosthetic valve infections caused by gram-negative bacilli. Late-onset infections caused by streptococci usually respond to antimicrobial therapy alone and do not require valve replacement.

The mortality in early-onset infection is 60% to 80%, and in late-onset endocarditis it is 40%. Congestive heart failure secondary to valve dehiscence or myocardial abscesses and cerebral arterial emboli are the leading causes of death. Because the effects of a prosthetic valve infection can be devastating, prevention is important. A prophylactic antistaphylococcal agent should be administered just before operation and during the perioperative period while the long lines are present (usually for 2 to 3 days postoperatively). Prophylaxis is indicated as well for procedures associated with transient bacteremias, such as dental work, genitourinary manipulations, or any surgery through a contaminated area. Antimicrobial prophylaxis for other procedures, such as sigmoidoscopy or gastrointestinal roentgenography, is controversial. (N.M.G.)

## Bibliography

Alsip SG, et al. Indications for cardiac surgery in patients with infective endocarditis. *Am J Med* 1985;78(Suppl 6B):138.
*Use a point system to determine the need for surgery. Surgery is indicated for moderate-to-severe heart failure, fungal etiology, persistent bacteremia, or unstable prosthesis.*
Blumberg EA, et al. Persistent fever in association with infective endocarditis. *Clin Infect Dis* 1992;15:983.
*Causes of fever in patients with endocarditis and persistent fever included myocardial abscess (27%), drug fever (19%), other nosocomial infections (19%), persistent infection (24%), other (8%), and unknown (15%).*
Calderwood SD. Risk factors for the development of prosthetic valve endocarditis. *Circulation* 1985;72:31.
*One third of the cases had an early onset, and two thirds occurred late.*
Chen TT, Schapiro JM, Loutit J. Prosthetic valve endocarditis due to *Legionella pneumophila. J Cardiovasc Surg* 1996;37:631–633.
*A rare cause of culture-negative endocarditis.*
Conte JE, et al. Antibiotic prophylaxis and cardiac surgery. *Ann Intern Med* 1972; 76:943.
*Compared a single dose of intraoperative cephalothin with preoperative plus intraoperative and postoperative cephalothin. There was no difference in infection rates.*
Daniel WG, et al. Improvement in the diagnosis of abscesses associated with endocarditis by transesophageal echocardiography. *N Engl J Med* 1991;324:795.
*The transesophageal approach was superior to transthoracic echocardiography, but a negative study result does not exclude a complication in a patient with a prosthetic valve.*
Dismukes WE, et al. Prosthetic valve endocarditis: analysis of 38 cases. *Circulation* 1973;48:365.

*Staphylococci (both* S. aureus *and* S. epidermidis*) are the most common organisms causing early-onset infections; streptococci are the leading causes among late-onset cases.*

Douglas JL, Cobbs CG. Prosthetic valve endocarditis. In: Kaye D, ed. *Infective endocarditis,* 2nd ed. New York: Raven Press, 1992.
*A review emphasizing an approach to diagnosis and management.*

Durack DT, Lukes AS, Bright DK, Duke Endocarditis Service. New criteria for diagnosis of infective endocarditis: utilization of specific echocardiographic findings. *Am J Med* 1994;96:200–209.
*Criteria to improve accuracy of diagnosis.*

Everett ED, Hirschmann JV. Transient bacteremia and endocarditis prophylaxis. A review. *Medicine (Baltimore)* 1977;56:61.
*An extensive review of the incidence of and organisms associated with bacteremia secondary to various procedures or manipulations. The authors favor prophylactic antimicrobials for patients with prosthetic valves who undergo dental procedures, urologic manipulations, upper gastrointestinal endoscopy, sigmoidoscopy, liver biopsy, or barium enema.*

Fang G, et al. Bacteremia in patients with prosthetic cardiac valves. *Ann Intern Med* 1993;119:560.
*The most frequent source of bacteremia for a patient with nosocomial endocarditis was an intravascular catheter, wound, or skin infection.*

Giladi M, et al. Microbiological cultures of heart valves and valve tags are not valuable for patients without infective endocarditis who are undergoing valve replacement. *Clin Infect Dis* 1997;24:884–888.
*When endocarditis is not suspected, cultures of heart valves or prosthetic valve tags are not indicated.*

John MDV, et al. *Staphylococcus aureus* prosthetic valve endocarditis: optimal management and risk factors for death. *Clin Infect Dis* 1998;26:1302–1309.
*In patients with* S. aureus *infection, valve replacement during the treatment of infection was associated with reduced mortality.*

Karchmer AW, Archer GL, Dismukes WE. *Staphylococcus epidermidis* causing prosthetic valve endocarditis: microbiologic and clinical observations as guides to therapy. *Ann Intern Med* 1983;98:447.
*Most (87%) isolates of* S. epidermidis *were methicillin-resistant. Therapy of choice consists of vancomycin, plus rifampin with or without an aminoglycoside.*

Karchmer AW, Gibbons GW. Infections of prosthetic heart valves and vascular grafts. In: Bisno AL, Waldvogel FA, eds. *Infections associated with indwelling medical devices,* 2nd ed. Washington, DC: American Society for Microbiology, 1994:213–249.
*Review.*

Karchmer AW, et al. Late prosthetic valve endocarditis. Clinical features influencing therapy. *Am J Med* 1978;64:199.
*The occurrence of any two of three features (nonstreptococcal etiology, a new regurgitant murmur, and moderate-to-severe congestive heart failure) carried a high mortality. Surgery should be strongly considered.*

Kluge RM, et al. Sources of contamination in open heart surgery. *JAMA* 1974;230:1415.
*A variety of organisms, including diphtheroids and* S. epidermidis, *were frequently (71%) isolated in cultures obtained from the operative sites.*

Lytle BW, et al. Surgery for acquired heart disease. Surgical treatment of prosthetic valve endocarditis. *J Thorac Cardiovasc Surg* 1996;111:198–210.
*The risk for PVE is about 3% after the first year and 1% per year thereafter. Mortality with surgery for PVE has declined, with a survival rate of 82% at 5 years and 60% at 10 postoperative years.*

Mayer KH, Schoenbaum SC. Evaluation and management of prosthetic valve endocarditis. *Prog Cardiovasc Dis* 1982;25:43.
*Early surgical intervention is recommended in most cases of PVE, except for late-onset streptococcal disease.*

Melgar GR, et al. Fungal prosthetic valve endocarditis in 16 patients. *Medicine* 1997; 76:94–103.
*Amphotericin B plus surgery resulted in a 67% survival rate, but relapse may occur that requires long-term suppression therapy.*

Meyer DJ, Gerding DN. Favorable prognosis of patients with prosthetic valve endocarditis caused by gram-negative bacilli of the HACEK group. *Am J Med* 1988;85:104.
*A group of fastidious gram-negative rods that includes* Haemophilus *species,* Actinobacillus actinomycetemcomitans, Cardiobacterium hominis, Eikenella corrodens,
*and* Kingella *species.*

Mugge A, et al. Echocardiography in infective endocarditis: reassessment of prognostic implications of vegetation size determined by the transthoracic and transesophageal approach. *J Am Coll Cardiol* 1989;14:631.
*Vegetations were detected in 86% of patients by means of transesophageal echocar-
diography, compared with only 36% by the transthoracic technique.*

Mullany CJ, et al. Early and late survival after surgical treatment of culture-positive
active endocarditis. *Mayo Clin Proc* 1995;70:517–525.
*Overall mortality was 26%. A higher mortality was seen in patients with an abscess
at surgery (40%) and with an increased serum creatinine (40%).*

Nasser RM, et al. Incidence and risk of developing fungal prosthetic valve endocarditis after nosocomial candidemia. *Am J Med* 1997;103:25–32.
*Among patients with candidemia and a prosthetic heart valve, evidence of PVE never
developed in 75%, 16% had endocarditis at the time of the fungemia, and 9% had a
late onset of endocarditis.*

Nettles RE, et al. An evaluation of the Duke criteria in 25 pathologically confirmed
cases of prosthetic valve endocarditis. *Clin Infect Dis* 1997;25:1401–1403.
*The Duke diagnostic criteria had a sensitivity of 76% in cases of endocarditis that
were confirmed pathologically.*

Nguyen MH, et al. *Candida* prosthetic valve endocarditis: prospective study of six
cases and review of the literature. *Clin Infect Dis* 1996;22:262–267.
*In patients unable to tolerate surgery, antifungal therapy followed by chronic sup-
pression may be effective (46%).*

Pazin GJ, et al. Determination of site of infection in endocarditis. *Ann Intern Med* 1975;
82:746.
*Quantitative blood cultures from various cardiac chambers may indicate the site of
infection.*

Sande MA, et al. Sustained bacteremia in patients with prosthetic cardiac valves.
*N Engl J Med* 1972;286:1067.
*Discusses the diagnostic dilemma of sustained bacteremia without endocarditis ver-
sus endocarditis.*

Schulz R, et al. Clinical outcome and echocardiographic findings of native and prosthetic valve endocarditis in the 1990s. *Eur Heart J* 1996;17:281–288.
*Vegetations were detected by transesophageal echocardiography in 80% of episodes
of PVE. This finding compares with a yield of only 15% for transthoracic echocardiography.*

Tornos P, et al. Clinical outcome and long-term prognosis of late prosthetic valve endocarditis: a 20-year experience. *Clin Infect Dis* 1997;24:381–386.
Staphylococcus aureus *infection had a mortality rate of 67%; streptococcal infection,
6%; other causes, 23%.*

Weinstein L, Rubin RH. Infective endocarditis 1973. *Prog Cardiovasc Dis* 1973;16:239.
*Review.*

Wilson WR, et al. Prosthetic valve endocarditis. *Ann Intern Med* 1975;82:751.
*The incidence of prosthetic valve infections was low. In this series, most infections
occurred more than 2 months after surgery.*

Wilson WR, et al. Antibiotic treatment of adults with infective endocarditis due to
streptococci, enterococci, staphylococci, and HACEK microorganisms. *JAMA* 1995;
274:1706–1713.
*Guidelines for therapy.*

Wolff M, et al. Prosthetic valve endocarditis in the ICU. Prognostic factors of overall
survival in a series of 122 cases and consequences for treatment decision. *Chest*
1995;108:688–694.
*In patients with* S. aureus *PVE, survival was higher (45%) in those who received
medical-surgical therapy compared with only antibiotics (0).*

## 48. PROLONGED FEVER AND GENERALIZED LYMPHADENOPATHY

Prolonged fever with generalized lymphadenopathy is a symptom complex common to many different disease entities. Distinct categories of illness, such as infection, malignancy, rheumatologic disorders, and drug hypersensitivity, may all present with fever and lymph node enlargement.

Initial evaluation of the patient will require a detailed history. Clinical clues may be found in the symptoms themselves, an epidemiology system review, or the social or occupational history. Fungal diseases such as histoplasmosis and coccidioidomycosis may be suggested by exposure history and geographic setting. A history of contact with sheep, or employment in a slaughterhouse, or drinking unpasteurized milk requires that brucellosis be considered. Contact with ticks or rodents suggests the possibility of tularemia. Contact with cats might be a clue to cat scratch disease or toxoplasmosis. The patient should be asked about exposure to tuberculosis or travel to areas where trypanosomal or leishmanial organisms are endemic. A detailed history of sexual activities and risk factors for AIDS needs to be obtained. Secondary syphilis and lymphogranuloma venereum can also cause fever and diffuse lymphadenopathy. Symptoms of joint pain and rash and other manifestations of connective tissue diseases must also be assessed. Drugs such as phenytoin, carbamazepine, and paraaminosalicylic acid can cause fever and lymphadenopathy.

On physical examination, it must be determined whether lymph node enlargement is localized or generalized. Localized adenopathy in the neck suggests pharyngitis or intraoral infection. Careful examination of the face, ears, throat, and mouth will follow. Hodgkin's disease may present as cervical adenopathy. Enlarged posterior cervical nodes may be caused by scalp infection or systemic disease, such as toxoplasmosis. If axillary adenopathy is the finding, examination of the breast and arms is most important. Cat scratch fever, staphylococcal and streptococcal infection, sporotrichosis, and lymphoma can cause isolated axillary adenopathy. Isolated inguinal adenopathy is not uncommon in the general population but may be caused by infections of the genitalia or perineum.

Generalized adenopathy, particularly when accompanied by night sweats and weight loss, should suggest the diagnosis of AIDS in any high-risk patient. Lymphoma may present as generalized adenopathy, but only at an advanced stage. As noted, many infectious processes, including infectious mononucleosis, toxoplasmosis, and cat scratch fever, present with generalized lymphadenopathy.

The laboratory evaluation of fever and generalized adenopathy proceeds according to clinical clues. All patients should have a CBC count, with review of a blood smear for atypical lymphocytes and other abnormal cells. If the patient appears toxic, blood cultures should be obtained to rule out subacute endocarditis, tularemia, or brucellosis. A serologic test for Epstein-Barr virus (EBV), Venereal Disease Research Laboratory (VDRL) test for syphilis, IgM determination for toxoplasmosis, and HIV serology for AIDS will be indicated. A complement fixation test for cytomegalovirus (CMV) should be drawn, and titers greater than 128 are suggestive of infection with this agent. Some authors have recommended that EBV, HIV, and CMV infection and toxoplasmosis be ruled out first, with the investigation then proceeding to diseases caused by other agents. Agglutinin tests for brucellosis and tularemia and serology for histoplasmosis and coccidioidomycosis are obtained based on the index of suspicion for these processes. Antinuclear antibody and rheumatoid factors may be supportive of a diagnosis of systemic lupus erythematosus or Still's disease. A chest x-ray film showing hilar adenopathy will require evaluation for tuberculosis, sarcoidosis, or lymphoma.

Definitive diagnosis may require lymph node biopsy. Slap et al. studied 123 young patients who had undergone biopsy of enlarged peripheral lymph nodes. In 42% of the cases, biopsy results led to specific treatment. Patients found to have granuloma or tumor were more likely to have abnormal findings on chest x-ray films, lymph node greater than 2 cm in diameter, a history of night sweats or weight loss, and a hemoglobin level of less than 10 g/dL. Patients with a recent history of ear, nose, and throat symptoms were less likely to have a biopsy result that led to specific therapy.

When a lymph node biopsy is performed in a patient with generalized adenopathy, the node should be selected with care. Excisional biopsy is generally preferred; however, for fluctuant nodes, needle aspiration may be sufficient for diagnosis. Inguinal nodes should be avoided for biopsy because they frequently show nonspecific reactive hyperplasia. Supraclavicular nodes and scalene nodes have the highest yield. The node itself should be divided between the pathology and microbiology laboratories.

About 20% of patients in one series were given a specific diagnosis based on the results of subsequent biopsy. In patients subsequently found to have lymphoma, 90% had a diagnosis made within 8 months of the first biopsy. When a definitive diagnosis cannot be made by biopsy, careful follow-up is required. If the patient is anemic, bone marrow biopsy may be considered. If the patient has an associated hepatitis, liver biopsy is indicated.

Several processes that cause both fever and generalized adenopathy have become better defined:

1. Angioimmunoblastic lymphadenopathy is characterized by fever, hepatosplenomegaly, polyclonal hypergammaglobulinemia, and Coombs-positive hemolytic anemia. It frequently evolves into malignant lymphoma. The disease may cause a false-positive result on HIV serology by enzyme-linked immunosorbent assay (ELISA).

2. The etiologic agents in cat scratch disease are now well defined. In 1983, a small pleomorphic bacterium was demonstrated in sections of a lymph node by Warthin-Starry stain. In 1988, a gram-negative bacterium and cell wall variants were isolated from lymph nodes of 10 patients. Two organisms have now been cultured from lymph nodes of infected patients. They are *Bartonella henselae* (formerly *Rochalimaea henselae*) and *Afipia felis*. Both are members of the class of Proteobacteria.

3. Bacillary angiomatosis is an opportunistic infection seen most frequently in AIDS patients, although immunocompetent patients have also been afflicted. The disease usually presents with angiomatous skin lesions, but fever and lymphadenopathy may be presenting signs. Organisms have been identified in tissue by the Warthin-Starry method. *Bartonella quintana* and *B. henselae* can be grown from skin lesions, and patients have serologic evidence of *Bartonella* infection.

4. Whipple's disease usually presents with steatorrhea, weight loss, and abdominal pain; however, fever and lymphadenopathy may be the most prominent presenting features. Relman et al. found the organism to be a gram-positive actinomycete, which was named *Tropheryma whippelii*. Trimethoprim-sulfamethoxazole has been shown to be superior to tetracycline in inducing clinical remission.

5. The definitive diagnosis of sarcoidosis continues to be difficult. Lymph node biopsy will show granuloma with whorls of epithelioid cells surrounding multinucleated giant cells. True caseation is unusual. The Kveim-Siltzbach reaction is rarely used because it lacks precision; standardization and antigen are not readily available. Serum angiotensin I-converting enzyme is elevated in about 70% of all cases. The enzyme may be elevated in tuberculosis and leprosy but not in lymphoma. Other tests, such as lysozyme and metalloendopeptidase, are promising but not in routine use for diagnosis of sarcoid. Scanning of lung or parotid gland with gallium 67 may be useful in detecting unsuspected organ involvement in the patient who presents with fever and generalized lymphadenopathy. (S.L.B.)

### Bibliography

Alkan S, et al. Dual role for *Afipia felis* and *Rochalimaea henselae* in cat scratch disease. *Lancet* 1995;345:385.
  *The authors isolated both* B. henselae *and* A. felis *from the lymph nodes of patients with cat scratch disease.*
Bujak JS, et al. Juvenile rheumatoid arthritis presenting in the adult as fever of unknown origin. *Medicine (Baltimore)* 1973;52:431.
  *Generalized significant lymphadenopathy may occur in febrile adults with Still's disease (juvenile rheumatoid arthritis).*
Case records of the Massachusetts General Hospital. Weekly clinicopathological exercises. Case 30-1977. *N Engl J Med* 1977;297:206.

*A discussion of the pathology of Hodgkin's disease, toxoplasmosis, angioimmunoblastic lymphadenopathy, and Lennert's lesion.*

De Vriese AS, et al. Carbamazepine hypersensitivity syndrome: report of four cases and review of the literature. *Medicine* 1995;74:144.

*A syndrome of fever, rash, and lymphadenopathy occurs between 1 week and 3 months after the drug is taken. A patch test and lymphocyte transformation tests have been used to confirm the diagnosis.*

English CK, et al. Cat-scratch disease: isolation and culture of the bacterial agent. *JAMA* 1988;259:1347.

*A gram-negative organism was isolated from the lymph nodes of 10 patients with cat scratch disease.*

Feurle GE, Marth T. An evaluation of antimicrobial therapy for Whipple's disease. Tetracycline vs. trimethoprim-sulfamethoxazole. *Dig Dis Sci* 1994;39:1643.

*In a retrospective study, trimethoprim-sulfamethoxazole was better than tetracycline in inducing remission and treating central nervous system disease.*

Greenfield S, Jordan MC. The clinical investigation of lymphadenopathy in primary care practice. *JAMA* 1978;240:1388.

*Provides an algorithm for the investigation of lymphadenopathy. Recommends serology for toxoplasmosis, EBV, and CMV before extensive workup.*

Holmes GP, et al. A cluster of patients with a chronic mononucleosis-like syndrome: is Epstein-Barr virus the cause? *JAMA* 1987;257:2297.

*Describes an outbreak of 134 cases of fever, lymphadenopathy, and fatigue. The relationship of symptoms to EBV was unclear.*

Horwitz CA, et al. Heterophil-negative infectious mononucleosis and mononucleosis-like illnesses. *Am J Med* 1977;63:947.

*A diagnosis of mononucleosis-like syndrome was made in 43 patients. Thirty cases were caused by CMV based on serology findings.*

Koehler JE, et al. Isolation of *Rochalimaea* species from cutaneous and osseous lesions of bacillary angiomatosis. *N Engl J Med* 1992;327:1625.

*B. henselae and B. quintana were cultured directly from skin lesions of patients with bacillary angiomatosis. Originally named Rochimalaea, the organism was transferred to the genus Bartonella a year later.*

Montoya JG, Remington JS. Studies on the serodiagnosis of toxoplasmic lymphadenitis. *Clin Infect Dis* 1995;20:781.

*Compares the newer serologic tests with traditional tests in the diagnosis of toxoplasmic lymphadenopathy. The ELISA result was positive for IgM antibodies in the first 3 months of illness.*

Relman DA, et al. Identification of the uncultured bacillus of Whipple's disease. *N Engl J Med* 1992;327:293.

*T. whippelii is described as the etiologic agent of Whipple's disease, which can present as generalized adenopathy.*

Rosenfeld S, et al. Syndrome simulating lymphosarcoma induced by diphenylhydantoin sodium. *JAMA* 1961;176:491.

*A syndrome consisting of fever, joint swelling, facial edema, generalized aches and pains, and adenopathy was associated with phenytoin sodium therapy.*

Saltzstein SL, Ackerman IV. Lymphadenopathy induced by anticonvulsant drugs and mimicking clinically and pathologically malignant lymphomas. *Cancer* 1959;12:164.

*Phenytoin may cause prolonged fever and lymphadenopathy.*

Schroer KR, Fransilla KO. Atypical hyperplasia of lymph nodes. A follow-up study. *Cancer* 1979;44:1155.

*Results of some biopsies were nondiagnostic in patients later found to have lymphoma.*

Sinclair S, Beckman E, Ellman L. Biopsy of enlarged superficial lymph nodes. *JAMA* 1974;228:602.

*Thirty-seven percent of patients had lymphoma, 10% had carcinoma, and 5% had tuberculosis.*

Slap GB, Brooks JSJ, Schwartz JS. When to perform biopsies of enlarged peripheral lymph nodes in young patients. *JAMA* 1984;252:1321.

*Reviews records of 123 young patients to determine which had biopsy results that led to specific therapy. Those with abnormal findings on chest x-ray films, a node greater than 2 cm, night sweats, or weight loss benefited from biopsy diagnosis.*

Straus SE. The chronic mononucleosis syndrome. *J Infect Dis* 1988;157:405.
*Excellent review of EBV as a cause of chronic symptomatology.*

Wear DJ, et al. Cat scratch disease: a bacterial infection. *Science* 1983;221:1403.
*Demonstration of organisms in lymph node biopsy by Warthin-Starry stain.*

Weinstein L, Weinstein AJ. The pathophysiology and pathoanatomy of reactions to antimicrobial agents. *Adv Intern Med* 1974;19:109.
*A clinical picture resembling infectious mononucleosis (sore throat, generalized lymphadenopathy, splenomegaly, lymphocytosis, and the presence of cells resembling typical Downey cells) is an uncommon manifestation of an allergic response to paraaminosalicylic acid.*

Wilson KH, et al. Phylogeny of the Whipple's disease-associated bacterium. *Lancet* 1991;338:474.
*Intracellular organisms of Whipple's disease were studied by polymerase chain reaction. The organism was similar to* Rhodococcus *species and weakly related to* mycobacteria.

Wood TA, Frenkel EP. The atypical lymphocyte. *Am J Med* 1967;42:923.
*A syndrome that resembles infectious mononucleosis is produced by paraaminosalicylate; it usually occurs 3 to 6 weeks after therapy starts.*

## 49. FEVER AND SKIN RASH

The acutely ill, febrile patient with a generalized skin rash presents a diagnostic challenge; the list of disorders in the differential diagnosis is extensive and includes both infectious and noninfectious causes. The skin is capable of reacting only in a limited way, and disease may be manifested by macules or papules; vesicles, bullae, or pustules; or purpuric macules, papules, or vesicles. The clinical features of the various disorders causing a skin rash are similar, and one infection may readily mimic another. Misdiagnosis and delay in starting specific therapy can be disastrous in patients with Rocky Mountain spotted fever, toxic shock syndrome (TSS), or meningococcal or staphylococcal bacteremia. It is critical to make a presumptive etiologic diagnosis rapidly and identify treatable infections for which immediate therapy is required to prevent death.

### Diagnostic Procedures

Certain diagnostic procedures can be used to obtain a diagnosis in the acutely ill, febrile patient with a rash. Skin lesions can be aspirated, and the material obtained should be examined with Gram's stain. Gram-positive organisms in clusters are staphylococci, and gram-negative diplococci are either meningococci or gonococci. Organisms can sometimes be seen by Gram's-staining a smear of the buffy coat. Meningococci can also be identified by latex particle agglutination tests of the serum, cerebrospinal fluid, or other body fluids. A Tzanck preparation is useful in the diagnosis of a number of vesiculobullous disorders. This test consists of several steps: (a) selecting an intact vesicle, (b) swabbing the lesion with 70% isopropyl alcohol, (c) opening the vesicle with a scalpel blade, (d) scraping the base very gently to avoid bleeding, (e) placing the specimen on a glass slide, and (f) staining it with Giemsa or Wright's stain. Multinucleated, syncytial giant cells are present with varicella-zoster viral infection and herpes simplex but are absent in vaccinia and variola. A dark-field examination of material from a mucous membrane or skin lesion may reveal spirochetes. A cutaneous biopsy can be helpful in identifying rickettsiae; it provides material for an immunofluorescence technique that produces results before the results of serologic tests are positive. A vasculitis secondary to a noninfectious cause can also be identified by a cutaneous punch biopsy. Acute serum (at the time of presentation and 2 weeks later) should be drawn and frozen for various serologic tests. In addition, several sets of blood cultures are prepared, as well as cultures of throat, urine, and other tissues and fluids as indicated. Table 49-1 lists some of the conditions in which fever and a generalized rash may be prominent symptoms.

## Toxic Shock Syndrome

In 1978, an illness was described in seven children ages 8 to 17 years. It was characterized by high fever, generalized erythroderma, hypotension, and conjunctival hyperemia, with involvement of the kidneys, liver, and gastrointestinal system. This disease was called toxic shock syndrome (TSS) and was attributed to toxins produced by *Staphylococcus aureus*. The illness was similar to staphylococcal scarlet fever, which had been described in 1927. Not until late in 1979 and 1980, however, did the syndrome attract widespread attention when studies demonstrated a statistically significant association between use of tampons and the development of TSS. The peak incidence to date occurred in August 1980, when 135 cases were reported to the Centers for Disease Control (CDC). The number of new cases reported to the CDC has declined to approximately 20 per month. The majority of cases are nonmenstrual and occur in patients with staphylococcal infections associated with wounds, vaginal delivery, or cesarean section. In addition to patients with staphylococcal skin and soft-tissue infections, patients with primary staphylococcal bacteremia are at risk for TSS. Rarely, cases are associated with the use of vaginal contraceptive diaphragms.

Table 49-1.  Conditions in which rash and fever are prominent

| Type of lesion | Microbial agents and related diseases |
| --- | --- |
| Maculopapular lesions | Viruses: measles, rubeola, rubella, enterovirus (echovirus, coxsackievirus), arbovirus, infectious hepatitis, infectious mononucleosis (cytomegalovirus, Epstein-Barr virus), human herpesvirus 6, parvovirus B19, HIV |
| | Bacteria: scarlet fever, typhoid fever, secondary syphilis, rat-bite fever, leptospirosis, erysipeloid, toxic shock syndrome, Lyme disease, ehrlichiosis |
| | Rickettsiae: Rocky Mountain spotted fever (early), murine (endemic) typhus, scrub typhus |
| | Other: drug reactions, pityriasis rosea, collagen diseases (e.g., systemic lupus erythematosus), toxoplasmosis, trichinosis, rheumatic fever, mucocutaneous lymph node syndrome, acute graft-versus-host disease |
| Vesicles, bullae, or pustules | Viruses: varicella, herpes zoster, herpes simplex, variola, enterovirus (coxsackievirus), smallpox, monkey pox |
| | Bacteria: toxic epidermal necrolysis, impetigo |
| | Other: drug reactions, erythema multiforme, rickettsial pox |
| Petechial or purpuric lesions | Viruses: atypical measles |
| | Bacteria: bacteremia (meningococcal, gonococcal, streptococcal, or staphylococcal) |
| | Rickettsiae: Rocky Mountain spotted fever, epidemic typhus |
| | Other: drug reactions, allergic vasculitis, malaria |

*Diagnosis*

The diagnosis of TSS still requires use of the CDC case definition because no laboratory test has been developed to confirm the diagnosis. The initial CDC case definition has been modified to include orthostatic dizziness as evidence of hypotension and staphylococcal bacteremia. *S. aureus* isolated from patients with TSS can be studied for the production of toxic shock syndrome toxin 1 (TSST-1) and staphylococcal enterotoxins A and B. The absence of antibody to the toxin indicates susceptibility to the development of TSS. These toxins appear to activate T cells, resulting in the production of macrophage-derived mediators such as interleukin-1 and tumor necrosis factor, which cause shock-like symptoms. The toxins interact with cells of the immune system and act as superantigens.

The diagnosis of TSS should be considered in any patient, particularly a postoperative or postpartum patient, and any menstruating woman who has unexplained fever, hypotension, and a diffuse rash resembling sunburn. Initially, the rash may be absent in patients with hypotension and may appear only after fluid replacement, or it may go unnoticed or be attributed to the flush of fever. The surgical wound infection often appears clinically trivial, and the patient may be discharged from the hospital before the onset of toxic shock symptoms. The menstrually related disease typically begins abruptly during the menstrual period. Sore throat or vomiting and diarrhea may be prominent complaints and suggest other diagnoses, such as group A streptococcal pharyngitis or gastrointestinal infection.

Criteria to establish a diagnosis of TSS are listed in Table 49-2. Neurologic examination usually reveals a confused, disoriented patient without focal symptoms. Until a specific laboratory test is developed, cases of mild toxic shock are excluded by the strict case definition. A vaginal examination should be performed to remove any tampon and obtain cultures for *S. aureus*. Normally, 10% of women have vaginal cultures

Table 49-2. Case criteria for toxic shock syndrome

Fever: temperature >38.9°C (102°F)

Rash: diffuse macular erythroderma; desquamation 1 to 2 weeks after onset of illness, particularly of palms and soles

Hypotension: systolic blood pressure <90 mm Hg for adults or below fifth percentile by age for children less than 16 years of age; orthostatic drop in diastolic blood pressure >15 mm Hg from lying to sitting; orthostatic syncope or orthostatic dizziness

Multisystem involvement with three or more of the following:

Gastrointestinal: vomiting or diarrhea at onset of illness

Muscular: severe myalgia or creatine phosphokinase level at least twice the upper limit of normal

Mucous membrane: vaginal, oropharyngeal, or conjunctival hyperemia

Renal: blood urea nitrogen (BUN) or creatinine level at least twice the upper limit of normal, or urinary sediment with pyuria (>5 leukocytes per high-power field) in the absence of urinary tract infection

Hepatic: total bilirubin, SGOT, SGPT levels twice the upper limit of normal

Hematologic: platelets <100,000/μL

Central nervous system: disorientation or alteration in consciousness without focal neurologic signs when fever and hypotension are absent

Negative results for the following tests, if performed:

Blood, throat, or cerebrospinal fluid cultures (blood culture may be positive for *Staphylococcus aureus*)

Rise in titer in Rocky Mountain spotted fever, leptospirosis, or rubeola

SGOT, serum aspartate transaminase; SGPT, serum alanine transaminase.

positive for *S. aureus,* but 98% of vaginal cultures are positive in patients with menstrually associated TSS.

*Treatment*
Acute management of a patient with TSS requires aggressive treatment for shock with massive IV fluids (up to 12 L/d) and vasopressors to maintain blood pressure and renal output. In a retrospective study, use of high-dose corticosteroids for 3 days reduced the severity of illness and duration of fever if they were administered within 2 to 3 days of TSS onset, but there was no difference in mortality. High doses (400 mg/kg) of IV immune globulin given as a single dose may be useful, as high levels of TSST-1 antibody are present in commercial sera. Immune globulin is preferred to corticosteroids. A β-lactamase-resistant penicillin such as nafcillin should be administered to eradicate staphylococci and lessen the chance of recurrence. Rifampin, which may be useful to eradicate the staphylococcal carrier state, is given in combination with nafcillin or dicloxacillin if nafcillin administration alone fails to eliminate the organism. The recurrence rate is 2% to 30%, depending on the study and criteria for TSS. The case-fatality rate is about 5%. Women who have had TSS should not resume using tampons until more is known about the disease. Recurrent disease is more common with menstrual than nonmenstrual cases.

Numerous reports have described a life-threatening illness caused by group A streptococci that mimics TSS. Several streptococcal exotoxins (including streptococcal pyrogenic exotoxins A, B, and C) activate T cells, resulting in the production of various cytokines, such as tumor necrosis factor and interleukin-6. Various clinical manifestations include bacteremia, hypotension, pneumonia, myositis, and fasciitis. Patients may have renal failure, adult respiratory distress syndrome, and delirium or confusion; they lack the typical rash of scarlet fever or staphylococcal TSS. Petechial or maculopapular rashes may occur. Penicillin is the drug of choice, and clindamycin should be used in the penicillin-allergic patient.

## Rocky Mountain Spotted Fever
*Diagnosis*
Several life-threatening illnesses are included in the differential diagnosis of patients with fever and a petechial or purpuric rash. Rocky Mountain spotted fever should be suspected in any patient living where this disease is endemic. A seasonal variation—most cases are seen from April to October—corresponds to the tick season and recreational exposure. In states with a warmer climate, the disease can occur throughout the year. The history of a tick bite can be elicited in about 75% of patients. The incubation period is 3 to 12 days. The illness begins with a nonspecific syndrome of headache, malaise, myalgias, and fever. The rash, which is the most characteristic feature, is usually delayed until the fourth day of fever (but ranges from the second to sixth day). The initial lesions are on the wrists, ankles, palms, and soles. After 6 to 12 hours, the rash spreads centripetally to the trunk and face. At first, the rash is macular and blanches with pressure, but it becomes maculopapular and petechial or purpuric after 2 to 3 days.

The pathologic changes, such as thrombus formation, are a result of rickettsial invasion of the endothelial cells of blood vessels. Disseminated intravascular coagulation and thrombocytopenia also account for the clinical observations. In addition to the rash, which occurs in 90% of patients, nonpitting edema is common, especially in the periorbital area. Other features are intense headache, myalgias with muscle tenderness, nausea, vomiting, constipation, and sometimes splenomegaly or hepatomegaly. Neurologic complications (stiff neck, mental confusion, seizures, hemiplegia, coma) may occur. Myocarditis, hepatitis, and interstitial pneumonitis are occasionally seen. The WBC count and differential are normal, in contrast to the findings of leukocytosis in meningococcal infection. Thrombocytopenia is common.

A presumptive diagnosis must be made and specific antimicrobial therapy started based solely on the clinical observations, as the results of complement fixation and the Weil-Felix test usually are not positive until the eighth to twelfth day of the illness. With an immunofluorescence test, rickettsiae can be identified in a skin biopsy specimen as early as the fourth day of illness.

*Treatment*
Therapy with tetracycline or parenteral chloramphenicol is started and continued until improvement occurs (usually for 5 afrebrile days). A response is seen in 24 to 48 hours if treatment is begun before the sixth day of illness. Sulfonamides can make the illness worse. Usually, by the end of the second week of illness, rickettsial antibodies can be detected by complement fixation or the more sensitive indirect fluorescent antibody and microagglutination tests. Polymerase chain reaction may be used to identify the organism, but this procedure is not readily available at most centers.

## Kawasaki Disease
Kawasaki disease, or mucocutaneous lymph node syndrome, is an illness of unknown cause. High fever lasting at least 5 days and an erythematous rash are prominent symptoms. The disease occurs predominantly in children under the age of 5 years, with a peak incidence between 1 and 2 years of age. The disease rarely occurs in persons more than 8 years old. Outbreaks continue to occur in the United States, particularly in the winter and spring. Person-to-person transmission has not been demonstrated. The case-fatality rate is 1% to 2%. Therapy consists of aspirin, other antiplatelet drugs (e.g., dipyridamole), and IV immunoglobulin.

*Lyme Disease*
Lyme disease is caused by a spirochete, *Borrelia burgdorferi,* which is transmitted by various ixodid ticks. In the United States, the disease occurs most frequently in areas where *Ixodes scapularis* or *Ixodes pacificus* can be found. The disease has been described in many other countries around the world. After an incubation period of about 1 week, with a range of 3 to 32 days, the characteristic skin lesion, erythema migrans, appears. Fever is usually low-grade and intermittent and is reported in half the patients. The fever may be high (up to 40°C) and persistent in children. Multiple skin lesions can develop, and erythema migrans usually lasts 2 to 3 weeks. Intense headache, malaise, fatigue, and regional lymphadenopathy are frequent early clinical features. Weeks to months later, neurologic manifestations, including meningoencephalitis, cranial nerve palsies (particularly of the facial nerve), and motor and sensor radiculoneuropathy, develop in 10% of patients. Neurologic abnormalities may persist for months but usually resolve completely. Weeks after onset, cardiac symptoms develop in 8% of patients, most commonly various degrees of atrioventricular block. Still later, weeks to several years after onset, migratory arthritis develops in some patients. Arthritis usually begins months after the onset of Lyme disease, affects primarily the large joints, such as the knees, and in 10% of patients becomes chronic, with destruction of cartilage and bone. (The diagnosis of Lyme disease is discussed in Chapter 40.)

## Differential Diagnosis
A guide to the differential diagnosis of fever and a skin rash is given in Table 49-1; it includes treatable infectious disease emergencies (e.g., Rocky Mountain spotted fever, meningococcal or staphylococcal septicemia, and TSS). Failure to institute appropriate therapy based on the epidemiologic history and results of rapid diagnostic tests, such as the Gram's stain, can be disastrous. (N.M.G.)

## Bibliography
Ackerman AB, Miller RC, Shapiro L. Gonococcemia and its cutaneous manifestations. *Arch Dermatol* 1965;91:227.
  *Illustrates lesions.*
Anderson LJ, Torok TJ. The clinical spectrum of human parvovirus B19 infections. In: Remington JS, Swartz MN, eds. *Current clinical topics in infectious diseases.* Cambridge, MA: Blackwell Science, 1991.
  *In adults, rash and arthralgias often occur. The arthritis can be present without a rash.*
Baker RC, et al. Fever and petechiae in children. *Pediatrics* 1989;84:1051.
  *Of children with fever and petechiae, 7% had meningococcal disease.*
Bergman SJ, Kundin WD. Scrub typhus in South Vietnam. *Ann Intern Med* 1973; 79:26.

*The characteristic features are fever (100%), adenopathy (85%), eschar (46%), and maculopapular eruption (34%).*
Bodey GP. Dermatologic manifestations of infections in neutropenic patients. *Infect Dis Clin North Am* 1994;8:655–675.
*Review. Sweet's syndrome, or acute febrile neutrophilic dermatosis, is often misdiagnosed as cellulitis.*
Burns JC, et al. Clinical and epidemiologic characteristics of patients referred for evaluation of possible Kawasaki disease. *J Pediatr* 1991;118:680.
*Measles, group A β-hemolytic streptococcal infection, and drug reaction may mimic Kawasaki disease.*
Cale DF, McCarthy MW. Treatment of Rocky Mountain spotted fever in children. *Ann Pharmacol* 1997;31:492–494.
*Doxycycline can be given safely to children less than 9 years of age for Rocky Mountain spotted fever.*
Case records of the Massachusetts General Hospital (case 26-1973). *N Engl J Med* 1973;288:1400.
*Discusses the differential diagnosis of an acutely ill patient with a rash and fever.*
Case records of the Massachusetts General Hospital (case 16-1978). *N Engl J Med* 1978;298:957.
*Presentation of the case of a fish cutter with fever and a skin rash caused by* Erysipelothrix rhusiopathiae *(erysipeloid).*
Case records of the Massachusetts General Hospital (case 27-1985). *N Engl J Med* 1985;313:36.
*Discussion of fever, rash, and pulmonary infiltrates in a veterinarian with tularemia.*
Case records of the Massachusetts General Hospital (case 30-1990). *N Engl J Med* 1990;323:254.
*Discussion of a patient with fever and pustular skin lesions (neutrophilic dermatosis, or Sweet's syndrome).*
Case records of the Massachusetts General Hospital (case 32-1997). *N Engl J Med* 1997;337:1149–1156.
*A fatal case of Rocky Mountain spotted fever.*
Centers for Disease Control. Follow-up on toxic shock syndrome. *MMWR Morb Mortal Wkly Rep* 1980;29:441.
*Case definition.*
Chambers HF, Korzoniowski OM, Sande MA. *Staphylococcus aureus* endocarditis: clinical manifestations in addicts and nonaddicts. *Medicine (Baltimore)* 1983;62:170.
*A murmur was absent in about 25% of addicts on the initial presentation.*
Cherry JD. Contemporary infectious exanthems. *Clin Infect Dis* 1993;16:199–207.
*Pictures of classic exanthems. Epidemiologic clues (e.g., season) are key to diagnosis.*
Clinicopathological Conference. A 54-year-old woman with fevers, arthralgias, myalgias, and rash. *Am J Med* 1988;85:84.
*A discussion of leukocytoclastic vasculitis (allergic).*
Clinicopathologic Conference. Abdominal pain, fever, and rash in a 39-year-old male. *Am J Med* 1994;97:300–306.
*Diagnosis of Henoch-Schönlein purpura by skin biopsy in an adult with fever, abdominal pain, and rash.*
Duma RJ, et al. Epidemic typhus in the United States associated with flying squirrels. *JAMA* 1981;245:2318.
*Clinical features include headache, fever, myalgias, and rash.*
Dumler JS, Bakken JS. Human ehrlichioses: newly recognized infections transmitted by ticks. *Annu Rev Med* 1998;49:201–213.
*In this tick-borne disease, rash is present in up to one third of patients. Treatment with doxycycline usually results in cure.*
Dumler JS, Taylor JP, Walker DH. Clinical and laboratory features of murine typhus in south Texas, 1980 through 1987. *JAMA* 1991;266:1365.
*The features often include fever, headache, chills, myalgias, and rash.*
Fichtenbaum CJ, Peterson LR, Weil GJ. Ehrlichiosis presenting as a life-threatening illness with features of the toxic shock syndrome. *Am J Med* 1987;95:351.
*Patients with ehrlichiosis may fulfill the criteria for TSS, including a rash and conjunctival hemorrhage or erythema.*

Gentry LO, Zeluff B, Kielhofner MA. Dermatologic manifestations of infectious diseases in cardiac transplant patients. *Infect Dis Clin North Am* 1994;8:637–654.
*A skin lesion in a transplant recipient may be a primary infection site or indicate another, occult focus of infection.*

Gersony WM. Diagnosis and management of Kawasaki disease. *JAMA* 1991;265:2699.
*Reviews cardiovascular features. Although coronary artery aneurysms were noted in 20% of patients, aneurysms may also occur in other arteries, most often axillary, iliac, or renal.*

Haynes RE, Sanders DV, Cramblett HG. Rocky Mountain spotted fever in children. *J Pediatr* 1970;76:685.
*Classic. A clinical diagnosis requiring empiric therapy.*

Hill WR, Kinney TD. The cutaneous lesions in acute meningococcemia. *JAMA* 1947;134:513.
*Discusses the clinical and pathologic features of meningococcal skin lesions.*

Kain KC, Schulzer M, Chow AW. Clinical spectrum of nonmenstrual toxic shock syndrome (TSS): comparison with menstrual TSS by multivariate discriminant analyses. *Clin Infect Dis* 1993;16:100.
*S. aureus from patients with nonmenstrual TSS produced TSST-1 with a frequency comparable with that of strains from patients with menstrual TSS (62% vs. 84%). Nonmenstrual TSS was often nosocomial.*

Kato H, et al. Long-term consequences of Kawasaki disease. A 10- to 21-year follow-up study of 594 patients. *Circulation* 1996;94:1379–1385.
*The incidence of coronary aneurysms in acute Kawasaki disease was 25%, with half of cases showing regression.*

Kennedy NJ, Duncan AW. Acute meningococcaemia: recent advances in management (with particular reference to children). *Anaesth Intensive Care* 1996;24:197–216.
*Review. No vaccine is available for group B meningococci.*

Kingston ME, Mackey D. Skin clues in the diagnosis of life-threatening infections. *Rev Infect Dis* 1986;8:1.
*Examination of a Gram's-stained smear of a scraping from the base of an ulcer or of a skin biopsy specimen may establish the diagnosis. Cutaneous manifestations are illustrated in color.*

Kirk JL, et al. Rocky Mountain spotted fever: a clinical review based on 48 confirmed cases, 1943–1986. *Medicine (Baltimore)* 1990;69:35.
*Review. The classic triad of fever, headache, and rash were present in only 62% of patients. Two thirds of patients noted an exposure to ticks.*

Lee VTP, Chang AH, Chow AW. Detection of staphylococcal enterotoxin B among toxic shock syndrome (TSS) and non–TSS-associated *Staphylococcus aureus* isolates. *J Infect Dis* 1992;166:911.
*Staphylococcal enterotoxin B was found in 62% of patients with nonmenstrual TSS who were negative for TSST-1.*

Levin S, Goodman LJ. An approach to acute fever and rash (AFR) in the adult. In: Remington JS, Swartz MN, eds. *Current clinical topics in infectious diseases.* Boston: Blackwell Science, 1995:19–75.
*Comprehensive review.*

Litwack KD, Hoke AW, Borchardt KA. Rose spots in typhoid fever. *Arch Dermatol* 1972;105:252.
*Illustrates rose spots.*

Mackowiak PA, LeMaistre CF. Drug fever: a critical appraisal of conventional concepts. *Ann Intern Med* 1987;106:728.
*Fever patterns were not helpful, and a rash was present in only 18% of patients.*

Marrack P, Kappler J. The staphylococcal enterotoxins and their relatives. *Science* 1990;241:705.
*Various staphylococcal toxins, TSS toxin, and streptococcal toxins activate T cells, resulting in the production of mediators such as interleukin-1 and tumor necrosis factor.*

Martin DB, et al. Atypical measles in adolescents and young adults. *Ann Intern Med* 1979;90:877.
*Rash may be vesicular, petechial, and purpuric.*

Mawhorter SD, et al. Cutaneous manifestations of toxoplasmosis. *Clin Infect Dis* 1992;14:1084.
*Acute toxoplasmosis may be associated with fever and a maculopapular rash.*
Melish ME. Kawasaki syndrome. *Pediatr Rev* 1996;17:153–162.
*Peak incidence occurs between the ages of 1 and 2 years, with 80% of cases seen in children less than 4 years of age.*
Miller JQ, Price TR. The nervous system in Rocky Mountain spotted fever. *Neurology* 1972;22:561.
*Most frequent findings were headache and lethargy. Cerebral spinal fluid pleocytosis, usually less than 50 cells per cubic millimeter, may occur.*
Parsonnet J. Nonmenstrual toxic shock syndrome: new insights into diagnosis, pathogenesis and treatment. In: Remington JS, Swartz MN, eds. *Current clinical topics in infectious diseases.* Boston: Blackwell Science, 1996: 1–20.
*Review. Testing for TSST-1 and its antibody may be helpful in menstrual but not in nonmenstrual cases of TSS.*
Perez CM, et al. Adjunctive treatment of streptococcal toxic shock syndrome using intravenous immunoglobulin: case report and review. *Am J Med* 1997;102:111–113.
*IV immunoglobulin was useful for streptococcal TSS.*
Procop GW, et al. Immunoperoxidase and immunofluorescent staining of *Rickettsia rickettsii* in skin biopsies. A comparative study. *Arch Pathol Lab Med* 1997;121:894–899.
*Immunoperoxidase and immunofluorescent staining of skin biopsy specimens were useful in diagnosing Rocky Mountain spotted fever (senstivity of 73% and specificity of 100%).*
Pruksananonda P, et al. Primary human herpesvirus 6 infection in young children. *N Engl J Med* 1992;326:1445.
*An important cause of an acute febrile illness in young children.*
Reingold AI, et al. Nonmenstrual toxic shock syndrome. *Ann Intern Med* 1982;96 (Pt 2):871.
*Clinical features are identical to those seen in menses-related cases, but the epidemiology differs.*
Sexton DJ, Corey GR. Rocky Mountain "spotless" and "almost spotless" fever: a wolf in sheep's clothing. *Clin Infect Dis* 1992;15:439.
*Rash may be absent or minimal in male and black patients, making the diagnosis difficult in these populations.*
Shands KN, et al. Toxic shock syndrome in menstruating women. *N Engl J Med* 1980; 303:1436.
*Classic. Associated TSS with tampon use and isolated* S. aureus *from vaginal cultures.*
Shrestha M, Grodzicki RL, Steere AC. Diagnosing early Lyme disease. *Am J Med* 1985;78:235.
*Blood cultures were positive for the spirochete in one of 40 patients (2.5%).*
Silpapojakul K, et al. Scrub and murine typhus in children with obscure fever in the tropics. *Pediatr Infect Dis J* 1991;10:200.
*Scrub typhus in children was characterized by fever, diarrhea, vomiting, and hepatosplenomegaly. Rash was rare.*
Spach DH, et al. Tick-borne diseases in the United States. *N Engl J Med* 1993;329:936.
*Illustrated review. To remove a tick, use a tweezer and pull slowly.*
Steere AC, et al. Lyme carditis: cardiac abnormalities of Lyme disease. *Ann Intern Med* 1983;99:8.
*The most common abnormality is atrioventricular block of various degrees, especially complete heart block.*
Steere AC, et al. Treatment of the early manifestations of Lyme disease. *Ann Intern Med* 1983;99:22.
*Penicillin is an alternative drug for treating early Lyme disease.*
Steere AC, et al. The early clinical manifestations of Lyme disease. *Ann Intern Med* 1983;99:76.
*Color pictures of erythema chronicum migrans.*
Steere AC, et al. The spirochetal etiology of Lyme disease. *N Engl J Med* 1983;308:733.
*Isolated the spirochete from the blood, skin lesions, and cerebrospinal fluid of patients, and also from the ticks.*

Stevens DL. Invasive group A *Streptococcus* infections. *Clin Infect Dis* 1992;14:2.
  *Review. Discusses virulence factors and clinical features.*
Stevens DL. Streptococcal toxic shock endrome. *Emerging Infect Dis* 1995;1:69–78.
  *Review.*
Stevens DL. The toxic shock syndromes. *Infect Dis Clin North Am* 1996;10:727–746.
  *Review of streptococcal and staphylococcal TSS.*
Stevens DL, et al. Severe group A streptococcal infections associated with a toxic
  shock-like syndrome and scarlet fever toxin A. *N Engl J Med* 1989;321:1.
  *Patients with this life-threatening illness did not have the typical rash of scarlet fever
  or the erythroderma of staphylococcal TSS. Petechial and maculopapular rashes
  were noted.*
Stevens FA. The occurrence of *Staphylococcus aureus* infection with a scarlatiniform
  rash. *JAMA* 1927;88:1957.
  *Classic.*
Todd JK. Therapy of toxic shock syndrome. *Drugs* 1990;39:856.
  *Reviews management of TSS.*
Todd J, et al. Toxic shock syndrome associated with phage group 1 staphylococci.
  *Lancet* 1978;2:1116.
  *Classic.*
Todd JK, et al. Corticosteroid therapy for patients with toxic shock syndrome. *JAMA*
  1984;252:3399.
  *Corticosteroid therapy may be beneficial, but the trial was not controlled.*
Toews WH, Bass JW. Skin manifestations of meningococcal infection. *Am J Dis Child*
  1974;127:173.
  *Color pictures. Mortality was high (44%) in patients with purpuric or ecchymotic skin
  lesions.*
Torok TJ. Parvovirus B19 and human disease. *Adv Intern Med* 1992;37:431.
  *Review.*
Toxic shock syndrome. *Ann Intern Med* 1982;96:831.
  *Entire issue on TSS.*
Van Nguyen O, Nguyen EA, Weiner LB. Incidence of invasive bacterial disease in chil-
  dren with fever and petechiae. *Pediatrics* 1984;74:77.
  *Twenty percent of patients with fever and petechiae had bacterial infections.*
Walker DH. Rocky mountain spotted fever: a seasonal alert. *Clin Infect Dis* 1995;20:
  1111–1117.
  *A history of a tick exposure with a 3- to 12-day incubation period is key to diagnosis.*
Wolfson JS, Sober AJ, Rubin RH. Dermatologic manifestations of infections in
  immunocompromised patients. *Medicine (Baltimore)* 1985;64:115.
  *Diagnosis is usually established by skin biopsy for culture and histologic examina-
  tion. The gross appearance of the skin lesions is of limited value.*
Woodward TE, et al. Prompt confirmation of Rocky Mountain spotted fever: identification of rickettsiae in skin tissues. *J Infect Dis* 1976;134:297.
  *An immunofluorescence technique identified rickettsiae in a skin biopsy specimen in
  4 hours.*
Working Group on Severe Streptococcal Infections. Defining the group A streptococcal toxic shock syndrome. *JAMA* 1993;269:390–391.
  *Cases are defined by isolation of group A streptococci from a sterile site, presence of
  hypotension, and presence of two or more of the following: renal impairment, coagulopathy, liver abnormalities, acute respiratory distress syndrome, tissue necrosis,
  and an erythematous rash.*

## 50. FEVER AND THE RENAL TRANSPLANT RECIPIENT

Infection is the primary cause of death (41%) following renal transplantation (the
other causes being cardiovascular problems, 20%; suicide, 15%; gastrointestinal problems, 13%; neoplasms, 4%; and various other disorders, 7%). Nevertheless, there has
been a substantial decrease in the frequency of infection, which can be attributed to

improved surgical techniques, more precise immunosuppressive regimens, better matching of donor and recipient organs, improved harvesting and preservation of donor organs, and prompt diagnosis and treatment of infections. Since the introduction of cyclosporine, an 11-amino acid, cyclic polypeptide antirejection agent, the incidence of infection has decreased even further. In a randomized, prospective trial of cyclosporine versus azathioprine for immunosuppression in renal allograft recipients, the incidence of all infections in the cyclosporine-treated patients was approximately half that in the azathioprine-treated patients. The number of bacterial infections was similar in the two groups, but viral infections, particularly cytomegalovirus (CMV) infections, occurred in a significantly greater number of azathioprine-treated than cyclosporine-treated patients. There was no significant difference, however, between the two treatment groups in the actuarial patient and graft survival rates.

Other drugs for immunosuppression to decrease the dosage of corticosteroids used include a monoclonal pan-T-cell antibody (OKT3), tacrolimus (FK506), and mycophenolate. With improved immunosuppression, the rate of fungal infections has decreased from 45% to 5% in recent years.

Rubin and associates categorized the most common types of infection in renal transplant recipients according to time of onset in the period after transplantation. During the first month after transplantation, the chief considerations are wound, pulmonary, urinary tract, and IV line-related infections caused by the usual bacterial pathogens. Hepatitis B and herpes simplex virus infections are also common during this period. Opportunistic infections are rare during the first month after transplantation, and their occurrence suggests either an unusual nosocomial exposure or an infection that was present but unrecognized in the period before transplantation, with symptomatic disease resulting from immunosuppressive therapy, surgical manipulation, or both.

Opportunistic infections become manifest 1 to 6 months after transplantation. Infections caused by CMV, Epstein-Barr virus, varicella-zoster virus, hepatitis C and other hepatitis virus agents, *Nocardia, Listeria,* fungi, *Toxoplasma,* and *Pneumocystis carinii,* and serious bacterial infections related to the surgical procedure are common at this time. Among these pathogens, CMV predominates. During this period, the infections are probably a consequence of the intensive immunosuppressant therapy; CMV itself is immunosuppressive.

In the late post-transplantation period, 6 months or more after the transplantation, cryptococcal meningitis is seen. Cryptococcal infections usually begin more than 1 year after transplantation. Other infections observed in the late period are CMV infection, chorioretinitis, urinary tract infection, chronic viral hepatitis, and the usual community-acquired infections, such as pneumococcal pneumonia.

Fever in a renal transplant recipient may indicate an infectious or noninfectious cause. Important noninfectious causes of fever are allograft rejection, malignancy, drug fever, and pulmonary emboli. When a renal transplant patient has a fever, the clinician should initiate an exhaustive evaluation to determine any clues to its cause. Symptoms and signs other than fever help to localize the site of infection. Clues to the presence of infection are often subtle in a renal transplant recipient. Headache, even without a stiff neck, indicates the possibility of meningitis. Travel history and place of residence are important factors if coccidioidomycosis, histoplasmosis, or parasitic disease is suspected and diagnosed. The possibility of drug fever must always be considered. The clinician should order blood, urine, and other cultures based on the clinical clues. Signs of rejection should be assessed by measuring changes in renal function. Other useful studies include urinalysis, chest roentgenography, CBC count, acute and convalescent serologies, and cultures of the urine and buffy coat for CMV. Computed tomography and ultrasound examinations are useful to evaluate the transplant site and detect any other occult intraabdominal disease.

Infection is responsible for approximately 75% of fevers. Of these infections, viruses are the most frequent cause, responsible for more than half (55%) of all febrile episodes. Of the viral agents, CMV is by far the most frequent and can be found alone or in combination with other viruses. Most CMV disease occurs between 14 days and 4 months after transplantation, and only 17% of the febrile episodes observed more than 1 year after transplantation are associated with CMV infection. Bacterial and fungal infections are responsible for 14% and 5% of febrile episodes, respectively. The other important cause of fever is rejection, which accounts for 13% of post-transplantation fever. Infection with HIV can occur, and screening for this agent should be carried out in donors as well as recipients.

Bacterial wound and urinary tract infections occur frequently in renal transplant recipients. Immunosuppressive drugs often obscure the usual symptoms and signs of a wound infection and may make the diagnosis difficult. In recent years, the incidence of wound infections has decreased dramatically because of increased technical and surgical expertise and, possibly, the use of antimicrobial prophylaxis. The diagnosis of a wound infection can be established by aspiration of the wound or by ultrasonic or computed tomographic examination of the site. Ultrasonography may not differentiate an abscess from a lymphocele or seroma. Lymphoceles can become secondarily infected, and the collection must be drained.

Urinary tract infections are the most common bacterial infections in renal transplant recipients. The incidence varies from 35% to 79% in some reports, and approximately 60% of the bacteremias originate from the transplant. Urinary tract infections in the first 3 months after the transplantation are often associated with pyelonephritis and bacteremia. Infections that occur after months are generally benign and respond to conventional 10- to 14-day courses of antimicrobials. Trimethoprim-sulfamethoxazole (TMP-SMX), given as one double-strength tablet at bedtime for 4 months, significantly decreased the incidence of urinary tract infection in one test group compared with a control group that received placebo. In another study in which TMP-SMX was used twice daily for 1 year, the incidence of bacterial infections was reduced, especially infections of the urinary tract and bacteremias. Use of TMP-SMX may also prevent *P. carinii* pneumonia, listeriosis, and nocardiosis.

Infection with CMV occurs in most (60% to 96%) patients after renal transplantation. Three patterns of disease are described: primary disease, reactivation disease, and superinfection. Primary disease occurs in a seronegative renal transplant recipient who receives an allograft from a seropositive donor. The virus is transmitted with the donor kidney, and immunosuppressive therapy activates the latent virus. In reactivation disease, endogenous latent virus is reactivated during immunosuppressive therapy in an already seropositive transplant recipient. Superinfection occurs in a seropositive renal transplant recipient and involves acquisition of another CMV strain from the donor kidney. Patients with superinfection are usually symptomatic.

Most infections begin 1 to 4 months after transplantation, and approximately 25% of the infections are symptomatic. The effects of the virus can be categorized as follows: (a) clinical symptoms and signs, (b) depression of host defenses leading to superinfection by other pathogens, and (c) allograft rejection. The clinical manifestations of CMV infection are fever, malaise, arthralgias, pneumonitis, hepatitis, abdominal pain, diarrhea, gastrointestinal bleeding, and leukopenia. Splenomegaly and lymphadenopathy are generally absent. Chorioretinitis is an important, late-occurring symptom of CMV infection. Infection with CMV is rarely fatal when it occurs alone, but when it is complicated by another infection, the outcome is often fatal. The virus can have devastating effects on the renal transplant recipient. Various strategies have been used to prevent CMV infection in transplant recipients, including use of acyclovir, ganciclovir, and high-titer anti-CMV immunoglobulin. The results are encouraging, but further studies are needed to define the optimal prophylactic regimen for renal transplant recipients.

CNS infections occur in about 10% of renal transplant recipients. The CNS is second only to the lungs as a site of infection by opportunistic pathogens. Three pathogens are responsible for about 90% of the infections: *Listeria monocytogenes, Cryptococcus neoformans,* and *Aspergillus fumigatus.* Fever and headache are the most common symptoms and are often the only clues present. A minority of cases have nuchal rigidity. All renal transplant recipients with fever and headache should have a lumbar puncture analysis. Computed tomography should precede the lumbar puncture if papilledema or any focal neurologic finding is present. The use of OKT3 to reverse graft rejection following renal transplantation has been associated with an aseptic meningitis syndrome characterized by fever, headache, and an altered mental status. In this syndrome, patients have a cerebrospinal fluid pleocytosis with negative cultures.

Fever and pulmonary infiltrates in a renal transplant recipient, as in any other immunocompromised host, suggest many diagnoses, both infectious and noninfectious, and an organized approach to establish a causative diagnosis is imperative. Pulmonary infection is a major cause of mortality in renal transplant recipients. Noninfectious causes, such as pulmonary emboli and pulmonary edema, account for about 25% of the cases in one report. Clues to the cause can be obtained from assessing the course of illness and the chest roentgenographic pattern. For example, fungi and *Nocardia* produce cavitation, and the infiltrates generally develop over several weeks. Common infecting pathogens, such as *Streptococcus pneumoniae* and influenza virus, are still seen more often than opportunistic pathogens, except for CMV, and must always be considered in a patient with community-acquired pneumonia. CMV infection occurs during the 1- to 4-month interval after transplantation. In one report, mixed infections were noted in 40% of patients. If the expectorated sputum fails to yield a diagnosis, more invasive techniques are required. Treatment should be based on the specific cause. (N.M.G.)

## Bibliography

Ahsan N, Blanchard RL, Mai ML. Gastrointestinal tuberculosis in renal transplantation: a case report and review. *Clin Transplant* 1995;9:349–352.
*Review. Consider extrapulmonary tuberculosis in a renal transplant patient with fever.*

Arduino R, Johnson P, Miranda A. Nocardiosis in renal transplant recipients undergoing immunosuppression with cyclosporine. *Clin Infect Dis* 1993;16:505–512.
*Lung involvement predominates. Drug interaction between cyclosporine and TMP-SMX may require use of another agent for therapy of* Nocardia *infection (e.g., imipenem, amikacin, minocycline, or amoxicillin-clavulanic acid).*

Bencini PL, et al. Cutaneous manifestations in renal transplant recipients. *Nephron* 1983;34:79.
*Twelve percent of the skin lesions were precancerous or cancerous.*

Brayman KL, et al. Analysis of infectious complications occurring after solid-organ transplantation. *Arch Surg* 1992;127:38.
*Infection remains the most frequent cause of death after renal transplantation. Most life-threatening infections were noted in the first 4 months after transplantation.*

Case records of the Massachusetts General Hospital (case 24-1984). *N Engl J Med* 1984;310:1584.
*Fever and pancytopenia in a renal transplant recipient from Venezuela. Diagnosis is disseminated histoplasmosis.*

Dowling JN, et al. Infections caused by *Legionella micdadei* and *Legionella pneumophila* among renal transplant recipients. *J Infect Dis* 1984;149:703.
*Renal transplant recipients are at increased risk for* Legionella *infection at certain transplant centers.*

Ettinger NA, Trulock EP. Pulmonary considerations of organ transplantation. Parts 1 and 2. *Am Rev Respir Dis* 1991;143:1386 and 1991;144:213,433.
*Review.*

Farrugia E, Schwab TR. Management and prevention of cytomegalovirus infection after renal transplantation. *Mayo Clin Proc* 1992;67:879.
*CMV disease usually occurs within 2 to 6 months after transplantation.*

Fisher J, Tuazon CU, Geelhoed GW. Mucormycosis in transplant patients. *Am Surg* 1980;46:315.
*An unusual cutaneous complication.*

Fishman JA, Rubin RH. Infection in organ-transplant recipients. *N Engl J Med* 1998; 338:1741–1751.
*Review. CMV is the most important pathogen affecting transplant recipients. Diagnosis is made with tests for antigenemia, polymerase chain reaction assays, or tissue biopsy.*

Fox BC, et al. A prospective, randomized, double-blind study of trimethoprim-sulfamethoxazole for prophylaxis of infection in renal transplantation: clinical efficacy, absorption of trimethoprim-sulfamethoxazole, effects on the microflora, and the cost-benefit of prophylaxis. *Am J Med* 1990;89:255.
*After removal of the catheters, long-term prophylaxis, for at least 1 year, was effective in reducing infections in renal transplant patients.*

Gantz NM, et al. Listeriosis in immunosuppressed patients: a cluster of eight cases. *Am J Med* 1975;58:637.
*An unusual outbreak. Therapy for meningitis should be given for 3 weeks to prevent relapse.*
Green M, et al. Comparison of intravenous ganciclovir followed by oral acyclovir with intravenous ganciclovir alone for prevention of cytomegalovirus and Epstein-Barr virus disease after liver transplantation in children. *Clin Infect Dis* 1997;25: 1344–1349.
*Two weeks of IV ganciclovir alone was effective CMV prophylaxis in liver transplant recipients.*
Hadley S, Karchmer AW. Fungal infections in solid-organ transplant recipients. *Infect Dis Clin North Am* 1995;9:1045–1074.
*Review. Infection, particularly fungal infection, is the major cause of mortality in patients undergoing a solid-organ transplant.*
Hooper DC, Pruitt AA, Rubin RH. Central nervous system infection in the chronically immunosuppressed. *Medicine (Baltimore)* 1982;61:166.
*Three major pathogens accounted for more than 75% of CNS infections:* Cryptococcus neoformans, Listeria monocytogenes, *and* Aspergillus fumigatus.
John GT, et al. A timetable for infections after renal transplantation in the tropics. *Transplantation* 1996;61:970–972.
*In the tropics (India), the infections noted were similar to those seen outside the tropics except for an increase in cases of tuberculosis.*
Kontoyiannis DP, Rubin RH. Infection in the organ transplant recipient. An overview. *Infect Dis Clin North Am* 1995;9:811–822.
*Review. Infections result from technical problems (e.g., wound hematoma), epidemiologic exposures (e.g., Aspergillus species), and net state of immunosuppression (e.g., CMV infection, drugs to prevent rejection).*
Lichtenstein IH, MacGregor RR. Mycobacterial infections in renal transplant recipients: report of five cases and review of the literature. *Rev Infect Dis* 1983;5:216.
*Review. Almost half of the patients had disseminated infections.*
Lloveras J, et al. Mycobacterial infections in renal transplant recipients. Seven cases and a review of the literature. *Arch Intern Med* 1982;142:888.
*Tuberculosis occurred in fewer than 1% of renal transplant recipients. Joint and subcutaneous tissue infections predominated.*
Martin MA, et al. Nosocomial aseptic meningitis associated with administration of OKT3. *JAMA* 1988;259:2002.
*The pathogenesis of this syndrome is unknown. No meningeal signs or focal defects were noted.*
Martinez-Marcos F, et al. Prospective study of renal transplant infections in 50 consecutive patients. *Eur J Clin Microbiol Infect Dis* 1994;13:1023–1028.
*During the first year after transplantation, urinary tract infections, especially asymptomatic bacteriuria, were most common.*
Mayoral JL, et al. Diagnosis and treatment of cytomegalovirus disease in transplant patients based on gastrointestinal tract manifestations. *Arch Surg* 1991;126:202.
*Clinical symptoms in patients with invasive CMV disease involving the gastrointestinal tract included abdominal pain (79%), fever (36%), diarrhea (21%), and gastrointestinal bleeding (21%).*
Paterson DL, Singh N. Interactions between tacrolimus and antimicrobial agents. *Clin Infect Dis* 1997;25:1430–1440.
*Tacrolimus (FK506) is metabolized by the cytochrome P-450 3A system, and any antimicrobial drug that inhibits or induces these enzymes can alter levels of tacrolimus. Tacrolimus can cause nephrotoxicity.*
Peterson PK, et al. Cytomegalovirus disease in renal allograft recipients: a prospective study of the clinical features, risk factors and impact on renal transplantation. *Medicine (Baltimore)* 1980;59:283.
*Review of CMV. Fever was present in 95% of patients.*
Peterson PK, et al. Fever in renal transplant recipients: causes, prognostic significance and changing patterns at the University of Minnesota Hospital. *Am J Med* 1981; 71:345.

*Viral infections, primarily CMV infections, were responsible for more than 50% of the episodes.*

Peterson PK, et al. Infectious diseases in hospitalized renal transplant recipients: a prospective study of a complex and evolving problem. *Medicine (Baltimore)* 1982; 61:360.
*Review.*

Ponticelli C, et al. Randomized study with cyclosporine in kidney transplantation: 10-year follow-up. *J Am Soc Nephrol* 1996;7:792–797.
*Cyclosporine allows better graft survival than azathioprine at a 10-year follow-up.*

Ramsey PG, et al. The renal transplant patient with fever and pulmonary infiltrates: etiology, clinical manifestations, and management. *Medicine (Baltimore)* 1980;59:206.
*Mortality of 50% reported.*

Reyna J. Head and neck infection after renal transplantation. *JAMA* 1982;247:3337.
*Symptoms and causes were similar to those found in normal hosts.*

Rolfe MW, Strieter RM, Lynch JP III. Nocardiosis. *Semin Respir Med* 1992;13:216.
*Review. Single or multiple nodular chest lesions, along with a pleural effusion (33%), occur commonly.*

Rubin RH. Infection in the organ transplant recipient. In: Rubin RH, Young LS, eds. *Clinical approach to infection in the compromised host,* 3rd ed. New York: Plenum Publishing, 1994.
*A comprehensive review.*

Rubin RH, Tolkoff-Rubin NE. Antimicrobial strategies in the care of organ transplant recipients. Minireview. *Antimicrob Agents Chemother* 1993;37:619–624.
*Review of prophylaxis. Use fluconazole for asymptomatic candiduria in diabetic renal transplant patients.*

Rubin RH, et al. Infection in the renal transplant recipient. *Am J Med* 1981;70:405.
*Infections categorized according to time of onset in this classic article.*

Scroggs MW, et al. Causes of death in renal transplant recipients. *Arch Pathol Lab Med* 1987;111:983.
*Infection remains the leading cause of death, but the rates have diminished because of more selective immunosuppression.*

Stamm AM. Listeriosis in renal transplant recipients: report of an outbreak and review of 102 cases. *Rev Infect Dis* 1982;4:665.
*The major manifestations of the disease are meningitis (50%) and primary bacteremia (30%).*

Stephan RN, Munschauer CE, Kumar A. Surgical wound infection in renal transplantation: outcome data in 102 consecutive patients without perioperative systemic antibiotic coverage. *Arch Surg* 1997;132:1315–1319.
*Incidence of wound infection was only 2%.*

Stevens DA, et al. Laboratory evaluation of an outbreak of nocardiosis in immunocompromised hosts. *Am J Med* 1981;71:928.
*Air and dust samples were positive for* Nocardia. *This is a common problem in* Aspergillus *infection but extremely unusual with* Nocardia.

Stone RM. Case records of the Massachusetts General Hospital (case 31-1997). *N Engl J Med* 1997;337:1065–1074.
*Fever and diffuse pulmonary infiltrates 5 months after renal transplantation. Diagnosis was lymphoma.*

Tolkoff-Rubin NE, Rubin RH. The infectious disease problems of the diabetic renal transplant recipient. *Infect Dis Clin North Am* 1995;9:117–130.
*Diabetic renal transplant recipients have the same infections as nondiabetic patients, plus infections resulting from vascular compromise (e.g., foot infections).*

Tolkoff-Rubin NE, et al. A controlled study of trimethoprim-sulfamethoxazole prophylaxis of urinary tract infection in renal transplant recipients. *Rev Infect Dis* 1982;4:614.
*TMP-SMX is effective for prophylaxis of urinary tract infection.*

Toogood GJ, Roake JA, Morris PJ. The relationship between fever and acute rejection or infection following renal transplantation in the cyclosporin era. *Clin Transplant* 1994;8:373–377.
*Fever in the first 2 weeks is more likely caused by rejection rather than infection.*

Wagener MM, Yu VL. Bacteremia in transplant recipients: a prospective study of demographics, etiologic agents, risk factors, and outcomes. *Am J Infect Control* 1992;20:239.

*The urinary tract (58%) was the most frequent source for a bacteremia in renal transplant recipients. Mortality was 11%.*

Weiland D, et al. Aspergillosis in 25 renal transplant patients. *Ann Surg* 1983;622:198.

*Sputum culture failed to yield the organism in 60% of patients.*

Wheat, LJ et al. Histoplasmosis in renal allograft recipients. Two large urban outbreaks. *Arch Intern Med* 1983;143:703.

*A diagnosis of histoplasmosis is suspected in renal transplant recipients with prolonged unexplained fever in endemic areas. Results of chest roentgenography are often negative.*

Wilson JP, et al. Nocardial infections in renal transplant recipients. *Medicine (Baltimore)* 1989;68:38.

*Review. Overall mortality was 25% but 42% in patients with CNS disease.*

---

## 51. FEVER FOLLOWING TRAVEL ABROAD

About 10% of international travelers will experience a febrile illness either during their travels or within 2 weeks of returning from abroad. Travelers who present with febrile illnesses to their primary care physicians offer difficult diagnostic challenges. The geographic distribution of exotic diseases is complex, and the signs and symptoms of imported infections are rarely unique. Discounting the importance of international travel, especially if the trip was brief, patients may neglect to volunteer salient aspects of the epidemiologic history. In addition, travelers in whom a febrile or gastrointestinal disorder develops may be given empiric antimicrobial therapy that can suppress the clinical manifestations of the illness or impair the microbiologic evaluation; for example, antimicrobials can eliminate the bacteremia associated with typhoid fever but not eradicate the infection.

Changes in the natural history of disorders that were once prevalent in the United States can contribute to confusion in the diagnosis of the foreign traveler's illness. For example, most persons born before 1957 are likely to have had measles and therefore are usually protected from that infection; persons born after that date who did not have natural infection or who received an ineffective vaccine are susceptible to measles, which remains common in many underdeveloped countries of the world. Measles, therefore, must be considered in the differential diagnosis of the traveler with fever, cough, and a rash on the palms and soles.

The possibility of noninfectious disorders also exists in the febrile traveler. For example, the older person with cardiovascular disease is at risk to experience thrombophlebitis with pulmonary embolism as the result of sitting in a cramped position during a prolonged flight (so-called "economy class syndrome"). Similarly, the pyrexic patient taking trimethoprim-sulfamethoxazole for a diarrheal illness may have drug fever.

Detailed descriptions of the geographic distribution, modes of transmission, and clinical manifestations of exotic diseases can be found in a number of textbooks of tropical medicine (see annotated references); the liberal use of reference material is essential in evaluating the febrile traveler. The clinician must also realize that a number of uncommon bacterial (typhoid fever, ehrlichiosis, plague), rickettsial (Q fever, scrub typhus), fungal (histoplasmosis, coccidioidomycosis), and parasitic (babesiosis) diseases can be acquired by travel within the United States. Conversely, although Rocky Mountain spotted fever is often considered endemic only to the United States, the disease occurs in regions of Canada, Mexico, Colombia, and Brazil. Thus, the question, *Unde venis?* ("Where do you come from?") remains an essential component of the history of patients with febrile illnesses of obscure origin.

About 25% of travelers to the tropics who return with a febrile illness will remain without a diagnosis despite extensive evaluations and will experience a resolution of their fever within 1 to 2 weeks. The fact that some pyrexial illnesses are benign and self-limited and the realization that the international traveler is also at risk to acquire common diseases should temper diagnostic zeal and serve to focus the evaluation; thus, the differential diagnosis of the person who presents in January with fever, headache, malaise, and myalgias following a trip to Africa must include influenza as well as malaria. Similarly, the possibility of infectious mononucleosis exists in the young adult who has vacationed abroad and is found to have fever, lymphadenopathy, and a splenomegaly. The sexually promiscuous person who has been abroad and presents with fever is at risk to have a number of exotic diseases as a consequence of international travel as well as underlying infection with HIV. Indeed, high-risk behavior abroad, such as sexual intercourse with prostitutes, can result in the acquisition of HIV, and the fever experienced on returning home may represent a manifestation of primary HIV infection.

## Approach to the Febrile Traveler
*History*
The initial encounter with a traveler who has fever will dictate the speed and direction of the subsequent medical evaluation; therefore, a detailed history and thorough physical examination are essential to elicit clues that can provide insight into the cause of the patient's illness. The interval between the trip abroad and the onset of symptoms should be determined. Many infections become clinically apparent within 21 days of exposure. Relatively short-incubation disorders include malaria, bacterial infections (typhoid fever, plague, relapsing fever, acute brucellosis, tularemia, septicemic melioidosis, septicemic glanders), chlamydial and rickettsial diseases (psittacosis, scrub typhus, epidemic typhus), and viral illnesses (dengue, yellow fever, poliomyelitis, and the hemorrhagic fevers—Lassa fever, Crimean-Congo fever, Omsk hemorrhagic fever). The aseptic meningoencephalitides (Venezuelan equine encephalitis, lymphocytic choriomeningitis, East African trypanosomiasis) will also present within 3 weeks. In contrast, chronic brucellosis, tuberculosis, Q fever, malaria, schistosomiasis, trichinosis, filariasis, visceral leishmaniasis, amebic abscess, cysticercosis, and West African trypanosomiasis can become apparent months or years after the patient has left an endemic region. Hepatitis (A, B, C, E) and HIV infection may also become manifest more than 3 weeks after exposure.

The existence of a periodicity to the patient's fever should be determined; however, with the exception of relapsing fever (borreliosis), in which the patient is typically febrile for 3 to 4 days and afebrile for a similar length of time, characteristic patterns are uncommon. Fever that occurs every other day or every third day is highly suggestive of malaria, but these cycles are usually absent in the traveler with imported infection. On occasion, the fever associated with visceral leishmaniasis (kala-azar) may have a periodicity mimicking that of malaria.

A complete travel history should be obtained, including a list of the countries visited and the specific regions toured; the importance of this information is illustrated by the fact that malaria is generally not associated with travel to Mexico, but the disease is present outside cities and resorts along Mexico's southwestern coast. Moreover, the significance of short visits must not be overlooked; for example, voyagers to highly endemic areas can contract malaria during transient stops in airports or seaports, and bartonellosis (Oroya fever) can develop in travelers to Peru, Ecuador, or Colombia following brief excursions into the Andes mountains.

Many infections are acquired by ingesting contaminated food, and so the patient's dietary practices and preferences should be detailed. The traveler to less well-developed countries who enjoys indigenous food and drink is at risk to acquire salmonellosis, toxoplasmosis, trichinosis, or cysticercosis from inadequately cooked meat; salmonellosis, shigellosis, leptospirosis, amebiasis, giardiasis, dracunculiasis, or hepatitis A from contaminated ice cubes or drinking water; brucellosis, salmonellosis, campylobacteriosis, or tuberculosis from unpasteurized milk or milk products, including cheese and ice cream; and salmonellosis, hepatitis A, fish tapeworm infection, angiostrongyliasis, or infection with liver or lung flukes from raw or undercooked fish or shellfish.

Although food-borne disease is often associated with the poor sanitation prevalent in Third World countries, visitors to industrialized nations and to urban areas of developing countries are also at risk. For example, an outbreak of typhoid fever has been reported among vacationers at a tourist resort in Switzerland, and brucellosis remains a threat to visitors to Mexico and Spain who eat unpasteurized goat cheese.

Because arthropods represent common vectors for the transmission of infections, a history of insect contact or bites should be secured. Among the arthropods associated with the transmission of disease are mosquitoes (malaria, dengue, filariasis, yellow fever, Rift Valley fever), fleas (plague, murine typhus), lice (epidemic typhus, relapsing fever), blackflies (onchocerciasis), mites (rickettsialpox, scrub typhus), and ticks (tularemia, relapsing fever, Crimean-Congo hemorrhagic fever, and the spotted fever group of rickettsial infections, including Rocky Mountain spotted fever, boutonneuse fever, African tick-bite fever and Queensland tick typhus). Contact with rodents—and, in some cases, potential arthropod vectors—suggests plague, leptospirosis, lymphocytic choriomeningitis, Lassa fever, Venezuelan equine encephalitis, rickettsialpox, and both the spotted fever and typhus groups of rickettsial diseases. Exposure to farm animals indicates the possibility of brucellosis, tuberculosis, salmonellosis, tularemia, glanders, anthrax, psittacosis, and Q fever.

Wading, bathing, swimming, or boating in fresh water in endemic regions (the Caribbean, South America, Africa, the Middle East, Japan, China, and the Philippines) suggests a diagnosis of schistosomiasis. Many travelers with diseases transmitted by these arthropod and environmental vectors do not provide a history of exposure; thus, the absence of highly suggestive historical information does not exclude the possibility of the illnesses.

The patient's history should include a review of the travel precautions that were taken, including vaccinations and chemoprophylaxis for malaria or traveler's diarrhea. Few of the usually recommended vaccines are totally effective in preventing disease; for example, the typhoid vaccines are 60% to 80% effective in protecting against the disease, and they do not confer long-term immunity. Similarly, even strict adherence to malaria chemoprophylaxis, which occurs infrequently, does not guarantee that *Plasmodium* species will not return with the international traveler. Chloroquine may not be adequate to prevent infection with *Plasmodium vivax* or *Plasmodium ovale,* and the drug does not protect against chloroquine-resistant *Plasmodium falciparum,* which is prevalent in regions of Panama, South America, India, Southeast Asia, East Africa, and the Indonesian archipelago.

The patient's sexual and gastrointestinal histories are other important elements of the initial evaluation. A complaint of persistent diarrhea would suggest intestinal parasites, such as *Entamoeba histolytica,* and invasive bacterial pathogens, including *Salmonella* species, *Shigella* species, and *Aeromonas hydrophila,* which has been identified as a cause of traveler's diarrhea that can persist for months. In addition, diarrhea can be a prominent symptom in patients with malaria. The exposure of a group of travelers to a common source of infection can result in a cluster of patients with disease; therefore, travel agents and other members of tour groups should be contacted to determine if fellow travelers have become ill. Information derived in this manner may not only facilitate the evaluation of the traveler with enigmatic fever but may also be of importance to public health agencies.

*Physical Examination*
Meticulous and repeated physical examinations are essential in evaluating the febrile traveler. A pulse that is inappropriately slow for the degree of concomitant temperature elevation (i.e., pulse-temperature deficit) can be a manifestation of typhoid fever, Q fever, psittacosis, scrub typhus, or anicteric leptospirosis. Conversely, a tachycardia that persists when the patient is afebrile suggests viral, rickettsial, or parasitic myocarditis—the latter caused by trichinosis, toxoplasmosis, Chagas' disease, or African trypanosomiasis. Bilateral periorbital swelling is a clue to the diagnosis of trichinosis and Rocky Mountain spotted fever, and unilateral periorbital swelling in the traveler to South America indicates Chagas' disease. Conjunctival injection may indicate leptospirosis or Rocky Mountain spotted fever; an ulcerating, purulent conjunctivitis in a patient with regional lymphadenitis suggests oculoglandular tularemia. A severe tonsillitis with pseudomem-

branes and lymphadenopathy in the traveler who consumed meat from wild animals is a sign of tularemia.

A cutaneous ulcer is characteristic of tularemia, anthrax, glanders, mycotic disease (blastomycosis, sporotrichosis), mycobacterial infection (*Mycobacterium ulcerans, Mycobacterium marinum*), cutaneous leishmaniasis, and dracunculiasis. An eschar is suggestive of a rickettsial illness (scrub typhus, rickettsialpox, boutonneuse fever, Queensland tick typhus, North Asian tick typhus). Skin nodules are often seen in patients with bartonellosis, cysticercosis, or onchocerciasis; travelers with cutaneous myiasis have nodules that drain purulent material, but these patients usually do not have fever or other constitutional symptoms. A skin rash is characteristic of secondary syphilis, relapsing fever, plague, meningococcemia, gonococcemia, rat-bite fever, leptospirosis, glanders, rickettsial disease, toxoplasmosis, and a number of viral illnesses, including rubella, measles, acute HIV infection, the hemorrhagic fevers, dengue, and denguelike illnesses (chikungunya, O'nyong-nyong fever). The rash associated with syphilis, rubella, and measles can occur on the palms and soles. Rose spots, which are small (2 to 4 mm) erythematous maculopapular lesions, suggest typhoid fever; unfortunately, rose spots are infrequently present (10%) in patients with the illness. A generalized vesicular rash is expected in chickenpox or rickettsialpox. Multiple pustular or necrotic cutaneous lesions in a patient with chest radiographic findings compatible with tuberculosis suggest melioidosis. Recurrent or upper-extremity cellulitis that spreads in a centrifugal fashion is a cardinal manifestation of paroxysmal inflammatory filariasis.

Lymphadenopathy is common in patients with secondary syphilis, HIV infection, plague, tularemia, tuberculosis, glanders, histoplasmosis, South American blastomycosis, scrub typhus, lymphogranuloma venereum, rubella, Chagas' disease, toxoplasmosis, visceral leishmaniasis (kala-azar), filariasis, African trypanosomiasis, and onchocerciasis. Posterior auricular or posterior cervical adenopathy and a skin rash are highly suggestive of rubella and toxoplasmosis. Liver tenderness, hepatomegaly, or splenomegaly is an expected finding in patients with typhoid fever, brucellosis, relapsing fever, leptospirosis, Rocky Mountain spotted fever, chronic Q fever, psittacosis, viral hepatitis (A, B, C, E), yellow fever, malaria, toxoplasmosis, visceral leishmaniasis (kala-azar), amebic abscess, schistosomiasis, flukes, and visceral larva migrans.

An abnormal mental status or signs of meningitis may be important clues to the presence of relapsing fever, leptospirosis, rickettsial disease (especially Rocky Mountain spotted fever), psittacosis, tuberculosis, viral encephalitis, malaria, or African trypanosomiasis. Seizures are characteristic of cysticercosis, and they can occur in patients with paragonimiasis or schistosomiasis caused by *Schistosoma japonicum*.

*Laboratory Evaluation*

The preliminary laboratory evaluation should include a CBC count with differential analysis. A marked anemia with fragmented RBCs on the peripheral smear might indicate hemolysis secondary to malaria or bartonellosis (Oroya fever). A hypochromic microcytic anemia can result from chronic gastrointestinal blood loss produced by hookworm infestation. An eosinophilia suggests schistosomiasis, filariasis, liver or lung flukes, or intestinal helminths (hookworm, *Strongyloides, Ascaris, Trichuris*); a marked eosinophilia (>50%) indicates extraintestinal parasitic disease (trichinosis, visceral larva migrans, or the autoinfection syndrome of strongyloidiasis). Although eosinophilia occurs between paroxysmal attacks of filariasis, the finding may be absent during acute episodes. Liver function studies may reveal hepatocellular dysfunction, which is found in typhoid fever, leptospirosis, relapsing fever, Q fever, viral hepatitis (A, B, C, E), yellow fever, malaria, and toxoplasmosis. The liver function tests may also reveal an elevated alkaline phosphatase or other evidence of obstruction, characteristic of secondary syphilis, amebic abscess, hydatid cyst, liver flukes, schistosomiasis, and visceral larva migrans. Renal failure with hepatitis and aseptic meningitis indicates a possibility of leptospirosis.

An infiltrate on chest radiograph is expected in patients with pneumonic melioidosis, Q fever, psittacosis, tuberculosis, fungal infection (histoplasmosis, blastomycosis), or Legionnaires' disease, which can be acquired through travel abroad. Pneumonia in the patient with synovitis, orchitis, or meningoencephalitis may be a sign of brucellosis. The presence of pulmonary infiltrates in a patient with eosinophilia suggests paragonimiasis, strongyloidiasis, or ascariasis. Plague and anthrax are very unusual and highly lethal causes of pneumonia in travelers. An isolated, right-sided pleural effusion is an important clue to the presence of an amebic liver abscess.

A sputum analysis of patients with abnormal chest radiographic findings might include a wet preparation to detect yeast (*Histoplasma capsulatum, Paracoccidioides brasiliensis*) and acid-fast staining to identify mycobacteria (*Mycobacterium tuberculosis*). The sputum from travelers to regions where melioidosis is endemic (Southeast Asia and adjacent countries) should be carefully reviewed for the presence of *Burkholderia (Pseudomonas) pseudomallei*, which is a small, poorly staining, gram-negative bacillus. Lower respiratory tract secretions from voyagers to Korea, Japan, Taiwan, central China, the Philippines, West Africa, and certain regions of Thailand and South America should be searched for the characteristic operculated egg of *Paragonimus westermani*, which is the most common species associated with human paragonimiasis. Both melioidosis and paragonimiasis can closely mimic pulmonary tuberculosis.

Identified in 30% to 40% of cases, malaria represents the most common cause of pyrexia among febrile travelers returning from the tropics. Obviously, blood smears are an essential component of the initial laboratory evaluation of any voyager who has visited a region in which malaria is endemic. Several smears should be obtained during a 2- to 3-day period, and they should be carefully reviewed by an experienced hematologist, pathologist, or tropical medicine expert. A blood smear can reveal bacteremia (*Bartonella bacilliformis* or *Yersinia pestis*) or parasitemia (*Plasmodium* species, *Trypanosoma* species, *Leishmania* species, *Wuchereria bancrofti,* or *Brugia malayi*). Because some microfilaria exhibit nocturnal periodicity, blood for smears from patients who travel to endemic regions of filariasis (regions of the Caribbean and South America, Southeast Asia, and East and West Africa) should be obtained after sundown; patients from the South Pacific who are infected with *W. bancrofti* have maximal parasitemia during daytime hours. Concentration techniques or diethylcarbamazine provocation may be necessary to detect microfilaria.

Several blood cultures should be performed. In general, the bacteria that produce blood-borne infection in the international traveler can usually be isolated with commercially available culture media. To increase the probability that relatively fastidious bacteria, such as *Brucella* species, will be isolated, the clinical microbiology laboratory should hold blood cultures for 4 to 6 weeks. A number of bacterial pathogens cannot be recovered by using routine microbiologic media; for example, a semisolid medium (e.g., Fletcher's medium) is usually required for the isolation of *Leptospira* species, and selective media (e.g., cysteine-glucose-blood agar) and special containment facilities are necessary for the recovery of *Francisella tularensis*. A careful microscopic examination of stools must be performed to detect intestinal parasites. An evaluation of a minimum of three fresh fecal specimens is usually required to exclude the presence of ova or parasites. Catharsis-induced or "purged" stools are superior to other specimens for the detection of these organisms. Stool culture should also be performed to detect the presence of bacterial pathogens.

Serologic tests can be pivotal to the diagnosis of a number of exotic diseases, including brucellosis, relapsing fever, melioidosis, glanders, leptospirosis, tularemia, Q fever, psittacosis, rickettsial disease, lymphogranuloma venereum, viral infection, South American blastomycosis, toxoplasmosis, amebiasis, trichinosis, cysticercosis, schistosomiasis, and visceral larva migrans. Accordingly, 5 to 10 mL of serum should be obtained early in the patient's course and stored frozen; a second aliquot should be obtained 2 to 4 weeks later, and both samples are then sent for testing. A serologic diagnosis usually requires the demonstration of a seroconversion or a fourfold rise in antibody titer.

The subsequent medical evaluation is guided by the results of the history, physical examination, and preliminary laboratory data. A bone marrow biopsy for culture and histologic evaluation should be considered early in the assessment of the traveler with persistent fever, progressive weight loss, or other significant constitutional symptoms. The bone marrow culture may identify *Salmonella* species or *Brucella* species in patients with sterile blood cultures, and the histologic review may reveal findings consistent with mycobacterial infection (tuberculosis), fungal disease (histoplasmosis), or a parasitic disorder (leishmaniasis). The other tissues from which biopsy specimens may be needed to establish a diagnosis include lymph nodes (tuberculosis, toxoplasmosis, leishmaniasis), liver (tuberculosis, schistosomiasis, leishmaniasis), muscle (trichinosis, toxoplasmosis), and rectum (schistosomiasis). In addition, the biopsy of cutaneous lesions, such as ulcers, may be required to obtain sufficient material for histologic and microbiologic evaluation. Biopsy specimens of skin lesions in patients with suspected Rocky Mountain spotted fever can be stained with an immunofluorescent antibody technique that permits rapid diagnosis.

*Treatment*
As with other patients with persistent and perplexing fever, indiscriminate antimicrobial trials should be avoided. Nevertheless, in the critically ill patient, empiric therapy may be life-saving; such therapy must be based on the patient's travel history, which should provide epidemiologic clues to the most likely offending agents. The traveler to a region of endemic *P. falciparum* must receive treatment for malaria; in general, these patients should be assumed to be infected with chloroquine-resistant strains. Chloramphenicol or ciprofloxacin should be included in most empiric antimicrobial regimens for the toxic traveler; although perhaps they are not the drugs of choice, these agents possess activity against a variety of pathogens capable of producing a fatal illness, such as *Salmonella* species (typhoid fever), *Brucella* species (brucellosis), *Borrelia recurrentis* (relapsing fever), *B. bacilliformis* (Oroya fever), *Burkholderia (Pseudomonas) pseudomallei* (melioidosis), *Bacillus anthracis* (anthrax), *Y. pestis* (plague), *F. tularensis* (tularemia), *Rickettsia rickettsii* (Rocky Mountain spotted fever), *Rickettsia prowazekii* (epidemic typhus), and *Rickettsia tsutsugamushi* (scrub typhus). The initiation of empiric therapy does not eliminate the need to identify the source of the patient's illness. The gravity of the clinical situation that precipitates the empiric use of antimicrobials demands a specific diagnosis; thus, the medical evaluation of the seriously ill traveler must be expedited.

*Infection Control*
Stringent infection control measures may be necessary in the hospitalized febrile traveler. In most circumstances, specific findings will determine which infection control guidelines are necessary; these findings include pulmonary infiltrates and skin rashes suggestive of communicable disorders, such as chickenpox, measles, and the viral hemorrhagic fevers. When the cause of the patient's illness is unknown and the travel history includes exposure to communicable diseases (typhoid fever, viral hepatitis, dengue, yellow fever), the patient should be placed in a private room, and health care workers must adhere to the appropriate precautions. In selected cases, the patient will require respiratory ("droplet") or strict isolation, at least until the cause of the illness is known or until the possibility of readily transmissible disorders is excluded. (A.L.E.)

**Bibliography**
Boreham RE, Relf WA. Imported malaria in Australia. *Med J Aust* 1991;155:754.
  *In this review of 146 cases of imported malaria, the authors find that only 11.6% of the patients were taking the recommended prophylactic drugs.*
Castellani PM, et al. Six cases of travel-associated Legionnaires' disease involving four countries. *Infection* 1992;20:73.
  *Legionnaires' disease can be acquired as a consequence of travel to Europe and elsewhere.*
Centers for Disease Control. Imported dengue—United States, 1995. *MMWR Morb Mortal Wkly Rep* 1995;45:988.
  *The authors note a substantial increase in the incidence of dengue in the Caribbean, Central America, and Mexico and a corresponding rise in the number of imported cases.*
Cossar JH, et al. A cumulative review on travelers, their experience of illness and the implications of these findings. *J Infect* 1990;21:27.
  *In this extensive analysis, the authors note that many travelers lacked protective antibodies against a number of infectious illnesses, including typhoid and diphtheria, and that the travel agent was the most frequently consulted source of pretravel health advice.*

Doherty JF, et al. Fever as the presenting complaint of travelers returning from the tropics. *OJM* 1995;88:277.

*In a review of 587 febrile patients, the authors report that malaria (42%), diarrheal illness (6.5 %), and dengue (6%) represented the most common diagnoses; in 25% of the cases, however, a specific diagnosis could not be established.*

Liu LX, Weller PF. Approach to the febrile traveler returning from Southeast Asia and Oceania. *Curr Clin Top Infect Dis* 1992;12:138–164.

*A comprehensive review of the illnesses leading to pyrexia in patients returning from these regions.*

Magill AJ. Fever in the returned traveler. *Infect Dis Clin North Am* 1998;12:445.

*A very well-referenced review.*

Markowitz LE, et al. International measles importations United States, 1980–1985. *Int J Epidemiol* 1988;17:187.

*Nonimmune travelers who acquire measles abroad can precipitate outbreaks of the disease in the United States.*

Ryan CA, Hargrett-Bean NT, Blake PA. *Salmonella typhi* infections in the United States, 1975–1984: increasing role of foreign travel. *Rev Infect Dis* 1989;11:1.

*In a review of 2,666 reported cases of typhoid fever, the authors note that 62% were imported, most frequently from Mexico or India.*

Strickland GT. *Hunter's tropical medicine*, 6th ed. Philadelphia: WB Saunders, 1984.

*A classic reference textbook in tropical medicine.*

Svenson JE, et al. Imported malaria. Clinical presentation and examination of symptomatic travelers. *Arch Intern Med* 1995;155:861.

*In this retrospective review of imported malaria at two hospital-based tropical disease centers, the authors note that chemoprophylaxis was prescribed for only 46% of the patients and that only half of those travelers took the medication as prescribed. They also report that almost 90% of the patients with* P. falciparum *malaria presented within 6 weeks following their return from travel; in contrast, almost one third of the patients with* P. vivax *malaria presented 6 months following their trips.*

Warren KS, Mahmoud AAF. *Tropical and geographical medicine*, 2nd ed. New York: McGraw-Hill, 1990.

*This comprehensive textbook can provide substantial assistance in the evaluation of the febrile traveler.*

Wilson ME. *A world guide to infections: diseases, distribution, diagnosis.* New York: Oxford University Press, 1991.

*The unique format of this detailed textbook provides succinct discussions, by specific geographic region, of many infectious diseases.*

Wyler DJ. Evaluation of cryptic fever in a traveler to Africa. *Curr Clin Top Infect Dis* 1992;12:329.

*An excellent discussion of the assessment of the patient with enigmatic fever following a trip to Africa, plus concise descriptions of some exotic illnesses.*

---

## 52. HYPERPYREXIA AND HYPERTHERMIA

---

For centuries, fever has been recognized as a cardinal sign of disease, and recent scientific studies have provided substantial insight into the mechanisms contributing to a rise in body temperature. The effectiveness of the systems involved in thermoregulation explains why body temperatures in excess of 41°C (106°F) are unusual in adults. By considering the limited number of conditions associated with extreme elevations of body temperature, reviewing the epidemiologic history, and focusing on the physical examination, the clinician can usually establish a correct diagnosis. Further, because useful therapies exist for all the disorders associated with hyperpyrexia and hyperthermia, a prompt diagnosis can be expected to result in a greater likelihood that the patient will survive the event. Central to the approach to any patient with a temperature above 41°C is a recognition that both the underlying condition and the exaggerated temperature can produce substantial morbidity or death.

In the healthy adult, body temperature is maintained within a narrow range (37°C ± 1°C) by mechanisms that balance the rates of heat production and dissipation and that compensate for environmental changes predisposing to heat gain or loss. "Thermosensors" in the anterior hypothalamus play a pivotal role in maintaining homeostasis by receiving information via the brainstem from the skin and viscera and effecting adjustments through the posterior hypothalamus "set point." Input from the posterior hypothalamus through the brainstem results in changes in the activity of the endocrine, musculoskeletal, and autonomic nervous systems; these alterations, in turn, produce adjustments in body temperature. A number of neurotransmitters and modulators within the central nervous system (CNS), including dopamine, serotonin, pros-z taglandins, acetylcholine, and neuropeptides, contribute to temperature regulation. Basal heat production, which is modulated by thyroid hormones and catecholamines, is a product of essential metabolic processes. The rate of heat production can be increased up to 10-fold by shivering or intense physical exercise. Changes in dermal blood flow, which is regulated through cholinergic nerve activity, permit heat conservation (vasoconstriction) or facilitate heat dispersion (vasodilation). Finally, heat can be transferred from the skin to the atmosphere by a number of mechanisms, especially evaporation (sweating).

Induced by infectious disease, fever (or pyrexia) represents a disorder of thermoregulation in which the hypothalamic set point of the host rises, resulting in a rise in temperature produced by peripheral vasoconstriction and shivering. The elevated body temperature appears to enhance host defenses against a variety of viral, bacterial, and mycobacterial pathogens. Rarely exceeding 41°C, the temperature elevation associated with infection is mediated by the products of monocytes and other cells ("endogenous pyrogens"), including interleukin-1, interleukin-6, and tumor necrosis factor. These cytokines induce the synthesis of prostaglandin $E_2$ by endothelial cells within the CNS, resulting in the "resetting" of the hypothalamus and a rise in body temperature. The generation of interleukin-1 and the other endogenous pyrogens is usually triggered by "exogenous pyrogens"; these include components of bacterial cell walls, such as lipopolysaccharide (endotoxin) from gram-negative bacilli, and toxins, such as the staphylococcal toxic shock toxin and the streptococcal pyrogenic exotoxins.

In contrast to an increased body temperature resulting from infection, hyperthermia represents a condition in which regulatory mechanisms fail to compensate for heat gain; in this circumstance, the hypothalamic set point remains unchanged. Temperatures in excess of 42.2°C (108°F) are not uncommon in hyperthermal states, and they tend to be self-perpetuating. More important, because enzyme denaturation, protein coagulation, and lipid liquefaction in the brain and other vital organs tend to commence at about 42°C (107.6°F), sustained hyperthermia is ultimately injurious to the patient. Patients may experience a rise in body temperature that is precipitated by an infectious illness but exaggerated by inadequacies in heat-dissipating mechanisms; for example, temperatures higher than 41°C are occasionally observed in quadriplegic patients with autonomic nervous system dysfunction and common infections, such as pyelonephritis. Thus, a distinction between hyperpyrexia and hyperthermia may be difficult to appreciate in some cases. Of note, hyperthermia enhances the tumoricidal activity of ionizing radiation, chemotheraputic drugs, and perhaps radioimmunotherapy agents; indeed, the use of local hyperthermia (i.e., intravesicular and intraperitonal) in combination with radiotherapy and chemotherapy to treat malignancies is under active investigation.

## Hyperpyrexia

Fortunately, infectious diseases are not commonly associated with hyperpyrexia. For example, in studies of large numbers of adults who were treated during the preantimicrobial era for lobar pneumonia and other serious infections, temperatures of 41°C or higher were noted in fewer than 5% of recordings. Because the clinical characteristics of patients with extreme pyrexia were not detailed in these older reports, the factors beyond infection that may have contributed to the high temperatures are not known. In more contemporary surveys of febrile patients, extreme pyrexia has been observed in patients with pneumonia, gram-negative bacteremia, staphylococcal bacteremia, pyelonephritis, and malaria. In many cases, the hyperpyrexia is associated with both infection and impaired thermoregulation caused by heatstroke, extensive burns, paraplegia, quadriplegia, and other diseases of the CNS. Extreme pyrexia does not appear to produce an increased risk for immediate death; however, many patients who survive the febrile episode subsequently succumb to underlying diseases. Among infants and young children, temperatures higher than 41°C have been observed in fewer than 1% of patients presenting to emergency departments for evaluation. Between 12% and 50% of children with hyperpyrexia will have serious bacterial infections, including pneumonia, bacteremia, and meningitis; these infections are usually caused by *Streptococcus pneumoniae, Haemophilus influenzae,* group B streptococci, or *Escherichia coli.*

In summary, although uncommon, hyperpyrexia can be a manifestation of infection in adults (and children). Consequently, if the etiology of a substantial temperature elevation is unclear at presentation, blood cultures and other routine tests to detect bacterial infection should be obtained promptly, and empiric antimicrobial therapy should be initiated. In the adult, the initial therapy should cover gram-negative bacilli (*E. coli, Klebsiella pneumoniae*) and *Staphylococcus aureus;* accordingly, a fluoroquinolone, a third-generation cephalosporin, aztreonam, or an aminoglycoside plus oxacillin or vancomycin would be appropriate. The selection of specific agents will be guided by a variety of factors, including the setting in which the pyrexia evolved (community-acquired vs. nosocomial illness), nature of underlying diseases, results of Gram's stains of clinical specimens, drug allergy history, and presence of abnormal or changing renal function.

### Hyperthermia
*Neuroleptic Malignant Syndrome*

The neuroleptic malignant syndrome represents a condition that can be confused with sepsis. An idiosyncratic reaction first described in the 1960s, the disorder remains an occasionally unrecognized and potentially lethal complication of neuroleptic drug therapy. Several observations indicate that a reduction in dopaminergic activity within the CNS plays a central role in precipitating the syndrome. First, the drugs associated with the disorder are known to be antidopaminergic, and the potential for a drug to induce the illness appears to parallel its activity as a dopamine antagonist. Second, the symptoms of the disorder can be explained by dopamine receptor blockade within the hypothalamus and basal ganglia. Finally, the manifestations of the syndrome can be treated with bromocriptine, a potent dopamine agonist. The hyperthermia appears to result from changes in the hypothalamic set point and an increase in heat production caused by a generalized contraction of muscles.

The factors that precipitate the neuroleptic malignant syndrome in susceptible persons remain poorly defined. Nevertheless, underlying conditions, such as organic brain disease, dehydration, and exhaustion, seem to predispose patients to the disorder; on occasion, an intercurrent infectious illness, such as a urinary tract infection, appears to trigger the hyperthermal episode. The importance of these precipitating factors is illustrated by the fact that most patients who experience the syndrome will not have a recurrence when rechallenged with neuroleptics.

The neuroleptic malignant syndrome usually occurs in association with the use of a dopamine-blocking agent, including a butyrophenone (haloperidol), thioxanthene (thiothixene), or phenothiazine (fluphenazine, chlorpromazine, thioridazine, perphenazine, trimeprazine, prochlorperazine); haloperidol, alone or in combination with other medications, represents the most frequently identified offending drug. Finally, the syndrome can also evolve following the withdrawal of dopamine agonists (amantadine, levodopa, carbidopa) and during treatment with dopamine-depleting drugs (tetrabenazine, α-methyltyrosine). The syndrome can appear soon after initiation of neuroleptic therapy or following dosage adjustments in patients on long-term treatment. The disorder typically occurs in patients given therapeutic doses of the drugs. Although usually seen in patients with serious psychiatric disease (schizophrenia, manic-depressive illness), the syndrome has also been reported in normal patients given neuroleptic agents as part of preinduction anesthesia or for the management of sedative-hypnotic withdrawal.

Abrupt in onset and rapidly progressing during 24 to 72 hours, the neuroleptic malignant syndrome usually begins with the appearance of involuntary movements and generalized "lead pipe" or "plastic" muscular rigidity. Dystonic movements, tremors, and facial grimacing are prominent signs. Dysarthria, dysphagia, and sialorrhea result from hypertonicity of the pharyngeal muscles. Catatonic behavior can be present. The level of consciousness fluctuates and ranges from an alert mutism to stupor or coma. Signs of autonomic dysfunction include pallor, tachycardia, labile blood pressure, profuse diaphoresis, and urinary incontinence. Hyperthermia characteristically follows the occurrence of extrapyramidal rigidity. The laboratory abnormalities are nonspecific but commonly include a leukocytosis and an elevated serum creatine phosphokinase, the latter resulting from myonecrosis induced by intense and sustained muscle contractions. Myoglobinuria can lead to acute renal failure.

Lethal catatonia should be included in the differential diagnosis of the psychiatric patient with an abnormal mental status and hyperthermia. Patients with lethal catatonia typically have a history of intense excitement, anxiety, or physical activity lasting for weeks; the initial symptoms are hallucinations, delusions, and self-destructive or assaultive behavior. The activity of the patient with lethal catatonia precludes adequate nutrition and hydration, and it leads to exhaustion. Thus, in lethal catatonia, psychosis precedes the onset of the catatonic state. In contrast to lethal catatonia, the neuroleptic malignant syndrome develops over hours to days, and the condition is not associated with severe excitement or anxiety. Because the therapy of lethal catatonia may include neuroleptic agents, the importance of excluding a diagnosis of neuroleptic malignant syndrome is apparent.

Malignant hyperthermia represents a second condition that can present with manifestations similar to those of the neuroleptic malignant syndrome. A disorder of skeletal muscle, malignant hyperthermia occurs in genetically susceptible persons. The illness is characterized by generalized muscular contractions, which produce rigidity, hyperthermia, rhabdomyolysis, hyperkalemia, and shock. Malignant hyperthermia is precipitated by exposure to halogenated inhalational anesthetics or depolarizing agents such as succinylcholine; these substances induce changes in skeletal muscle membranes, resulting in an excessive calcium influx and sustained contraction. Therapy for malignant hyperthermia is directed at relaxing the contracting muscles, and dantrolene sodium is the drug of choice.

Although the definitive therapy for the neuroleptic malignant syndrome has not been established, a number of interventions appear useful in treating the condition. The offending drugs should be withdrawn, and supportive measures should be initiated, including hydration and external cooling. Dantrolene sodium, a peripheral muscle relaxant, reduces the spasticity and related symptoms. Dantrolene can be administered by mouth or nasogastric tube at a dose of 50 to 200 mg/d or intravenously at a dose of 0.8 to 10 mg/kg daily; the initial IV dose should be 2 to 3 mg/kg daily. Bromocriptine, a dopamine agonist, usually produces a rapid resolution of all clinical manifestations of the illness; bromocriptine can be given orally or by nasogastric tube at a dose of 2.5 to 10 mg three to four times daily. On occasion, therapy with both dantrolene sodium and bromocriptine has been used with success. However, even with drug therapy, complete resolution of the problem can require 9 to 10 days. Patients who received a depot neuroleptic (fluphenazine) are at risk to experience a relapse of the syndrome; thus, they may require prolonged therapy. Pneumonia, pulmonary emboli, and soft-tissue infections can complicate the neuroleptic malignant syndrome, and these intercurrent problems should be suspected when fever persists or recurs in patients apparently cured of the disorder.

The mortality rate for patients with the neuroleptic malignant syndrome is 5% to 20%; recent case-control studies have indicated that dantrolene and bromocriptine have reduced fatality rates by approximately 50%. Because of an increased awareness of the problem and a reduced use of IM neuroleptics, the incidence of the syndrome appears to be declining. In the majority of cases, the neurologic recovery is complete; on occasion, cognitive defects secondary to CNS damage persist.

*Heatstroke*

The most common cause of hyperthermia in adults is heatstroke, a life-threatening condition that is precipitated by environmental factors and results from a failure of heat-dissipating mechanisms, especially sweating. At ambient temperatures above 35°C (95°F), heat loss becomes dependent on the evaporation of sweat. The rate of evaporation is influenced by the relative humidity and air movement; thus, as the humidity rises and air flow decreases, sweating becomes less efficient, and the body temperature tends to increase. Heat cramps and heat exhaustion are milder clinical syndromes produced by excessive environmental heat. Heatstroke typically occurs when someone is suddenly exposed to unusually hot and humid conditions for more than 48 hours. Epidemic heatstroke is observed in cities that experience cold winters followed by hot weather and high humidity during the late spring or early summer. Among the conditions that enhance susceptibility to heatstroke are advanced age, alcoholism, heart disease, obesity, incidental infection, and certain medications, especially anticholinergics and major tranquilizers (phenothiazines, butyrophenones). Military personnel, laborers, athletes, and other young adults who exercise strenuously in hot, moist environments are at risk for the development of exertional heatstroke; risk factors for this condition include heavy clothing or protective equipment, drugs that impair heat loss (including illegal agents, such as cocaine and amphetamines), obesity, poor physical condition, and volume depletion.

Most patients with heatstroke experience prodromal symptoms, such as headache, dizziness, weakness, nausea, and a feeling of warmth, for 2 to 4 days before seeking medical attention. Up to 75% of patients notice decreased sweating shortly before hospitalization. The primary manifestations of heatstroke are hyperthermia, hot and dry skin, and CNS disturbances, including delirium, stupor, and coma. Hypotension, electrolyte disturbances, renal dysfunction, and coagulation abnormalities are common findings. Rhabdomyolysis and lactic acidosis can be prominent in patients with exertional heatstroke; acute hepatic necrosis can also occur. Infection is an uncommon precipitant of heatstroke; however, pneumonia has been found at presentation in some elderly heatstroke victims, and gram-negative bacilli (*E. coli, Klebsiella, Pseudomonas*) and *S. aureus* have been isolated from these patients. On rare occasion, meningitis will also be present.

The cornerstone of therapy for heatstroke remains external, whole-body cooling. Patients should be immersed in cold water or packed in ice and massaged. These aggressive cooling measures can usually be discontinued when the core body temperature falls below 39.4°C (103°F). Ice water lavage or enemas are not recommended. Phenothiazines should not be used to control shivering, and dantrolene sodium plays no role in the management of patients with this condition. Because pooling of blood in cutaneous vessels may contribute to hypotension, fluid should be administered judiciously during the period of external cooling; if the blood pressure does not rise as the body temperature falls and following the infusion of normal saline, a Swan-Ganz catheter should be inserted to permit a more accurate assessment of fluid requirements. Complications of heatstroke, including seizures, cardiac arrhythmias, metabolic acidosis, hyperkalemia, and renal failure, also require prompt identification and therapy. Aged patients with heatstroke must be carefully evaluated for concomitant pyogenic infection, especially pneumonia. Patients who survive heatstroke can have residual neurologic sequelae; these include focal defects, such as cerebellar dysfunction or hemiplegia, and a decline in intellectual capacity, ranging from a mild confusional state to a frank dementia.

*Other Conditions*

Resembling exertional heatstroke in etiology, cocaine-associated hyperthermia appears to be triggered by a myriad of drug-related phenomena, including exaggerated physical exercise, increased sympathetic activity, impaired heat loss, and seizures. Obtundedness, rhabdomyolysis, renal failure, coagulopathy, acidosis, and hepatic injury are characteristic. External cooling represents the cornerstone of therapy. Amphetamines, phenylpropanolamine, mescaline, and phencyclidine are other illicit drugs that are associated with hyperthermia. On occasion, salicylate overdose can produce temperatures in excess of 41°C; serum salicylate levels in these cases are typically greater than 1,000 g/mL.

A few other conditions are associated with substantial temperature elevations. Temperatures above 41°C may be the primary manifestation of factitious disease. A factitious illness should be suspected in a young female patient who is a student, nurse, or medical technologist and who has an enigmatic illness that is characterized by extreme temperature elevations without concomitant tachycardia, warm skin, diaphoresis, or signs of serious systemic illness. To achieve the dramatic temperature elevations that guarantee medical attention, patients with factitious fever often heat the thermometer by exposing it to a lamp or immersing it in hot water. Finally, tetanus, the toxic shock syndrome, CNS diseases (tumors, encephalitis, hemorrhage), and endocrine disorders (thyroid storm, pheochromocytoma) will occasionally produce temperatures exceeding 41°C. (A.L.E.)

## Bibliography

Allen GC, Rosenberg H. Pheochromocytoma presenting as acute malignant hyperthermia—a diagnostic challenge. *Can J Anaesth* 1990;37:593.
*Surgical anesthesia can trigger a pheochromocytoma-related crises.*

Bennett MH, Wainwright AP. Acute thyroid crisis on induction of anaesthesia. *Anaesthesia* 1989;44:28.
*Hyperthyroidism and hyperthermia can be precipitated by anesthesia.*

Bonadio WA, Grunske L, Smith DS. Systemic bacterial infections in children with fever greater than 41°C. *Pediatr Infect Dis J* 1989;8:120.
*In this retrospective review of 108 children with temperatures greater than 41°C evaluated in an emergency department, 12% had serious bacterial infections, including 3% with meningitis.*

Castillo E, Rubin RT, Holsboer-Trachsler E. Clinical differentiation between lethal catatonia and neuroleptic malignant syndrome. *Am J Psychiatry* 1989;146:324.
*A detailed and extensively referenced discussion of these distinct but potentially confused conditions.*

Chan TC, Evans SD, Clark RF. Drug-induced hyperthermia. *Crit Care Clin* 1997;13:785.
*The authors provide a review of malignant hyperthermia, neuroleptic malignant syndrome, sympathomimetic poisoning, and anticholinergic toxicity.*

Delaney KA. Heatstroke. Underlying processes and life-saving management. *Postgrad Med* 1992;91:379.
*A contemporary review of the problem and its management.*

Dinarello CA. Thermoregulation and the pathogenesis of fever. *Infect Dis Clin North Am* 1996;10:433.
*A contemporary review of the mechanisms involved in the generation of fever, with emphasis on cytokines and the acute-phase response.*

Dubois EF. Why are fever temperatures over 106°F rare? *Am J Med Sci* 1949;117:361.
*In an analysis of 357 patients with serious infectious diseases, only 4.3% of 1,761 temperature recordings were 41°C or higher.*

Freund PR, Sharar SR. Hyperthermia alert caused by unrecognized temperature monitor malfunction. *J Clin Monit* 1990;6:257.
*The failure of electronic thermometers or monitoring devices can produce very high temperature recordings.*

Graham BS, et al. Nonexertional heatstroke. Physiologic management and cooling in 14 patients. *Arch Intern Med* 1986;146:87.
*Treated with a standard protocol that included the use of ice, a tepid water spray, massage, and a fan, the patients experienced rapid cooling, a low mortality rate, and complete neurologic recovery.*

Hantson P, et al. Hyperthermia complicating tricyclic antidepressant overdose. *Intensive Care Med* 1996;22:453.
*The authors describe a middle-aged patient whose core body temperature rose above 43°C following an amitryptyline overdose.*

Heiman-Patterson TD. Neuroleptic malignant syndrome and malignant hyperthermia: important issues for the medical consultant. *Med Clin North Am* 1993;77:477.
*The author provides a useful approach to the patient suspected of having these conditions.*

Juul A, Skakkebaek NE. Growth hormone deficiency and hyperthermia. *Lancet* 1991;338:887.
*Growth hormone deficiency is associated with reduced sweating, a condition that can lead to hyperthermia.*

Keck P, Pope H, McElroy S. Declining frequency of neuroleptic malignant syndrome in a hospital population. *Am J Psychiatry* 1991;148:880.
*The investigators document a significant fall in the incidence of the disorder at one psychiatric center; they attribute the decline in attack rate to a reduction in the use of IM neuroleptics.*

Milroy CM, et al. Pathology of deaths associated with ecstasy and eve misuse. *J Clin Pathol* 1996;49:149.
*The amphetamine derivatives, ecstasy and eve, can cause hyperthermia, liver necrosis, cerebral and cardiac injury, and death.*

Plattner O, et al. Efficacy of intraoperative cooling methods. *Anesthesiology* 1997;87:1089–1095.
*In this study with six healthy volunteers, the authors compared heat transfer and cooling rates with five techniques (circulating water mattress, forced cold air, gastric lavage, bladder lavage, and immersion in ice water); immersion in ice water slurry produced the most rapid rate of heat loss and the largest decrease in core body temperature.*

Pope H, et al. Neuroleptic malignant syndrome: long-term follow-up of 20 cases. *J Clin Psychiatry* 1991;52:208.
*Of 20 patients who experienced the disorder, 11 resumed neuroleptic therapy and had no recurrence, which indicates that factors beyond the drugs contributed to evolution of the syndrome.*

Rosenberg J, et al. Hyperthermia associated with drug intoxication. *Crit Care Med* 1986;14:964.
*The authors describe 12 patients with hyperthermia resulting from intoxication with stimulants, anticholinergics, salicylates, or combinations of these drugs; five died, and four had severe neurologic sequelae.*

Rosenberg MR, Green M. Neuroleptic malignant syndrome. *Arch Intern Med* 1989;149:1927.
*This detailed analysis of the published data concerning the efficacy of dantrolene and bromocriptine concludes that the addition of either agent to supportive management shortens the time to clinical response from 6.8 days to approximately 1 day.*

Sakkas P, et al. Drug treatment of neuroleptic malignant syndrome. *Psychopharmacol Bull* 1991;27:381.
*In this retrospective analysis, the mortality rate for the controls was found to be 21%; for patients treated with dantrolene or bromocriptine, the rates were 8.6% and 7.8%, respectively.*

Simon HB. Extreme pyrexis. *JAMA* 1976;236:2419.
*Of 28 patients with hyperpyrexia seen at the Massachusetts General Hospital between 1970 and 1975, 71% had an infectious illness, usually caused by a gram-negative bacillus.*

Simon HB. Hyperthermia. *N Engl J Med* 1993;329:483.
*An overview of the physiology of temperature regulation and a discussion of selected conditions associated with hyperthermia.*

van Harten PN, Kemperman CJ. Organic amnestic disorder: a long-term sequel after neuroleptic malignant syndrome. *Biol Psychiatry* 1991; 29:407.
*The authors review long-lasting cognitive impairments experienced by some patients with neuroleptic malignant syndrome.*

Walter FG, et al. Marijuana and hyperthermia. *J Toxicol Clin Toxicol* 1996;34:217.
*The authors report the first case of hyperthermia associated with marijuana use and jogging.*

## 53. FEVER IN THE GRANULOCYTOPENIC PATIENT

Granulocytopenia is associated with conditions as diverse as hematologic malignancy and its treatment, adverse reactions to medications, selected infections, and hereditary disorders. Although fever can be associated with any of these, it is most feared when complicating leukemia and other hematologic malignancies.

Granulocytopenia *per se* is associated with infections caused by *Staphylococcus aureus,* selected enteric gram-negative bacilli, (especially *Escherichia coli* and *Klebsiella* species), *Pseudomonas aeruginosa, Candida* species, and *Aspergillus* species. Hairy-cell leukemia, indwelling Foley or IV catheters, and chemotherapy are associated with risks for other pathogens. In the 1990s, such risks have especially been noted with indwelling IV lines and have resulted in a major increase in the number of gram-positive infections identified. These may be associated with coagulase-negative staphylococci, diphtheroids, and *viridans* streptococci. Often, these organisms are resistant to commonly employed β-lactam antibiotics. On occasion, fever can be explained by noninfectious processes (underlying malignancy, recent administration of pyrogens, or drug fever), but often it is a consequence of infections that not only are associated with considerable morbidity in the leukemic patient but are also the most important cause of death.

Although at least 40% of patients with fever and neutropenia demonstrate no source of infection, they may clinically improve with antibiotics. The likelihood of response to initial antibiotics reaches 95% for those with neutropenia of less than 7 days' duration, but it is only 32% in those with fever and neutropenia for longer than 2 weeks. The risk for infection varies directly with both duration of granulocytopenia and rate of decline, and inversely with the absolute granulocyte count. With regard to acute leukemia, infections are noted more commonly during relapse and when granulocyte counts are below $100/mm^3$.

Fever above 101°F for more than 2 hours that is not associated with the administration of known pyrogens represents infection until proved otherwise.The diagnosis of infection in the granulocytopenic host is made difficult by subtleties of signs and symptoms. Frank pus is rarely encountered because polymorphonuclear leukocytes are necessary for its production. Host responses to infection may be blunted, but pain and fever are usually preserved. Thus, the afebrile patient is unlikely to be infected. Patients with pharyngitis may have pain and erythema without exudate. Skin and anorectal infections demonstrate erythema and local pain but usually lack prominent local heat, swelling, exudate, fluctuation, or regional adenopathy. Urinary tract infections often occur in the absence of irritative voiding symptoms (dysuria, frequency, urgency) and pyuria. Classic hallmarks of pneumonia (cough, sputum production, rales, and clinical consolidation) are frequently not observed. As a general rule, fever attributable to leukemia, drugs, and other noninfectious causes is usually not associated with rigors or hypotension. Alternatively, shaking chills or a "toxic" appearance indicates probable infection, possibly bacteremia.

### Evaluation

Evaluation begins with a comprehensive history and physical examination. The history can provide evidence of localized discomfort. Sore throat associated with fever and pharyngeal ulceration caused by antineoplastic drugs may be early signs of bacteremia resulting from *P. aeruginosa* or infection with herpes simplex. Dysphagia suggests esophagitis caused by *Candida* species, herpes simplex, or other potential pathogens. Painful defecation can alert the physician to perirectal cellulitis or phlegmon, often involving *P. aeruginosa* and anaerobes. Fever, vomiting, abdominal pain, and abdominal tenderness may be symptoms of typhlitis (inflammation of the cecum) or pseudomembranous colitis from either underlying leukemia or antibiotics.

Physical examination should be meticulous and repeated often. Special attention should be directed toward painful or erythematous skin and anorectal lesions, pharyngeal erythema, periodontal inflammation, sinus tenderness, and rales. Skin lesions of ecthyma gangrenosum (classically, necrotic centers with surrounding areolae, but having many variants) indicate probable gram-negative bacteria, often *P. aeruginosa*. Such lesions provide sources for biopsy and culture, often yielding rapid bacteriologic information. Periodontal infection is manifested by local tenderness and fever accompanied by minimal signs and symptoms of inflammation. Careful attention should be paid to indwelling lines. Redness and swelling may be the only indications of infection. Up to 50% of line-related bacteremias may present without localized clinical evidence of infection.

Urine cultures, several sets of blood cultures, and chest roentgenography are indicated in the initial assessment. However, because of granulocytopenia, Gram's stains (of urine, sputum, other specimens) may fail to demonstrate polymorphonuclear leukocytes. With pneumonia, radiographic evidence is usually present, although findings may be subtle. The presence of lung necrosis generally indicates pneumonia associated with gram-negative enteric bacilli, *S. aureus,* or *Aspergillus* or *Mucor.* Other cultures and x-ray imaging should be obtained as clinically indicated. Routine surveillance cultures of nasal secretions, stool, and other specimens are not generally recommended.

The bacteriology of infections in the granulocytopenic patient includes facultative gram-positive and gram-negative organisms. Anaerobes are uncommonly implicated, except in anorectal infections, where they predominate and require specific therapy. Gram-negative pathogens commonly demonstrated include *E. coli, Klebsiella* species, *Enterobacter,* and *P. aeruginosa.* The frequent use of indwelling venous access devices has been associated with a resurgence of gram-positive infections caused by *S. aureus, Staphylococcus epidermidis,* streptococci, and occasionally others. Fungal infections are usually noted in patients who are maintained for a long time on broad-spectrum antimicrobials and have prolonged neutropenia. Although *Aspergillus* and *Candida* species have been classically implicated, recent studies demonstrate the possibility of infection with diverse organisms that include *Trichosporon beigelii, Fusarium* species, *Geotrichum candidum,* and *Pseudallescheria boydii.* Infection with these more unusual species is often associated with sinusitis, deep-organ involvement, or fungemia. Risk factors for adverse outcome include prolonged neutropenia and organ involvement.

### Therapy

Selected neutropenic patients with fever may be safely managed as outpatients. This concept has been promulgated in part because of the availability of oral antipseudomonal antibiotics, and the availability of an infrastructure that allows for IV therapy outside the hospital. Table 53-1 summarizes the risk stratification of patients with fever and neutropenia. Table 53-2 summarizes the indications for outpatient therapy of febrile neutropenic patients. Forty percent to 60% of patients fall into the category of those who can be safely treated outside the hospital. Patients at low risk for adverse outcome from fever and leukopenia generally do not have uncontrolled cancer and concurrent associated problems requiring hospitalization. In the absence of these features, complications were noted in only 2% of patients, and mortality approached zero. On the basis of similar parameters, patients may be safely discharged to home to complete therapy with either IV or oral antibiotics. All patients receiving outpatient therapy should live within a reasonable distance of the medical center where treatment is being administered. Some centers require this to be no more than 30 miles. Daily follow-up by telephone is indicated, and the patients must have accessibility to a health care provider.

Treatment of the febrile neutropenic outpatient may be with either oral or parenteral antibiotics. Fluoroquinolones (generally ciprofloxacin or ofloxacin) have been

Table 53-1.  Risk stratification for febrile, neutropenic patients

| Risk group | Features | Morbidity/mortality |
|---|---|---|
| I | Develops in hospital | Mortality, 13% |
| II | Outpatients with hypotension, altered sensoria, respiratory failure, bleeding | Serious complications in 40%; mortality, 12% |
| III | Outpatients without comorbidity but with uncontrolled cancer | Serious complication in 25%; mortality, 18% |
| IV | Stable outpatients | Serious complications in 3%; mortality, 0% |

Table 53-2.  Patients with fever and neutropenia: candidates for outpatient therapy

Patients lack:

Hypotension (blood pressure <90 systolic)
Tachypnea (respiratory rate >30/min)
Renal insufficiency (serum creatinine >2.5, or creatinine clearance <50 mL/min)
Hyponatremia (serum sodium <128 mg/dL)
Altered liver function tests (serum transaminases >4 times normal)
Uncontrolled hypercalcemia
Altered sensorium

the primary oral antibiotics studied, either alone or in conjunction with either clindamycin or amoxicillin-clavulanate. Response rates of approximately 90% have been noted in many studies after appropriate cultures have been obtained. The optimal antimicrobial therapy is unknown.

A recent retrospective investigation demonstrated that the average patient receives approximately five agents per course, which entails greatly excessive use (based on bacteriologic and clinical indications of infection) and expense and enhances the potential for renal and hepatic toxicity. Selection of an initial antimicrobial therapy should be based on such factors as local pathogens and their antimicrobial susceptibilities, allergy and organ failure, and adjunctive medications. Initial therapy should consist of broad-spectrum bactericidal agents. Controversy continues regarding combination therapy versus monotherapy. Numerous studies now demonstrate the efficacy of broad-spectrum antibiotics (imipenemcilastatin, meropenem, ceftazidime, cefepime) as monotherapy in the uncomplicated patient. However, many centers continue to recommend combinations that include double β-lactams (e.g., ceftazidime plus piperacillin) or β-lactams plus aminoglycosides (e.g., piperacillin or ceftazidime plus gentamicin, tobramycin, or amikacin). If aminoglycosides are employed, a loading dose of more than 2 mg/kg should be used to optimize initial levels. Use of 5-7 mg/kg as a single daily dose should be strongly considered. When *P. aeruginosa* is strongly considered (e.g., based on epidemiology, presence of ecthyma gangrenosum), two effective antipseudomonal agents are always indicated.

The need for vancomycin in the initial regimen remains controversial. Initial data strongly suggested it was not needed. However, this issue is undergoing reassessment as the role of serious gram-positive infection increases (primarily because of the use of long-standing invasive IV devices in many patients) and methicillin-resistant staphylococci become more frequently encountered. Vancomycin should be employed in the initial antibiotic regimen at institutions where fulminant gram-positive infections have been observed. It may be used when the likelihood of catheter-related infection is high, in patients in whom fever and neutropenia develop while they are on quinolone prophylaxis, in patients known to be colonized with methicillin-resistant *S. aureus* or highly penicillin-resistant *Streptococcus pneumoniae,* or in critically ill patients when failure to cover a pathogen could lead to rapid death.

After initial treatment, 3 days are generally needed to define etiology and response to therapy. Further management strategies are guided by these parameters.

Vancomycin should be discontinued from an initial regimen if cultures fail to substantiate its need. If clinical improvement is noted and cultures define a pathogen, therapy should be optimized, but broad-spectrum therapy should be continued. If the patient improves in the absence of a defined organism, therapy should be maintained for at least a week. Stable, compliant patients who can be monitored as outpatients can be switched to oral antibiotics (quinolone, cefixime).

Failure to improve within 3 to 5 days requires meticulous reassessment of the patient and usually an antimicrobial change. Occult sites of infection should be sought. Computed tomography scanning of the abdomen with percutaneous sampling of collections is expeditious and reasonably well tolerated. A recent review of the role of radionuclide imaging in immunosuppressed patients points out the benefits and pitfalls of these modalities. Gallium may not be picked up at infection sites in neutropenic patients, and its accumulation in the bowel may make for difficult interpretations. Most radionuclide modalities take several days for complete evaluations, and this limits their usefulness in critically ill patients.

If no site of infection can be identified after 5 to 7 days, empiric addition of amphotericin B is indicated. The maximum dose is 0.5 to 1.0 mg/kg per day. Up to 50% of patients will respond clinically to this treatment, although the source of infection may not be identified. The results of fungal antigen detection tests are not reliable, and blood cultures are positive in fewer than 40% of patients with fungal infections documented by other means. Fluconazole remains a controversial alternative to amphotericin; it could be used with care in patients who are at hospitals where problems with *Aspergillus* and *Mucor* are limited, have not received prior fluconazole prophylaxis, and are unlikely to tolerate amphotericin B. However, a recent pilot study comparing fluconazole with amphotericin B in patients with antibiotic-resistant neutropenic fever demonstrated a poorer response with fluconazole and a significantly higher tendency toward the development of invasive fungal disease. Several forms of liposomal amphotericin B have been approved for use in the United States. All have the advantage of allowing higher dosing with enhanced safety—typically up to 5 mg/kg versus 1 mg/kg with amphotericin B. Their major role appears to be in the management of mold infections (*Aspergillus* and *Mucor*) and of patients in whom significant intolerance to amphotericin has developed. Their high price precludes routine use at this time.

For patients who do not clinically respond to initial antimicrobial therapy, current recommendations do not include careful discontinuation of therapy within the first week. However, some would cautiously curtail antimicrobials if the patient is stable and without clinical infection. With the addition of amphotericin B, broad-spectrum antimicrobials should be modified to delete aminoglycosides to decrease the likelihood of nephrotoxicity. Antiviral therapy with acyclovir (herpes simplex, herpes zoster) or ganciclovir (cytomegalovirus) is indicated for proven or suspected infections but is not recommended empirically.

Antimicrobial chemotherapy is generally continued until granulocyte counts have risen above 500 to 1,000/mm$^3$. Alternatively, treatment may be carefully terminated in selected patients who are clinically stable and without signs of infection.

Colony-stimulating factors, such as granulocyte colony-stimulating factor (G-CSF) and granulocyte-macrophage colony-stimulating factor (GM-CSF), have been employed to shorten the duration of neutropenia following chemotherapy for solid tumors and hematologic malignancies. Several studies have now demonstrated decreased antimicrobial needs, decreased hospital stays, and shortened neutropenic periods when colony-stimulating factors are employed. However, mortality related to infection has not been shown to be reduced. Additionally, most patients respond favorably without them, and they are expensive. Colony-stimulating factors should be considered in selected patients with severe infection, a poor likelihood of rapid marrow recovery, and a poor response to appropriate antimicrobials.

Bacteremia associated with indwelling venous access devices can often be treated without removal of the device. Indications for removal include "tunnel" infections, infections caused by fungi or *Corynebacterium jeikeium,* failure to respond, or clinical relapse.

Focal hepatic candidiasis usually presents with ongoing fever in the face of resolving neutropenia. Abdominal pain, nausea, and diarrhea occasionally may be noted. Focal hepatic candidiasis often presents as a manifestation of more widespread disease. Striking elevations of the serum alkaline phosphatase have been noted. Hepatic defects are sometimes detected on computed tomography or ultrasonography, but the yield is higher without neutropenia. Liver biopsy confirms the diagnosis, but cultures may be negative if prior antifungal therapy has been rendered. Prolonged intensive parenteral therapy with amphotericin B (total dose >2 g) is the preferred treatment. Several recent studies with fluconazole demonstrate its utility for this syndrome. Dosages have been 100 to 400 mg daily for a median of 30 weeks. Fluconazole has also been used for patients who have failed amphotericin B therapy or have demonstrated intolerable side effects from that agent. (R.B.B.)

### Bibliography

Crawford J, et al. Reduction by granulocyte colony-stimulating factor of fever and neutropenia induced by chemotherapy in patients with small-cell lung cancer. *N Engl J Med* 1991;315:164–170.

*This is one of several published studies on the efficacy of colony-stimulating factors in aborting fever and neutropenia in cancer patients who are receiving chemotherapy. This double-blind placebo-controlled investigation demonstrated that G-CSF decreases fever and infection in patients receiving chemotherapy for small-cell carcinoma of the lung. Fever and neutropenia were noted in 77% of controls but in only 40% of those who received G-CSF. Duration of cell counts below 500/mm³ was 6 days (control) versus 1 day (G-CSF). Number of infections, duration of hospitalization, and need for antimicrobials were all significantly decreased in the G-CSF group.*

EORTC International Antimicrobial Therapy Cooperative Group and the National Cancer Institute of Canada—Clinical Trials Group. Vancomycin added to empirical combination antibiotic therapy for fever in granulocytopenic cancer patients. *J Infect Dis* 1991;163:951–958.

*Febrile neutropenic patients were randomized to receive ceftazidime plus amikacin with or without vancomycin for empiric therapy. The outcome of patients with gram-positive bacteremias was not improved by the addition of vancomycin, and no patients with gram-positive bacteremia in the absence of vancomycin died within the first 3 days. Patients who received vancomycin had greater nephrotoxicity. The authors do not feel that vancomycin is a required part of an initial regimen but could be safely used later if infection caused by a susceptible pathogen is identified.*

Glenn J, et al. Anorectal infections in patients with malignant diseases. *Rev Infect Dis* 1988;10:42–52.

*This is a retrospective review of approximately 60 patients with anorectal infection documented at a tertiary care cancer hospital. The infection itself was associated with death in fewer than 10% of cases. Most cases were associated with a polymicrobial flora that often involved anaerobes. More than 50% of cases were successfully managed with medical therapy alone. Treatment with an aminoglycoside and an antianaerobic agent was usually employed. Indications for surgery included presence of necrotic material, fluctuance, and failure to respond to antimicrobials.*

Holleran WM, Wilbur JR, DeGregorio MW. Empiric amphotericin B therapy in patients with acute leukemia. *Rev Infect Dis* 1985;7:619–624.

*This excellent overview of several aspects of fungal infections in acute leukemia addresses risk factors, clinical presentation, and justification for empiric therapy with amphotericin B. Clinical response is often noted. Dosing should maximize at 0.5 mg/kg per day, and treatment is generally discontinued on recovery of granulocytes.*

Hughes WT, et al. 1997 Guidelines for the use of antimicrobial agents in neutropenic patients with unexplained fever. *Clin Infect Dis* 1997;25:551–573.

*The Infectious Diseases Society of America published this first in a series of guidelines to aid clinicians in decision making. This document addresses most of the important issues in the management of the febrile neutropenic patient and provides excellent treatment strategies and algorithms that are easy to follow. It also provides alternatives based on the literature. This is an excellent single reference on the subject.*

Malik IA, et al. Feasibility of outpatient management of fever in cancer patients with low-risk neutropenia: results of a prospective randomized trial. *Am J Med* 1995;98:224–231.

*One hundred subjects were inpatients or outpatients. Results demonstrated equal efficacy statistically; however, 21% of the outpatients required hospitalization. Carefully chosen patients with fever and leukopenia can be safely managed outside the hospital. The best antibiotic is not determined. Use of a quinolone should be reserved for those who have not received these agents as prophylaxis.*

Powderly WG, et al. Amphotericin B-resistant yeast infection in severely immunocompromised patients. *Am J Med* 1988;84:826–832.

*Recent isolates of* Candida *species from immunocompromised patients may be more resistant to amphotericin B than similar isolates from patients who are immunocompetent. When resistance is encountered, the outcome is dismal. These findings stress the need for better sensitivity testing of antifungal agents and the availability of suitable alternatives to amphotericin B.*

Ramphal R, et al. Clinical experience with single-agent and combination regimens in the management of infection in the febrile neutropenic patient. *Am J Med* 1996;100(6A):83S–89S.

Cefepime is a fourth-generation cephalosporin similar to ceftazidime but with enhanced stability against selected enteric bacilli and better gram-positive activity. Febrile neutropenic patients were randomized to receive either cefepime as monotherapy or combination antibiotic therapy. Bacterial infections were documented in 40% of patients in both groups. Outcomes as measured by fever resolution, need for alternative therapies, and survival were similar in both groups. This is another study demonstrating that for most febrile neutropenic patients, monotherapy is sufficient. There are now several appropriate agents from which to choose. I would still employ combination therapy for patients at high risk for infection with P. aeruginosa (i.e., those with ecthyma gangrenosum lesions, known positive blood cultures), but in most other instances monotherapy will suffice.

Rolston KV, Rubenstein EB, Freifeld A. Early empiric antibiotic therapy for febrile neutropenic patients at low risk. *Infect Dis Clin North Am* 1996;10:223–237.
*The authors present an excellent summary of the indications and choices for antibiotic therapy in the low-risk patient. Options run from therapy without hospitalization, to early switch from IV to oral antibiotics, to use of home IV therapy. Determinants of low-risk patients are provided.*

Rubin RH, Fischman AJ. Radionuclide imaging of infection in the immunocompromised host. *Clin Infect Dis* 1996;22:414–422.
*The authors provide a succinct report on the advantages and pitfalls of radionuclide imaging in immunosuppressed patients. Such processes are of limited value in the diagnosis of infections below the diaphragm, and in the presence of neutropenia. They can occasionally be useful in patients with chest infections and may help target further studies in patients with unexplained fevers.*

Talcott JA, et al. The medical course of cancer patients with fever and neutropenia. *Arch Intern Med* 1988;148:2561–2568.
*This interesting retrospective analysis of patients with fever and neutropenia attempts to identify populations that may require less intensive care and evaluation. The authors conclude that in many patients complications are unlikely to develop; the risk factors include concurrent morbidities and uncontrolled cancer.*

## 54. FEVER OF UNKNOWN ORIGIN

In 1961, Petersdorf and Beeson defined the clinical syndrome of fever of unknown origin (FUO) as continuous fever of at least 3 weeks' duration, with temperatures of 101°F or more, that remains unexplained despite 1 week of complete investigation. Using this definition, the authors studied 100 patients at a university teaching hospital. This study, which divided the causes of FUO into infections, malignancy, and rheumatic diseases and described drug fevers, factitious fevers, and cranial arteritis as additional diagnoses, demonstrated that patients may often present with atypical manifestations of common diseases. The authors recommended no one battery of tests and discouraged therapeutic trials unless treatment was directed at a particular disease. Biopsy specimens were frequently required for specific diagnosis.

Petersdorf and colleagues looked again at FUO between the years 1970 and 1980. This second study, of 105 patients, was somewhat different from the initial one of 20 years earlier:

1. Neoplastic disease became the most common cause of FUO. Most neoplastic cases were secondary to Hodgkin's or non-Hodgkin's lymphoma. In these cases, peripheral lymphadenopathy was absent, and disease was confined to retroperitoneal nodes or the liver. Patients were usually elderly. Not all recent studies support the high incidence of malignancy. Knockaert et al., in a study from Belgium, found tumor to be a less important cause of FUO in a 1980–1989 prospective series.

2. Bacterial endocarditis, which caused 5 of 100 cases of FUO in the first study, did not occur in any patient during the 1970–1980 study. Better culture methods, echocar-

diography, and appreciation of the causes of culture-negative endocarditis may explain this change. Tuberculosis also became less common. Biliary tract infection continued to be an important cause of FUO, even in an era of better imaging techniques.

3. Rheumatic fever was a cause of FUO in only one patient in the second study, compared with six patients in the first. However, rheumatic fever has reemerged in some parts of the United States in the past several years; young clinicians who are unfamiliar with the disease might overlook it as a cause of fever.

4. Systemic lupus erythematosus is no longer a cause of FUO owing to better serologic methods.

5. Cytomegalovirus caused FUO in four patients in the second study and in none in the first. Patients presented with a mononucleosis-like syndrome, had self-limited disease, and had often undergone transfusion or coronary artery bypass surgery.

Continued technologic improvements make some types of FUO less common. Progress in transesophageal echocardiography has made endocarditis increasingly less common as a cause of FUO. Improved methods of computed tomography (CT) and magnetic resonance imaging (MRI) make it possible for most intraabdominal abscesses to be diagnosed in less than 3 weeks. Better serologic tests have made most collagen vascular diseases less likely to become FUOs.

There are relatively few important new causes of FUO. Cunha describes histiocytic necrotizing adenitis (Kikuchi's syndrome) and hypergammagobulinemia IgD syndrome, but these diseases are rare.

As noted by Cunha, the workup of a patient with FUO is now usually performed on an outpatient basis. Although procedures such as bone marrow biopsy, transesophageal echocardiography, liver biopsy, and CT or MRI are now easily performed in an outpatient setting, the overall evaluation must be organized in a logical order and completed in a timely manner. Factors such as the overall toxicity of the patient, vital signs during febrile episodes, and rate of weight loss may help determine whether the workup requires a period of hospitalization. In general, basic aspects of the evaluation, such as history and physical examination, CBC count, erythrocyte sedimentation rate, blood cultures, liver function tests, and urinalysis, should be completed before hospitalization.

The rising incidence of tuberculosis in the United States will likely be reflected in more cases of this disease presenting as FUO. The enhancing or boosting phenomenon in serial tuberculin testing will help exclude false-negative tests. Elderly patients in particular may have a positive purified protein derivative (PPD) test result when given a second test 1 week after a negative result on the first test. When tuberculosis presents as an FUO, it will usually be associated with miliary disease. Disseminated pulmonary lesions may be so small that they are not appreciated on chest x-ray films. This is particularly likely to occur in the elderly.

Extrapulmonary tuberculosis may also present as FUO, although better imaging techniques should help in the diagnosis. Sterile pyuria in a patient with an FUO should suggest renal tuberculosis. In some cases, the urinary sediment may be unremarkable but the urine culture is positive. Tuberculosis of mesenteric lymph nodes may present without abdominal pain but can be diagnosed by abdominal CT scan. Tuberculosis of the endometrium and fallopian tubes usually causes fever and menstrual irregularities. Tuberculous pericarditis should be suggested by changing cardiac silhouette on chest x-ray films, with confirmation of pericardial effusion on echocardiogram.

The literature on the FUO syndrome has recognized that the problem varies with the patient population studied. Durack and Street have redefined FUO to include (a) classic FUO, (b) nosocomial FUO, (c) neutropenic FUO, and (d) HIV-associated FUO. FUO that develops in a hospitalized patient, although not well studied, requires a different approach than does classic FUO. The history and physical examination, particularly in the ICU setting, may be less reliable, making clinical diagnosis more difficult. Diseases causing FUO may include pulmonary embolism, transfusion-related hepatitis or cytomegalovirus infection, drug fever, IV line infection, intubation-related sinusitis, or *Clostridium difficile* colitis. FUO in neutropenic patients requires a modification in definition. These fevers of unknown cause occur abruptly and tend not to be prolonged, as patients usually respond to treatment or succumb to infection. Unlike the treatment of classic FUO, empiric treatment of neutropenic FUO must be begun quickly. Most cases of FUO in neutropenic patients are bacterial infections without an obvious source. Disseminated candidemia and aspergillosis are also common. Careful, repeated physical examination, including examination of the anorectal area, is important. FUO is extremely common in AIDS patients, although it has not been studied well as an entity. Fever may be caused by HIV infection itself. *Mycobacterium avium-intracellulare* infection, tuberculosis, and cytomegalovirus infection are among the common causes of FUO in AIDS patients, often taking weeks to declare themselves as clinical entities. *Salmonella* infection, fungal infection, and lymphoma are also well described.

Several studies have assessed FUO in the elderly patient population (Table 54-1). Giant-cell arteritis was responsible in 16% of elderly patients with classically defined FUO in one study. This syndrome may include headaches, transient visual loss, and polymyalgia rheumatica symptoms. Respiratory tract symptoms of cough, sore throat, and hoarseness have been more recently described. The temporal artery may be tender, nodular, and pulseless. Often in the FUO patient, these symptoms are not prominent and may be absent altogether. The erythrocyte sedimentation rate is almost always very high in giant-cell arteritis; however, an elevated erythrocyte sedimentation rate is common in many cases of FUO. Temporal biopsy is the diagnostic intervention of choice when the disease is suspected. Results of empiric therapy with steroids may be dramatic and is indicated when vision is threatened. However, a definitive diagnosis is necessary to justify long-term steroid therapy.

Biliary tract and intraabdominal infection are also common causes of FUO in the elderly. Hepatic abscess, cholecystitis, and empyema of the gallbladder may present with fever alone, particularly in the debilitated patient.

Weinstein has described the clinically benign FUO syndrome. These patients may have persistent fever that is clinically unimportant. Temperature elevation may be minimal or reach 102°F to 104°F. Despite persistent fever, patients generally appear well nourished. Malaise and aching joints are common for patients with low-grade fever. Diurnal variations, ovulation, use of tobacco and chewing gum, and exercise can cause these low-grade fevers. In patients who appear well but have a high-grade fever, drugs, occupational exposures, and metabolic disorders may be causative.

Another subcategory of FUO has been defined by Knockaert. Some patients have recurrent or episodic fevers that may last months or years. Subacute cholangitis, chronic prostatitis, adults Still's disease, and familial Mediterranean fever are common diagnoses in these patients.

Mackowiak has reviewed the characteristics of drug-induced fever, an increasingly common problem. Fifty-one episodes of drug fever and 97 cases from the literature were analyzed. Hectic fever patterns and shaking chills were common. Rashes were seen in only 18% of patients and eosinophilia in 22%. The time between initiation of the drug and development of fever averaged 8 days. Patients tended to tolerate drug fever well, and exaggerated or dangerous reactions did not develop when the patients were rechallenged. Antimicrobials appear to be becoming a more common cause of drug fever in several studies.

When FUO is studied in a community hospital, the etiologies may be somewhat different than in a referral hospital. Pulmonary emboli and alcoholic hepatitis may cause prolonged fever in this setting, whereas illnesses such as familial Mediterranean fever will be rare. One recent study finds AIDS and Lyme disease to be causes of FUO in a community hospital.

Table 54-1.  Causes of fever of unknown origin in the elderly

---

Giant-cell arteritis
Intraabdominal abscess
Lymphoma
Tuberculosis
Pulmonary emboli
Drug fever

---

Recent literature on the FUO syndrome has focused on the role of imaging in diagnosis. Schmidt et al., using granulocyte scintigraphy with indium 111, studied 32 patients who had at least 3 weeks of unexplained fever. Focal infections were identified in five patients—four with abdominal infection and one with dental abscess. Intestinal activity was observed in one patient found to have Whipple's disease. McNeil et al. prospectively compared CT, ultrasound, and gallium imaging in patients thought to have a focal source of sepsis. The diagnoses of the patient population studied were uncertain after standard diagnostic evaluation. All three modalities had a similar ability to detect sepsis, but sensitivity was increased by the use of any two. Rowland and Del Bene studied the impact of CT in the workup of FUO. They found that CT reduced the incidence of biopsy of normal tissue, with CT of the abdomen often correctly directing the investigation to laparotomy.

Several authors have proposed algorithms and standard workup for FUO. However, history, physical examination, and clinical judgment will continue to dictate a patient-oriented approach to the diagnosis of this syndrome. (S.L.B.)

## Bibliography

Brusch JL, Weinstein L. Fever of unknown origin. *Med Clin North Am* 1988;72:1247.
  *Basic review of FUO that includes many clinical insights and contains an interesting section on miscellaneous causes.*
Chang JC. NSAID test to distinguish between infectious and neoplastic fever in cancer patients. *Postgrad Med* 1988;84:71.
  *Nonsteroidal antiinflammatory drugs are helpful in distinguishing FUO of malignancy from that of infection; they have an antipyretic effect only in tumor patients.*
Chang JC. Neoplastic fever: a proposal for diagnosis. *Arch Intern Med* 1989;149:1728.
  *Proposes criteria for the diagnosis of fever caused by cancer. Some would disagree with the use of empiric antimicrobial therapy in the FUO setting.*
Chang JC, Gross HM. Utility of naproxen in the differential diagnosis of fever of undetermined origin in patients with cancer. *Am J Med* 1984;76:597.
  *Of 15 patients with neoplastic fever, 14 responded to naproxen. None of five cases of infectious fever resolved.*
Cunha BA. Fever of unknown origin. *Infect Dis Clin North Am* 1996;10:111.
  *Updates the causes of FUO and describes the ambulatory workup appropriate for most patients. Categorizes diseases by laboratory abnormality, history, and physical examination clues.*
Dinarello CA, Wolff SM. Molecular basis of fever in humans. *Am J Med* 1982;72:799.
  *Insights into the pathogenesis of fever are useful in the understanding of FUO.*
Drenth JPH, et al. Hyperimmunoglobulinemia D and periodic fever syndrome. *Medicine* 1994;73:133.
  *This syndrome presents with prolonged fevers, arthritis of large joints, and rash. Serum levels of IgD are greater than 100 U/mL.*
Durack DT, Street AC. Fever of unknown origin reexamined and redefined. In: Remington JS, Swartz MN, eds. *Current clinical topics infectious disease.* New York: McGraw-Hill, 1990.
  *Redefines FUO based on patient group. Categories of FUO include classic, nosocomial, neutropenic, and FUO in HIV-positive patients.*
Gartner JC Jr. Fever of unknown origin. *Adv Pediatr Infect Dis* 1992;7:1.
  *Reviews series of FUO cases among children.*
Ghose MK, Shensa S, Lerner PI. Arteritis of the aged (giant-cell arteritis) and fever of unexplained origin. *Am J Med* 1976;60:429.
  *Giant-cell arteritis may present with prolonged fever but without headache, visual disturbance, or arthralgias.*
Gleckman R, Crowley M, Esposito A. Fever of unknown origin: a view from the community hospital. *Am J Med Sci* 1977;274:21.
  *In a community hospital, pulmonary emboli and alcoholic hepatitis were common causes of prolonged fever.*
Hurley DL. Fever in adults. What to do when the cause is not obvious. *Postgrad Med* 1983;74:232.
  *Provides a practical approach to evaluation of FUO and concludes that each patient's illness will dictate a specific diagnostic approach.*

Jacoby GA, Swartz MN. Fever of undetermined origin. *N Engl J Med* 1973;289:1407.
*Good overview of etiologic classification of FUO.*

Kauffman CA, Jones PG. Diagnosing fever of unknown origin in older patients. *Geriatrics* 1984;39:46.
*Excellent review of FUO in elderly patients. Giant-cell arteritis, biliary tract infection, and drug fever are particularly important in this group.*

Kazanjian PH. Fever of unknown origin: review of 86 patients treated in community hospitals. *Clin Infect Dis* 1992;15:968.
*AIDS and Lyme disease caused FUO in a recent community hospital study.*

Kerttula Y, Hirvonen P, Pettersson T. Fever of unknown origin: a follow-up investigation of 34 patients. *Scand J Infect Dis* 1983;15:185.
*Five-year follow-up of 34 patients with FUO from a hospital in Finland.*

Knockaert DC. Diagnostic strategy for fever of unknown origin in the ultrasonography and computed tomography era. *Acta Clin Belg* 1992;47:100.
*Attempts to provide a standard approach to the FUO workup.*

Knockaert DC, et al. Fever of unknown origin in the 1980s. An update of the diagnostic spectrum. *Arch Intern Med* 1992;152:51.
*Large, prospective study of FUO from Belgium, 1980–1989. Malignancy occurred in only 7% of patients.*

Knockaert DC, Vaneste LJ, Bobbaers HJ. Recurrent or episodic fever of unknown origin. Review of 45 cases and review of the literature. *Medicine* (Baltimore) 1993;72:184.
*Long-standing recurrent fevers have a smaller differential diagnosis. Bacterial infections include chronic biliary tract or prostatic infection. Still's disease, familial Mediterranean fever, Crohn's disease, and lymphoma are examples of this type of FUO.*

Larson EB, Featherstone HJ, Petersdorf RG. Fever of undetermined origin: diagnosis and follow-up of 105 cases, 1970–1980. *Medicine (Baltimore)* 1982;61:269.
*Follow-up study by Petersdorf group (see also Petersdorf RG, Beeson PM, 1961). Neoplastic disease was the most common cause of FUO.*

Larson TS, et al. Respiratory tract symptoms as a clue to giant-cell arteritis. *Ann Intern Med* 1984;101:594.
*Sixteen patients with giant-cell arteritis had symptoms of cough, sore throat, or hoarseness.*

Mackowiak PA. Southwestern Internal Medicine Conference. Drug fever: mechanisms, maxims and misconceptions. *Am J Med Sci* 1987;294:275.
*Excellent detailed review of the clinical picture of drug fevers. Some findings go against standard teachings on drug fever.*

McNeil BJ, et al. A prospective study of computed tomography, ultrasound, and gallium imaging in patients with fever. *Radiology* 1981;139:647.
*Prospective study compared three imaging modalities in workup of unexplained fever and found all equally sensitive in diagnosis of focal disease.*

Mellors JW, et al. A simple index to identify occult bacterial infection in adults with acute unexplained fever. *Arch Intern Med* 1987;147:666.
*Several features in patients with unexplained fever predict bacterial infection: age above 50 years, diabetes, WBC above 15,000/mm³, and band count above 1,500/mm³.*

Murray HW, et al. Urinary temperature: a clue to early diagnosis of factitious fever. *N Engl J Med* 1977;296:23.
*Urinary temperature can be used to diagnose factitious fever.*

Musher DM. Fever of unknown origin: diagnostic principles. *Hosp Pract* 1982;17:89.
*Excellent description of the traditional case-by-case approach to the diagnosis of FUO.*

Musher DM, et al. Fever patterns: their lack of clinical significance. *Arch Intern Med* 1979;139:1225.
*Fever patterns were not helpful in assessing the etiology of fever on an infectious disease consultation service.*

Petersdorf RG. Fever of unknown origin. *Arch Intern Med* 1992;152:21.
*Petersdorf's most recent reflections on FUO (see also Petersdorf RG, Beeson PM, 1961; Larson EB, Featherstone HJ, Petersdorf RG, 1982.) Patients with a diagnosis of FUO should rarely die.*

Petersdorf RG, Beeson PM. Fever of unexplained origin: report of 100 cases. *Medicine (Baltimore)* 1961;40:1.
*Initial, classic paper that defined FUO, its etiologies, and diagnostic approach.*

Pizzo PA, Lovejoy FH, Smith DH. Prolonged fever in children: review of 100 cases. *Pediatrics* 1975;5:468.
*Children are more likely to have viral and collagen inflammatory causes of FUO than are adults.*
Quinn MJ, et al. Computed tomography of the abdomen in evaluation of patients with fever of unknown origin. *Radiology* 1980;136:407.
*Results of 29% of 78 CT scans were positive in FUO patients.*
Rowland MD, Del Bene VE. Use of body computed tomography to evaluate fever of unknown origin. *J Infect Dis* 1987;156:408.
*Documents role of CT in the workup of FUO.*
Schmidt KG, et al. Indium 111 granulocyte scintigraphy in the evaluation of patients with fever of undetermined origin. *Scand J Infect Dis* 1987;19:339.
*Indium scintigraphy was very useful in 5 of 32 patients with unexplained fever.*
Smith JW. Southwestern Internal Medicine Conference. Fever of undetermined origin: not what it used to be. *Am J Med Sci* 1986;292:56.
*Includes 80 cases seen at Dallas Veterans Administration Medical Center between 1979 and 1985. Solid tumors, the most common cause of FUO, responded to nonsteroidal antiinflammatory agents.*
Weinberger A, Kesler A, Pinkhas J. Fever in various rheumatic diseases. *Clin Rheumatol* 1985;4:258.
*Describes the pathophysiology of fever in patients with rheumatologic diseases.*
Weinstein L. Clinically benign fever of unknown origin: a personal retrospective. *Rev Infect Dis* 1985;7:692.
*Description of both low-grade and high-grade fever with a benign course. Fever resulting from occupational exposure, such as polymer fume fever, can be high-grade.*
Welsby PD. Pyrexia of unknown origin 60 years on. *Postgrad Med* 1985;61:887.
*British perspective on FUO in the elderly, including role of foreign travel.*
Wolff SM, Fauci AS, Dale DC. Unusual etiologies of fever and their evaluation. *Ann Rev Med* 1975;26:277.
*Discussion includes brief overview of each major category of disease, including granulomatous hepatitis.*
Young EJ, Fainstain V, Musher DM. Drug-induced fever: cases seen in the evaluation of unexplained fever in a general hospital population. *Rev Infect Dis* 1982;4:69.
*Antimicrobial agents were responsible for most cases of drug fever.*

## 55. CHRONIC FATIGUE SYNDROME

Fatigue remains an extremely common complaint of persons seeking medical care. This complaint was reported by 20% to 25% of patients in general medical clinics. Despite the high frequency of fatigue, a standardized blood test or instrument to measure it does not exist. Fatigue is the hallmark of the chronic fatigue syndrome (CFS); as defined in 1988, fatigue must be "new, persistent, or relapsing" and "associated with a 50% reduction in a patient's premorbid activity for a period of at least 6 months." Fatigue is a frustrating complaint for both patients and practitioners because no laboratory tests are available to confirm or quantify this symptom. Patients are usually initially seen by their family practitioner or internist and often are referred for diagnosis and management to a neurologist, psychiatrist, or infectious disease specialist. The subject of CFS continues to evoke intense controversy in the medical profession and in the media. Researchers disagree on the causative role of psychiatric disorders in this illness. Some investigators report that depression and other psychiatric disorders are responsible for more than 80% of cases of CFS. Other investigators, in Australia, noted no increase in predisposing psychiatric disorders in patients with this syndrome when they were compared with matched controls. There also appears to be a close relationship between CFS and fibromyalgia, and patients often fulfill the case definition for both illnesses.

Despite the high frequency of fatigue in the general population, CFS as defined by the Centers for Disease Control (CDC) may be uncommon. In a study from Australia, the prevalence of CFS was 37.1 cases per 100,000 residents, a rate similar to that for multiple sclerosis. In a community survey in five U.S. cities, an estimate of the prevalence of CFS was 7 cases per 100,000 persons. A similar rate (1.8 to 6 cases per 100,000) was noted in the CDC surveillance study from four U.S. cities. In a recent community survey in the state of Washington, the prevalence of CSF ranged from 75 to 267 cases per 100,000 persons. There is a female predominance, and most patients are between the ages of 20 and 50 years. People of all socioeconomic groups are affected. The majority of patients report an acute rather than a gradual onset of their illness.

The diagnosis of CFS is difficult and remains one of exclusion. There is no laboratory test to confirm the diagnosis; results of routine laboratory tests are normal, and the sedimentation rate is not elevated. An evaluation to exclude other disorders should be based on the patient's history and epidemiologic exposures. A Lyme or HIV serology is indicated only if an appropriate epidemiologic history suggests these illnesses. Similarly, an antinuclear antibody or rheumatoid factor test should be ordered only if the patient has joint complaints. Results of selected immunologic tests may be abnormal in patients with CFS, but such tests are indicated only for research purposes. They are not of value in confirming the diagnosis, and their added cost is not justified. Although symptoms of the so-called yeast connection or *Candida* hypersensitivity syndrome overlap those of CFS, there is no evidence that the "yeast syndrome" exists, and testing for *Candida* antibodies is not indicated.

Diminished cortisol excretion has been noted in patients with CFS when they are compared with controls. This may be secondary to a deficiency of either corticotropin-releasing hormone or another stimulus of the pituitary-adrenal axis. In contrast to patients with CFS, patients with primary depression may show an increase in cortisol secretion. Although CFS is similar to depression in some aspects, these two disorders are associated with different hormonal abnormalities.

An association between CFS and neurally mediated hypotension has been noted. Many patients with CFS (30% to 89%) will have abnormal results on a tilt-table test, and in an uncontrolled trial, they responded to salt loading, fludrocortisone, β-adrenergic blockers, and disopyramide alone or in combination. Magnetic resonance imaging of the brain may show multiple foci of high signal intensity in the white matter of patients with CFS in comparison with controls. The meaning of these findings is unknown, and magnetic resonance imaging of the brain is not useful as a diagnostic test. The role for other tests, such as single-proton emission computed tomography, sleep studies, or positron emission tomography, is unknown; consequently, these tests should be considered experimental in evaluating a patient with CFS. Patients complain of multiple cognitive defects, but various neuropsychologic tests have not been of value in documenting these abnormalities. Although fatigue is a hallmark of this syndrome, no myopathy has been identified. Similarly, patients often complain of weakness yet demonstrate normal muscle strength on testing.

The CDC case definition is currently the most accepted basis for diagnosing CFS, although two other definitions have been proposed by investigators in Australia and the United Kingdom. The CDC diagnosis requires that a patient have unexplained persistent fatigue for 6 months that is new, not caused by exertion, and not relieved by rest, and that results in a substantial reduction in previous levels of activity. In addition to the severe unexplained fatigue, four or more of the symptoms listed in Table 55-1 should be present concurrently for at least 6 months. This revised case definition, published in 1994, deleted the physical signs and required fewer symptoms to be present for fulfillment of the diagnosis in an attempt to eliminate patients with a somatization disorder. Patients with severe fatigue for 6 months but fewer than four other symptoms are classified as having idiopathic chronic fatigue. At a National Institutes of Health-sponsored conference on CFS, it was proposed that patients with prior psychoses or behavioral disorders, such as psychotic depression, bipolar disorder, schizophrenia, or substance abuse, be excluded, as well as patients with any prior chronic medical illness. In contrast, patients with fibromyalgia or prior infectious diseases that have been adequately treated and are not associated with chronicity, such as toxoplasmosis, should be included.

Table 55-1. Symptoms of chronic fatigue syndrome
(four symptoms required for diagnosis)

Impaired memory or concentration that interferes with work, social, or personal activities

Sore throat

Tender lymph nodes

Muscle pain

Arthralgias

New headaches

Unrefreshing sleep

Postexertion exhaustion lasting more than 24 hours for activities previously tolerated

The etiology of CFS remains unknown. It is unlikely that Epstein-Barr virus or human herpesvirus 6 is involved as a causative agent. Conflicting evidence exists regarding the importance of enteroviruses in the disease. In one report that used polymerase chain reaction methodology, enteroviral RNA was identified more often in muscle biopsy specimens from patients with CFS than in specimens from controls. Other investigators were unable to implicate enteroviruses as an etiologic agent. One report suggested that CFS was the result of a retroviral infection, but researchers at the CDC failed to identify HTLV-II, a retrovirus, in the blood of patients with CFS. It appears unlikely that a single pathogen is involved in all cases of CFS. It is hoped that future research will help clarify both the etiology and pathogenesis of this syndrome. Multiple agents, both infectious and noninfectious, may be involved in precipitating the illness.

Multiple drugs have been advocated to treat patients with CFS, but few regimens have been subjected to well-designed case-control studies. Acyclovir has no beneficial effect in treating patients with this illness. IV immunoglobulin is not helpful. One investigator who used high-dose IV immunoglobulin found a benefit while patients were receiving the drug; another researcher found no significant improvement in treated patients compared with those who received placebo. Another study was performed by the same investigator who found a benefit for immunoglobulin, but in a repeated study, no difference was noted between IV immunoglobulin and placebo.

A controlled trial has failed to document a benefit for nystatin therapy for the yeast connection syndrome. A mixture of liver extract, folic acid, and cyanocobalamin also appears to have no value in therapy. Further information is needed to classify the role of IM magnesium sulfates, essential fatty acids, and ampligen in managing patients with this illness. Ampligen, or poly(I):poly(C12U), is an RNA drug with possible antiviral and immunomodulatory activity. Transfer factor has been studied and does not appear to be useful. Low doses of amitriptyline (10 to 20 mg) at bedtime help improve sleep. Various nonsteroidal antiinflammatory drugs, such as naproxen, are beneficial for muscle and joint complaints. Cyclobenzaprine, a drug closely related to the tricyclic antidepressants, helps alleviate muscle and joint complaints and improves sleep. Nonsedating antihistamines may be useful to manage the allergic symptoms that occur more frequently in patients with CFS than in controls. Antidepressants such as fluoxetine or desipramine are extremely beneficial, although one controlled trial found no benefit with fluoxetine. A patient's response to an antidepressant, however, does not indicate that CFS is a psychiatric illness. A randomized, double-blind, placebo-controlled trial found no benefit with normal replacement doses of hydrocortisone in comparison with placebo. In an uncontrolled study of patients with a positive tilt-table test result, salt loading, fludrocortisone, β-adrenergic blockers, and disopyramide alone or in combination were beneficial. A small, controlled trial of fludrocortisone versus placebo found no benefit with the drug, and a larger trial is in progress. Although controlled studies are lacking, some CFS patients who suffer from anxiety or a panic disorder note benefit from medicines such as alprazolam, clonazepam, or buspirone. A graduated exercise program combined with cognitive behavior therapy has been associated with complete recovery in 28% of patients and improvement in 70%.

Because there is no specific therapy for CFS, emotional support is critical. Exotic, untested remedies should be avoided. Patients should be followed to continue to exclude other medical problems. (N.M.G.)

## Bibliography

Bennett RM, Clark SC, Walczyk J. A randomized, double-blind, placebo-controlled study of growth hormone in the treatment of fibromyalgia. *Am J Med* 1998;104:227–231.
*An improvement in symptoms and a decrease in the number of tender points after daily injections of growth hormone for 9 months.*

Bombardier CH, Buchwald D. Outcome and prognosis of patients with chronic fatigue vs. chronic fatigue syndrome. *Arch Intern Med* 1995;155:2105–2110.
*Sixty-four percent of patients with CFS improved, but only 2% reported complete recovery.*

Bou-Holaigah I, et al. The relationship between neurally mediated hypotension and the chronic fatigue syndrome. *JAMA* 1995;274:961–967.
*An abnormal tilt-table test result was found in 89% of patients with CFS. Symptoms improved in most patients with therapy for neurally mediated hypotension.*

Buchwald D, et al. Chronic fatigue and the chronic fatigue syndrome: prevalence in a Pacific Northwest health care system. *Ann Intern Med* 1995;123:81–88.
*In a community survey, the prevalence of CFS ranged from 75 to 267 cases per 100,000 persons.*

Buchwald D, et al. Functional status in patients with chronic fatigue syndrome, other fatiguing illnesses, and healthy individuals. *Am J Med* 1996;101:364–370.
*Based on results of the short-form General Health Survey (SF-36), functional status was impaired in patients with CFS and chronic fatigue.*

Buchwald D, et al. Viral serologies in patients with chronic fatigue and chronic fatigue syndrome. *J Med Virol* 1996;50:25–30.
*Viral serologies for 13 common viruses were not useful in evaluating patients with CFS.*

Butler S, et al. Cognitive behavior therapy in the chronic fatigue syndrome. *J Neurol Neurosurg Psychiatry* 1991;54:153.
*When cognitive behavior therapy was used, 70% of patients improved and 26% noted complete recovery.*

Deale A, et al. Cognitive behavior therapy for chronic fatigue syndrome: a randomized controlled trial. *Am J Psychiatry* 1997;154:408–414.
*Cognitive behavior therapy was more effective than relaxation therapy in this trial.*

Demitrack MA, et al. Evidence for impaired activation of the hypothalamic-pituitary-adrenal axis in patients with chronic fatigue syndrome. *J Clin Endocrinol Metab* 1991;73:1224.
*A mild glucocorticoid deficiency was noted, possibly resulting from a deficiency of corticotropin-releasing hormone.*

Freeman R, Komaroff AL. Does the chronic fatigue syndrome involve the autonomic nervous system? *Am J Med* 1997;102:357–364.
*Abnormal measures of sympathetic and parasympathetic nervous system function.*

Fukuda K, Gantz NM. Management strategies for chronic fatigue syndrome. *Federal Practitioner* 1995;12:12–17.
*A review of diagnosis and therapy.*

Fukuda K, et al., International Chronic Fatigue Syndrome Study Group. *Ann Intern Med* 1994;121:953–959.
*The revised case definition requires severe fatigue plus at least four concurrent symptoms to be present for 6 months.*

Fulcher KY, White PD. Randomised controlled trial of graded exercise in patients with the chronic fatigue syndrome. *BMJ* 1997;314:1647–1652.
*A 12-week graded exercise program was more effective than relaxation and flexibility treatment for patients with CFS. A benefit was still noted 1 year later.*

Gaudino EA, Coyle PK, Krupp LB. Post-Lyme syndrome and chronic fatigue syndrome. *Arch Neurol* 1997;54:1372–1376.
*Patients with post-Lyme syndrome had more cognitive deficits than patients with CFS.*

Goldenberg DL, et al. High frequency of fibromyalgia in patients with chronic fatigue seen in a primary care practice. *Arthritis Rheum* 1990;33:381.
*In a study of women with severe fatigue for more than 6 months, 59% fulfilled criteria for chronic fatigue, 70% had symptoms of fibromyalgia, and 30% had neither.*

Goldenberg D, et al. A randomized, double-blind crossover trial of fluoxetine and amitriptyline in the treatment of fibromyalgia. *Arthritis Rheum* 1996;39:1852–1859.
*Fluoxetine and amitriptyline in combination were better than placebo in treating patients with fibromyalgia.*

Holmes GP, et al. Chronic fatigue syndrome: a working case definition. *Ann Intern Med* 1988;108:387.
*For a clinician to establish the diagnosis of CFS, the patient must fulfill two major criteria and eight minor criteria (symptoms and signs). Original definition.*

Jacobson SK, et al. Chronic parvovirus B19 infection resulting in chronic fatigue syndrome: case history and review. *Clin Infect Dis* 1997;24:1048–1051.
*Chronic parvovirus B19 infection may cause CFS, which resolved with administration of immune globulin.*

Joyce J, Hotopf M, Wessely S. The prognosis of chronic fatigue and chronic fatigue syndrome: a systematic review. *OJM* 1997;90:223–233.
*Ninety percent of adults failed to recover after the diagnosis of CFS.*

Kane RL, Gantz NM, DiPino RK. Neuropsychological and psychological functioning in chronic fatigue syndrome. *Neuropsychiatry Neuropsychol Behav Neurol* 1997;10:25–31.
*On neuropsychologic testing, impaired attention and memory were noted in this controlled study.*

Khan AS, et al. Assessment of a retrovirus sequence and other possible risk factors for the chronic fatigue syndrome. *Ann Intern Med* 1993;118:241.
*A retrovirus, HTLV-II, was not identified in these patients with CFS.*

Komaroff AL, Buchwald DS. Chronic fatigue syndrome: an update. *Annu Rev Med* 1998;49:1–13.
*Review.*

Kroenke K, Jackson JL, Chamberlin J. Depressive and anxiety disorders in patients presenting with physical complaints: clinical predictors and outcome. *Am J Med* 1997;103:339–347.
*Patients with physical complaints often have an associated depressive or anxiety disorder (29%).*

Landay AL, et al. Chronic fatigue syndrome: clinical condition associated with immune activation. *Lancet* 1991;338:707.
*The authors noted an increase in CD8-cell subsets with immune activation markers.*

Lane TJ, Manu P, Matthews DA. Depression and somatization in the chronic fatigue syndrome. *Am J Med* 1991;91:335.
*An unrecognized psychiatric disorder such as depression or somatization may mimic CFS.*

Levine PH. Epidemiologic advances in chronic fatigue syndrome. *J Psychiatr Res* 1997; 31:7–18.
*A review of CFS epidemiology risk factors include female sex and physical or psychologic stress.*

Lloyd A, et al. A double-blind, placebo-controlled trial of intravenous immunoglobulin therapy in patients with chronic fatigue syndrome. *Am J Med* 1990;89:561.
*High-dose IV immunoglobulin was helpful in reducing symptoms.*

Lloyd AR, et al. Immunologic and psychologic therapy for patients with chronic fatigue syndrome: a double-blind, placebo-controlled trial. *Am J Med* 1993;94:197.
*Lack of response to therapy with transfer factor with or without cognitive behavior therapy.*

Manu P, Lane TJ, Matthews DA. The frequency of the chronic fatigue syndrome in patients with symptoms of persistent fatigue. *Ann Intern Med* 1988;109:554.
*Depression and other psychiatric diagnoses were responsible for more than 80% of the cases evaluated.*

Matthews DA, Manu P, Lane TJ. Evaluation and management of patients with chronic fatigue. *Am J Med Sci* 1991;302:269.

*Common diagnoses of patients referred for evaluation of CFS included depression, an anxiety disorder, or a somatization disorder. Evaluation was based on a structured psychiatric interview, the Diagnostic Interview Schedule.*

Mawle AC, et al. Immune responses associated with chronic fatigue syndrome: a case-control study. *J Infect Dis* 1997;175:136–141.
   *No differences in immune function were noted between CFS cases and controls.*

McKenzie R, Straus SE. Chronic fatigue syndrome. *Adv Intern Med* 1995;40:119–153.
   *Review.*

Natelson BH, et al. Randomized, double-blind, controlled placebo phase in trial of low-dose phenelzine in the chronic fatigue syndrome. *Psychopharmacology* 1996;124: 226–230.
   *In this placebo-controlled trial, phenelzine, a monamine oxidase inhibitor, was effective.*

Peakman M, et al. Clinical improvement in chronic fatigue syndrome is not associated with lymphocyte subsets of function or activation. *Clin Immunol Immunopathol* 1997;82:83–91.
   *No relationship between clinical improvement and immune status.*

Peterson PK, et al. A controlled trial of intravenous immunoglobulin G in chronic fatigue syndrome. *Am J Med* 1990;89:554.
   *IV immunoglobulin was not beneficial.*

Peterson PK, et al. A preliminary placebo-controlled crossover trial of fludrocortisone for chronic fatigue syndrome. *Arch Intern Med* 1998;158:908–914.
   *Low-dose fludrocortisone (0.1 to 0.2 mg) was no better than placebo in reducing symptoms of patients with CFS.*

Price RK, et al. Estimating the prevalence of chronic fatigue syndrome and associated symptoms in the community. *Public Health Rep* 1992;107:514.
   *Although 23% of patients noted fatigue, CFS was rare (7.4 cases per 100,000) when the Diagnostic Interview Schedule was used to assess patients.*

Salit IE, and Vancouver Chronic Fatigue Syndrome Consensus Group. *J Rheumatol* 1996;23:540–544.
   *CFS is a heterogeneous disorder that needs further study.*

Scheffers MK, et al. Attention and short-term memory in chronic fatigue syndrome patients: an event-related potential analysis. *Neurology* 1992;42:1667.
   *Although patients with CFS have multiple cognitive complaints, no gross deficits in perception, attention, or short-term memory were noted according to the tests used.*

Schluederberg A, Straus SE, Grufferman S. Considerations in the design of studies of chronic fatigue syndrome. *Rev Infect Dis* 1991;13 (Suppl 1):S1.
   *Entire issue focuses on approach to CFS study design and research.*

Schluederberg A, et al. Chronic fatigue syndrome research: definition and medical outcome assessment. *Ann Intern Med* 1992;117:325.
   *Clarified use definition. Patients with prior psychotic depression, bipolar disorder, schizophrenia, or substance abuse should be excluded. Include patients with fibromyalgia.*

Sharpe M. Chronic fatigue syndrome. *Psychiatr Clin North Am* 1996;19:549–573.
   *Review. Both pathophysiologic changes and psychologic factors are important.*

Sharpe M, et al. Cognitive behaviour therapy for the chronic fatigue syndrome: a randomized controlled trial. *BMJ* 1996;312:22–26.
   *Seventy-three percent of patients given cognitive behavior therapy improved, compared with only 27% of those who received regular medical care.*

Sharpley A, et al. Do patients with pure chronic fatigue syndrome (neurasthenia) have abnormal sleep? *Psychosom Med* 1997;59:592–596.
   *Although patients with CFS complain of unrefreshing sleep, results of the majority of sleep studies are normal.*

Straus SE, et al. Acyclovir treatment of the chronic fatigue syndrome: lack of efficacy in a placebo-controlled trial. *N Engl J Med* 1988;319:1692.
   *The response to both acyclovir and placebo was favorable, with no statistical difference between the agents.*

Vercoulen JH, et al. Prognosis in chronic fatigue syndrome: a prospective study on the natural course. *J Neurol Neurosurg Psychiatry* 1996;60:489–494.

*Only 20% of patients reported improvement or recovery when followed for 18 months.*

Vercoulen JH, et al. Randomised, double-blind, placebo-controlled study of fluoxetine in chronic fatigue syndrome. *Lancet* 1996;347:858–861.

*Fluoxetine was not helpful in this randomized controlled trial.*

Vollmer-Conna U, et al. Intravenous immunoglobulin is ineffective in the treatment of patients with chronic fatigue syndrome. *Am J Med* 1997;103:38–43.

*IV immunoglobulin was not effective in a randomized placebo-controlled trial.*

Wessely S, et al. Psychological symptoms, somatic symptoms, and psychiatric disorder in chronic fatigue and chronic fatigue syndrome: a prospective study in the primary care setting. *Am J Psychiatry* 1996;153:1050–1059.

*A current psychiatric disorder was reported in 75% of patients with CFS.*

Wessely S, et al. The prevalence and morbidity of chronic fatigue and chronic fatigue syndrome: a prospective primary care study. *Am J Public Health* 1997;87:1449–1455.

*The point prevalence of CFS when the 1994 CDC case definition was used was 2.6%, and it decreased to 0.5% if psychologic disorders were excluded.*

Wolfe F, et al. Health status and disease severity in fibromyalgia. *Arthritis Rheum* 1997;40:1571–1579.

*Patients with fibromyalgia, managed by experts, had persistent symptoms such as pain, fatigue, and sleep disturbances during a 7-year follow-up.*

# XII. IMMUNITY

## 56. MANAGEMENT OF THE PATIENT WITH SUSPECTED β-LACTAM ALLERGY

Despite more than 40 years of clinical use, penicillin remains an important agent for many types of infection. Currently, parenteral β-lactam antibiotics (penicillins, cephalosporins, cephamycins, carbapenems, and monobactams) comprise the largest group of parenteral antimicrobials administered to hospitalized patients. Similarly, oral β-lactams are frequently used for outpatients with a wide variety of presumably treatable infections, and they have more recently been extensively employed as step-down therapy for patients being switched from parenteral antibiotics in preparation for hospital discharge. They remain popular because of reasonable safety, dosing flexibility, ease of administration (few drug-drug interactions), and an excellent spectrum of activity with proven efficacy in many clinical situations.

Allergy is a major problem associated with the use of β-lactams, and these agents may be the most common cause of drug allergy. Although rates of immediate allergy among penicillins have historically been felt to be similar, a recent investigation suggests that allergy to ampicillin may be the most common. Allergy to other cephalosporins, carbapenems, and carbacephems has been less well studied. Up to 20% of hospitalized patients claim to be penicillin-allergic. This rate is much higher than what has been demonstrated in clinical studies and is substantially higher than the rates associated with most other antimicrobials, with the possible exception of the sulfonamides. Because of similarities in structure among various types of β-lactams, it is not surprising that cross-allergenicity has been described. This issue was initially complicated because early cephalosporins were probably contaminated by penicillin. Some data have suggested that allergy may be targeted to specific side chains, and thus allergy to amoxicillin but not to penicillin has been reported. However, a recent investigation assessing the risk for cross-allergenicity between amoxicillin and cefadroxil (which share side chains) demonstrated that almost 90% of persons allergic to the former tolerated the latter.

Rates of allergy to cephalosporins in patients with and without penicillin allergy are thought to be 5% to 16% and 1% to 3%, respectively. Regarding penicillin, early investigations suggested that 0.7% to 10% of patients receiving this agent had allergic reactions, with a fatality rate below 0.002%. The first reported case of anaphylaxis was in 1946 and the first reported death in 1949. Administration of parenteral penicillin is more likely to be associated with fatalities, probably because of the higher doses employed. However, more recent data demonstrate no difference in rate of allergy between high oral doses and similar doses administered parenterally. Additionally, the risk for penicillin allergy is higher in persons with a history of previous reaction. Allergy may nonetheless develop in persons without documented prior β-lactam exposure, for reasons that include prior exposure through foods and other environmental factors. Risk is lower in children and the elderly, with fatal outcomes more common in the latter group. A history of atopy is not an independent risk factor for penicillin allergy. Signs of allergy may persist for weeks after discontinuation of the offending agent.

Anaphylaxis to penicillin occurs in 0.01% of those who receive this agent, with a mortality rate of 9%. Alternatively, urticaria can be noted in up to 5% of patients receiving penicillin, even in the absence of known allergy. Neither penicillins nor cephalosporins cause significant cross-allergenicity with monobactams (i.e., aztreonam). This fact provides *de facto* data that the allergenic moiety does not reside within the β–lactam ring itself.

Many patients carry the label "penicillin-allergic" for obscure reasons. The problem is confounded because many adverse reactions to these compounds are not associated with true allergic mechanisms (although they may be reproducible), and such reactions are associated with little further risk on repeated administration. Examples include the maculopapular rash that occurs many days into the course of β-lactam administration, or the severe maculopapular rash that develops in patients with mononucleosis on administration of ampicillin. Table 56-1 summarizes known allergic mechanisms and their associated clinical manifestations. Problems associated with overemphasis of allergy include the use of secondary antibiotics that may be more expensive, toxic, and less reliable.

The role of skin testing for β-lactam allergy is controversial, with the problem complicated by a lack of available antigens for the cephalosporins and the commercial availability of only the major determinant for penicillin. Skin testing is indicated for patients who may need penicillin yet whose history of immediate reaction is uncertain. Only about 10% of patients labeled as penicillin-allergic will react to skin tests.

After administration, penicillin is broken down into the penicilloyl group (major determinant) and other derivatives (minor determinants). Most immediate reactions are the result of IgE antibodies reacting against the latter. Alternatively, later urticarial reactions usually are associated with IgE antibody activity against the major determinant. In patients without a reaction to major or minor determinants, IgE-mediated penicillin allergies are unlikely to develop. However, these tests have no value in determining the likelihood of other reactions.

The clinician who is considering the use of a β-lactam antimicrobial in a patient with presumed allergy needs to determine (a) the likelihood of true allergy and the conditions surrounding the initial adverse reaction, (b) the possibility of using an alternative β-lactam, (c) the availability of suitable alternative agents if a β-lactam is contraindicated, and (d) the role of desensitization if a β-lactam must be employed despite immediate allergy. It is incumbent on the clinician to assess the true history of presumed β-lactam allergy and to document the reaction and its relationship to the product.

True allergy must be differentiated from adverse reaction and toxicity. Stories such as, "My mother was allergic, and she told me that I could be allergic," and "My stomach became upset when I took penicillin," and "I got diarrhea when I took ampicillin," are examples of clinical situations where there is not a need for alternative agents. Indeed, the true clinical significance of many of the untoward reactions associated with unknown or idiopathic mechanisms is undetermined, and many such patients can receive the offending agent. The problem of defining true allergy is further confounded by the fact that selected adverse reactions may occur simultaneously with the administration of a β-lactam but are not related to the product itself. Examples include procaine or vasovagal reaction, pain at the site of injection, and the Jarisch-Herxheimer reaction. Procaine-induced adverse reactions rapidly follow accidental IV injection of procaine penicillin and can include agitation, hallucinations, seizures, and hypertension. Problems tend to subside within minutes. The Jarisch-Herxheimer reaction is most often noted following the administration of penicillin for spirochetal disease (most commonly syphilis) and is related to the release of endotoxin from dying organisms. Manifestations include fever, rigors, and other constitutional symptoms and generally begin several hours after the first dose of drug.

Table 56-1. Mechanisms of antimicrobial allergy

| Mechanism | Syndrome |
| --- | --- |
| Immediate, IgE antibody | Anaphylaxis, laryngeal edema, early urticaria |
| Cytotoxic antibody | Hemolysis |
| Antigen-antibody complexes | Serum sickness |
| T cell | Contact dermatitis (often related to skin exposure) |
| Idiopathic/unknown | Maculopapular rash, late drug eruptions, eosinophilia, drug fever, interstitial nephritis |

From Saxon A, et al. Immediate hypersensitivity reactions to β-lactam antibiotics. *Ann Intern Med* 1987; 107:204–215.

The majority of patients with reactions to β-lactams have late maculopapular rashes associated with unknown mechanisms. These are unlikely to cause severe reactions on readministration of a β-lactam product, and therefore an alternative β-lactam can be safely utilized. As an example, the patient in whom a maculopapular reaction developed on day 5 of parenteral nafcillin can be safely treated with cefazolin, and the outpatient with a similar history of allergy to dicloxacillin can be managed with an oral cephalosporin. Although data are scarcer, patients with most other forms of non–IgE-mediated reactions can probably also be managed with alternative β-lactams. Examples include serum sickness, interstitial nephritis, and drug fever.

Patients with a history of an immediate reaction to a β-lactam antimicrobial should, if possible, not be treated with any of these products. Fortunately, the current antimicrobial armamentarium allows alternative strategies for most infections. Table 56-2 summarizes alternative agents for selected infections when a β-lactam is contraindicated. The route, dose, and duration of therapy depend on the site and severity of the infection.

Rarely, a patient who has had an immediate reaction to a β-lactam requires treatment with the offending agent, and in these instances desensitization should be performed. Examples include gonococcal endocarditis, enterococcal endocarditis (vancomycin-resistant organism), and selected forms of syphilis and Lyme borreliosis during pregnancy. Desensitization appears to work by binding IgE antibodies so that interaction with mast cells is prevented. Many authorities recommend that desensitization be performed following informed consent and in a carefully controlled environment, such as an ICU. Desensitization consists of administering progressively larger doses of penicillin (or another agent). There is no need for antihistamine-corticosteroid premedication. Table 56-3 provides an oral desensitization regimen that can be employed so long as the patient can reliably absorb oral medications. The typical interval between doses is at least 20 minutes; intradermal injections should be carefully observed for wheal/flare reactions. Once a final dose has been reached, it must be administered according to standard dosing regimens without doses being missed. The best data demonstrate that approximately one third of persons undergoing desensitization have mild reactions, either during desensitization or during active treatment. The risk for IgE-mediated reactions during desensitization is low. Mild allergic reactions seen during desensitiza-

Table 56-2. Alternative antimicrobials when β-lactams are contraindicated

| Organism | Alternative antibiotic |
|---|---|
| *Staphylococcus aureus* | Vancomycin, clindamycin |
| Streptococci (excluding enterococci) | Vancomycin, clindamycin, erythromycin, selected quinolones |
| Spirochetes | Tetracycline, erythromycin |
| Oral anaerobes | Clindamycin |
| Enteric gram-negative bacilli | Quinolones, TMP-SMX, aminoglycoside, aztreonam |
| Gonococci* | Selected quinolones, tetracycline |
| *Pasteurella multocida* | Tetracycline, selected quinolones |
| Enterococci** | Vancomycin |
| *Listeria monocytogenes* | TMP-SMX |
| Actinomycetes | Clindamycin, chloramphenicol |
| Clostridia | Clindamycin, chloramphenicol |
| *Haemophilus influenzae* | Tetracycline, TMP-SMX, selected quinolones |
| *Neisseria meningitidis* | Chloramphenicol, selected quinolones |

TMP-SMX, trimethoprim-sulfamethoxazole.
* Infective endocarditis may require desensitization.
** Endocarditis requires addition of aminoglycoside.

Table 56-3. Oral desensitization of β-lactam-allergic patients

| Dose No. | Dose (mg/mL) | Amount (mL) | Dose given (mg) |
|---|---|---|---|
| 1 | 0.5 | 0.1 | 0.05 |
| 2 | 0.5 | 0.2 | 0.1 |
| 3 | 0.5 | 0.4 | 0.2 |
| 4 | 0.5 | 0.8 | 0.4 |
| 5 | 0.5 | 1.6 | 0.8 |
| 6 | 0.5 | 3.2 | 1.6 |
| 7 | 0.5 | 6.4 | 3.2 |
| 8 | 5.0 | 1.2 | 6.0 |
| 9 | 5.0 | 2.4 | 12.0 |
| 10 | 5.0 | 4.8 | 24.0 |
| 11 | 50 | 1.0 | 50 |
| 12 | 50 | 2.0 | 100 |
| 13 | 50 | 4.0 | 200 |
| 14 | 50 | 8.0 | 400 |

Adapted from Weiss ME, Adkinson NF, Jr. Chapter 18. In: Mandell GL, Bennett JE, Dolin R, eds. *Principles and practice of infectious disease,* 4th ed. New York: Churchill Livingstone, 1995: 272–278.

tion require that the offending dose be repeated until tolerated. More severe reactions require active management, and the dose of the offending product should be decreased by at least 90%.

In summary, the initial management of a patient with a suspected allergy to β-lactam antimicrobials requires a careful evaluation of the type of reaction and its immunologic basis. Many patients with late (generally on a poorly defined immunologic basis) reactions can be successfully treated with alternative β-lactams or even with the offending antibiotic. Those with immediate or rapidly progressive reactions can generally be managed with alternative antimicrobials. For patients with defined IgE-mediated reactions who must be treated with the offending agent, desensitization is usually successful. (R.B.B.)

### Bibliography
Anne S, Reisman RE. Risk of administering cephalosporin antibiotics to patients with histories of penicillin allergy. *Ann Allergy* 1995;74:167–170.
*Available data were reviewed to assess the risks of administering cephalosporins to patients allergic to penicillin. Few data demonstrated a likelihood of cross-allergenicity. The authors are not convinced that skin testing provides any useful data, and conclude that penicillin allergy does not predict allergy to cephalosporins.*
Chisholm CA, et al. Penicillin desensitization in the treatment of syphilis during pregnancy. *Am J Perinatol* 1997;14:553–554.
*The authors conducted a retrospective study of 16 patients who required penicillin desensitization for syphilis during pregnancy. The oral regimen was equally effective, and the cost was approximately 40% of the cost of parenteral desensitization. The authors conclude that oral desensitization is as effective as parenteral desensitization and less expensive.*
Pichichero ME, Pichichero DM. Diagnosis of penicillin, amoxicillin and cephalosporin allergy: reliability of examination assessed by skin testing and oral challenge. *J Pediatr* 1998;132:137–143.
*Approximately 250 children or adolescents with clinically documented allergies to β-lactams were studied prospectively by skin testing and oral rechallenge. Of these, only one third demonstrated an IgE-mediated reaction on skin testing or oral challenge. None of the patients with negative test results demonstrated a significant reaction on oral rechallenge. The authors conclude that true allergy is overdiagnosed based on prior history, and that skin testing is indicated to rule out allergy. With negative test results, oral rechallenge is safe.*

Sastre J, et al. Clinical cross-reactivity between amoxicillin and cefadroxil in patients allergic to amoxicillin and with good tolerance of penicillin. *Allergy* 1996;51:383–386.
*The authors investigated 16 patients with allergy to amoxicillin but without clinical intolerance to penicillin to assess the role of the side chain on the former as a moiety for allergy. Patients with amoxicillin allergy were given cefadroxil, which contains the same side chain. Only 12% demonstrated immediate reactions, which shows that the side chain is not the target of hypersensitivity.*

Saxon A, et al. Immediate hypersensitivity reactions to β-lactam antibiotics. *Ann Intern Med* 1987;107:204–215.
*This conference discusses the types of allergic reactions and provides an excellent overview of the chemistry of the β-lactams and the relationship to allergy and skin testing. It is the best recent review of the topic.*

Weiss ME, Adkinson NF. β-Lactam allergy. In: Mandell GL, Bennett JE, Dolin R, eds. *Principles and practice of infectious diseases,* 4th ed. New York: Churchill Livingstone, 1995.
*This excellent summary of issues related to β-lactam antimicrobial allergy provides historic material, a sound rationale for penicillin testing, and several tables for penicillin desensitization, including one for oral desensitization.*

# XIII. NOSOCOMIAL INFECTIONS

## 57. POSTOPERATIVE FEVER

In the numerous discussions of the problem of postoperative fever, certain causes of fever, such as atelectasis or wound or urinary tract infection, are associated with a variety of surgical procedures. Others, such as mediastinitis or a prosthetic graft infection following the insertion of a heart valve, are specific for the particular type of operation performed. Occasionally, the fever represents an infectious disease problem unrelated to the surgical procedure, such as acute cholecystitis after a hernia repair. Any major surgical procedure can produce a fever for a few days after the operation. This is usually a low-grade, self-limited fever, and no cause is determined. However, a localized or systemic infectious disease is always a consideration, especially with a high, persistent, or recurrent fever.

In evaluating a patient with postoperative fever, it is helpful to note the temporal relationship of the fever to the operation. Causes of fever during the procedure or within the first 24 hours include malignant hyperthermia, transfusion reactions, atelectasis, aspiration pneumonia, wound infection, drug reactions, or endocrine disorders such as acute adrenal insufficiency, thyroid storm, or pheochromocytoma. Malignant hyperthermia is a rare but life-threatening cause in which high fever occurs immediately after the introduction of anesthesia. It is triggered by halogenated inhalational anesthetics such as enflurane, isoflurane, and the muscle relaxant succinylcholine. The disorder is dominantly inherited, and a family history of fatal reactions associated with anesthesia may be the only clue present. High fever and muscle rigidity occur, resulting from elevated cytoplasmic calcium levels triggered by various anesthetic agents. The disorder is diagnosed by a muscle biopsy and an *in vitro* muscle contracture test. In the future, genetic testing will play a role in diagnosis. Therapy consists of supportive measures and dantrolene. Another disorder that can cause fever is the neuroleptic malignant syndrome. Fever also occurs commonly with blood transfusions. Although these reactions are usually self-limited, they may represent red cell or granulocyte incompatibility or contamination of the blood with microorganisms. Atelectasis, although this is controversial, may be the most frequent cause identified for fever during the first 24 hours and responds to vigorous chest physiotherapy. The aspiration of a foreign body such as a denture should be excluded. Although wound infections are usually detected after several days, those caused by group A streptococci or *Clostridium* organisms may present during the first 24 hours.

Fever may begin after the initial 24 to 48 postoperative hours. The possibilities are numerous, but five causes are most frequent: infection in an IV site, wound, or urinary tract; deep venous thrombosis; or a pulmonary source. Two uncommon but potentially lethal infections should be considered when a patient has high fever in the initial 24 to 48 hours after surgery: toxic shock syndrome associated with *Staphylococcus aureus* or a group A streptococcal wound infection or bowel perforation. After an abdominal operation, an unnoticed injury to the bowel or an anastomotic leak may cause high fever and shock. In patients with toxic shock syndrome, there may be only minimal signs of a wound infection, and the clinical picture is characterized by fever, diarrhea, erythroderma, and shock.

"Third-day surgical fever" has been used to describe fever occurring on the third postoperative day as a result of an infection at the IV site. Such fevers are not limited to the third day and may result from contaminated IV fluid as well as infection at the catheter site. Inflammation may be absent from the IV site, making the diagnosis more difficult. Therapy consists of removing the catheter, culturing its tip, and obtaining several blood cultures.

Most wound infections are seen from 4 to 10 days after an operation. Increased warmth, redness, pain, and tenderness, along with purulent drainage, may be detected. A Gram's stain and culture of the discharge should identify the etiologic agent. Adequate drainage and antimicrobials are usually required. A urinary tract infection should be suspected in any patient who has an indwelling catheter or has undergone urinary tract instrumentation. Although urinary tract infection occurs infrequently, the source of the fever may be in the prostate; thus, rectal examination should not be neglected. Fever developing 5 to 7 days or longer after an operation should always raise the possibility of deep venous thrombosis. An asymptomatic presentation, except for fever, can occur. The lungs are the other common site of infection. Atelectasis, aspiration, bacterial pneumonia, and pulmonary embolism are the most likely possibilities. Atelectasis with or without pleural effusion may be a clue to an intraabdominal abscess beneath the diaphragm. Another cause of postoperative fever is antimicrobial-associated colitis caused by *Clostridium difficile*. The onset is usually 4 to 9 days after operation. Diarrhea, abdominal pain and tenderness, and fever are often present. Some patients have little or no diarrhea and present with fever and abdominal pain. Fecal leukocytes are present in the stool in half the patients, and the diagnosis is confirmed by identifying *C. difficile* toxin in the stool.

Fever with an onset at least 24 hours after an operation suggests other causes, such as complications associated with anesthesia, hepatitis, infection with cytomegalovirus (CMV) or Epstein-Barr virus, malaria transmitted via the blood, sterile or infected hematomas, drugs, and infections unrelated to the operation (e.g., acute cholecystitis). Halothane, which is rarely used, may cause postoperative fever, although this is infrequent. Chemical and bacterial meningitides are other reported febrile complications that may occur with spinal anesthesia. Transmission of CMV is not restricted to patients after open heart surgery, and CMV infection can develop after any blood transfusion. Fever developing 2 to 4 weeks after an operation and accompanied by atypical lymphocytes is a clue to mononucleosis. Hepatitis C is the major cause of transfusion hepatitis, but fever is usually absent. Drugs are an important noninfectious cause of persistent postoperative fever, especially in patients on antimicrobials, quinidine, procainamide, allopurinol, or medications for sleep. However, drug fever may be caused by any drug, and the associated rash and eosinophilia may be absent. Finally, always consider the possibility of an infection unrelated to an operation, such as acute cholecystitis caused by biliary stones, acalculous cholecystitis, pancreatitis, or hospital-acquired influenza.

In addition to the complications that can occur with various surgical procedures, the cause of the fever may be closely related to the particular kind of operation performed. An intraabdominal, subphrenic hepatic abscess or pancreatitis may develop after abdominal surgery. A pelvic operation may be complicated by septic pelvic thrombophlebitis, pelvic abscess, or cellulitis. After cardiovascular surgery, sternal osteomyelitis, endocarditis, mediastinitis, or the postcardiotomy syndrome are diagnostic considerations. Similarly, in neurosurgical, orthopedic, and other surgical specialty operations, the causes of fever may be unique to the procedure. Only after analysis of the patient's complaints, the physical and laboratory findings, and the fever onset and its relationship to surgery in general or the particular operation can the cause of the fever become apparent. (N.M.G.)

## Bibliography

Abraham RB, et al. Malignant hyperthermia susceptibility: anaesthetic implications and risk stratification. *QJM* 1997;90:13–18.
*Review. A rare autosomal dominant trait resulting in fever and rhabdomyolysis.*

Adair JC, et al. Aseptic meningitis following cardiac transplantation: clinical characteristics and relationship to immunosuppressive regimen. *Neurology* 1991;41:249.
*Use of OKT3 may cause fever and aseptic meningitis in patients after cardiac transplantation.*

Adelson-Mitty J, Fink MP, Lisbon A. The value of lumbar puncture in the evaluation of critically ill, non-immunosuppressed surgical patients: a retrospective analysis of 70 cases. *Intensive Care Med* 1997;23:749–752.
*In surgical patients who are not immunosuppressed and have no history of recent head trauma or neurosurgery, a lumbar puncture has a low yield.*

Altemeier WA, McDonough JJ, Fuller WD. Third-day surgical fever. *Arch Surg* 1971; 103:158.
*Septic thrombophlebitis related to IV infusion catheters is emphasized.*

Appleberg M. The value of the postoperative temperature chart as an aid to the diagnosis of deep-vein thrombosis. *S Afr Med J* 1976;50:2149.
*The three major causes for fever were wound sepsis, urinary infection, and deep-vein thrombosis.*

Bartlett JG, Gorbach SL, Finegold SM. The bacteriology of aspiration pneumonia. *Am J Med* 1974;56:202.

*The importance of anaerobes in aspiration pneumonia is stressed. A mixture of anaerobes and aerobes was common in hospital-acquired infections.*

Bell DM, et al. Unreliability of fever and leukocytosis in the diagnosis of infection after cardiac valve surgery. *J Thorac Cardiovasc Surg* 1978;75:87.

*These two tests were not useful in distinguishing infected from uninfected patients after cardiac valve surgery.*

Bennett SN, et al. Postoperative infections traced to contamination of an intravenous anesthetic, propofol. *N Engl J Med* 1995;333:147–154.

*Postoperative fever and a bloodstream infection were caused by contamination of a multidose vial of an anesthetic agent, propofol.*

Bertorini TE. Myoglobinuria, malignant hyperthermia, neuroleptic malignant syndrome and serotonin syndrome. *Neurol Clin* 1997;15:649–671.

*Review.*

Borger MA, et al. Deep sternal wound infection: risk factors and outcomes. *Ann Thorac Surg* 1998;65:1050–1056.

*Male sex and diabetes were risk factors for deep sternal wound infections.*

Clancy CJ, Nguyen MH, Morris AJ. Candidal mediastinitis: an emerging clinical entity. *Clin Infect Dis* 1997;25:608–613.

*A rare cause of mediastinitis. An intraoperative sternal culture for Candida should not be readily dismissed as a contaminant.*

Clarke DE, Kimelman J, Raffin TA. The evaluation of fever in the intensive care unit. *Chest* 1991;100:213.

*Review.*

Craven DE, Steger KA, Barber TW. Preventing nosocomial pneumonia: state of the art and perspectives for the 1990s. *Am J Med* 1991;91:44S.

*A review of pathogenesis and prophylaxis.*

Cruse PJE, Foord R. A 5-year prospective study of 23,649 surgical wounds. *Arch Surg* 1973;107:206.

*A comprehensive study of wound infections.*

Drew WL, Miner RC. Transfusion-related cytomegalovirus infection following noncardiac surgery. *JAMA* 1982;247:2389.

*Consider this diagnosis in a postoperative patient with fever in the presence or absence of atypical lymphocytes 3 weeks after a blood transfusion.*

Durand ML, et al. Acute bacterial meningitis in adults. *N Engl J Med* 1993;328:21.

*Recent neurosurgery (45%) or the presence of a neurosurgical device (21%) such as a shunt were the major predisposing factors in patients with nosocomial meningitis.*

Eason E, Aldis A, Seymour RJ. Pelvic fluid collections by sonography and febrile morbidity after abdominal hysterectomy. *Obstet Gynecol* 1997;90:58–62.

*The presence of pelvic fluid as determined by endovaginal ultrasound was not helpful in determining the cause of fever after abdominal hysterectomy.*

Engoren M. Lack of association between atelectasis and fever. *Chest* 1995;107:81–84.

*Fever should not be attributed to atelectasis in patients who have undergone cardiac surgery.*

Fischer SA, et al. Infectious complications in left ventricular assist device recipients. *Clin Infect Dis* 1997;24:18–23.

*The mean onset of infection of a left ventricular assist device was 23 days after implantation. Cure of infection did not always require removal of the device.*

Fitzgerald RH, et al. Deep-wound sepsis following total hip arthroplasty. *J Bone Joint Surg Am* 1977;59:847.

*An extensive review of hip infections that may present during the immediate postoperative period or after several years. A spontaneously draining hematoma with hip pain and an elevated sedimentation rate are clues to an early hip infection.*

Galicier C, Richet H. A prospective study of postoperative fever in a general surgery department. *Infect Control* 1985;6:487.

*The rate of postoperative fever was about 14% and was unrelated to the classification of the surgical procedure.*

Garibaldi RA, et al. Evidence for the non-infectious etiology of early postoperative fever. *Infect Control* 1985;6:273.
*Most of the causes of fever during the first 48 hours after surgery were not infectious in origin.*

Gaynes R, et al. Mediastinitis following coronary artery bypass surgery: a 3-year review. *J Infect Dis* 1991;163:117.
*Risk factors for infection included prolonged duration of surgery (>210 minutes), low preoperative levels of serum albumin (<3.0 g/dL), and a resident with a positive nasal culture for methicillin-resistant S. aureus.*

Gerding DN, et al. *Clostridium difficile*-associated diarrhea and colitis. *Infect Control Hosp Epidemiol* 1995;16:459–477.
*Review. Treat symptomatic patients with metronidazole or vancomycin for 10 days.*

Green SL, Sarubbi FA. Risk factors associated with postcesarean section febrile morbidity. *Obstet Gynecol* 1977;49:686.
*Causes of fever included endometritis (43%), urinary tract infection (19%), wound infection (11%), pneumonia (2%), and unknown sources (26%).*

Gur E, et al. Clinical-radiological evaluation of poststernotomy wound infection. *Plast Reconstr Surg* 1998;101:348–355.
*Computed tomography is useful in the detection and staging of poststernotomy infections.*

Henle W, et al. Antibody responses to the Epstein-Barr virus and cytomegaloviruses after open heart and other surgery. *N Engl J Med* 1970;282:1068.
*The postperfusion syndrome may result from the transfusion of blood with CMV or, less often, Epstein-Barr virus.*

Holt HM, et al. Infections following epidural catheterization. *J Hosp Infect* 1995; 30:253–260.
*Infection, both local at the catheter exit site or generalized (e.g., meningitis), can complicate epidural catheterization. Most frequent causative organisms included coagulase-negative staphylococci (41%), S. aureus (35%), and gram-negative bacilli.*

Howard RJ. Finding the cause of postoperative fever. *Postgrad Med* 1989;85:223.
*Review.*

Iaizzo PA, Wedel DJ, Gallagher WJ. *In vitro* contracture testing for determination of susceptibility to malignant hyperthermia: a methodologic update. *Mayo Clin Proc* 1991;66:998.
*Muscle tissue from persons susceptible to malignant hyperthermia have lower contracture thresholds (in vitro contracture test) for halothane and caffeine than does normal muscle.*

Ishikawa S, et al. Management of postoperative fever in cardiovascular surgery. *J Cardiovasc Surg* 1998;39:95–97.
*Only 28% of patients with postoperative fever had a bacteriologic cause.*

Johnson LB. The importance of early diagnosis of acute acalculous cholecystitis. *Surg Gynecol Obstet* 1987;164:197.
*Fever is often the initial finding, and normal liver function test results should not exclude the diagnosis. An ultrasound study showing a thickening of the gallbladder (≥3 mm) was helpful in the diagnosis.*

Johnson S, et al. Prospective, controlled study of vinyl glove use to interrupt *Clostridium difficile* nosocomial transmission. *Am J Med* 1990;88:137.
*Hand carriage of C. difficile is an important factor in the transmission of this disease.*

Kirsh MM, et al. Postpericardiotomy syndromes. *Ann Thorac Surg* 1970;9:158.
*A review of the postcardiotomy and postperfusion syndromes.*

Langdale LA. Infectious complications of blood transfusions. *Infect Dis Clin North Am* 1992;6:731.
*A discussion of transfusion-related pathogens, including HIV, with an estimated risk of 1/153,000 U transfused.*

Lee Y-H, Kerstein MD. Osteomyelitis and septic arthritis: a complication of subclavian venous catheterization. *N Engl J Med* 1971;285:1179.
*Osteomyelitis and septic arthritis are potential risks following subclavian vein catheterization.*

Le Gall JR, et al. Diagnostic features of early high postlaparotomy fever: a prospective study of 100 patients. *Br J Surg* 1982;69:452.
*Of patients with fever of 39°C 10 days after laparotomy, half had an intraabdominal focus.*

Lerner PI, Sampliner JE. Transfusion-associated cytomegalovirus mononucleosis. *Ann Surg* 1977;185:406.
*This complication is not limited to patients with extracorporeal circulation; it can occur following blood transfusions in many situations.*

Loeber B, Swenson RM. Bacteriology of aspiration pneumonia. *Ann Intern Med* 1974; 81:329.
*The bacteriology of community-acquired and hospital-acquired aspiration pneumonia differs and reflects pharyngeal colonization.*

Mellors JW, et al. A simple index to estimate the likelihood of bacterial infection in patients developing fever after abdominal surgery. *Am Surg* 1988;54:558.
*After abdominal surgery, only 16% of patients with postoperative fever had a bacterial infection.*

Nathens AB, Chu PTY, Marshall JC. Nosocomial infection in the surgical intensive care unit. *Infect Dis Clin North Am* 1992;6:657.
*Review. Frequent ICU-acquired pathogens include* Staphylococcus epidermidis, Candida, Pseudomonas, *and* Enterococcus.

O'Grady NP, et al. Practice guidelines for evaluating new fever in critically ill adult patients. *Clin Infect Dis* 1998;26:1042–1059.
*Review. Fever in the initial 48 hours after surgery is usually noninfectious.*

Ottinger LW. Acute cholecystitis as a postoperative complication. *Ann Surg* 1976; 184:162.
*Acute cholecystitis may be a cause of fever following an operation for unrelated disease. An atypical presentation is emphasized, with a mortality of 47%.*

Perry JW, et al. Wound infections following spinal fusion with posterior segmental spinal instrumentation. *Clin Infect Dis* 1997:24:558–561.
*Most wound infections were caused by gram-negative aerobic bacilli. Removal of the hardware (rods or wires) was not required for cure.*

Pien FD, Ho PWL, Fergusson DJG. Fever and infection after cardiac operation. *Ann Thorac Surg* 1982;33:382.
*Fever after the third postoperative day suggests an infectious etiology.*

Rader DL, et al. Cytomegalovirus infection in patients undergoing noncardiac surgical procedures. *Surg Gynecol Obstet* 1985;160:13.
*The interval between surgery and the onset of fever ranged from 12 to 31 days (mean, 21 days) in patients with a CMV infection.*

Rello J, et al. Nosocomial respiratory tract infections in multiple-trauma patients. Influence of level of consciousness with implications for therapy. *Chest* 1992;102:525–529.
*In multiple-trauma patients, the most common causes of pneumonia were* S. aureus *(46%),* Haemophilus influenzae *(20%), enteric gram-negative bacilli (22%), and* Streptococcus pneumoniae *(9%).*

Robson MC, Krizek TJ, Heggers JP. Biology of surgical infections. *Curr Probl Surg* 1973;10:1–62.
*Classic. A monograph on surgical wound infections.*

Sarubbi FA, Vasquez JE. Spinal epidural abscess associated with the use of temporary epidural catheters: report of two cases and review. *Clin Infect Dis* 1997;25:1155–1158.
*Fever and localized back pain may be caused by an abscess associated with an epidural catheter.*

Scheld WM, Mandell GL. Nosocomial pneumonia: pathogenesis and recent advances in diagnosis and therapy. *Rev Infect Dis* 1991;13:S743.
*Review of diagnosis and therapy issues.*

Schlenker JD, Hubay CA. The pathogenesis of postoperative atelectasis. *Arch Surg* 1973;107:846.
*This is an early, noninfectious cause of postoperative fever.*

Schoenbaum SC, Gardner P, Shillito J. Infections in cerebrospinal fluid shunts: epidemiology, clinical manifestations, and therapy. *J Infect Dis* 1975;131:543.
*Shunt replacement and antimicrobials are usually required for cure.*

Shapira OM, et al. Unexplained fever after aortic valve replacement with cryo-preserved allografts. *Ann Thorac Surg* 1995;60:S151–S155.
*Unexplained fever was noted in 26% of patients undergoing allograft aortic valve replacement after the third postoperative day. It lasted 24 to 48 hours and resolved without antibiotics.*

Siegel SE, et al. Transmission of toxoplasmosis by leukocyte transfusion. *Blood* 1971; 37:388.
*Toxoplasma was transmitted to four patients with leukemia by granulocyte trans-fusions.*

Soto-Hernandez JL, et al. Secondary adrenal insufficiency manifested as an acute febrile illness. *South Med J* 1989;82:384.
*In this case report, fever 5 weeks after surgery was caused by adrenal insufficiency.*

Sullivan NM, et al. Clinical aspects of bacteremia after manipulation of the genito-urinary tract. *J Infect Dis* 1973;127:49.
*In bacteremia of patients undergoing urologic procedures, antimicrobials are indi-cated only if an antecedent infection is present.*

Talmore M, Li P, Barie PS. Acute paranasal sinusitis in critically ill patients: guide-lines for prevention, diagnosis, and treatment. *Clin Infect Dis* 1997;25:1441–1446.
*Computed tomography of the paranasal sinus is the best test for diagnosis. Sinusitis develops in about 25% of nasally endotracheally intubated patients.*

Verkkala K, et al. Fever, leucocytosis, and C-reactive protein after open heart surgery and their value in the diagnosis of postoperative infections. *Thorac Cardiovasc Surg* 1987;35:78.
*After open heart surgery, a temperature above 38°C after the sixth postoperative day suggests an infectious etiology.*

Warshaw AL. Diagnosis of starch peritonitis by paracentesis. *Lancet* 1972;2:1054.
*Starch granules demonstrated by iodine staining of ascitic fluid may be the cause of fever, pain, and abdominal tenderness 1 to 4 weeks after an operation.*

Wenzel RP. Nosocomial candidemia: risk factors and attributable mortality. *Clin Infect Dis* 1995;20:1531–1534.
*About half of the cases of* Candida *fungemia are caused by species other than* C. albicans.

Wolfe JE, Bone RC, Ruth WE. Effects of corticosteroids in the treatment of patients with gastric aspiration. *Am J Med* 1977;63:719.
*No beneficial effect was noted in a controlled study. Gram-negative pneumonia occurred more frequently in the steroid-treated patients, which suggests a harmful effect.*

Wynne JW, Modell JH. Respiratory aspiration of stomach contents. *Ann Intern Med* 1977;87:466.
*Reviews the pathophysiology and therapy of gastric aspiration.*

Yeung RSW, Buck JR, Filler RM. The significance of fever following operations in chil-dren. *J Pediatr Surg* 1982;17:347.
*Of the children studied, postoperative fever developed in 28.5%, but in only 1.6% was infection responsible for the fever.*

---

## 58.  URINARY CATHETER-RELATED INFECTIONS

The urinary catheter is an extremely useful device but a nosocomial infection hazard. More than four decades ago, in an editorial entitled "Case against the Catheter," the importance of the urinary catheter was noted and its dangers emphasized. Today, the urinary tract is still the most common site of nosocomial infection, accounting for approximately 40% of infections.

The two most effective measures to prevent nosocomial urinary tract infections—decreasing the duration of catheterization and use of a closed, sterile drainage system—were described three decades ago. Approximately 85% of cases of urinary tract infections are catheter-associated, and another 5% follow other types of urologic instrumentation, such as cystoscopy. Prevalence studies show that about 10% of patients in acute care hospitals have a urinary catheter; in an ICU, the rate of urinary catheter use is even higher.

Nosocomial urinary tract infections vary from asymptomatic conditions that resolve spontaneously on catheter removal to infections associated with complications that include pyelonephritis, bacteremia, perinephric abscess, renal stones, renal failure, and death. Bloodstream invasion occurs at a rate of nearly 3% among cases of nosocomial bacteriuria. The rate of bacteremia in patients with a *Serratia* urinary tract infection was four times that of patients with nosocomial urinary tract infections caused by other organisms. Bacteremia developed in men with nosocomial urinary tract infections twice as often as in women. In fact, the urinary tract is the most common portal of entry for bacteria in patients with gram-negative bacteremia. The mortality rate of bacteremia from a catheter-associated urinary tract infection is estimated to be 10% to 30%. In one study, the mortality was three times higher among patients with nosocomial bacteriuria than in uninfected controls, although bacteremias were not documented in the group with the increased mortality rate. In a subsequent study, a marked reduction was noted in the frequency of infections and death rate after introduction of a catheter bag drainage system that did not disconnect at the junction of the catheter and collection tube. Other investigators in a case-control study found no relationship between nosocomial urinary tract infections and death.

## Risk Factors

A number of factors are associated with an increased rate of catheter-associated nosocomial bacteriuria, including female sex, age above 50 years, and the presence of a rapidly progressive, fatal underlying illness. Using an aseptic technique during catheter insertion and maintaining a closed, sterile drainage system are key factors in determining the incidence of bacteriuria. The average rate of acquisition of bacteriuria is 5% to 10% for each day of catheterization; thus, after 10 days, about 50% of patients have bacteriuria. Breaks in the closed drainage system and improper care of the drainage bag occurred in 30% of catheterized patients. Other investigators found that in patients whose urinary catheters had sealed catheter-drainage tube junctions that could not be disconnected, the rate of infection was nearly three times lower than in patients assigned to catheters with unsealed junctions.

Systemic antimicrobials can decrease the rate of bacteriuria but are effective only for the initial 4 days of catheterization. When infection does occur in patients receiving systemic antimicrobials, however, the organisms isolated are generally more resistant. Having more than one patient with a urinary catheter in a room is another risk factor. This is especially a problem if one patient already has bacteriuria, because the hands of medical personnel have been shown to spread organisms from one drainage bag to another.

## Pathogenesis

Organisms appear to enter the urinary tract by one of three routes: (a) from the urethra into the bladder by way of the catheter, (b) at the urethral meatus around the catheter, or (c) by an intraluminal route from the drainage bag or the junction between the catheter and collecting tube during a disconnection. The majority of infections result when bacteria ascend from the periurethral area by means of a thin layer of fluid on the outside of the catheter at the catheter-meatal junction or by the intraluminal route during disconnection of the junction between the catheter and the collection tube. Studies have emphasized the importance of the meatal route in the pathogenesis of bacteriuria; 70% of catheterized patients acquire bacteriuria with the same organism isolated from the urethral meatus before the development of bacteriuria. In another study assessing the importance of prior urethral and rectal colonization in the pathogenesis of catheter-associated bacteriuria, prior urethral colonization was observed in 67% of women and 29% of men in whom bacteriuria developed. Antecedent rectal colonization was noted in 78% of women and 29% of men. In catheterized women, the majority of episodes of bacteriuria develop through the periurethral route, and the source is usually the rectal flora. In contrast, in male patients, most infections develop via the intraluminal route; the source of bacteria is not the rectum but rather cross-infection. This study suggests that different prevention strategies may be needed for male and female patients.

### Etiology

*Escherichia coli* is the most common cause of nosocomial bacteriuria, accounting for about one third of infections. Other common pathogenic agents are *Proteus* species (15%), *Klebsiella* species (10%), *Pseudomonas* species (10%), *Enterobacter* species (5%), enterococci (10% to 15%), and *Candida* (5%). Other organisms, such as *Serratia* and *Providencia,* account for the remaining 7% to 12%. In general, the organisms responsible for nosocomial bacteriuria are more resistant to antimicrobials than are the strains that cause community-acquired infections. The patient's own gastrointestinal flora is the source of many gram-negative bacilli that cause catheter-associated infections. Outbreaks of nosocomial urinary tract infections have been linked to contaminated rectal thermometers, cystoscopes, irrigation solutions, and disinfectants. Medical personnel who do not wash their hands after caring for each patient can transmit gram-negative bacilli from one urinary drainage bag to another.

### Diagnosis

The diagnosis of a nosocomial urinary tract infection in a catheterized patient is based on a urine culture showing significant bacteriuria. Formerly, counts of more than $10^5$ colony-forming units (CFU) per milliliter were required to establish a diagnosis; however, according to a study by Maki and associates, counts as low as $10^2$ CFU/mL are probably significant and should not be ignored. Low-level counts of bacteria or *Candida* in the urine usually increase within 3 days to concentrations above $10^5$ CFU/mL. When a urinary tract infection is responsible for fever, pyuria (more than five white cells per high-power field) should be present. One or more organisms per oil-immersion field in a Gram's-stained drop of unspun urine may provide a clue to the identity of the pathogen and help guide the initial selection of antimicrobial therapy. Polymicrobial bacteriuria occurs in about 75% of patients with long-term indwelling urethral catheters, with a mean of more than two organisms per specimen. The duration of bacteriuric episodes varies with each species. Gram-positive organisms such as coagulase-negative staphylococci persist for about 1 week, whereas *Providencia stuartii* may be present for 10 weeks or longer. Routine bacteriologic monitoring of urine from asymptomatic catheterized patients, however, is not a cost effective approach to decrease or predict the frequency of symptomatic, catheter-related urinary tract infections.

The clinical features of nosocomial bacteriuria in a catheterized patient vary; the patient may have no symptoms or may have chills, fever, flank pain, oliguria, disseminated intravascular coagulation, or shock. Lower urinary tract symptoms such as frequency and dysuria are absent. In elderly catheterized patients, manipulation and change of the urinary catheter are frequent predisposing factors of urosepsis. In this group of patients, gastrointestinal complaints may predominate and direct attention away from the urinary tract.

### Treatment

All patients with a symptomatic, catheter-related urinary tract infection should be treated with a drug to which the causative organism is susceptible. If possible, the catheter should be removed or changed. The optimal duration of therapy is unknown, and the patient should be treated at least until the symptoms resolve if the catheter remains in place. For patients with a secondary bacteremia, which indicates a renal or prostatic source, drugs should be used that provide adequate levels in both urine and serum. Patients who have candiduria without candidemia may respond to catheter removal alone, amphotericin B bladder irrigation, or fluconazole. If clinical evidence of systemic candidiasis is lacking and there is no indication that pyelonephritis is present, then amphotericin B bladder irrigation may be tried if the catheter cannot be removed. Amphotericin B bladder irrigation consists of infusion of 5 to 10 mg of amphotericin B in 250 mL of sterile water into the bladder once daily; the catheter is cross-clamped for 1 hour. The appropriate duration of therapy is unknown, but 2 to 7 days is usually adequate. Most *Candida* organisms are susceptible to less than 1 µg of amphotericin B per milliliter, and the concentrations achieved with the suggested mixture are 20 to 40 μ/mL. Amphotericin B can also be given by continuous bladder irrigation over 12 hours; 25 mg of drug in 500 mL of 5% dextrose in water or sterile water is infused at a rate of 42 mL/h. In patients without renal insufficiency, fluconazole can be given at a dosage of 200 mg orally followed by 100 mg once daily for 4 days. Fluconazole is preferred for therapy of candiduria.

Generally, patients with catheter-associated bacteriuria who are asymptomatic do not require therapy because of the risk of selecting for resistant organisms. One exception may be patients with asymptomatic bacteriuria and a prosthetic graft or heart valve; such patients are at risk for seeding of the foreign body. The most effective measure is to remove the catheter and, if the urine culture remains positive, then treat the patient. In patients without prosthetic devices, the management of catheter-acquired bacteriuria after catheter removal is controversial. In one report, patients often became symptomatic after the catheter was removed. A single dose of oral trimethoprim-sulfamethoxazole (TMP-SMX) after catheter removal was usually effective in preventing symptomatic disease, particularly in patients less than 65 years old.

Recommendations by the Centers for Disease Control to prevent catheter-related bacteriuria are listed in Table 58-1. Using a closed, sterile drainage system and enforcing hand washing before and after a urinary catheter or drainage bag is handled are two measures to prevent nosocomial bacteriuria. The use of meatal disinfectants such as a povidone-iodine solution or silver sulfadiazine cream, antimicrobial-impregnated catheters, silver oxide-coated catheters, antibacterial urethral lubricants, and antibacterial bladder irrigation has failed to decrease the incidence of bacteriuria. The addition of disinfectants such as hydrogen peroxide to the drainage bag is not effective in reducing the incidence of catheter-related bacteriuria.

The value of prophylactic systemic antimicrobials in preventing or delaying bacteriuria remains unclear. The possible benefits must be balanced against cost, adverse

Table 58-1. Summary of recommendations for prevention of catheter-associated urinary tract infections

**Strongly recommended for adoption**
  Educate personnel in correct techniques of catheter insertion and care.
  Catheterize only when necessary.
  Emphasize hand washing.
  Use aseptic technique and sterile equipment to insert catheter.
  Secure catheter properly.
  Maintain closed sterile drainage.
  Obtain urine samples aseptically.
  Maintain unobstructed urine flow.

**Moderately recommended for adoption**
  Periodically reeducate personnel in catheter care.
  Use smallest-bore catheter that is suitable.
  Avoid irrigation unless necessary to prevent or relieve obstruction.
  Refrain from daily meatal care with either povidone-iodine solution or soap and
    water.
  Do not change catheters at arbitrarily fixed intervals.

**Weakly recommended for adoption**
  Consider alternative techniques of urinary drainage before using an indwelling
    urethral catheter.
  Replace the collecting system when sterile closed drainage has been breached.
  Spatially separate infected and uninfected patients with indwelling catheters.
  Avoid routine bacteriologic monitoring.

Adapted from Centers for Disease Control Working Group. Guidelines for prevention of catheter-associated urinary tract infections. In: *Guidelines for the Prevention and Control of Nosocomial Infections.* Atlanta: U.S. Department of Health and Human Services, Public Health Service, 1981.

effects, and selecting for resistant flora. In one study, there was no benefit from the use of TMP-SMX to reduce the incidence of urinary tract infections in patients with long-term indwelling catheters. Resistant organisms such as *Pseudomonas aeruginosa* and *P. stuartii* were identified more often in the antimicrobial-treated group than in the control group. For selected patients, condom catheters can be used to prevent nosocomial bacteriuria. Condoms, however, can produce gangrene and serve as reservoirs for resistant bacteria. The technique of intermittent catheterization appears effective, but controlled studies evaluating this approach are necessary. Hospital-acquired urinary tract infections cause considerable patient suffering and economic loss, and new approaches to dealing with this common problem are needed. (N.M.G.)

### Bibliography

Beeson PB. Case against the catheter. *Am J Med* 1958;24:1.
*Classic.*
Breitenbucher RB. Bacterial changes in the urine samples of patients with long-term indwelling catheters. *Arch Intern Med* 1984;144:1585.
*Neither monthly cultures nor prophylactic TMP-SMX was of value.*
Bryan CS, Reynolds KL. Hospital-acquired bacteremic urinary tract infection: epidemiology and outcome. *J Urol* 1984;132:494.
*Mortality was 31% and related to the severity of the underlying disease.*
Burke JP, Larsen RA, Stevens LE. Nosocomial bacteriuria: estimating the potential for prevention by closed sterile urinary drainage. *Infect Control* 1986;7:96.
*Bacteriuria, particularly in female patients, was associated with improper suspension of the drainage bag.*
Burke JP, et al. Prevention of catheter-associated urinary tract infections: efficacy of daily meatal care regimens. *Am J Med* 1981;70:655.
*Daily meatal care was of no benefit in preventing bacteriuria.*
Classen DC, et al. Daily meatal care for prevention of catheter-associated bacteriuria: results using frequent applications of polyantibiotic cream. *Infect Control Hosp Epidemiol* 1991;12:157.
*Use of an antimicrobial cream containing polymyxin B, neomycin, and gramicidin applied to the urethral meatus three times daily did not reduce the rate of bacteriuria.*
Daifuku R, Stamm WE. Association of rectal and urethral colonization with urinary tract infection in patients with indwelling catheters. *JAMA* 1984;252:2028.
*Women with catheter-related bacteriuria have a rectal source more often than men do.*
Ehrenkranz NJ, Alfonso BC. Failure of bland soap handwash to prevent hand transfer of patient bacteria to urethral catheters. *Infect Control Hosp Epidemiol* 1991;12:654.
*In an experimental study, hand washing with a bland soap did not prevent transfer of bacteria from the groin to the catheter. Use of an isopropyl alcohol hand rinse was more effective in preventing hand transfer of gram-negative bacteria.*
Filice GA, et al. Nosocomial febrile illnesses in patients on an internal medicine service. *Arch Intern Med* 1989;149:319.
*Pneumonia and urinary tract infection were the two most common causes for nosocomial fever in patients on the medical service.*
Fisher JF, Newman CL, Sobel J. Yeast in the urine: solutions for a budding problem. *Clin Infect Dis* 1995;20:183–189.
*Patients with candiduria should be evaluated for possible candidemia or a deep-seated infection.*
Garibaldi RA, et al. Factors predisposing to bacteriuria during indwelling urethral catheterization. *N Engl J Med* 1974;291:215.
*Risk factors are outlined. Antimicrobials were effective during the initial 4 days of catheterization.*
Garibaldi RA, et al. Meatal colonization and catheter-associated bacteriuria. *N Engl J Med* 1980;303:316.
*Bacteria can often be isolated in the periurethral space before the development of bacteriuria.*
Garibaldi RA, et al. An evaluation of daily bacteriologic monitoring to identify preventable episodes of catheter-associated urinary tract infection. *Infect Control* 1982; 3:466.

*Daily urine cultures do not reduce the incidence of symptomatic, catheter-related urinary tract infections.*

Gleckman R, et al. Catheter-related urosepsis in the elderly: a prospective study of community-derived infections. *J Am Geriatr Soc* 1982;30:255.
*Usually a polymicrobial infection. A traumatic catheter event often precedes the acute symptomatic episode.*

Haley RW, et al. The nationwide nosocomial infection rate. *Am J Epidemiol* 1985; 121:159.
*Nosocomial urinary tract infections accounted for 42% of all infections.*

Hamory BH, Wenzel RP. Hospital-associated candiduria: predisposing factors and review of the literature. *J Urol* 1978;120:444.
*Key risk factors include increased duration of catheterization and use of multiple antimicrobials.*

Harding GKM, et al. How long should catheter-acquired urinary tract infection in women be treated? A randomized, controlled study. *Ann Intern Med* 1991;114:713.
*After catheter removal, asymptomatic bacteriuria frequently becomes symptomatic. Single-dose therapy with oral TMP-SMX was effective after short-term catheter use.*

Hirsh DD, Fainstein V, Musher DM. Do condom catheter collecting systems cause urinary tract infections? *JAMA* 1979;242:340.
*Cooperative patients with condom catheters had lower rates of urinary tract infections than did patients with indwelling catheters.*

Huth TS, et al. Randomized trial of meatal care with silver sulfadiazine cream for the prevention of catheter-associated bacteriuria. *J Infect Dis* 1991;165:14.
*Meatal care with silver sulfadiazine cream did not reduce the rate of bacteriuria.*

Jacobs LG, et al. Oral fluconazole compared with bladder irrigation with amphotericin B for treatment of fungal urinary tract infections in elderly patients. *Clin Infect Dis* 1996;22:30–35.
*Both amphotericin B bladder irrigation and oral fluconazole were effective treatments for patients with candiduria.*

Johnson ET. The condom catheter: urinary tract infection and other complications. *South Med J* 1983;76:579.
*Long-term use of a condom catheter drainage system was associated with urinary tract infections and penile complications.*

Johnson JR, et al. Prevention of catheter-associated urinary tract infection with a silver oxide-coated urinary catheter: clinical and microbiologic correlates. *J Infect Dis* 1990;162:1145.
*Overall, no reduction in the rate of bacteriuria was noted with use of the silver oxide-coated catheter except for women not receiving antimicrobials.*

Krieger JN, Kaiser DL, Wenzel RP. Urinary tract etiology of bloodstream infections in hospitalized patients. *J Infect Dis* 1983;148:57.
*Bacteremia developed in almost 39% of patients with nosocomial bacteriuria.*

Kunin CM, Finkelberg Z. Evaluation of an intraurethral lubricating catheter in prevention of catheter-induced urinary tract infections. *J Urol* 1971;106:928.
*Classic. Ineffective approach to preventing urinary tract infections.*

Kunin CM, McCormack RC. Prevention of catheter-induced urinary tract infections by sterile closed drainage. *N Engl J Med* 1966;274:1155.
*Classic.*

Leu HS, Huang CT. Clearance of funguria with short-course antifungal regimens: a prospective, randomized, controlled study. *Clin Infect Dis* 1995;20:1152–1157.
*Spontaneous clearance rate in the control group was 40%. Systemic regimens with amphotericin B or oral fluconazole were more effective than local irrigation with amphotericin B.*

Maki DG, et al. Nosocomial urinary tract infection with *Serratia marcescens:* an epidemiologic study. *J Infect Dis* 1973;128:579.
*An infected, catheterized patient should not share a room with another catheterized patient.*

Platt R, et al. Mortality associated with nosocomial urinary tract infection. *N Engl J Med* 1982;307:637.
*Nosocomial bacteriuria was associated with a threefold increase in mortality.*

Platt R, et al. Reduction of mortality associated with nosocomial urinary tract infections. *Lancet* 1983;1:893.
*Fewer infections and deaths were noted in the patients whose bladder catheters had preconnected, sealed junctions.*

Platt R, et al. Prevention of catheter-associated urinary tract infection: a cost-benefit analysis. *Infect Control Hosp Epidemiol* 1989;10:60.
*Analysis supporting the use of sealed-junction catheters.*

Riley DK, et al. A large, randomized clinical trial of a silver-impregnated urinary catheter: lack of efficacy and staphylococcal superinfection. *Am J Med* 1995;98: 349–356.
*Silver-coated catheters were not effective in preventing bacteriuria.*

Saint S, Elmore JG, Sullivan SD, Emerson SS, Koepsell TD. The efficacy of silver alloy-coated urinary catheters in preventing urinary tract infection: a meta-analysis. *Am J Med* 1998;105(3): 236–41.

Sanford JP. The enigma of candiduria: evolution of bladder irrigation with amphotericin B for management—from anecdote to dogma and a lesson from Machiavelli. *Clin Infect Dis* 1993;16:145.
*Guidelines for treating candiduria.*

Stamm WE. Catheter-associated urinary tract infections: epidemiology, pathogenesis, and prevention. *Am J Med* 1991;91(Suppl 3B):65S.
*Comprehensive review.*

Stark RP, Maki DG. Bacteriuria in the catheterized patient. *N Engl J Med* 1984; 311:560.
*Quantitative cultures showing fewer than $10^5$ CFU per milliliter are significant.*

Thompson RL, et al. Catheter-associated bacteriuria. *JAMA* 1984;251:747.
*Instillation of hydrogen peroxide into the drainage bag did not prevent bacteriuria.*

Warren JW. Catheter-associated bacteriuria in long-term care facilities. *Infect Control Hosp Epidemiol* 1994;15:557–562.
*Review. Closed catheter drainage is the only effective method to prevent bacteriuria.*

Warren JW. Catheter-associated urinary tract infections. *Infect Dis Clin North Am* 1997;11:609–622.
*Review.*

Warren JW, Muncie HL, Hall-Craggs M. Acute pyelonephritis with bacteriuria during long-term catheterization: a prospective clinicopathological study. *J Infect Dis* 1988; 158:1341.
*Among long-term elderly patients, acute inflammation of the kidneys was noted at autopsy in 38% of those with a urinary catheter, and in 5% of those without a catheter.*

Warren JW, et al. Antibiotic irrigation and catheter-associated urinary tract infections. *N Engl J Med* 1978;299:570.
*Antimicrobial irrigation is not effective in preventing bacteriuria.*

Warren JW, et al. A prospective microbiologic study of bacteriuria in patients with chronic indwelling urethral catheters. *J Infect Dis* 1982;146:719.
*Of patients with long-term indwelling catheters, 98% had bacteriuria, which was usually polymicrobial (77%).*

---

## 59. HOSPITAL-ACQUIRED (NOSOCOMIAL) PNEUMONIA

---

Hospital-acquired (nosocomial) infections are those occurring after at least 48 hours of hospitalization; they affect 5% to 6% of all hospitalized patients. This rate is at least three times higher for adult patients in ICUs. In most studies, pneumonia is the second or third most common type identified, accounting for 13% to 18% of all cases, occurring at rates of 4 to 7/1,000 hospitalizations. Nosocomial pneumonia develops in up to 25% of patients in an ICU, and the incidence of pneumonia in mechanically ventilated patients may approach 30/100 patients. If adjusted for "ventilator days," the rates are approximately 15/1,000 ventilator days for medical or surgical patients.

Looked at slightly differently, estimated rates of ventilator-associated nosocomial pneumonia are 1% to 3% per day of intubation/ventilation. Mortality from nosocomial pneumonia is 30% to 50%, and pneumonia is the most common fatal nosocomial infection. The problem is especially severe in the elderly and in intubated and ventilated patients. Rates of 17/1,000 patient-days have been noted in this age group, compared with fewer than 2/1,000 patient-days in persons under the age of 50 years.

Approximately 17% of all nosocomial pneumonias occur in the 1% of patients who are ventilated. Patients with endotracheal tubes or tracheostomies are at risk because these devices bypass respiratory tract host defense mechanisms and allow bacteria to be deposited directly into the lower respiratory tract. Additionally, secretions may pool in the subglottic area above the endotracheal cuff and slowly leak into the lower respiratory tract. Best estimates are that approximately 137,000 deaths may be attributable to this condition annually.

Other overlapping high-risk groups for nosocomial pneumonia are patients in intensive care units (ICUs) and persons undergoing thoracic or thoracoabdominal surgery. Reasons include analgesia, sedation, and pain from thoracotomy tubes.

### Bacteriology and Pathogenesis

Historically, the most common causes of nosocomial pneumonia were considered to be Enterobacteriaceae (most often *Escherichia coli, Enterobacter* species, *Klebsiella* species, and *Serratia* species), *Staphylococcus aureus,* and other gram-negative bacilli (e.g., *Pseudomonas aeruginosa*). Certain species of enteric gram-negative rods often predominate in individual hospitals. Depending on the study and the diagnostic test performed, more than one pathogen may be found in up to 60% of patients. Such observations have important implications for therapy. Data based on transtracheal aspiration techniques and anaerobic bacteriology demonstrate the potentially important role of anaerobes, *Haemophilus influenzae,* and *Streptococcus pneumoniae.* In almost 50% of cases, mixed infection was documented and often involved anaerobes. *S. pneumoniae* and *H. influenzae* are more likely to be noted early in hospitalization (especially in immunocompetent patients with trauma) and in patients who have not received prior antimicrobials. *Legionella* species have also been reported as causes of both sporadic and epidemic cases of hospital-acquired pneumonia. Many cases occur in heavy smokers, those with chronic obstructive lung disease, and persons with underlying disorders of cell-mediated immunity. Nosocomial pneumonias associated with viruses, such as respiratory syncytial virus and influenza virus, among others, have been less thoroughly investigated, in part because of difficulties with cultures.

Up to 25% of ICU patients become colonized with resident gram-negative bacilli within 24 hours, and this increases to approximately 50% after 4 to 5 days. Sources of bacteria are often the patient's own upper respiratory tract flora. Historically, respiratory therapy equipment was incriminated, but this problem is now less important. Exogenous factors associated with nosocomial pneumonia include the hands of hospital personnel and occasionally tap water and other liquids. Contaminated hands were a contributory factor in a recent outbreak of nosocomial legionellosis. Factors associated with colonization include antimicrobial therapy, underlying illnesses, acidosis, coma, and endotracheal intubation. The percentage of colonized patients in whom clinical pneumonia developed was 23%, versus only 3% for those who were not colonized. Other sources of organisms that may predispose to nosocomial pneumonia include the stomach.

### Diagnosis

The diagnosis of nosocomial pneumonia is often difficult, not least because communication with the patient may be impossible. In the presence of endotracheal tubes or tracheostomy, purulent secretions may be indicative of local irritation rather than true infection, and for similar reasons, polymorphonuclear leukocytes may be present on Gram's-stained endotracheal material. Cultures of lower respiratory tract secretions obtained through endotracheal tubes or tracheostomies (blind bronchial sampling) may reveal potential pathogens that possibly reflect only colonization or tracheobronchitis (a clinical entity with far less severe implications). Fever and leukocytosis can develop in a severely ill patient for many reasons other than lower respiratory tract infection. Alternatively, the patient with pneumonia may fail to have a fever or elevated WBC count for reasons that include old age, renal failure, or effects of medication. Well-defined infections may be unaccompanied by fever in up to 30% of cases. Similarly, roentgenography of the chest may prove unreliable. Among the numerous other causes for pulmonary infiltrates are infarct, congestive heart failure, and malignancy. Autopsies performed on patients with adult respiratory distress syndrome suspected of having nosocomial pneumonia have failed to corroborate clinical and radiographic findings in up to 30% of cases.

The diagnosis of nosocomial pneumonia in the intubated/ventilated patient is controversial. Recommendations have ranged from empiric antibiotic therapy through initial invasive procedures that include flexible fiberoptic bronchoscopy with protected brush (FFPB) and quantitative bacteriology or bronchoalveolar lavage (BAL) with quantitative bacteriology. Endpoints that differentiate true pathogens from contaminants are more than $10^3$ (FFPB) and more than $10^4$ (BAL) organisms per milliliter. An endotracheal aspirate is a relatively simple specimen to obtain; however, its role in the diagnosis of nosocomial pneumonia has been controversial. Although some data demonstrate a failure to identify pathogens in up to 40% of cases, others consider the absence of gram-negative bacilli or gram-positive cocci, which is consistent with *S. aureus,* to be reliable information in helping to determine the bacteriology of ventilator-associated pneumonia. Additionally, two recent studies have employed quantitative bacteriology of endotracheal aspirates, with more than $10^5$ to $10^6$ organisms per milliliter as a cutoff. Corroboration with "gold standards" was approximately 70%. A recent prospective investigation of ventilator-associated pneumonia utilized FFPB, BAL, and quantitative endotracheal aspirates, with mortality as the endpoint. There was no mortality advantage when data from FFPB or BAL were utilized in comparison with data available from quantitative endotracheal aspirates. Furthermore, antibiotics were changed more often in patients in whom FFPB and BAL were carried out. It is the opinion of the author that endotracheal aspiration with quantification is evolving into the most cost effective method of diagnosing nosocomial pneumonia in ventilated patients and should be performed before changes in antibiotics are made.

Blood cultures should be obtained from all patients, although positive results may be noted in only about 5% of cases. In general, a diagnosis of nosocomial pneumonia should be strongly considered when the following are present: (a) new or worsening pulmonary infiltrates of uncertain origin; (b) purulent pulmonary secretions in association with polymorphonuclear leukocytes and organisms seen with Gram's stain; (c) an appropriate clinical course, usually associated with respiratory decompensation; and (d) fever and leukocytosis. In practice, it is often necessary to treat critically ill patients as if they had pneumonia even if not all the criteria are fulfilled. Endotracheal aspiration with quantitative bacteriology may evolve into the simplest and most valuable study to identify likely pathogens.

## Management

Respiratory support, treatment of ancillary conditions (congestive heart failure, adult respiratory distress syndrome), and antimicrobial therapy are the cornerstones of management. Antimicrobials should be administered in full therapeutic doses, generally intravenously, with consideration of any organ failure. Recent recommendations from the American Thoracic Society suggest that antibiotics be chosen based on risks for "severe" pneumonia, underlying host conditions, and time of onset of nosocomial pneumonia. Patients at risk for severe nosocomial pneumonia include those who require care in a critical care unit, show rapid radiologic progression of pneumonia, have acute renal failure requiring dialysis, or are in shock or respiratory failure. Early pneumonia is that which occurs within the first 5 days of hospitalization. Underlying conditions that need to be assessed include risk for aspiration, underlying structural lung disease, and risks for legionellosis. Table 59-1 provides antibiotic recommendations based on core pathogens. Table 59-2 expands antibiotic recommendations when mitigating factors are present.

Table 59-1. Management of patients with mild/moderate nosocomial pneumonia, no unusual risk factors, onset anytime, or patients with severe nosocomial pneumonia and early onset

| Likely (core) organisms | Appropriate antibiotics |
|---|---|
| Enteric gram-negative bacilli (*E. coli, Klebsiella* species, *Enterobacter* species, *Serratia, Proteus* species)<br>*Streptococcus pneumoniae*<br>*Haemophilus influenzae*<br>Methicillin-sensitive *Staphylococcus aureus* | Either second-generation cephalosporin or nonpseudomonal third-generation cephalosporin or β-lactam–β-lactamase inhibitor combination.<br>If allergic to β-lactam: flouroquinolone or clindamycin plus aztreonam. |

In most conditions, a single effective antibiotic suffices for treatment. Two agents may be indicated for pneumonia caused by *P. aeruginosa* or *Enterobacter* species (when treatment includes selected cephalosporins), and for empiric therapy when precise organism identification is not available. When legionellosis is considered, either a macrolide or quinolone should be included in the antibiotic regime. Third-generation cephalosporins, imipenem-cilastatin, ticarcillin-clavulanate, and parenteral quinolones are probably all effective against susceptible gram-negative pathogens. Aminoglycosides remain valuable agents for many enteric gram-negative bacilli and *P. aeruginosa*. Regimens of single daily doses of 5 to 7 mg/kg are generally more efficacious and may be safer than the more classic regimens in which doses are administered thrice daily. For considerations of *P. aeruginosa* (e.g., severe nosocomial pneumonia) two effective agents are advised. Clinicians may employ double β-lactam therapy or regimens that include a quinolone. Gram-positive nosocomial pneumonias can be treated with a single appropriate antimicrobial.

The optimal length of therapy for nosocomial pneumonia is unknown. At least 10 days of effective therapy is generally employed. Patients with lung abscess, empyema, and other suppurative complications will require longer courses. Those with pneumonia caused by *Legionella pneumophila* are generally treated for up to 21 days. Use of quinolones may allow selected patients to complete prolonged courses with oral medications. Staphylococcal pneumonia should be treated parenterally for at least 2 weeks. Patients who are bacteremic with *S. aureus* often require at least 4 weeks of parenteral therapy.

Table 59-2. Management of patients with mild/moderate nosocomial pneumonia and risk factors

| Organism based on risk factor | Core antibiotics plus |
|---|---|
| Anaerobes (recent abdominal surgery, witnessed aspiration) | Clindamycin or β-lactam–β-lactamase inhibitor +/– vancomycin (until methicillin-resistant *S. aureus* ruled out). |
| *Staphylococcus aureus* (coma, head trauma, diabetes mellitus, renal failure) | |
| *Legionella* (high-dose corticosteroids) | Erythromycin +/– rifampin (or quinolone alone). |
| *Pseudomonas aeruginosa* (prolonged ICU stay, corticosteroids, prior antibiotics, structural lung disease) | Aminoglycoside or ciprofloxacin plus one of the following: imipenem-cilastatin, aztreonam, or cefepime β-lactam–β-lactamase inhibitor. |

Endotracheal administration of aminoglycosides (generally gentamicin or tobramycin) is valuable in selected patients. It should be considered for persons with gram-negative bacillary or *P. aeruginosa* pneumonia who are receiving parenteral gentamicin or tobramycin. This adjunctive mode of administration provides excellent levels of drug within bronchial secretions and is generally well tolerated. Dosage is typically 40 mg of gentamicin or tobramycin administered endotracheally every 8 hours. Patients are positioned to allow distribution to the area of pneumonia. A recent blinded, placebo-controlled trial demonstrated enhanced microbiologic eradication of the offending pathogen(s). Other studies suggest improved clinical outcomes as well.

## Prevention

Endotracheal tubes and other equipment that bypass normal respiratory defenses should be used judiciously. Postoperative patients should be given cough and deep-breathing exercises, and it is sensible to position patients so as to decrease vomiting. Somnolent patients should be turned regularly. Endotracheal or tracheostomy tubes should be suctioned as necessary. Routine treatment of colonizing bacteria in the absence of clinical or radiographic lower respiratory tract infection is not indicated. Such therapy enhances the emergence of resistant organisms and the potential for clinical infection. Adherence to infection control procedures, including hand washing and appropriate equipment management, is mandatory.

An association between upper gastrointestinal tract colonization and nosocomial pneumonia is now established. Organisms located within the stomach may be aspirated. Colonization with gram-negative bacilli is enhanced by elevations in gastric pH, as may be noted with the use of medications (antacids and histamine$_2$ antagonists) that prevent stress bleeding. Sucralfate (which does not alter gastric pH) appears more effective in preventing colonization and respiratory infection than antacids and histamine$_2$ antagonists. Reasons include a preserved lower pH and a direct antibacterial action of the drug. Other measures that attempt to decrease aspiration of upper gastrointestinal tract contents include the use of jejunostomy tubes for long-term feeding and acidification of enteral feedings.

Selective digestive tract decontamination has been studied, with conflicting results. Intraoral plus nasogastric mixtures of amphotericin B, polymyxin E, and tobramycin (or variants) have been employed in selected patients at high risk for nosocomial pneumonia. These products are administered several times daily throughout the ICU stay. IV cefotaxime has also been used during the first 3 days. Although many data demonstrate decreased oropharyngeal and upper gastrointestinal tract colonization as well as decreased rates of nosocomial pneumonia, mortality rates do not generally change, and this procedure is not currently considered a standard of care.

Occasional outbreaks of nosocomial pneumonia caused by a specific pathogen may occur in hospital areas such as an ICU. Prophylactic administration of aerosolized polymyxin B has been shown to be effective in decreasing both transmission and infection with *P. aeruginosa* during respiratory outbreaks with this pathogen. All at-risk persons entering the ICU should receive the aerosol for several weeks after the last isolate. However, prolonged prophylaxis results in higher mortality rates from pneumonia caused by pathogens resistant to polymyxin. Thus, the routine use of this aerosol as a preventive measure is not encouraged.

It is unlikely that the availability of more potent antimicrobials will result in a decline in the morbidity or mortality of nosocomial pneumonia. Improving host defenses, adherence to infection control policies and procedures, and preventing colonization with potential pathogens, however, may prove to be beneficial. (R.B.B.)

## Bibliography

American Thoracic Society. Hospital-acquired pneumonia in adults: diagnosis, assessment of severity, initial antimicrobial therapy, and preventative strategies. *Am J Respir Crit Care Med* 1995;153:1711–1725.

*Conclusions of a consensus panel. Provides recommendations for the management of nosocomial pneumonia, including antibiotic decision making based on severity of disease, time of onset of nosocomial pneumonia, and risk factors for specific pathogens. Some of the recommendations are somewhat outdated, as newer antibiotics are now available, such as the newer fluorinated quinolones, meropenem, and cefepime.*

Bartlett JG, et al. Bacteriology of hospital-acquired pneumonia. *Arch Intern Med* 1986; 146:868–871.
*One of the few studies of the etiology of nosocomial pneumonia that employed transtracheal aspiration and anaerobic bacteriology. The subjects were a Veterans Administration population having no association with endotracheal intubation and ventilation. A diverse group of organisms was identified, including many anaerobes, common bacteria (S. pneumoniae and H. influenzae), and enteric gram-negative bacilli. At least two organisms were identified in almost 50% of patients.*

Brown RB, et al. Double-blind study of endotracheal tobramycin in the treatment of gram-negative bacterial pneumonia. *Antimicrob Agents Chemother* 1990;34:269–272.
*This blinded, prospective investigation assessed the role of endotracheal tobramycin in addition to standardized parenteral antimicrobial therapy for patients with gram-negative bacillary pneumonia. Microbiologic cure was enhanced in patients who received endotracheal antimicrobials, but clinical efficacy was no different. No significant adverse reactions occurred.*

Chastre J, Fagon JY, Trouillet JL. Diagnosis and treatment of nosocomial pneumonia in patients in intensive care units. *Clin Infect Dis* 1995;21(Suppl 3):S226–S237.
*An excellent summary article that deals with the problems of diagnosing nosocomial pneumonia in this patient population. The authors prefer FFPB with quantitative bacteriology, attempt to perform the procedure before initiating new antibiotic treatments, and withhold antibiotics if results are negative.*

Craven DE, Steger KA. Epidemiology of nosocomial pneumonia. New perspective of an old disease. *Chest* 1995;108 (Suppl):1S–16S.
*The authors present an excellent overview of nosocomial pneumonia, with special reference to bacteriology and risk factors for specific pathogens.*

Driks MR, et al. Nosocomial pneumonia in intubated patients given sucralfate as compared with antacids or histamine type 2 blockers. *N Engl J Med* 1987;317:1376–1382.
*An excellent study comparing two methods commonly employed to prevent stress ulceration in ICU patients. It demonstrates that sucralfate, not primarily associated with elevating gastric pH, was less likely to result in gastric colonization with enteric gram-negative bacilli and was associated with a lower incidence of nosocomial pneumonia.*

Fish DN, et al. An update on nosocomial pneumonia: treatment, prevention, and future directions. *Infect Med* 1992;9:27–28,33,37–42,44–46.
*This review stresses antimicrobial therapy of nosocomial pneumonia based on likely pathogens. Provides good pharmacokinetic and pharmacodynamic data and gives doses of often-employed antimicrobials and regimens.*

Sanchez-Nieto JM, et al. Impact of invasive and noninvasive quantitative culture sampling on outcome of ventilator-associated pneumonia. *Am J Respir Crit Care Med* 1998;157:371–376.
*The authors conducted an open, prospective, randomized study in 51 ventilated patients to determine if they could identify benefits of invasive diagnostic procedures in the management of ventilator-associated pneumonia. In one group, decision making was based on results of either FFPB or BAL (both with quantitative bacteriology), whereas in the second group it was based on endotracheal aspiration with quantitative bacteriology. There was no difference in mortality with the invasive procedures, but there were more changes in antibiotic treatment. The authors conclude that they could not identify benefits of the more invasive procedures in this pilot study.*

Tablan OC, et al., and the Hospital Infection Control Practices Advisory Committee. Guidelines for prevention of nosocomial pneumonia. *Infect Control Hosp Epidemiol* 1994;15:587–627.

*This Centers for Disease Control and Prevention document represents an excellent overview of the problem of nosocomial pneumonia and the methods available for prevention. Recommendations are stratified on the basis of strength of available data.*

---

## 60. MANAGEMENT OF THE EMPLOYEE WITH A NEEDLESTICK INJURY

---

Accidental needle punctures are a frequent hospital problem and a threat to the health of medical personnel. The reported rate is approximately 19 sharp injuries per 100 employees annually. Many needlestick injuries are not reported; in one study, 90% went unreported. Needlestick injuries account for nearly one third of all work-related accidents in the hospital and are second only to musculoskeletal injuries as a cause of work-related illness. Of the reported needlesticks, about 90% occur among nursing personnel, housekeepers, and laboratory technicians. Registered nurses experience at least half of all needlestick injuries. The nursing activities during which most of the needlesticks occur are recapping needles, drawing blood, and administering an injection or infusion. Among housekeeping personnel, needlesticks usually result from handling trash containing improperly disposed needles. Laboratory workers report that most of the needle punctures happen while they are drawing blood and recapping needles. IV systems without needles have decreased the rate of sharp injuries. However, needlesticks still occur because compliance with these devices may be only 50%.

Serious disease and considerable cost can result from needlestick injuries. Transmission of HIV, hepatitis B virus (HBV), and hepatitis C virus (HCV) poses the greatest risk associated with accidental needlesticks for hospital personnel. Other examples of infection that can be transmitted by needlestick punctures are tetanus, tuberculosis, syphilis, malaria, and Rocky Mountain spotted fever. Postexposure prophylaxis, however, should be directed at preventing only HIV, HBV, and HCV infection, not the other illnesses. Except for HIV infection and viral hepatitis, the frequency of transmission of potentially transmissible diseases from a needle puncture is extremely low and is at the level of a case report.

Before the 1980s, the major fear of a health care provider following a needlestick was the development of hepatitis B. The risk for transmitting hepatitis B from an infected patient to a susceptible health care provider following a sharp injury was estimated to be 5% to 35%. The risk for HIV transmission after a percutaneous exposure is about 0.3% to 0.4%. The widespread use of hepatitis B vaccine and the availability of postexposure hepatitis B immune globulin (HBIG) has reduced considerably the risk and fear of acquiring hepatitis B following a sharp injury. Today, the greatest concern of health care providers is to prevent the acquisition of HIV infection as the result of a sharp injury or cutaneous or mucous membrane exposure. Hospital personnel practices have been transformed with the use of double gloving, waterproof gowns, protective eye wear, and face shields. It is estimated that between 27 and 46 HIV seroconversions occur annually per 100,000 hospital personnel at risk. Surgeons and emergency medicine physicians at large urban centers may be at even greater risk. Efforts to reduce the occupational risk for acquiring HIV infection should encompass the following measures:

1. Improve the reporting rates of sharp injuries.

2. Realize that the risk for acquiring HIV infection is lowest for cutaneous and mucous membrane exposures and highest for transfusions and IM inoculations.

3. Evaluate the source patient for HIV and obtain a baseline serum on the exposed health care worker.

4. Consider using postexposure chemoprophylactic treatment of high-risk exposures. Early initiation (within 1 to 2 hours) of prophylaxis is recommended, although failures have occurred when the drug was begun as soon as 30 minutes to 12 hours after an exposure. Zidovudine has been relatively well tolerated, but long-term effects are unknown (Table 60-1).

5. Direct efforts at reducing sharp injuries and developing safer devices.

Table 60-1. Recommendations for chemoprophylaxis after occupational exposure to HIV, by type of exposure and source material

| Type of exposure | Source material* | Antiretroviral prophylaxis[†] | Antiretroviral regimen[§] |
|---|---|---|---|
| Percutaneous | Blood[¶] | | |
| | Highest risk | Recommended | ZDV + 3TC + IDV |
| | Increased risk | Recommended | ZDV + 3TC, ± IDV |
| | No increased risk | Offer | ZDV + 3TC |
| | Fluid containing visible blood, other potentially infectious fluid,[††] or tissue | Offer | ZDV ± 3TC |
| | Other body fluid (e.g., urine) | Not offer | |
| Mucous membrane | Blood | Offer | ZDV + 3TC, ± IDV |
| | Fluid containing visible blood, other potentially infectious fluid,[††] or tissue | Offer | ZDV, ± 3TC |
| | Other body fluid (e.g., urine) | Not offer | |
| Skin, increased risk;[§§] | Blood | Offer | ZDV + 3TC, ± IDV |
| | Fluid containing visible blood, other potentially infectious fluid,[††] or tissue | Offer | ZDV, ± 3TC |
| | Other body fluid (e.g., urine) | Not offer | |

* Any exposure to concentrated HIV (e.g., in a research laboratory or production facility) is treated as percutaneous exposure to blood with highest risk.
[†] *Recommend* – Postexposure prophylaxis (PEP) should be recommended to the exposed worker. *Offer* – PEP should be offered to the exposed worker. *Not offer* – PEP should not be offered because these are not occupational exposures to HIV.
[§] Regimens: zidovudine (ZDV), 200 mg three times a day; lamivudine (3TC), 150 mg two times a day; indinavir (IDV), 800 mg three times a day. Prophylaxis is given for 4 weeks.
[¶] *Highest risk* – BOTH larger volume of blood (e.g., deep injury with large-diameter hollow needle previously in source-patient's vein or artery, especially involving an injection of source-patient's blood) AND blood containing a high titer of HIV (e.g., source with acute retroviral illness or end-stage AIDS; viral load measurement may be considered, but its use in relation to PEP has not been evaluated). *Increased risk*—EITHER exposure to larger volume of blood OR blood with a high titer of HIV. *No increased risk*—NEITHER exposure to larger volume of blood NOR blood with a high titer of HIV (e.g., solid suture needle injury from source-patient with asymptomatic HIV infection).
[††] Includes semen; vaginal secretions; cerebrospinal, synovial, pleural, peritoneal, pericardial, and amniotic fluids.
[§§] For skin, risk is increased by exposures involving a high titer of HIV, prolonged contact, an extensive area, or an area in which skin integrity is visibly compromised. For skin exposures without increased risk, the risk for drug toxicity outweighs the benefit of PEP.
Modified from Centers for Disease Control Update. Provisional Public Health Service recommendations for chemoprophylaxis after occupational exposure to HIV. *MMWR Morb Mortal Wkly Rep* 1996;45:1–5.

Hepatitis B can be transmitted by percutaneous inoculation (needlestick), mucous membrane inoculation, sexual intercourse with an infected person, or perinatally from an infected mother to her infant. Any of these routes can be classified as critical exposure. In a hospital, needlesticks and mucous membrane inoculation are the only routes of transmitting hepatitis. Blood that is positive for HBsAg (hepatitis B surface antigen) and HBeAg (hepatitis B early antigen) is infectious even at a dilution of $10^{-8}$. The presumption is that HBsAg does not cross intact skin but enters only at the site of broken skin.

HCV is an RNA virus that can be transmitted by a needlestick or sharp injury. The rate of seroconversion is about 2% (range, 0 to 7%). One study in which the polymerase chain reaction (PCR) technique was used found a seroconversion rate of 10% after a needlestick. Infection is rare after a mucous membrane or nonintact skin exposure. A case report describes the transmission of HCV following a blood splash to the conjunctiva. Figure 60-1 outlines guidelines for managing a possible HCV exposure. If the source is positive for HCV, then the serologic status of the exposed person must be determined. A variety of tests are available to detect HCV, including antibody enzyme immunoassay (EIA) and recombinant immunoblot assay (RIBA). The sensitivity of the new EIA is about 92%. If the EIA result is positive, then an RIBA is ordered. If the RIBA result is positive, then measure the HCV RNA with PCR. The PCR result can be positive for HCV RNA in 1 to 3 weeks after an exposure. Unfortunately, results of the PCR test for HCV RNA are frequently false-positive or false-negative. Persons exposed to an HCV-positive source should at present have a baseline EIA and liver function tests, and these should be repeated at 6 months. The role of interferon for HCV seroconversion is limited. Immune globulin (IG) is not beneficial (Fig. 60-1).

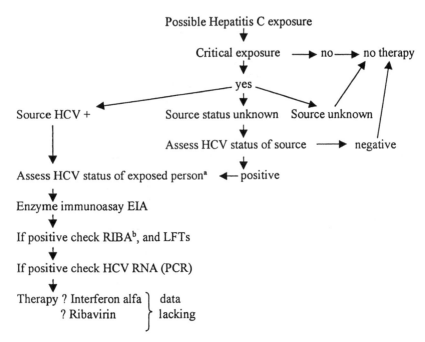

**Figure 60-1.** Management of a possible HCV exposure. [a]Assess HCV status of exposed person at baseline and repeat assessment at 3 months and 6 months. HCV RNA can be detected in the blood in 1 to 3 weeks by PCR, but false-positives and false-negatives occur. [b]RIBA, recombinant immunoblot assay.

A number of questions must be answered relating to the management of an employee who has recently had a needlestick injury:

1. *Has the employee had a critical exposure?* Critical exposures include percutaneous punctures and mucous membrane contact. Blood-to-hand contact does not require prophylaxis unless cuts are present on the hand. The skin is an excellent barrier against hepatitis B; however, dermatologic disease is extremely common in hospital employees, and if skin disease is present, then IG prophylaxis can be recommended depending on the hepatitis status of the blood source and the hepatitis B immunity of the employee. Stool contact does not constitute critical exposure unless the stool is from a patient who has gastrointestinal bleeding.

2. *What is the hepatitis status of the source of the inoculum?* If the source is found to be HBsAg-positive, the recipient of the needlestick should receive HBIG immediately unless immune. If the source is found to HBsAg-negative, there is little risk for transmission of hepatitis B, and prophylaxis to prevent hepatitis B is not indicated. If the source is found to be HBsAg-negative and positive for anti-HBc (antibody to hepatitis B core antigen), the source is probably not infectious for hepatitis B after a needlestick. Blood that is positive for anti-HBc, however, may be infectious when it is transfused, but the inoculum is considerably smaller after a needlestick than after a transfusion. Blood that is HBsAg-positive and positive for either HBeAg or anti-HBe (antibody to HBe antigen) must be considered infectious, although the risk is far greater if the blood is positive for both HBsAg and HBeAg. Table 60-2 outlines an approach to managing persons after a percutaneous (needlestick, laceration, or bite) or permucosal (ocular or mucous membrane) exposure to blood. The therapeutic decisions are based on the HBsAg status of the source blood and the anti-HBs status of the recipient of the exposure.

3. *What is the risk for hepatitis B following a needlestick if the blood status of the source is unknown and cannot be determined?* If the source is unknown, the risk for acquiring hepatitis B is extremely low (1/2,000), and HBIG prophylaxis is unnecessary for that exposure.

4. *What is the immune status of the recipient of the needlestick?* If the serologic test on the recipient shows evidence of immunity (blood positive for anti-HBs), HBIG is unnecessary. Usually, the serologic result of the source of the blood is available before the immune status of the recipient is known. Whether HBIG is administered or not depends on the test results.

5. *When should HBIG be administered?* As soon as the results of the HBsAg test on the blood source are available, HBIG can be given if the blood source is found to be HBsAg-positive. HBIG is effective if given within 7 days of the exposure, but the sooner it is administered, the more effective it probably will be.

6. *When should hepatitis C be suspected?* Hepatitis C should be suspected if the source of the blood (donor) has a history of unexplained chronic liver disease, has received several blood transfusions, has hemophilia, is on long-term hemodialysis, or is a drug addict. Hepatitis C has been transmitted by accidental needlestick or sharp injury; the average incidence of anti-HCV seroconversion was 1.8% (range, 0 to 7%).

7. *Is effective prophylaxis available to prevent hepatitis B after a critical exposure to HBsAg-positive blood?* Both IG and HBIG are effective in postexposure prophylaxis. One study showed that clinical type B hepatitis was reduced further with HBIG than with IG (2% vs. 8%); however, subclinical infection occurred more often with HBIG prophylaxis, and overall infection occurred equally in both groups. In another report, there was no difference in the percentages of patients in whom hepatitis developed between those who received normal-titer IG and those who received HBIG. Evidence of hepatitis B appeared after postexposure prophylaxis with IG or HBIG in 7% of patients. Despite these reports, most authorities recommend HBIG for those who sustain a needlestick with blood from an HBsAg-positive donor. A second dose of HBIG is given after 1 month if the recipient of the needlestick is found to be susceptible to hepatitis B (lacking anti-HBs at the time of the needlestick exposure) and has refused hepatitis vaccine. The use of HBIG or IG is not contraindicated in pregnancy. There is also no evidence that AIDS is transmitted with either IG or HBIG.

8. *Is IG effective in preventing hepatitis C after a needlestick exposure?* Current IG lacks protective antibody against HCV.

Table 60-2.  Recommendations for hepatitis B prophylaxis
following percutaneous or permucosal exposure

| Exposed person | Source | | |
|---|---|---|---|
| | HBsAg positive | HBsAg negative | Source not tested or unknown |
| Unvaccinated | HBIG × 1* and initiate HB vaccine | Initiate HB vaccine | Initiate HB vaccine |
| Previously vaccinated known responder (within 12 mo) | Test exposed for anti-HBs: (1) if adequate,** no treatment (2) if inadequate, HB vaccine booster dose and HBIG × 1 | No treatment | No treatment |
| Known non-responder | HBIG × 2, or HBIG × 1 plus HB vaccine | No treatment | If known high-risk source, treat as if source were HBsAg-positive |
| Response unknown | Test exposed for anti-HBs: (1) if inadequate,** HBIG × 1 plus HB vaccine booster dose (2) if inadequate, no treatment | No treatment | Test exposed for anti-HBs: (1) if inadequate** and known high-risk source, HB vaccine booster dose plus HBIG × 1 (2) if adequate, no treatment |

HB, hepatitis B; HBIG, hepatitis B immune globulin; RIA, radioimmunoassay; EIA, enzyme immunosorbent assay.
* HBIG dose 0.06 mL/kg IM.
** Adequate anti-HBs is ≥10 sample ratio units by RIA.
Modified from Centers for Disease Control. Immunization of health-care workers. Recommendations. *MWWR* 1997;46:23.

9. *What is the role of hepatitis B vaccine after a needlestick?* The HBIG is only about 75% effective, is very expensive ($150 per dose), and provides only temporary protection. Because of these considerations, hepatitis B vaccine can be given along with HBIG after a needlestick exposure if the recipient is negative for anti-HBs. A second dose of HBIG is unnecessary if the hepatitis B vaccine is administered. The response to hepatitis B vaccine is not impaired by concurrent administration of HBIG. A dose of vaccine is repeated after 1 month and 6 months.

10. *What is the therapy for a critically exposed recipient of blood that is HBsAg-positive who has received a single dose of vaccine?* A single dose of HBIG is indicated if the recipient has received only one dose of hepatitis B vaccine. If a person has received at least two doses of hepatitis B vaccine before a needlestick, no treatment is necessary if serologic tests show adequate levels of anti-HBs.

11. *How should a person who has received the complete hepatitis B vaccine series be managed following a percutaneous or other critical exposure to a source known to be HBsAg-positive?* First, test the person for the level of anti-HBs. If the antibody level is greater than or equal to 10 sample ratio units by radioimmunoassay, no treatment

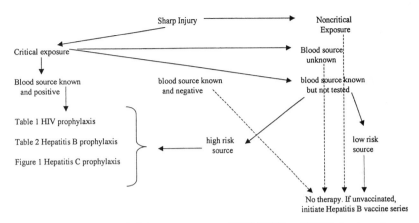

**Figure 60-2.** Recommended therapy to prevent HBV, HCV, and HIV infection after an exposure.

is necessary. If inadequate antibody levels are found, give one dose of HBIG and a booster dose of vaccine. If the person has had adequate anti-HBs levels within the past year, no treatment is necessary. The anti-HBs titer determination is repeated if the test was performed more than 1 year before. If the exposed person is known to have inadequate antibody levels, administer one dose of HBIG and one booster dose of hepatitis B vaccine.

12. *How many health care workers are infected yearly in the United States with HIV from an occupational exposure?* About five to 10 cases occur yearly. An acute retroviral illness develops in 75% of these cases.

13. *How long should postexposure prophylaxis be given?* The guidelines suggest a 4-week treatment period, but this is arbitrary. A shorter (1- to 2-week course) with a two- or three-drug regimen may be appropriate, but data are lacking.

14. *How long should a health care worker be monitored after exposure to detect HIV seroconversion?* Ninety-five percent of seroconversions occur within 6 months. If an exposed health care worker has a possible acute retroviral illness within the first 6 months, a high-risk exposure, an illness associated with impaired antibody production, or HCV infection, then a 1-year follow-up is indicated.

15. *When should postexposure prophylaxis be administered?* Preferably, start antiretroviral drugs within 1 to 2 hours. Indications for therapy are based on the type of exposure and source material.

A flowchart of therapy to prevent HBV, HCV, and HIV infection for the person who sustains a needlestick injury is presented in Fig. 60-2. (N.M.G.)

**Bibliography**
Bell DM, Gerberding JL. Human immunodeficiency virus (HIV) postexposure management of health care workers. *Am J Med* 1997;102:1–126.
*The entire issue is devoted to HIV postexposure management. The Public Health Service suggests that an exposed health care provider be followed for 6 months (e.g., 6 weeks, 12 weeks, and 6 months) to detect HIV seroconversion.*
Cardo DM, et al. A case-control study of HIV seroconversion in health care workers after percutaneous exposure. *N Engl J Med* 1997;337:1485–1490.
*Factors associated with an increased risk for HIV transmission include deep injury, injury with a device that is visibly contaminated with blood, procedures that involve inserting a needle into the source patient's artery or vein, and a terminally ill source patient.*

Centers for Disease Control and Prevention. Update: provisional Public Health Service recommendations for chemoprophylaxis after occupational exposure to HIV. *MMWR Morb Mortal Wkly Rep* 1996;45:468–472.
*Prophylaxis was associated with a 79% decreased risk for HIV seroconversion.*

Centers for Disease Control and Prevention. Immunization of health care workers: recommendations of the Advisory Committee on Immunization Practices (ACIP) and the Hospital Infection Control Practices Advisory Committee (HICPAC). *MMWR Morb Mortal Wkly Rep* 1997;46(RR18):3–10, 14–17, 22–23.
*Guidelines.*

Centers for Disease Control and Prevention. Evaluation of safety devices for preventing percutaneous injuries among health care workers during phlebotomy procedures, Minneapolis-St. Paul, New York City, and San Francisco, 1993–1995. *MMWR Morb Mortal Wkly Rep* 1997;46:21–25.
*Injuries associated with phlebotomy account for 39% of cases of HIV seroconversion. Use of safety devices can decrease the sharp injuries related to phlebotomy.*

Centers for Disease Control and Prevention. Evaluation of blunt suture needles in preventing percutaneous injuries among health care workers during gynecologic surgical procedures, New York City, March 1993–June 1994. *MMWR Morb Mortal Wkly Rep* 1997;46:25–29.
*Blunt rather than curved suture needles were associated with fewer sharp injuries.*

Centers for Disease Control and Prevention. Recommendations for follow-up of health care workers after occupational exposure to hepatitis C virus. *MMWR Morb Mortal Wkly Rep* 1997;46:603–606.
*Guidelines for the management of an HCV exposure.*

Centers for Disease Control and Prevention. Public Health Service guidelines for the management of health care worker exposures to HIV and recommendations for postexposure prophylaxis. *MMWR Morb Mortal Wkly Rep* 1998;47(RR7):1–33.
*Guidelines for HIV postexposure prophylaxis.*

Dienstag JL, et al. Hepatitis B vaccine in health care personnel: safety, immunogenicity, and indicators of efficacy. *Ann Intern Med* 1984;101:34.
*Ninety-seven percent of vaccine recipients responded to three doses of vaccine.*

Folin AC, Nordström GM. Accidental blood contact during orthopedic surgical procedures. *Infect Control Hosp Epidemiol* 1997;18:244–246.
*Blood exposure occurred in 11% of orthopedic procedures, mostly with skin contamination (79%) and percutaneous injury (13%).*

Gerberding JL, et al. Risk of exposure of surgical personnel to patients' blood during surgery at San Francisco General Hospital. *N Engl J Med* 1990;322:1788.
*Parenteral exposures occurred in 1.7% of operations. Risk was greatest with procedures lasting more than 3 hours, blood loss exceeding 300 mL, and major vascular and intraabdominal gynecologic surgery.*

Hoofnagle JH, et al. Passive-active immunity from hepatitis B immune globulin. *Ann Intern Med* 1979;91:813.
*Efficacy of HBIG documented.*

Ippolito G, et al. The risk of occupational human immunodeficiency virus infection in health care workers. *Arch Intern Med* 1993;153:1451.
*The rate of seroconversion was 0.25% after percutaneous exposure and 0.09% after mucous membrane contamination. The rate of seroconversion after HIV contamination of nonintact skin is even lower than with a mucous membrane exposure.*

Knodell RB, et al. Efficacy of prophylactic gamma globulin in preventing non-A, non-B posttransfusion hepatitis. *Lancet* 1976;1:557.
*Gamma globulin may be effective in reducing the severity of posttransfusion hepatitis C. Its value in preventing hepatitis C secondary to a needlestick is unknown. Gamma globulin used today has no role in the prevention of hepatitis C.*

Lawrence LW, et al. The effectiveness of a needleless intravenous connection system: an assessment by injury rate and user satisfaction. *Infect Control Hosp Epidemiol* 1997;18:175–182.
*Use of a needleless IV connection system was associated with about a 50% reduction in needlesticks.*

L'Ecuyer PB, et al. Randomized prospective study of the impact of three needleless intravenous systems on needlestick injury rates. *Infect Control Hosp Epidemiol* 1996;17:803–808.

*Needlestick injuries can occur despite the availability of needleless devices.*

Mangione CM, Gerberding JL, Cummings SR. Occupational exposure to HIV: frequency and rates of underreporting of percutaneous and mucocutaneous exposures by medical house staff. *Am J Med* 1991;90:85.

*Only 30% of sharp injuries were reported by the house staff.*

Manian FA, Meyer L, Jenne J. Puncture injuries due to needles removed from intravenous lines: should the source patient routinely be tested for blood-borne infections? *Infect Control Hosp Epidemiol* 1993;14:325.

*Testing of source blood is unnecessary in injuries caused by needles from peripheral IV lines and distal ports of central lines unless blood is seen.*

McCormick RD, et al. Epidemiology of hospital sharps injuries: a 14-year prospective study in the pre-AIDS and AIDS eras. *Am J Med* 1991;91(Suppl3B):301S–307S.

*Injuries occurred during disposal of used procedure trays (20%), administration of parenteral drugs (16%), surgery (16%), blood drawing (13%), and recapping of used needles (10%).*

Management of Hepatitis C. *NIH Consensus Statement* 1997;15:1–41.

*Review of hepatitis C.*

Noguchi S, et al. Early therapy with interferon for acute hepatitis C acquired through a needlestick. *Clin Infect Dis* 1997;24:992–994.

*Case reports of a short course of interferon used to treat two patients in whom HCV infection developed after a needlestick.*

O'Neill TM, Abbott AV, Radecki SE. Risk of needlesticks and occupational exposures among residents and medical students. *Arch Intern Med* 1992;152:1451.

*Only 9% of exposures were reported. Residents and students cited being too busy as the main reason for not reporting.*

Patel N, Tignor GH. Device-specific sharps injury and usage rates: an analysis by hospital department. *Am J Infect Control* 1997;25:77–84.

*Reported injury rates per 100,000 devices. Injury rates were 11.1/100,000 for butterfly needles and 8.5/100,000 for IV catheters.*

Petrosillo N, et al. The risks of occupational exposure and infection by human immunodeficiency virus, hepatitis B virus, and hepatitis C virus in the dialysis setting. *Am J Infect Control* 1995;23:278–285.

*In this dialysis unit, a seroprevalence survey revealed HIV antibody (0.1%), HBsA (5.1%), and HCV antibody (39.4%).*

Puro V, Petrosillo N, Ippolito G. Risk of hepatitis C seroconversion after occupational exposures in health care workers. *Am J Infect Control* 1995;23:273–277.

*Risk for HCV seroconversion after a hollow-bore needlestick was 1.2% and 0 after mucous membrane contamination.*

Resnic FS, Noerdlinger MA. Occupational exposure among medical students and house staff at a New York City Medical Center. *Arch Intern Med* 1995;155:75–80.

*Half of the surgical house officers, 27% of students, and 20% of medical house staff noted an exposure (sharp injury, mucous membrane, or broken skin) to a patient's blood within the past 6 months.*

Ridzon R, et al. Simultaneous transmission of human immunodeficiency virus and hepatitis C virus from a needlestick injury. *N Engl J Med* 1997;336:919–922.

*A rare example of delayed HIV seroconversion 9.5 months after a needlestick. Most cases (95%) of HIV seroconversion occur within 6 months.*

Tokars JI, et al. Surveillance of HIV infection and zidovudine use among health care workers after occupational exposure to HIV-infected blood. *Ann Intern Med* 1993;118:913.

*Rate of seroconversion after percutaneous exposure to HIV-infected blood was 0.36%. Failures of zidovudine prophylaxis have occurred.*

## 61. HEPATITIS C

Four million Americans are infected with the hepatitis C virus (HCV), and 30,000 new cases are expected annually. Hepatitis C is now responsible for 20% of all cases of hepatitis and causes about 10,000 deaths annually in the United States. It is the most common cause of chronic liver disease and is the most frequent reason for liver transplantation in the United States, accounting for 20% of all liver transplants. The disease will become even more of a problem during the next several decades, as most infected patients are currently in the third decade of life. Immunoprophylaxis is not available, but there is great hope that treatment can reduce the morbidity of the disease significantly. Non-A, non-B hepatitis was originally recognized more than 15 years ago, but the lack of a diagnostic test markedly limited knowledge and understanding of the disease. In a novel approach, Choo and colleagues in 1989 used molecular biology to clone HCV. These new techniques enabled the hepatitis C agent to be identified even though it could not be grown or serologically defined. Sensitive serologic tests are now available, and the risk for transfusion-related hepatitis is down to one case per 100,000 units transfused.

### Virology
HCV is an RNA virus of the flavivirus family. Its heterogeneous populations of viruses is now well-appreciated. HCV can be divided into subtypes by nucleotide sequences. Variations in these subtypes explain some of the variability in disease progression, response to therapy, and complexities of vaccine development.

### Epidemiology
Like hepatitis B, hepatitis C is perpetuated by the large reservoir of asymptomatic patients with the disease. Before 1989, hepatitis C was the major cause of post-transfusion hepatitis, and transfusion was the most important mode of transmission of the disease. HCV is now rarely caused by blood transfusion because of the development of sensitive serologic screening methods. Parenteral drug use now accounts for more than half of all HCV infections. Most of the additional cases occur in patients who received transfusions or were exposed to blood products before 1990. Body piercing and tattooing are likely to increase as causes of HCV, although no specific data are yet available on their importance in the transmission of HCV. The issue of sexually transmitted HCV remains controversial, but the Centers for Disease Control reports that 10% of patients with the disease had no risk factor other than sexual contact with a person who had hepatitis or sexual activity with multiple partners. HCV RNA has not been found in the semen of seropositive patients. The risk for transmission of HCV by sexual contact can be increased by coinfection with HIV or other sexually transmitted diseases.

Another mode of transmission appears to be frequent blood contact in persons employed in the medical or dental professions. Hemodialysis patients also appear to have an increased risk for HCV infection, with 10% to 30% of long-term hemodialysis patients affected. Infection from mother to infant is a possible mode of transmission, although this path is uncommon.

Current estimates are that in patients with a firm clinical diagnosis of post-transfusion hepatitis, about 80% are positive for anti-HCV. One group estimates the current risk for post-transfusion hepatitis to be one case per 100,000 units transfused, down from as high as 450 cases per 100,000 units transfused before 1986.

### Clinical Features
HCV RNA is present in the bloodstream 1 to 3 weeks after initial exposure. Liver injury usually develops in 7 to 8 weeks. Patients usually remain asymptomatic. A prodrome of nonspecific symptoms, such as malaise, fatigue, low-grade fever, and gastrointestinal symptoms, occur in one fourth of patients exposed. These symptoms are clinically indistinguishable from those of other forms of viral hepatitis. Fulminant liver failure is extremely rare. The rise in aminotransferases may well be the first evi-

dence of disease. Because most patients are totally asymptomatic, their being infected with HCV would be missed were enzyme monitoring not conducted. Several studies have shown that peak levels of alanine aminotransferase (ALT) are not as high in HCV infection as is commonly seen in HBV or HAV infection. HCV infection most commonly exhibits a fluctuating pattern of ALT activity, sometimes with such protracted periods of normal (or near-normal) levels that it becomes difficult to determine whether the acute disease has subsided or chronic hepatitis has developed. Prospective studies of transfusion recipients in whom HCV infection develops report the incidence of jaundice to be 15% to 25% in this population. In contrast, HBV infection more frequently causes overt jaundice. Infrequently reported features include microvesicular steatosis, eosinophilic changes, and sinusoidal cell activation. Perhaps the most significant and alarming feature of HCV infection is its propensity to progress to chronic liver disease. In about 80% of patients, chronic hepatitis with viremia develops.

Almost two thirds of patients have abnormal ALT levels, but as noted, most of these patients are symptomatic. Disease progression is variable, with cirrhosis of the liver developing in 20% of patients within 20 years. Hepatocellular carcinoma occurs in hepatitis C infection, probably as a result of inflammation and regeneration. Extrahepatic signs have included arthritis, keratoconjunctivitis, and lichen planus, and laboratory data may include mixed cryoglobulinemia. Patients with compensated cirrhosis have an excellent 5-year survival, about 91%.

## Differential Diagnosis

Acute hepatitis may be caused by several pathologic conditions, the most common of which are viral infections and ingestion of drugs or toxins such as isoniazid, acetaminophen, aspirin, methyldopa, propylthiouracil, halothane, sulfonamides, and nitrofurantoin. This variety makes serologic testing and medication history of paramount importance to the physician investigating hepatocellular disease. When the drug and toxin history are unrevealing, the following need to be excluded for accuracy of diagnosis: infection with viruses known to cause hepatitis (HAV, HBV, HCV, Epstein-Barr virus, cytomegalovirus, and, given the right setting, HIV and HEV), alcoholic liver disease, nonalcoholic steatohepatitis, Wilson's disease, hemochromatosis, $\alpha_1$-antitrypsin deficiency, congestive heart failure, severe hypotension, and biliary tree disease. Other known causes of elevations in ALT and aspartate aminotransferase in serum are autoimmune disease, obesity (fatty liver), exercise, thyroid disease, syphilis, and a poorly defined, nonviral hepatocyte injury associated with homologous blood transfusion.

## Methods of Detection

As in the investigation of any disease process, the initial steps should always be completion of a careful history and physical examination, with particular attention paid to risk factors for HCV and signs and symptoms of chronic liver disease. A history of prior transfusion of blood products, IV drug use, multiple sexual partners or sexual contact with a person known to have hepatitis, membership in a household with a known hepatitis case, and employment as a health care worker have all been suggested as risk factors.

Before 1989, testing for HAV, HBV, and HDV was available, but the agent of parentally acquired non-A, non-B hepatitis remained elusive. Fortunately, through major efforts of virologists, microbiologists, and immunologists, this period came to an end in 1989 when a radioimmunoassay, capable of detecting the presence in serum of antibody to the infectious cDNA clone belonging to HCV, became available. From these experiments followed the development of the enzyme-linked immunosorbent assay (ELISA) now widely used as a diagnostic tool for HCV infection. Enzyme immunoassays are now automated and inexpensive. Second-generation enzyme immunoassays (EIAs) are 92% to 95% sensitive. Depending on the population studied, 25% to 60% of blood donors with positive results by EIA will have positive results by the "gold standard" polymerase chain reaction (PCR) test.

Hence, the EIA has become an excellent screening test for HCV. A negative test result in a low-risk person rules out the disease. A positive EIA result needs to be confirmed by the recombinant immunoblot assay (RIBA). RIBA is a more specific test than the EIA, and a negative RIBA result means that the patient is very unlikely to have HCV infection. Patients who have positive EIA and RIBA results are very likely to be infected with HCV. An assay for HCV RNA by PCR can confirm viremia; however, a single PCR test result could be negative. These patients should be followed by repeated PCR testing and measurement of ALT levels. Patients who are candidates for antiviral therapy should undergo a liver biopsy to assess the severity of hepatitis. Quantitative testing for HCV RNA is not routinely necessary.

There are six genotypes and 30 subtypes of HCV RNA. Patients with serotypes 2 and 3 are more likely to respond to interferon alfa than patients with serotype 1. However, genotyping is not yet a standard approach to management, and patients with genotype 1 should not be excluded from treatment on that basis.

### Treatment

Although the response of patients with HBV infection to corticosteroids or immunosuppressive agents is well-known, little information is available about HCV in this regard. At least two studies, however, have shown that in liver disease caused by HCV, corticosteroids are of no benefit and may in fact worsen the clinical picture (as is true for HBV infection). A relentless, worldwide effort to identify a successful treatment for chronic hepatitis has included methods such as immunosuppression, immunostimulation with bacille Calmette-Guérin (BCG) or levamisole, the use of extracts from plants such as *Phyllanthus canarus,* and antiviral therapy with adenine arabinoside monophosphate (Ara-AMP), acyclovir, and interferon alfa. Interferon therapy has been most promising.

The interferons are a family of glycoproteins produced primarily by monocytes and transformed lymphocytes, usually in response to viral infections. Although not entirely understood, the interferons appear to act through immunomodulatory mechanisms by binding to specific cell receptors on infected cells and activating intracellular enzymes with several antiviral actions. Interferon also enhances both T-cell-mediated and natural killer cell cytotoxicity. Several types of interferon have been developed and made available through recombinant techniques. Of these, interferon alfa has definitively been shown to have anti-HCV activity. Randomized, double-blind, controlled trials in the United States have shown a complete response (normalization of ALT levels) in 48% of recipients and a partial response in another 14% after 24 weeks of interferon therapy. Most investigators agree that a dose approximating 3 million units three times weekly for 6 months is needed to obtain a response (complete or partial) in more than half of treated subjects (as many as 50% do not respond at all). Treatment is recommended for persons in whom cirrhosis is most likely to develop—including patients with persistently elevated ALT, those who test positive for HCV RNA, and those for whom liver biopsy shows portal bridging and fibrosis. Side effects of interferon alfa therapy generally are fatigue, malaise, weight loss, and mild leukopenia and thrombocytopenia. Unfortunately, a sustained response following cessation of therapy is not to be expected. Overall, only about 20% to 50% of patients treated with interferon alfa for 6 months appear to have a sustained response (one study reports a 10% sustained response rate). The benefit of larger doses or an extended treatment period, or both, remains unproven, as does the question of maintenance doses. The combination of interferon alfa and oral ribavirin has recently received FDA approval and appears to yield a more sustained response. (SLB)

### Bibliography

Alberti A. Diagnosis of hepatitis C: facts and perspectives. *J Hepatol* 1991;12:279.
   *Discusses the advantages of various diagnostic tests for HCV (ELISA, RIBA, RIBA-2, and PCR) and points to PCR as the "gold standard" indicator of infection.*
Alter MJ. Non-A, non-B hepatitis: sorting through a diagnosis of exclusion. *Ann Intern Med* 1989;110:583.
   *Two epidemiologically distinct types of non-A, non-B hepatitis are probably caused by different viruses. One type is transmitted parenterally, and the other by the fecal-oral route.*

Alter MJ. Clinical, virological and epidemiological basis for the treatment of chronic non-A, non-B hepatitis. *J Hepatol* 1990;11:S19.
*Changes in donor selection and transfusion practices with the advent of screening for non-A, non-B hepatitis have led to a decline in post-transfusion non-A, non-B infection—from 5% to 10% before 1985 to 2% to 4% in 1990.*

Alter MJ, et al. The natural history of community-acquired hepatitis C in the United States. *N Engl J Med* 1992;327:1899.
*The rate of chronic hepatitis among patients with community-acquired hepatitis C is high, but progression to liver failure is unusual.*

Bennett WG, et al. Estimates of the cost effectiveness of a single course of interferon-α2b in patients with histologically mild chronic hepatitis C. *Ann Intern Med* 1997;127:855.
*A metaanalysis of five prospective trials of interferon alfa in hepatitis C. Based on the natural history of hepatitis C, standard interferon therapy for 12 months should increase the life span of patients with hepatitis C at a reasonable cost, below that of some well-accepted interventions.*

Choo QL, et al. Isolation of cDNA clone derived from a blood-borne non-A, non-B hepatitis genome. *Science* 1989;244:359.
*Report of the cloning of the major virus responsible for blood-borne non-A, non-B hepatitis.*

Davis GL. Recombinant alpha-interferon treatment of non-A, non-B (type C) hepatitis: review of studies and recommendations for treatment. *J Hepatol* 1990;11:S72.
*ALT levels can be normalized in 38% of patients with hepatitis C by giving 2 to 3 million units of recombinant interferon alfa-2b three times per week; however, relapse rates are approximately 50% when the drug is stopped.*

Davis GL, et al. Treatment of chronic hepatitis C with recombinant interferon alpha: a multicenter randomized, controlled trial. *N Engl J Med* 1989;321:1501.
*Three million units of interferon alfa three times weekly for 24 weeks controls disease activity (normalizes ALT levels); however, relapse is common after treatment.*

Dewar TN. Non-A, non-B hepatitis. *West J Med* 1990;153:173.
*Outlines the experimental approach that has led to the identification and characterization of HCV and its role in non-A, non-B hepatitis, and summarizes what is known about preventing and treating the disease.*

DiBisceglie AM, Hoofnagle JH. GI drug column: antiviral therapy of chronic viral hepatitis. *Am J Gastroenterol* 1990;85:650.
*Interferon alfa is the most promising drug studied thus far in the treatment of chronic viral hepatitis.*

DiBisceglie AM, et al. Recombinant interferon alpha therapy for chronic hepatitis C: a randomized, double-blind, placebo-controlled trial. *N Engl J Med* 1989;321:1506.
*Recombinant interferon alfa reduced disease activity in chronic hepatitis C as assessed by serial testing of serum aminotransferase activities and histology of liver biopsy specimens.*

Donahue JG, et al. The declining risk of post-transfusion hepatitis C virus infection. *N Engl J Med* 1992;327:369.
*Because of blood donor screening, the risk for HCV transmission by transfusion of blood and blood products has decreased to 0.57% from 3.84% before 1986.*

Everhart JE, et al. Risk for non-A, non-B (type C) hepatitis through sexual or household contact with chronic carriers. *Ann Intern Med* 1990;112:544.
*Conclusive evidence of HCV transmission to family members or sexual contacts of adult patients with well-documented disease was not demonstrated in this study.*

Farrell GC. Treatment of chronic hepatitis C with alpha-interferon. *J Gastroenterol Hepatol* 1991;1:36.
*Clinical response to interferon alfa occurs in approximately 50% of hepatitis C patients; relapse rate following discontinuance of the drug varies from 40% to 80%.*

Garcia G, Gentry KR. Chronic viral hepatitis. *Med Clin North Am* 1989;73:971.
*Points out the common clinical problem of chronic viral hepatitis and reviews the treatment of chronic hepatitis B, delta hepatitis, and non-A, non-B viral hepatitis (hepatitis C).*

Gerber MA, et al. Histopathology of community-acquired chronic hepatitis C. *Mod Pathol* 1992;5:483.
*In this study, liver biopsy specimens of patients known to be HCV-positive showed chronic persistent hepatitis (45%), chronic active hepatitis (35%), and chronic lobular hepatitis (2%).*

Halfon P, et al. Indeterminate second-generation hepatitis C recombinant immunoblot test: detection of hepatitis C virus infection by polymerase chain reaction. *J Infect Dis* 1992;166:449.
*Most patients with indeterminate results on immunoblot tests for HCV had positive results on PCR tests. HIV-positive patients were often HCV-negative on PCR tests.*

Hess G. Treatment of chronic hepatitis C. *J Hepatol* 1991;1:17.
*Review article documents the effectiveness of interferon alfa in chronic hepatitis C and also points out its shortcomings.*

Hoofnagle JH, DiBisceglie AM. Treatment of chronic type C hepatitis with alpha interferon. *Semin Liver Dis* 1989;9:259.
*Treatment with interferon alfa (and possibly beta) in hepatitis C leads to a marked decrease in serum aminotransferases, which is sustained following discontinuance of the drug in approximately 50% of cases.*

Houghton M, et al. Molecular biology of the hepatitis C viruses: implications for diagnosis, development and control of viral disease. *Hepatology* 1991;14:381.
*HCV is a major etiologic agent in non-A, non-B hepatitis, and advances in the study of its molecular biology have implications for the diagnosis, treatment, and control of the disease.*

Hsia PC, Seeff LB. Non-A, non-B hepatitis: impact of the emergence of the hepatitis C virus. *Adv Intern Med* 1991;37:197.
*Reviews the history, prevalence, presentation, complications, and treatment of hepatitis C.*

Jacyna MR, Thomas HC. Parenterally acquired non-A, non-B hepatitis 10 years on: advances in diagnosis and therapy. *Postgrad Med J* 1990;66:1000.
*Twenty percent of patients with chronic non-A, non-B hepatitis have no detectable anti-HCV, which suggests that one or more other parenterally transmitted agents exist.*

Lumreras C, et al. Clinical, virological, and histologic evolution of hepatitis C virus infection in liver transplant recipients. *Clin Infect Dis* 1998;26:48.
*Prospective study to define the clinical course of hepatitis C in liver transplant patients. Hepatitis C was often associated with early graft hepatitis.*

Management of hepatitis C. *NIH Consensus Statement* 1997;15:1–41.
*Independent report of a consensus panel on the diagnosis and treatment of hepatitis C. Includes an updated bibliography.*

Marcellin P, et al. Long-term histologic improvement and loss of detectable intrahepatic HCV RNA in patients with chronic hepatitis C and sustained response to interferon-$\alpha$ therapy. *Ann Intern Med* 1997;127:825.
*Patients with hepatitis C who have been treated with interferon alfa and have persistently normal ALT levels with no HCV RNA after 6 months usually have a sustained response, histologic improvement, and no intrahepatic HCV RNA.*

Osmond DH, et al. Risk factors for hepatitis C virus seropositivity in heterosexual couples. *JAMA* 1993;269:361.
*Provides little evidence for sexual transmission of HCV.*

Pereira BJG, et al. Prevalence of hepatitis C virus RNA in organ donors positive for hepatitis C antibody and in the recipients of their organs. *N Engl J Med* 1992;327:910.
*Recipients of organs from HCV antibody-positive patients became infected with HCV.*

Phillips DL. What to do with the patient with a positive HCV antibody test. *Hawaii Med J* 1991;50:254.
*Describes the steps physicians might follow when antibody to HCV is identified in a patient.*

Sherlock S, Dushelko G. Hepatitis C virus updated. *Gut* 1991;21:966.
*Describes the methods of several investigators in their quest for a better definition of hepatitis C and for other potential non-A, non-B agents.*

Terada S, Katayama K. Minimal hepatitis C infectivity in semen. *Ann Intern Med* 1992;117:171.
*HCV RNA was not detected in the semen of seropositive patients.*

Van der Poel CL, et al. Confirmation of hepatitis C virus infection by new, four-antigen recombinant assay. *Lancet* 1991;337:317.
*This study finds the four-antigen RIBA to be a good confirmatory test for HCV infection in samples positive on C-100 ELISA; specificity of the four-antigen RIBA was confirmed by comparison with PCR testing, the gold standard.*

Weinstock HS, et al. Hepatitis C virus infection among patients attending a clinic for sexually transmitted diseases. *JAMA* 1993;269:392.
*HCV was not common in non-IV drug users presenting at a clinic for patients with sexually transmitted diseases.*

Williams AE, Dodd RY. The serology of hepatitis C virus in relation to post-transfusion hepatitis. *Ann Clin Lab Sci* 1990;20:192.
*The assay for anti-HCV is highly specific for the agent of non-A, non-B hepatitis, but the test is somewhat deficient for the diagnosis of acute-phase illness.*

Zonaro A, et al. Detection of serum hepatitis C virus RNA in acute non-A, non-B hepatitis. *J Infect Dis* 1991;163:923.
*Determination of HCV RNA by PCR can provide early information on the pathogen causing hepatitis. Viral RNA may be present before seroconversion.*

# XIV. ZOONOSES

## 62. HUMAN INFECTIONS FOLLOWING ANIMAL BITES

Animal bite injuries are common, accounting for about 1% of all emergency department visits and 10,000 hospital admissions. Dogs and cats are responsible for approximately 90% and 10%, respectively, of all animal bites, and these species are the focus of this chapter. However, the variety of animals causing bites is broad, and the spectrum of infections complicating these injuries is continually expanding; for example, "rat-bite fever," which is caused by *Spirillum minor* or *Streptobacillus moniliformis,* can complicate a rodent bite; "seal finger," an extremely painful condition that responds to tetracycline, can follow a seal bite; and the medical literature contains reports of *Acinetobacter* osteomyelitis following a hamster bite, *Aeromonas* soft-tissue infection resulting from a piranha bite, leptospirosis complicating a rat bite, tularemia transmitted by a squirrel bite, and *Vibrio* infection following a shark bite. Finally, bites can lead to substantial soft-tissue inflammation that can be confused with an infectious disease; the latter clinical scenario commonly follows the bite of the brown recluse spider (*Loxosceles*).

Although less common than dog bites, cat injuries are associated with a fivefold to 10-fold greater risk of infection. The increased infection rate following feline bites can be attributed, in part, to differences in the nature of the wound (puncture for cats vs. laceration for dogs) and to the higher rate of oropharyngeal carriage of *Pasteurella multocida* by cats (90% vs. 50% for dogs).

The majority of infections complicating animal bites involve the skin and subcutaneous tissues; however, animal bites can also lead to contiguous infections (osteomyelitis, septic arthritis), bacteremia with metastatic disease (endocarditis), and unusual conditions, such as cat scratch disease. Further, because bite injuries can be associated with the presence of bone fractures or foreign bodies, a radiographic study should be included in the initial evaluation of selected patients, such as children with dog bites of the hand.

Thorough local wound care is essential in patients presenting with an infected or uninfected animal bite. All wounds should be washed with large volumes of normal saline solution; the purpose of the cleansing is to reduce the number of viable bacteria inoculated during the attack and to remove dirt and other foreign material. Most authorities recommend that puncture wounds be irrigated under high pressure; other experts believe that high-pressure irrigation increases the extent of tissue injury. Similarly, most authorities recommend that all wounds be cleansed with a povidone-iodine solution; others suggest that disinfectant solutions aggravate the soft-tissue insult. Debridement of wounds, including punctures, should be performed under local anesthesia; devitalized skin and subcutaneous tissue must be removed, and involved contiguous structures, such as tendons, joint capsules, and bone, should be explored.

The surgical management of animal bite wounds is rarely straightforward. In general, wounds that are infected at presentation must be left open, and when located on cosmetically unimportant areas, they should be allowed to heal by secondary intention. When present on cosmetically important areas, infected bites can be cleansed, debrided, and packed, and if the infection resolves within 5 to 7 days, they can be revised and closed. Wounds that are open, a few hours old, uninfected at presentation, and amenable to thorough cleansing may be candidates for closure. Some authorities recommend that the primary closure of hand wounds be avoided, regardless of the age of the wound. Cat bites in cosmetically unimportant areas should not be closed; however, because of the rich vascularity and cosmetic importance of the face, many experts recommend that uninfected, fresh facial wounds be sutured primarily. Because of a high risk for infection, the closing of older wounds is not recommended.

Early in the evaluation of the patient with an animal bite, the need for tetanus and rabies immunoprophylaxis should be determined. Concern about the possibility of rabies has increased substantially along the East Coast since the epizootic among raccoons has spread from the mid-Atlantic states to New England. Bats and carnivorous wild animals (raccoons, skunks, foxes) are most likely to be infected with the virus. Any person who experiences an open wound following the bite of a carnivorous mammal should be considered at risk for rabies, unless brain tissue from the animal is negative for the virus on immunofluorescent staining. These wounds must be cleaned thoroughly with soap and water, and previously unvaccinated patients should be given passive and active immunization as soon as possible with human rabies immune globulin (HRIG) and the human diploid cell vaccine (HDCV), respectively. The recommended dose of HRIG is 20 IU/kg of body weight; if feasible, half of the dose should be infiltrated into the tissues around the wound and the balance administered intramuscularly into the gluteal area. The standard dose of HDCV is 1 mL given intramuscularly in the deltoid area at presentation and on days 3, 7, 14, and 28. HRIG and HDCV must not be administered in the same syringe or into the same anatomic site.

The decision concerning the need for antirabies immunoprophylaxis in the patient with a dog or other domestic animal bite will be guided by a number of factors, including the presence or absence of rabies in the region where the injury occurred, circumstances of the incident (provoked vs. unprovoked), and condition of the animal at the time of the attack (unknown, rabid or suspected rabid, healthy and available for observation). Although the animal's vaccination status should be determined, a history of rabies immunization does not exclude the possibility of the disease; indeed, deaths from rabies have occurred in travelers bitten outside the United States by dogs believed to have been immunized. The bites of squirrels, hamsters, chipmunks, rats, mice, rabbits, and hares almost never require antirabies prophylaxis. Additional details concerning postexposure rabies prophylaxis can be obtained from the Centers for Disease Control and state public health departments.

Microlobiologic data from studies of infected bites demonstrate that the lesions are usually polymicrobic, and that, on average, three bacteria can be isolated from each wound. The microbes most frequently isolated are *Staphylococcus aureus,* aerobic streptococci, *P. multocida,* and a variety of anaerobes, such as *Peptococcus* species, *Bacteroides* species, and *Fusobacterium* species. Although the antimicrobial therapy of infected wounds will be guided by the results of deep-tissue cultures, the initial regimen should have good activity against most of the pathogens listed, especially *P. multocida.* Most strains of *Pasteurella* are resistant to the semisynthetic penicillins (e.g., dicloxacillin), first-generation cephalosporins (e.g., cephalexin), clindamycin, and the aminoglycosides. In the outpatient setting, amoxicillin-clavulanate would be a rational choice, as it possesses good *in vitro* activity against all the pathogens usually associated with infected bite wounds. Penicillin-allegic patients with infected cat bites can be treated with doxycycline or ciprofloxacin, provided other contraindications are not present. Penicillin-allergic adults with infected dog bites can be given clindamycin plus a fluoroquinolone. In the inpatient setting, empiric therapy with ampicillin-sulbactam, ticarcillin-clavulanate, or penicillin plus oxacillin would provide the necessary coverage; the drug treatment can be modified as microbiologic information becomes available. In the penicillin-allergic patient, clindamycin plus doxycycline or a quinolone, which are agents with good *in vitro* activity against *P. multocida,* represent acceptable therapies. Of note, the potential toxicities of tetracyclines and quinolones limit their use in children. Erythromycin exhibits only moderate activity against *Pasteurella,* and life-threatening complications have evolved in patients with pasteurellosis treated with that agent; clarithromycin and azithromycin also have poor activity against the bacterium.

The role of prophylactic antimicrobials in patients with uninfected bite wounds remains controversial. Overall, the risk for infection in a wound that has been vigorously cleaned is low (about 10%); however, the risk appears to be substantially higher in hand lesions. In general, antimicrobials should be considered in patients who present within 12 to 24 hours and in circumstances in which the chances of infection are high or the consequences of infection would be great. Accordingly, prophylactic antimicrobials should be used in puncture wounds, especially cat bites; deep wounds of the hands; wounds involving joints or tendons; wounds in immunosuppressed persons; and perhaps facial wounds. Amoxicillin-clavulanate represents a rational choice; doxycycline alone or doxycycline plus clindamycin would be acceptable in the penicillin-allergic adult patient.

*Capnocytophaga canimorsus* (dysgonic fermenter-2, or DF-2) is a gram-negative bacillus that is carried in the oropharynx of about 25% of dogs and 15% of cats. In otherwise normal hosts, *C. canimorsus* rarely causes disease; however, the bacterium can cause a fulminant illness in splenectomized persons, alcoholics, and patients receiving corticosteroids. Usually following a dog bite, the *C. canimorsus* septicemia syndrome is characterized by fever, cellulitis, bacteremia, endocarditis, meningitis, disseminated intravascular coagulation, shock, renal failure, and peripheral gangrene. Penicillin represents the treatment of choice.

Patients with animal bites treated on an ambulatory basis should be seen within 24 to 48 hours in follow-up. Among patients with initially infected lesions, the response to antimicrobial treatment can be assessed, and the results of wound cultures can be reviewed; the evaluation will determine the need for additional surgical intervention or modifications in drug therapy. Among patients with initially uninfected wounds that are sutured, early follow-up is mandatory, as most infections following animal bites will become manifest within 24 to 48 hours of the injury. All sutures should be removed from infected lesions. As stated before, antimicrobial therapy will be guided by the results of wound cultures. (A.L.E.)

## Bibliography

Avner JR, Baker MD. Dog bites in urban children. *Pediatrics* 1991;88:55.
*Young children are at risk for bite injuries from pet dogs, especially German shepherds, pit bulls, rottweilers, and Doberman pinschers.*

Brakenbury PH, Muwanga C. A comparative double-blind study of amoxicillin-clavulanate vs. placebo in the prevention of infection after animal bites. *Arch Emerg Med* 1989;6:251.
*In this prospective study, the authors found that amoxicillin-clavulanate was superior to placebo in preventing infection in wounds 9 to 24 hours old; no significant difference was noted in wounds less than 9 hours old.*

Butt TS, et al. *Pasteurella multocida* infectious arthritis with acute gout after a cat bite. *J Rheumatol* 1997;24:1649.
*A geriatric patient who experienced a cat bite to the leg subsequently presented with septic and gouty arthritis.*

Capellan J, Fong IW. Tularemia from a cat bite: case report and review of feline-associated tularemia. *Clin Infect Dis* 1993;16:472.
*The authors describe a middle-aged man in whom ulceroglandular and pneumonic tularemia developed following a cat bite, and they review 14 previously reported cases of cat-associated tularemia.*

Centers for Disease Control. *Capnocytophaga canimorsus* sepsis misdiagnosed as plague—New Mexico, 1992. *MMWR Morb Mortal Wkly Rep* 1993;42:72.
*The article reports a patient with fatal C. canimorsus sepsis that was initially diagnosed as plague, and it summarizes some of the epidemiologic data derived from 200 human cases of disease caused by this pathogen.*

Dire DJ. Cat bite wounds: risk factors for infection. *Ann Emerg Med* 1991;20:973.
*In this prospective survey of 186 patients with 216 cat bites or scratches, the authors found that among the risk factors for infection were age over 50 years, a full-thickness lesion, and a long interval between injury and presentation. Among the subjects with bite injuries only and with uninfected wounds at presentation, infections were more likely to develop in patients with puncture or lower extremity wounds who did not receive prophylactic antimicrobials.*

Feder HM Jr, Shanley JD, Barbera JA. Review of 59 patients hospitalized with animal bites. *Pediatr Infect Dis J* 1987;6:24.
*In this review of pediatric and adult patients, the authors present the microbiology of infected wounds, noting that the Gram's stain of drainage from these lesions is not accurate in predicting results of cultures.*

Fishbein DB. Rabies. *Infect Dis Clin North Am* 1991;5:53.
*A thorough review of animal and human rabies in the United States, with discussions on preexposure and postexposure interventions.*

Francis DP, Holmes MA, Brandon G. *Pasteurella multocida*. Infections after domestic animal bites and scratches. *JAMA* 1975;233:42.
*P. multocida produces a rapidly evolving cellulitis, with most patients experiencing symptoms within 24 hours following the bite injury.*

Goldstein EJ. Bite wounds and infection. *Clin Infect Dis* 1992;14:633.
   *A thorough discussion of the microbiology and management of animal (and human) bite wounds.*
Hantson P, et al. Fatal *Capnocytophaga canimorsus* septicemia in a previously healthy woman. *Ann Emerg Med* 1991;20:93.
   *Although most serious infections caused by* C. canimorsus *(DF-2) occur in immunosuppressed patients, this report illustrates the capacity of the bacterium to produce a fatal illness in ostensibly fit persons.*
Hicklin H, Verghese A, Alvarez S. Dysgonic fermenter-2 septicemia. *Rev Infect Dis* 1987;9:884–890.
   *The clinical manifestations, course, and outcome of the dramatic infection caused by DF-2* (C. canimorsus) *are reviewed.*
Janda DH, et al. Nonhuman primate bites. *J Orthop Res* 1990;8:146.
   *Persons bitten by* Macaca *monkeys are at risk for a number of infections, including disease caused by* Herpesvirus simiae *(B virus), which can produce a fatal encephalomyelitis.*
Levin JM, Talan DA. Erythromycin failure with subsequent *Pasteurella multocida* meningitis and septic arthritis in a cat-bite victim. *Ann Emerg Med* 1990;19:1458.
   *Erythromycin and the newer macrolides have inadequate activity against* P. multocida.
McDonough JJ, Stern PJ, Alexander JW. Management of animal and human bites and resulting infections. *Curr Clin Topics Infect Dis* 1987;8:11.
   *This comprehensive review of the problem includes a discussion of the potential legal ramifications of treating animal bite wounds, such as the need to testify in a personal injury suit. To address that possibility, the authors emphasize the importance of meticulous documentation.*
Rollof J, Nordin-Fredriksson G, Holst E. *Pasteurella multocida* occurs in high frequency in the saliva of pet dogs. *Scand J Infect Dis* 1989;21:583.
   *In this survey of 21 pet dogs, 17 (81%) were found to harbor* P. multocida.
Shinall EA. Cat-scratch disease: a review of the literature. *Pediatr Dermatol* 1990;7:11.
   *A review of the clinical manifestations of the illness, with a discussion of the role of antimicrobials in normal and immunosuppressed patients.*
Talan DA, et al. Bacteriologic analysis of infected dog and cat bites. *N Engl J Med* 1999;340:85.
   *In a study of the microbiology of the infected wounds of 57 patients with cat bites and 50 patients with dog bites, the authors found an average of 5 bacterial isolates per culture.* Pasteurella *species were the microbes most frequently recovered from these patients and were isolated from 75% of patients with cat bites and 50% of those with dog bites.*
Valtonen M, et al. *Capnocytophaga canimorsus* septicemia: fifth report of a cat-associated infection and five other case. *Eur J Clin Microbiol Infect Dis* 1995;14:520.
   *Although usually associated with dog bites, the* C. canimorsus *sepsis syndrome can occur in susceptible patients following bites or the licking of skin ulcers.*
Weber DJ, et al. *Pasteurella multocida* infections: report of 34 cases and review of the literature. *Medicine* (Baltimore) 1984;63:133.
   *The clinical spectrum of infections associated with this microbe is reviewed.*
Wright JC. Reported cat bites in Dallas: characteristics of the cats, the victims and the attack events. *Public Health Rep* 1990;105:420.
   *In this survey, the author found that most cat bites are caused by stray female cats and that most victims are women.*

# XV. NEWLY APPRECIATED INFECTIONS

# 63. NEW AND INCREASINGLY RECOGNIZED PATHOGENS

During the last 5 years, scientists have discovered a number of new infectious organisms (including hepatitis G virus, *Chlamydia*-like microorganism Z, *Legionella*-like ameball pathogen, Cache Valley virus, and *Babesia* species) and have come to appreciate the expanded role of three additional pathogens [*Bartonella* (*Rochalimaea*) *quintana*, *Ehrlichia* species, and *Escherichia coli* 0157:H7].

Hepatitis G virus (an RNA virus of the genus *Flaviviridae*) is a blood-borne agent that frequently causes coinfection along with other hepatitis viruses. The majority of patients become chronic carriers, but there is no evidence that it causes chronic hepatitis, cirrhosis, or hepatocellular carcinoma. In addition, chronic infection with hepatitis G virus does not appear to affect the course, severity, or outcome of liver disease caused by hepatitis B or C virus. An unproven concern is that there may be an association between hepatitis G and aplastic anemia following acute hepatitis.

Microorganism Z is a *Chlamydia*-like bacterium that has been implicated in patients with community-acquired pneumonia. The illness attributed to microorganism Z is characterized by fever, a nonproductive cough, gastrointestinal symptoms, and a prompt response to erythromycin therapy. Identification of the infection requires isolation of the organism in tissue culture or serologic evidence of antibody.

In other patients with community-acquired pneumonia, infection appears to be caused by a *Legionella*-like ameball pathogen. The organism, a gram-negative bacterium known as Hall's coccus, is a nonculturable bacterial pathogen of amebae. The manifestations of pneumonia are not unique. Evidence of the organism's role in infection is established by serologic detection of a fourfold rise in antibody titer.

Cache Valley virus infection has been reported in a patient in North Carolina. This virus, a member of the family *Bunyaviridae*, caused encephalitis and multiple organ dysfunction. Presumably, the disease is transmitted through mosquito bites. The diagnosis requires viral isolation. There is no specific treatment, and therapy is supportive.

*Babesia*-like protozoal organisms that cause infections in humans, particularly patients who have undergone splenectomy, have been newly identified in the western United States (WA1) and in Missouri (MO1). These tick-transmitted disorders are characterized by fever, chills, headache, weakness, myalgia, nausea, and vomiting. The diagnosis is established by demonstration of the intraerythrocytic tetrad (Maltese cross) forms of merozoites and by detection with indirect immunofluorescence of antibody in acute- and convalescent-phase sera. Treatment consists of clindamycin with quinine, perhaps exchange transfusion of red cells, and, if indicated, hemodialysis.

*Bartonella* (*Rochalimaea*) *quintana*, a fastidious, slow-growing, gram-negative bacillus, shares with *Bartonella* (*Rochalimaea*) *henselae* the ability to cause bacillary angiomatosis, bacillary peliosis, relapsing fever, bacteremia, and endocarditis. *B. quintana* is transmitted by the body louse and appears to be an important cause of blood culture-negative endocarditis. Alcoholism and homelessness appear to be risk factors for the development of endocarditis. Attempts at isolation in blood cultures should include use of the lysis-centrifugation system and routine subculture on chocolate and freshly prepared blood agar in a carbon dioxide-enriched atmosphere. In addition to combination treatment with antibiotics (ampicillin or ceftriaxone with gentamicin), valve replacement is often required to cure the patient with *Bartonella* endocarditis.

Ehrlichiosis, a tick-borne disease that may be more common than Rocky Mountain spotted fever, is caused by two agents: *Ehrlichia chaffeensis,* the agent that causes human monocytic ehrlichiosis, and an *Ehrlichia* species (very nearly identical to *Ehrlichia equi*) that causes human granulocytic ehrlichiosis. Patients with ehrlichiosis experience fever, malaise, headache, myalgias, and on occasion rigors, nausea, vomiting, arthralgias, cough, confusion, and rash. Symptoms usually develop within 3 days to 1 week of a tick bite (between May and October). Ticks can transmit numerous pathogens (including *Borrelia burgdorferi, Babesia microti, Rickettsia rickettsii, Francisella tularensis*) in addition to *Ehrlichia* species, so that patients may experience coinfection or sequential infections; these can result in diagnostic confusion, uncharacteristic findings, and serologic cross-reactions, which contribute to diagnostic difficulty. Laboratory abnormalities can include thrombocytopenia, leukopenia, and elevated liver enzymes. Most patients will not demonstrate morulae (colonies of organisms within the cytoplasm of peripheral leukocytes), and treatment (consisting of 100 mg of doxycycline twice daily for 5 to 7 days) should be initiated when the disease is suspected, as fatalities have occurred from delayed therapy. The diagnosis is usually established by serologic testing (fourfold increase in indirect fluorescent antibody titer between acute and convalescent sera), although early antibiotic therapy can diminish the immune response, and there is a potential for serologic cross-reactions between *Ehrlichia* and other tick-borne pathogens. The polymerase chain reaction technique has been used for rapid detection of both human ehrlichiosis agents; however, this diagnostic test is not widely available.

Perhaps no pathogen has generated more media attention or occasioned more economic concerns recently than enterohemmorrhagic (0157:H7) *E. coli.* This organism produces both hemorrhagic colitis and hemolytic uremic syndrome. Initially identified as a contaminant of undercooked ground beef (ingested in fast-food restaurants), the organism has contaminated ham, roast beef, raw milk, yogurt, mayonnaise, apple cider, vegetables, salads, cantaloupe, and more recently alfalfa sprouts. At particular risk are elderly, bedridden persons.

Disease is caused by the toxin(s) elaborated by adherent *E. coli,* and it ranges from mild diarrhea to severe hemorrhagic colitis. The diarrhea can be accompanied by severe abdominal cramping, vomiting, and abdominal tenderness on examination. The most severe disease occurs in the proximal colon. Most patients do not have fever. Person-to-person transmission occurs, as in medical personnel caring for hospitalized patients.

The mainstay of diagnosis is culture of stool with confirmation by direct immuno-fluorescence to detect 0157 and H7 antigens. Treatment consists of fluid and electrolyte administration, monitoring for blood loss, and observation for hemolytic uremic syndrome. Antibiotic therapy has not decreased the length or severity of diarrhea, nor has it reduced progression to the hemolytic uremic syndrome. Antimotility agents are also not indicated.

The hemolytic uremic syndrome (acute renal failure, thrombocytopenia, microangiopathic hemolytic anemia) occurs approximately 1 week after the onset of diarrhea and is often associated with central nervous system complications. The syndrome occurs more commonly in persons who are elderly, bedridden, and/or in long-term care facilities. Therapy consists of dialysis and fluid and electrolyte management. There are no convincing data that treatment with a steroid, plasma infusion, IV immune globulin, or plasmapheresis is beneficial. (R.A.G.)

## Bibliography

Birtles RJ, et al. *Chlamydia*-like obligate parasite of free-living amoebae. *Lancet* 1997;349:925–926.
   *A gram-negative bacterium (Hall's coccus) related to Chlamydia appears to cause community-acquired pneumonia.*
Bonkovsky HL. The alphabet soup of viral hepatitis: is G a new flavor (or) in the mix? *World J Med* 1997;167:50–51.
   *A review of hepatitis G.*
Centers for Disease Control. Outbreaks of *Escherichia coli* 0157:H7 infection associated with eating alfalfa sprouts—Michigan and Virginia, June–July 1997. *MMWR Morb Mortal Wkly Rep* 1997;46:741–744.
   *Presumably, alfalfa seeds were contaminated with animal feces harboring E. coli 0157:H7.*
Centers for Disease Control. *Escherichia coli* 0157:H7 infections associated with eating a nationally distributed commercial brand of frozen ground beef patties and burgers—Colorado. *MMWR Morb Mortal Wkly Rep* 1997;46:777–778.
   *A massive recall of meat contaminated with E. coli 0157:H7.*
Drancourt M, et al. *Bartonella (Rochalimaea) quintana* endocarditis in three homeless men. *N Engl J Med* 1995;332:419–423.
   *B. quintana is a cause of endocarditis in homeless patients.*

File TM Jr. Etiology and incidence of community-acquired pneumonia. *Infect Dis Clin Pract* 1996;5(4 Suppl):S127–S135.
   Legionella-*like amebal pathogen as a potential cause of community-acquired pneumonia.*
Lieberman D, et al. Pneumonia with serological evidence of acute infection with the *Chlamydia*-like microorganism "Z." *Am J Respir Crit Care Med* 1997;156:578–582.
   *An illness characterized by fever, cough (nonproductive), gastrointestinal symptoms, and a prompt response to erythromycin.*
Raoult D, et al. Diagnosis of 22 new cases of *Bartonella* endocarditis. *Ann Intern Med* 1996;125:646–652.
   *Consider* Bartonella *in the evaluation of culture-negative endocarditis.*
Sexton DJ, et al. Life-threatening Cache Valley virus infection. *N Engl J Med* 1997; 336:547–549.
   *Cache Valley virus as a cause of severe encephalitis and multiorgan failure.*
Slutsker L, et al. *Escherichia coli* 0157:H7 diarrhea in the United States: clinical and epidemiologic features. *Ann Intern Med* 1997;126:505–513.
   *A comprehensive review of* E. coli *0157:H7 diarrhea.*
Spach DH, et al. *Bartonella (Rochalimaea) quintana* bacteremia in inner-city patients with chronic alcoholism. *N Engl J Med* 1995;332:424–428.
   B. quintana *as a cause of bacteremia and endocarditis in HIV-seronegative, homeless, inner-city patients with chronic alcoholism.*
Spach DH, et al. *Bartonella (Rochalimaea)* species as a cause of apparent "culture-negative" endocarditis. *Clin Infect Dis* 1995;20:1044–1047.
   B. quintana *as a cause of culture-negative endocarditis.*

# XVI. PROPHYLAXIS OF INFECTION IN TRAVELERS

# 64. PROPHYLAXIS OF INFECTIOUS DISEASES IN TRAVELERS

Travelers to foreign lands are at high risk to contract an infectious disease; in fact, 30% to 65% of international voyagers experience a diarrheal or systemic illness during or shortly following their stay abroad. Although the majority of these afflictions are of little consequence medically, a number of infections acquired by travelers can be life-threatening, especially when diagnosis is delayed because physicians may be unfamiliar with the manifestations of imported diseases. Thus, preventive measures are essential to increase the chances of illness-free travel and to reduce the likelihood that a serious disease will be acquired abroad.

Updated recommendations for chemoprophylaxis and immunoprophylaxis are published yearly by the *Medical Letter* and biannually by the Centers for Disease Control (CDC) in *Health Information for International Travel*, which can be purchased through the Superintendent of Documents, U.S. Government Printing Office, Washington, DC 20402 (202-512-1800). The CDC also maintains automated information services available at 888-232-3228 or on the Internet at www.cdc.gov. Finally, many medical centers have travelers' clinics, and reviews on the subject are regularly published; these contain useful information, including recommendations for medical travel kits, guidelines for insect avoidance, suggestions for preventing sexually transmitted diseases, and special information for travelers who are pregnant, disabled, or have chronic illnesses, including infection with HIV.

The clinician must realize that a number of exotic infections can be acquired within the boundaries of the continental United States, including plague (southwestern states), Rocky Mountain spotted fever (mid-Atlantic and south-central states), and relapsing fever (mountainous areas of the western states). Some infections potentially acquired through travel in the United States can produce catastrophic illnesses in patients with underlying conditions; for example, babesiosis (Shelter Island, New York; Nantucket Island, Massachusetts) in a splenectomized person and coccidioidomycosis (southwestern states) in a pregnant woman are potentially lethal diseases. The primary care physician, therefore, should review all travel plans and be prepared to provide specific advice for preventing travel-related illnesses.

## Sexually Transmitted Diseases

The advice that the physician offers to patients planning trips abroad should include a discussion of sexually transmitted diseases. Because business travelers or long-term residents of foreign countries often engage in sexual intercourse with native peoples, special attention must be paid to these groups. Sexual activity abroad places the traveler at risk for a variety of diseases, including gonorrhea, syphilis, chancroid, herpes simplex, and, most important, hepatitis B and infection with HIV. Travelers must be advised that abstinence is the only means of completely eliminating the risk for acquiring a sexually transmitted disease and that intercourse with male or female prostitutes must be avoided; the danger of sexual relations with prostitutes is highlighted by the fact that in some areas of the world, more than 50% of these persons are HIV-infected. Although the use of condoms reduces the risk for a sexually transmitted disease, it does not entirely eliminate the possibility of acquiring such an illness. Of note, condoms acquired abroad have a greater failure rate than do those purchased in the United States; thus, travelers who believe that they will need them should purchase an adequate supply before departure. Finally, female barrier contraceptives offer no protection from sexually transmitted diseases.

## Precautions in Eating and Drinking

Many of the infections acquired by the international traveler result from the ingestion of food or water contaminated by human feces. As a consequence, most water in less developed countries should be considered unfit for consumption or for use in personal hygiene activities, such as brushing teeth. A variety of treatments are available to render water safe for ingestion. Heating water to 65°C will eliminate all enteric bacterial pathogens, and heating to 100°C will disinfect water entirely. Halogenation with chlorine or iodine, contact inactivation with iodine resins, and filtration with sediment and microbial filters are other methods of generating water fit for consumption; preparations or devices for each of these methods are commercially available. If electricity is available, a small coil or beverage heater can be used to boil water for personal use.

Tap water that is too hot for hand washing is considered partially pasteurized and probably safe for brushing teeth, but it is not necessarily safe for drinking. In any case, hot tap water should be cooled without adding potentially contaminated ice cubes or colder water. Alcoholic beverages (e.g., beer, wine), drinks made with boiling water (e.g., tea, coffee), and carbonated beverages are usually safe to drink. Because of their acidic pH, carbonated beverages are bactericidal for common enteric pathogens, such as *Salmonella typhi.* Unless the purity of canned or bottled water and beverages can be ensured, the traveler cannot presume that their use will prevent illness; for example, bottled beverages have been implicated as the cause of an epidemic of typhoid fever, and bottled water has been linked to an outbreak of cholera.

Dairy products, including ice cream, should not be consumed because of potentially inadequate pasteurization and refrigeration. Fresh vegetables and fruits, such as lettuce and tomatoes, and food served by street vendors should be avoided. Because the treatment of vegetables with chemicals is either impractical or makes food inedible, boiling is usually necessary to ensure that cysts and pathogenic bacteria are killed. Fruits should be peeled before being eaten. Fish and meat must be cooked well and eaten while hot. Finally, bathing, swimming, and boating in fresh or brackish water must be restricted because of the risk for accidentally ingesting microbial pathogens and because of concern about schistosomiasis, which is endemic to portions of Africa, the Middle East, South America, the Caribbean, the Philippines, and Southeast Asia.

### Vaccinations

State and local health departments and the CDC can provide invaluable assistance in supplying up-to-date information on specific vaccine recommendations. In general, because some vaccines require multiple doses, immunization schedules should be established early to ensure optimal protection before the traveler departs. Live-virus vaccines must not be administered to immunocompromised patients, and the decision concerning their use in pregnant women should be individualized; for example, pregnant women who must travel to areas of endemic yellow fever should be vaccinated because the complications of yellow fever are assumed to be more severe than those associated with the vaccine. HIV-infected travelers should not receive the bacille Calmette-Guérin (BCG) vaccine or the live-attenuated polio vaccine, and patients with AIDS should not be given the yellow fever vaccine.

Regardless of destination, travelers should be fully immunized with routine vaccines, including those for diphtheria, tetanus, measles, and perhaps mumps and rubella. In addition, persons traveling to rural areas of the tropics may require updated immunization against polio. The hepatitis A vaccine is now recommended for susceptible travelers planning trips to any location outside the United States, Canada, Western Europe, Japan, Australia, or New Zealand. In general, a serologic response to the hepatitis A vaccine will occur within 2 weeks; if travel will be commencing within a few days and if the destination is in a highly endemic area, the patient can be given the hepatitis A vaccine plus a dose of human immune globulin.

Depending on the destination and the duration and purpose of travel, a number of other vaccinations may be necessary; these include the meningococcal, plague, rabies, and yellow fever vaccines. The oral live-attenuated typhoid vaccine should be offered to persons going to rural tropical regions or other areas where typhoid is endemic, including India, Pakistan, Chile, and Peru. Hepatitis B vaccine is recommended for persons traveling to highly endemic regions (Southeast Asia or sub-Saharan Africa), especially medical personnel and persons likely to have sexual contacts; persons at risk for hepatitis B can be identified by screening for the presence of antibodies to that virus. Cholera vaccine is not routinely recommended; however, some countries require proof of vaccination against cholera (as well as yellow fever) as a condition for entry. Specific information regarding vaccination requirements can be secured from the CDC or the *Medical Letter,* or through one of the references listed below. Required vaccinations must be recorded and validated by the stamp of an official vaccination center in the document "International Certificate of Vaccination"; public health departments can give the locations of these centers. Finally, smallpox vaccine is no longer required by any country.

## Prevention of Malaria

Malaria presents the most serious infectious threat to the international traveler. The number of imported civilian cases of malaria has increased steadily during the past two decades. The problem of imported malaria appears directly attributable to the fact that most travelers are not informed about the possibility of acquiring the disease or about the importance of chemoprophylaxis. Between 25% and 30% of visitors to malarious areas do not seek health information, and many travelers requesting guidelines for prevention from physicians are given incorrect advice. ("Take malaria prophylaxis if you want to." "Ask when you get down there.") As a consequence, fewer than 20% of persons traveling to regions of endemic malaria receive appropriate chemoprophylaxis.

Malaria is an illness caused by *Plasmodium* species, which is transmitted to humans through the bite of an infected female *Anopheles* mosquito. The disease is endemic in many areas of the world between 45 degrees north latitude and 45 degrees south latitude; these regions include Haiti, Central America, South America, sub-Saharan Africa, Southeast Asia, and the Middle East. The prevalence of malaria within these regions is not uniform and varies from year to year; annual reports published by the CDC and World Health Organization are indispensable for following changes in the distribution of the disease. Most importantly, detailed and up-to-date information can be obtained 24 hours a day through the CDC (770-488-7788 or 888-232-3228).

All visitors to areas of endemic malaria should receive chemoprophylaxis regardless of length of stay. Chloroquine remains the cornerstone of prophylaxis; adults should take chloroquine phosphate [300 mg base (500 mg salt)] once weekly, beginning 1 week before arrival at the malarious area and continuing during the entire stay and for 4 weeks after departure. Because routine malaria prophylaxis does not eliminate exoerythrocytic parasites, it may not prevent delayed attacks of disease caused by *Plasmodium vivax* or *Plasmodium ovale*. Therefore, some authorities recommend that primaquine [15 mg base (23.6 mg salt)] be given daily during the last 2 weeks of the course of chloroquine. Primaquine prophylaxis is controversial; in general, it is recommended primarily for persons (e.g., Peace Corps volunteers) who plan on extended stays in areas where *P. vivax* or *P. ovale* is endemic. In any case, primaquine is contraindicated for pregnant women, and because the drug can produce a hemolytic anemia in persons with glucose-6-phosphate dehydrogenase deficiency, candidates for primaquine should be screened for the disorder.

Chloroquine-resistant *Plasmodium falciparum* is found throughout the world, including countries in South America (Brazil, Colombia, Venezuela), sub-Saharan Africa, Southeast Asia, and Oceania. Because of serious adverse drug reactions and the emergence of resistant strains of malaria, Pyrimethamine sulfadoxine (Fansidar®) is no longer employed as a prophylactic agent. The CDC recommends that mefloquine [Lariam; 228 mg base (250 mg salt)] be taken once weekly, beginning 1 to 2 weeks before arrival and continuing during the stay and for 4 weeks after departure from the endemic area. About 10% of travelers given mefloquine will experience mild neuropsychiatric symptoms, including depression and dizziness, and those symptoms can lead to a discontinuation of the chemoprophylaxis. Unfortunately, mefloquine is not considered safe for use in pregnancy, and doxycycline, which is also effective in preventing infection by chloroquine-resistant *P. falciparum*, is similarly contraindicated in pregnancy. Of note, in portions of Cambodia, Thailand, and Myanmar (Burma), chloroquine and mefloquine resistance is prevalent, and travelers to those regions should receive doxycycline (100 mg daily) unless contraindicated.

In addition to being given antimalarial drugs, travelers should be informed that malaria-carrying *Anopheles* mosquitoes are active only during the hours of darkness and that precautions should be taken to minimize contact with the insects; these precautions include using screening or netting in non–air-conditioned sleeping quarters, avoiding outdoors activities from dusk to dawn, wearing long-sleeved shirts and long pants when outside in the evening, and applying repellent [diethyltoluamide (Deet) for skin, permethrin (Permanone) for clothing]. However, such precautions do not obviate the need for chemoprophylaxis. Patients should be advised that chemoprophylaxis is not 100% effective in preventing malaria and that symptoms consistent with malaria (i.e., chills, fever, headache, and malaise) should be promptly reported to a physician.

### Traveler's Diarrhea

Travelers' diarrhea is the most common malady experienced by international voyagers; it afflicts approximately 20% of all Americans abroad. The risk for traveler's diarrhea varies considerably by country; in one report, the attack rates among visitors to Mexico, Spain, Israel, France, and the United Kingdom were 38.8%, 25.6%, 15.4%, 12.9%, and 2.5%, respectively. Attack rates for travelers to Africa and South America exceed 30%. Travelers less than 30 years of age and those on package tours appear to be at greater risk. The difficulty of avoiding traveler's diarrhea is highlighted by epidemics among airline passengers and among clients at luxury hotels in endemic areas.

Because of the high attack rates and substantial disability associated with this illness, strategies have been devised to prevent it. Dietary discretion and restraint appear to be of little value. On the other hand, in controlled studies, a number of antimicrobial regimens have been found to be effective in preventing traveler's diarrhea, including ciprofloxacin (500 mg daily), norfloxacin (400 mg daily), ofloxacin (300 mg daily), and levofloxacin (500 mg daily). Voyagers who discontinue prophylactic antimicrobials before leaving an endemic region place themselves at risk to suffer a diarrheal illness. Large doses of bismuth subsalicylate (Pepto-Bismol; 60 mL or two tablets taken four times daily for the duration of exposure) also significantly reduce the likelihood of experiencing traveler's diarrhea; of note, bismuth subsalicylate is less effective than the fluoroquinolones or other antibiotics. Nevertheless, little enthusiasm for these prophylactic regimens exists. A major concern is that the widespread use of antimicrobials will encourage the emergence of drug-resistant pathogens. Further, antimicrobials are not innocuous drugs, and the use of the fluoroquinolones is precluded in pregnant women and children. Although bismuth subsalicylate is generally safe, the logistics of transporting the medicine and taking the necessary dose are formidable for the traveler seeking relaxation. Thus, the role of prophylactic regimens remains controversial. Some experts recommend prophylactic antimicrobials for selected travelers: athletes; military personnel; persons with a diminished gastric acid barrier to infection secondary to factors such as use of antacids or histamine$_2$ blockers; and patients with a significant underlying medical disorder, such as AIDS, diabetes mellitus, chronic renal disease, or congestive heart failure. The prophylactic regimen should be initiated 1 day before departure and continued for 2 days after returning.

Traveler's diarrhea usually appears early in the course of a stay abroad, typically within the first week. Clinically, the patient experiences the abrupt onset of diarrhea, which consists of four to five watery bowel movements daily and is associated with low-grade fever, malaise, anorexia, nausea, vomiting, and abdominal cramps. Without therapy, the disorder typically resolves within 2 to 4 days; however, the course may be protracted. Enterotoxigenic *Escherichia coli* is isolated from more than 50% of patients with traveler's diarrhea; thus, it is the organism most frequently associated with the illness. Other pathogens include invasive *E. coli*, *Campylobacter* species, *Shigella* species, *Salmonella* species, *Vibrio* species, *Giardia lamblia*, *Entamoeba histolytica*, and rotavirus. In addition, *Aeromonas hydrophila* and *Plesiomonas shigelloides* have been identified as causes of a protracted diarrheal illness in travelers.

The cornerstone of therapy for traveler's diarrhea is adequate hydration, preferably with oral solutions such as fruit juices that contain sugar (glucose or sucrose) and electrolytes. The antimotility agent loperamide (Imodium) can be helpful in controlling symptoms in patients with mild-to-moderate diarrhea. Because of the absence of data on clinical efficacy and because of high rates of side effects, anticholinergic drugs are not recommended.

In general, antimicrobials are required only for diarrhea caused by specific pathogens, such as *Shigella*. However, controlled studies have demonstrated that the initiation of antimicrobials at the onset of symptoms can reduce abdominal discomfort and decrease the number of unformed stools in patients with traveler's diarrhea. Thus, loperamide (loading dose of 4 mg followed by 2 mg after each loose bowel movement, to a maximum of 16 mg/d) plus a single dose of ciprofloxacin (750 mg), levofloxacin (500 mg), or ofloxacin (400 mg) will produce a reduction in the severity of symptoms in most patients within 24 hours.

If the diarrheal illness is associated with high fever, substantial constitutional symptoms, or bloody stools, the patient should be instructed to take ciprofloxacin (500 mg twice daily), levofloxacin (500 mg once daily), ofloxacin (300 mg twice dialy), or norfloxacin (400 mg twice daily) for 3 to 5 days; the use of loperamide in the patient with dysentery remains controversial, but many experts support its use to control cramps and fluid loss. Finally, bismuth subsalicylate can also be used to treat traveler's diarrhea, although the compound is less effective than loperamide and other therapies; because of widespread resistance, trimethoprimsulfamethoxazole is no longer utilized as a prophylactic or therapeutic agent for travel-associated diarrhea. In sum, self-initiated therapy appears to be an attractive alternative to prophylaxis, and most experts recommend it. Gastrointestinal symptoms that persist or progress require a medical evaluation.

## Medical Therapy Abroad

Travelers who require medical attention while abroad can contact travel agents, a U.S. or British embassy, or a U.S. military base for assistance in locating physicians and hospitals. Over-the-counter remedies and local medications should be avoided because they may contain multiple antimicrobials or potentially toxic compounds. Persons who plan to travel for extended periods or who are likely to need medical assistance because of advanced age or debilitating illness should be advised to join the International Association for Medical Assistance to Travelers (716-754-4883), a nonprofit organization that can provide a directory of hospitals and competent, English-speaking physicians in foreign countries. Finally, travelers should be warned that although most infections acquired abroad become manifest within a few weeks after return to the United States, some illnesses (e.g., malaria) may not produce symptoms for several months. (A.L.E.)

## Bibliography

Advice for travelers. *Med Lett* 1998;40:47.
*A concise summary with specific recommendations on traveler's diarrhea, immunizations, and malaria prophylaxis.*

DuPont HL, et al. Five versus 3 days of ofloxacin for traveler's diarrhea: a placebo-controlled study. *Antimicrob Agents Chemother* 1992;36:87.
*This double-blind study of 232 students who experienced diarrhea while visiting Mexico and were given a placebo or ofloxacin (300 mg twice daily) for 3 or 5 days demonstrated that the 3-day regimen was comparable with the 5-day course in producing clinical and microbiologic cures.*

Ericsson CD. Traveller's diarrhea. Epidemiology, prevention and treatment. *Infect Dis Clin North Am* 1998;12:285.
*A comprehensive review.*

Insect repellents. *Med Lett* 1989;31:45.
*A review of the safety and effectiveness of skin and clothing repellents likely to be used by travelers.*

Johnson PC, et al. Comparison of loperamide with bismuth subsalicylate for the treatment of acute traveler's diarrhea. *JAMA* 1986;255:757.
*In this study of 219 college students in Latin America, the investigators found that loperamide (a 4-mg initial dose followed by 2 mg for every loose stool, to a maximum of 16 mg/d) was as effective as bismuth subsalicylate in treating acute, nondysenteric traveler's diarrhea.*

Jong EC. Immunizations for international travel. *Infect Dis Clin North Am* 1998;12:249.
*The author provides detailed information concerning indications for and administration and efficacy of all vaccines potentially required for the traveler to foreign lands.*

Kemper CA, et al. Travels with HIV: the compliance and health of HIV-infected adults who travel. *Int J STD AIDS* 1997;8:44.
*In this retrospective study of 89 HIV-infected patients, the authors found that 45% traveled within the United States and 20%, abroad; more than 40% of the HIV-infected voyagers became ill either during or following their travels.*

Mileno MD, Bia FJ. The compromised traveler. *Infect Dis Clin North Am* 1998;12:369.
  *The authors provide a detailed review of the special precautions necessary for HIV-infected, asplenic, diabetic, organ transplant, and other immunocompromised voyagers.*
Petruccelli BP, et al. Treatment of traveler's diarrhea with ciprofloxacin and loperamide. *J Infect Dis* 1992;165:557.
  *In this study, 142 military personnel with traveler's diarrhea were given a single dose of ciprofloxacin (750 mg) with a placebo, or a single dose of ciprofloxacin (750 mg) with loperamide, or a 3-day course of ciprofloxacin (500 mg twice daily) plus loperamide. No significant differences in overall outcomes were noted, although patients randomized to the 3-day ciprofloxacin plus loperamide regimen had fewer liquid bowel movements.*
Sakmar TP. The traveler's medical kit. *Infect Dis Clin North Am* 1992;6:355.
  *The author provides detailed recommendations concerning items to be taken abroad to prevent or treat illness.*
Samuel BU, Barry M. The pregnant traveler. *Infect Dis Clin North Am* 1998;12:325.
  *The authors discusses a number of issues pertinent to the pregnant traveler and the fetus, including the risks of immunizations and malaria prophylaxis and the safety of commonly used antiinfective agents.*
Taylor DN, et al. Treatment of traveler's diarrhea: ciprofloxacin plus loperamide compared with ciprofloxacin alone. *Ann Intern Med* 1991;114:731.
  *In this double-blind, randomized study, 104 military personnel with traveler's diarrhea were given ciprofloxacin (500 mg twice daily for 3 days) plus either a placebo or loperamide (a 4-mg first dose, then 2 mg for every loose stool, up to a maximum of 16 mg/d). Treatment with ciprofloxacin plus loperamide resulted in a more rapid resolution of symptoms; however, at 48 hours, 90% of the subjects in both groups had improved or fully recovered.*

# XVII. TUBERCULOSIS

## 65. ROLE OF THE TUBERCULIN SKIN TEST

The clinician frequently must determine whether a patient has tuberculosis. Part of the evaluation involves tuberculin skin testing. Two preparations of tuberculin are available for use in the United States: old tuberculin (OT) and purified protein derivative (PPD).

Although several techniques are available, the most widely used are the intradermal PPD skin test (Mantoux procedure), with antigens of various strengths, and the tine test. Except for epidemiologic screening of low-risk groups, an intradermal PPD skin test rather than a tine test is used to decrease the problem of false-negatives. Three concentrations of PPD antigens are available: first strength [1 tuberculin unit (1 TU)], intermediate strength (5 TU), and second strength (250 TU). Testing should begin with the intermediate-strength preparation; a first-strength PPD is rarely, if ever, indicated. Tuberculin protein is absorbed by plastic, and the detergent polysorbate 80 is added to the diluent to prevent this reaction. After 48 to 72 hours, the extent of induration, not erythema, is determined by palpation and measured in millimeters. In the past, an area of induration of 10 mm or more was considered evidence of past or present infection with *Mycobacterium tuberculosis.* Reactions measuring 5 to 9 mm in a normal host usually represent prior infection with atypical mycobacteria that cross-react with PPD-S (*M. tuberculosis* preparation; purified protein derivative-standard). Prior infection with atypical mycobacteria can be demonstrated by skin testing with a battery of atypical antigens (available only for investigational studies). A person's largest reaction is to the infecting organism (dual skin test technique).

In 1990, the American Thoracic Society and the Centers for Disease Control revised the criteria defining a positive tuberculin skin test result in an effort to decrease the number of false-negatives in high-risk persons, such as those with HIV infection, and decrease the number of false-positives in low-risk groups. Three criteria were adopted for tuberculin reactivity based on risk factors for disease and the probability of having a true infection with *M. tuberculosis:*

1. A skin test reaction of 5 mm or more of induration is considered positive in persons likely to be infected with *M. tuberculosis,* such as persons with HIV disease, close contacts of infected patients, and those with chest roentgenographic findings consistent with old, healed tuberculosis.

2. A reaction of 10 mm or more of induration is considered positive in foreign-born persons from Asia, Africa, and Latin America; IV drug users; medically underserved, low-income groups; residents of long-term care facilities; and other immunosuppressed hosts, such as persons with silicosis, gastrectomy, chronic renal failure, diabetes mellitus, or underlying hematologic or other malignancies, or who are receiving high-dose corticosteroids or other cytotoxic therapy. Additionally, a reaction in employees of an institution where a person with tuberculosis would pose a risk to a large number of susceptible persons should be considered positive at 10 mm of induration. Also considered as a high-risk group are children less than 4 years of age.

3. A reaction of more than 15 mm of induration is positive in persons with no other risk factors (Table 65-1).

About 80% of normal hosts with active tuberculosis have a positive reaction to a 5-TU PPD test. The result of a 5-TU PPD skin test will be negative in 20% of seriously ill patients with active tuberculosis when first seen. In the evaluation of patients with suspected tuberculosis for delayed hypersensitivity, a number of factors can be considered that can explain false-negative tuberculin reactions (Table 65-2). A battery of skin test antigens is used to assess delayed-type hypersensitivity. Control antigens commonly used include mumps, *Candida,* and tetanus toxoid. If any amount of induration, but not erythema, is considered a positive reaction, about 60% of normal adult control subjects will react positively to each of these antigens. If three skin antigens are selected, 90% of normal subjects will react to at least one antigen. In addition to the

Table 65-1. Interpretation of purified protein derivative (PPD)
tuberculin skin test results

1. An induration of ≥5 mm is classified as positive in
   • persons who have HIV infection
   • persons who have had recent close contact with persons who have active TB
     (e.g., household contact)
   • persons who have fibrotic areas on chest radiographs (consistent with healed TB)
2. An induration of ≥10 mm is classified as positive in all persons who do not meet
   any of the criteria above but who have other risk factors for TB, including
   *High-risk groups—*
   • injecting drug users
   • persons who have other medical conditions (e.g., silicosis, gastrectomy or
     jejunoileal bypass, body weight ≥10% below ideal; chronic renal failure,
     diabetes mellitus, high-dose corticosteroid or other immunosuppressive
     therapy, malignancies)
   • children <4 years of age
   *High-prevalence groups—*
   • persons born in countries in Asia, Africa, the Caribbean, and Latin America
     that have a high prevalence of TB
   • persons from medically underserved, low-income populations
   • residents of long-term care facilities (e.g., correctional institutions and nursing
     homes)
3. An induration of ≥15 mm is classified as positive in persons who do not meet any of
   the above criteria (e.g., health care workers) unless other risk factors are present.

Modified from *MMWR Morb Mortal Wkly Rep* 1994;43(RR13):62.

Table 65-2. Reasons for false-negative tuberculin reactions

Technical errors
Measurement of skin induration
Faulty antigen or administration (rare)
Impaired cellular immunity
Nonspecific
Hypoalbuminemia (<2 g/dL)
Old age (>70 y)
Leukocytosis > 15,000/mm$^3$
Anemia
Fever
Azotemia
Drugs and other therapy
Immunosuppressive drugs (corticosteroids)
Irradiation
Live viral vaccines
Specific diseases
Viral infections and vaccines (e.g., rubella, infectious mononucleosis, mumps,
  influenza, HIV)
Overwhelming infection (e.g., tuberculosis, deep mycoses)
Sarcoidosis
Neoplasms (e.g., Hodgkin's disease, leukemia)
Too early for skin test conversion
Requires 3–6 weeks

Mantoux-type procedure for administering antigens to test delayed-type hypersensitivity, a multiple-puncture device (tinelike) is available that uses seven antigens. This device has two disadvantages: the amount of antigen injected into the skin is variable because of technical factors related to administration, and it is expensive.

A negative reaction to an intermediate-strength PPD skin test in patients who are not anergic does not exclude tuberculosis. It was found in one study that one third of patients with active tuberculosis who had a negative 5-TU PPD skin test result were not anergic. The question should be pursued further with a second-strength (250-TU) PPD skin test. A negative PPD (250-TU) test result and a positive result with one or more of the controls (anergy battery) constitute powerful evidence against tuberculosis. If the result of the 250-TU PPD test is negative and the result with the anergy battery is also negative, the possibility of tuberculosis still exists. A positive 250-TU PPD test result is less helpful, as it may signify nonspecific cross-reactivity to the atypical mycobacteria or a false-positive reaction resulting from the high concentration of tuberculin protein.

Another problem is to distinguish between a positive tuberculin reaction in a person who has received a bacille Calmette-Guérin (BCG) vaccination and one caused by an injection of *M. tuberculosis*. Tuberculin skin reactions caused by BCG vaccination wane with time, and large reactions are likely to indicate an infection with *M. tuberculosis*. In an adult who was given BCG vaccine as an infant, a tuberculin reaction of more than 10 mm of induration is unlikely to be caused by the BCG vaccine. It is more difficult to interpret the size of a tuberculin skin test reaction in an adult who received BCG vaccine after infancy.

Repeated tuberculin skin testing can also increase the reaction size from 5 to 9 mm to more than 10 mm. This boosting reaction can occur with skin tests performed from 1 to several weeks apart. In elderly subjects, the size of the tuberculin reaction decreases with age because of a waning of cell-mediated immunity to the tuberculin antigen. When elderly subjects are tested twice in a 3-week interval, a positive reaction may be detected on the second skin test as a result of immunologic recall. This must not be interpreted as a recent skin test conversion but as a false-negative skin test result on the initial tuberculin test. Progressive increase in the size of the tuberculin skin test reaction has been noted when a third and a fourth boosting test are used. Although the American Thoracic Society and Centers for Disease Control suggest that an increase of more than 10 mm of induration likely represents the occurrence of infection, in one study in the elderly, large increases were noted that did not indicate true conversions. Better tests are needed to identify persons at an increased risk for development of active disease. Rarely, an atypical mycobacterial infection will cause a reaction to the PPD-S skin test antigen that is larger than 10 mm.

A positive tuberculin skin test result in patients with suspected active tuberculosis together with negative results on acid-fast smears provides indirect evidence for the diagnosis pending cultures. A negative result on a properly performed tuberculin skin test, along with appropriately reacting controls, is evidence against the diagnosis in a normal host. (N.M.G.)

### Bibliography

Advisory Committee for Immunization Practices. Use of BCG vaccines in the control of tuberculosis: a joint statement by the ACIP and the Advisory Committee for Elimination of Tuberculosis. *MMWR Morb Mortal Wkly Rep* 1988;37:663.
*A positive skin test result in a BCG-immunized person need not be attributed to* M. tuberculosis *infection if the person is not in a high-risk group and has no history of exposure.*

American Thoracic Society and Centers for Disease Control. Diagnostic standards and classification of tuberculosis. *Am Rev Respir Dis* 1990;142:725.
*Guidelines for tuberculin skin testing and interpretation.*

Buoros D, et al. Palpation vs. pen method for the measurement of skin tuberculin reaction (Mantoux test). *Chest* 1991;99:416.
*Use either the palpation or pen method to measure tuberculin skin test reactivity.*

Centers for Disease Control. Guidelines for preventing the transmission of *Mycobacterium tuberculosis* in health-care facilities, 1994. *MMWR Morb Mortal Wkly Rep* 1994;43(RR13):1–132.

*Guidelines for interpreting tuberculin skin test results and methods to decrease transmission.*

Centers for Disease Control. Anergy skin testing and preventive therapy for HIV-infected persons: revised recommendations. *MMWR Morb Mortal Wkly Rep* 1997; 46(RR15):1–10.
*Guidelines for anergy testing. Anergy testing is no longer recommended as a routine component of screening for tuberculosis among HIV-infected persons.*

Centers for Disease Control. Tuberculin skin test survey in a pediatric population with high BCG vaccination coverage Botswana, 1996. *MMWR Morb Mortal Wkly Rep* 1997;46:846–851.
*A tuberculin skin test of ≥10 mm of induration is likely to be a consequence of tuberculous infection and not previous BCG vaccination.*

Comstock GW, Woolpert SF. Tuberculin conversions: true or false. *Am Rev Respir Dis* 1978;118:215.
*Describes the use of two tuberculin tests given at least 1 week apart to detect true but not necessarily recent conversions resulting from the booster phenomenon.*

Doto IL, Furcolow ML, MacInnis FE. Size of tuberculin reaction. *Arch Environ Health* 1971;23:392.
*The probability that reactivation tuberculosis will develop increases with the size of the skin test reactions.*

Edwards PQ. Tuberculin negative? *N Engl J Med* 1972;286:373.
*The causes of false-negative test results include anergic states, faulty antigenic material, improper administration, and errors in reading the reaction.*

Ferebee SH, Mount FW. Evidence of booster effect in serial tuberculin testing. *Am Rev Respir Dis* 1963;88:118.
*Because of "anamnestic recall," the area of induration may be increased on a repeated skin test.*

Franz ML, Carella JA, Galant SP. Cutaneous delayed hypersensitivity in a healthy pediatric population: diagnostic value of diphtheria-tetanus toxoids. *J Pediatr* 1976;88:975.
*Diphtheria toxoid (concentration 1:1,000) is useful for the assessment of delayed hypersensitivity.*

Galant SP, et al. Relationship between cutaneous delayed hypersensitivity and cell-mediated immunity *in vitro* responses assessed by diphtheria and tetanus toxoids. *J Allergy Clin Immunol* 1977;60:247.
*Cutaneous delayed hypersensitivity can be assessed with tetanus toxoid intradermally.*

Grabau JC, Burrows DJ, Kern ML. A pseudo-outbreak of purified protein derivative skin-test conversions caused by inappropriate testing materials. *Infect Control Hosp Epidemiol* 1997;18:571–574.
*False-positive tuberculin skin test results were caused by erroneously using a second-strength (250-TU) PPD skin test.*

Harrison BDW, Tugwell P, Fawcett IW. Tuberculin reaction in adult Nigerians with sputum-positive pulmonary tuberculosis. *Lancet* 1975;1:421.
*Lack of reaction to tuberculin skin test correlates with low serum albumin levels (< 2 g/dL).*

Heiss LI, Palmer DL. Anergy in patients with leukocytosis. *Am J Med* 1974;56:323.
*A discussion of the clinical conditions associated with anergy.*

Holden M, Dubin MR, Diamond PH. Frequency of negative intermediate-strength tuberculin sensitivity in patients with active tuberculosis. *N Engl J Med* 1971;285:1506.
*With 5 TU of polysorbate 80-stabilized PPD skin test antigen, 20% of results were negative.*

Howard TP, Solomon DA. Reading the tuberculin skin test: who, when, and how? *Arch Intern Med* 1988;148:2457.
*Patients' readings of their own skin tests are inaccurate.*

Huebner RE. The tuberculin skin test. *Clin Infect Dis* 1993;17:968.
*A review of administration, reading, and interpretation of tuberculin skin tests.*

Israel HL, Sones M. Sarcoidosis, tuberculosis, and tuberculin anergy. *Am Rev Respir Dis* 1966;94:887.

*The tuberculin skin test result was positive in patients with sarcoidosis who also had active tuberculosis.*

Johnson MP, et al. Tuberculin skin test reactivity among adults infected with human immunodeficiency virus. *J Infect Dis* 1992;166:194.
*Among HIV-positive persons, use a cut point of 5 mm or more of induration to increase the test sensitivity.*

Kent DC, Schwartz R. Active pulmonary tuberculosis with negative tuberculin reactions. *Am Rev Respir Dis* 1967;95:411.
*Negative results on intermediate-strength (5-TU) and second-strength (250-TU) PPD skin tests do not exclude the diagnosis.*

Levin S. The fungal skin test as a diagnostic hindrance. *J Infect Dis* 1970;122:343.
*Fungal skin tests (blastomycin, histoplasmin, and coccidioidin) should not be part of a workup for either fever of unknown origin or fungal infection.*

Lunn JA, Johnson AJ. Comparison of the tine and Mantoux tuberculin tests. *Br Med J* 1978;1:1451.
*Mantoux test results were positive in 35%, but the tine test result was positive in only 4%.*

Menzies R, Vissandjee B. Effect of bacille Calmette-Guérin vaccination on tuberculin reactivity. *Am Rev Respir Dis* 1992;145:621.
*In adults who have received BCG vaccine as infants, the tuberculin reactivity is usually less than 10 mm of induration.*

Palmer DL, Reed WP. Delayed-hypersensitivity skin testing. I. Response rates in a hospitalized population. *J Infect Dis* 1974;130:132.
*Positive skin tests (>5 mm induration at 48 hours) with mumps (68%),* Candida *(63%), and* Trichophyton *(62%) antigens; 89% of patients reacted to at least one of these antigens.*

Palmer DL, Reed WP. Delayed-hypersensitivity skin testing. II. Clinical correlates and anergy. *J Infect Dis* 1974;130:138.
*Anergy was associated with old age, immunosuppressive medications, malignancy, azotemia, leukocytosis, anemia, and fever.*

Present PA, Comstock GW. Tuberculin sensitivity in pregnancy. *Am Rev Respir Dis* 1975;112:413.
*Pregnancy has no effect on the tuberculin test.*

Reichman LB, O'Day R. The influence of a history of a previous test on the prevalence and size of reactions to tuberculin. *Am Rev Respir Dis* 1977;115:737.
*On retesting, a history of a positive tuberculin skin test result was confirmed in only 42% of patients. Severe reactions to the repeated test ("slough") were not a problem.*

Rhoades ER, Bryant RE. The effect of injection technique upon the size of the tuberculin reaction. *Am Rev Respir Dis* 1973;107:1089.
*The route of administration (intradermal or subcutaneous) has little effect on reaction size.*

Robertson JM, et al. Delayed tuberculin reactivity in persons of Indochinese origin: implications for preventive therapy. *Ann Intern Med* 1996;124:779–784.
*Some patients (26%) had a negative tuberculin skin test result at 48 to 72 hours that became positive at 6 days. This delayed response can be detected with the booster technique.*

Rooney JJ, et al. Further observations on tuberculin reactions in active tuberculosis. *Am J Med* 1976;60:517.
*Of patients who were seriously ill, 20% had a negative intermediate PPD skin test result. The majority (94%) reacted after the protein depletion was corrected.*

Sepkowitz KA, et al. Benefit of two-step PPD testing of new employees at a New York City hospital. *Am J Infect Control* 1997;25:283–286.
*Without use of the two-step testing technique, 10% of new employees would have been classified falsely as new tuberculin converters.*

Smith DT. Diagnostic and prognostic significance of the quantitative tuberculin tests. The influence of subclinical infections with atypical mycobacteria. *Ann Intern Med* 1967;67:919.
*Review. Lack of a reaction to second-strength PPD-S (250 TU) is strong evidence against tuberculosis; a reaction of 2 to 9 mm to PPD-S (5 TU) suggests an atypical infection.*

Sokal JE. Measurement of delayed skin-test responses. *N Engl J Med* 1975;293:501.
*A discussion of how to identify a positive reaction.*
Stead WW, To T. The significance of the tuberculin skin test in elderly persons. *Ann Intern Med* 1987;107:837.
*An increase of at least 12 mm in the size of a tuberculin skin test reaction is evidence of a new M. tuberculosis infection.*
Steele RW, et al. Screening for cell-mediated immunity in children. *Am J Dis Child* 1976;130:1218.
*Three fourths of children ages 6 weeks to 12 years reacted to* Candida *or tetanus toxoid skin test antigen.*
Stimpson PG, et al. Delayed-hypersensitivity skin testing for assessing anergy in the mid-South. *South Med J* 1976;69:424.
*When a battery of six antigens was used (mumps, PPD, histoplasmin, Candida, streptokinase-streptodornase, and Trichophyton), 95% of controls reacted.*
Webster CT, et al. Two-stage tuberculin skin testing in individuals with human immunodeficiency virus infection. *Am J Respir Crit Care Med* 1995;151:805–808.
*Use of two-stage tuberculin skin testing (booster technique) is of limited value in HIV-infected patients.*
Woeltje KF, et al. Tuberculosis infection and anergy in hemodialysis patients. *Am J Kidney Dis* 1998;31:848–852.
*Of hemodialysis patients, 16% had a positive tuberculin skin test result or history of tuberculosis and 32% were anergic.*

## 66. ISONIAZID CHEMOPROPHYLAXIS: INDICATIONS AND MANAGEMENT

Isoniazid (INH) chemoprophylaxis is preventive therapy for a subclinical tuberculous infection to prevent reactivation disease. Although the therapy of active pulmonary tuberculosis has improved considerably with highly effective short-course regimens, little progress has been made in INH preventive therapy.

Daily therapy with INH for 12 months has been the standard regimen for several decades. The major controversial issue concerns the recommendations of the American Thoracic Society and the Centers for Disease Control that all tuberculin skin test reactors between ages 21 and 35 years with no other risk factors should receive INH for 1 year. Using decision analysis, the authors concluded that young adults (ages 21 to 35 years) with a positive tuberculin skin test reaction and no additional risk factors should not take INH because the risk for INH-related hepatitis outweighs the benefits of preventive therapy. In the editorial that accompanied this report, Comstock concluded that the input values selected for decision analysis tipped the scales against INH prophylaxis. There is still a need for more data for this risk group.

An extensive controlled study involving almost 28,000 patients with positive Mantoux skin test reactions and fibrotic lesions detected by chest roentgenography was published in 1982 and provided important data on INH preventive therapy. In this study, patients were treated with either INH or placebo for 12, 24, or 52 weeks and were then followed for 5 years. Using data from this study to conduct a cost effectiveness analysis of the three treatment durations, Snider et al. (1986) concluded that a 24-week regimen was the most cost effective duration. A 12-week course of INH was felt to be inadequate, and the danger of a 24-week regimen was that patients might shorten their therapy even further. Other reports based on the application of decision-analysis techniques to the management of low-risk tuberculin reactors have failed to resolve the controversy.

A positive induration after testing with intermediate-strength (5 tuberculin units) purified protein derivative (PPD-S) stabilized with polysorbate 80 indicates recent or remote infection, usually with *Mycobacterium tuberculosis* (see Chapter 65). In the absence of evidence of active disease, a positive delayed-hypersensitivity reaction to tuberculosis means that the primary infection has been arrested by the host; thus, the tuberculin-positive person has viable tubercle bacilli that, although contained by acquired cellular immunity, may multiply in subsequent years with alterations in host-resistance factors. In fact, 92% of all new cases of active pulmonary tuberculosis represent reactivation disease in a small proportion (7%) of the tuberculin-positive population. The term INH chemoprophylaxis does not, in fact, indicate prophylaxis, but rather actual treatment of a subclinical infection to prevent the development of active tuberculosis. Single-drug therapy is effective because the number of organisms is small; thus, there is little chance of selecting out resistant mycobacteria.

## Efficacy

INH was commercially released in 1952, and since then numerous controlled studies have shown that a 12-month course of INH therapy is effective in preventing reactivation of disease in tuberculin reactors. The risk for active disease in a placebo group was found to be as many as 61 times that in patients treated with INH. Eighty percent of the active cases in a placebo group occurred within the first year after diagnosis, but the onset of active disease in the placebo group might be delayed as long as 8 years. The protective effect of INH is more impressive for children than for adults. Compliance is the key to the effectiveness of INH, and success rates approach 100% when the drug is given under direct supervision. One year of treatment is effective for at least 19 years and probably for the life of the patient. In summary, there is no controversy that INH chemoprophylaxis is effective for symptomless tuberculin reactors, tuberculin-positive household contacts, and persons with positive skin test reactions and inactive fibrotic lesions revealed by chest roentgenography.

## Isoniazid Hepatitis

The major disadvantage of INH is the risk for drug-induced hepatitis. The risk for hepatitis is age-related and is increased with daily alcohol consumption. This complication is extremely rare in a person under age 20 years but occurs in 2.1% to 4.3% of persons over the age of 50 years. Although the exact pathogenic mechanism of INH-associated hepatitis remains unknown, certain features are clear. Women may be at an increased risk for development of fatal INH hepatitis. Elevations in liver enzymes with or without symptoms develop in about 10% to 20% of those taking INH. In a small percentage (1%) of patients, jaundice and fatal hepatitis develop. The onset of the liver function abnormalities varies widely, from 1 week to 11 months after the start of treatment. Half the reactions occur within 2 months, mostly during the second month. Fatal hepatitis is more common in patients taking INH for at least 8 weeks than in those on therapy for a shorter period, and it often occurs in patients who continue therapy even after symptoms of hepatitis develop.

Symptoms of liver disease—anorexia, malaise, nausea, and vomiting—are low-sensitivity indicators of INH liver toxicity compared with liver function tests to detect INH hepatitis, and biochemical monitoring is required in patients over age 35 years. It is recommended that in subjects over age 35 years, determinations of transaminase levels and careful clinical assessments be performed at 1, 3, 6, and 9 months after the start of therapy. In persons under age 35 years, monthly evaluation of symptoms and signs of liver disease is adequate, and biochemical monitoring is not required unless adverse effects are detected by the clinical evaluation. In an asymptomatic person, a decision to discontinue INH should be made if the transaminase levels exceed five times the normal laboratory values. Only 7% of the patients in one large study had their INH treatments stopped because of symptoms or asymptomatic elevations of transaminase levels. Clinically, biochemically, and histologically, the liver injury is indistinguishable from viral hepatitis. Contrary to what was observed in earlier studies, the incidence is not increased in rapid acetylators. In fact, slow acetylators over age 35 years appear to be at an increased risk. The mechanism of the hepatitis appears to be conversion of INH to one or more toxic metabolites. The fatality rate is about 10% for icteric cases, and the illness is usually preceded by gastrointestinal symptoms. The majority of patients who have died of INH hepatitis continued to receive the drug despite clinical evidence of hepatitis.

## Decision to Use Isoniazid

The decision to treat a tuberculin reactor with INH is not an easy one to make and should be individualized. Active tuberculosis must be excluded, because usually four drugs are required. The clinician must weigh the risk for development of active tuberculosis and the consequences of infection in each patient. Children less than 5 years old and adolescents tend to have more serious disease than do older persons. Patients of low body weight are also at increased risk for tuberculous disease. Finally, the younger a tuberculin reactor is, the greater the number of years there are in which reactivation disease may occur. In a patient who has coexisting illnesses or is taking drugs with which adverse interactions are possible, deferring INH therapy should always be considered. INH should be deferred in pregnancy until the postpartum period, although women may be particularly vulnerable during this period and must be monitored closely if given this agent.

## Indications

Table 66-1 lists the indications for INH therapy in order of priority. All household contacts who are tuberculin-positive should receive INH unless active disease is documented, in which case two drugs are given. Children who are household contacts and are tuberculin-negative should be given INH for 3 months; a skin test is then repeated. If the test result remains negative and there is no further risk for exposure, INH can be discontinued. For tuberculin-negative adult household contacts, therapy with INH is optional, depending on the infectiousness of the source. Skin testing should be repeated after 3 months. Newly infected persons (documented to have a negative PPD skin test result within the past 2 years) should receive INH.

It is important to distinguish persons who are new, true tuberculin-positive reactors from those who are new positive reactors as a result of the booster phenomenon. The booster effect, which refers to an increase in the size of the tuberculin skin reaction as a consequence of serial tuberculin testing, can be demonstrated as early as 1 to 3 weeks

Table 66-1.  Indications for isoniazid therapy

---

Tuberculin-positive with HIV infection
Tuberculin-negative with HIV infection in high-risk group (e.g., drug users)
Tuberculin-positive household contacts
Tuberculin-negative household contacts—children
New tuberculin reactor*
Tuberculin-positive** with parenchymal scarring revealed on chest x-ray films
    (excluding isolated calcifications)
Tuberculin reactors with special circumstances:
    Underlying neoplasm such as Hodgkin's disease
    Prednisone (>15 mg/d) or its equivalent or other immunosuppressive drugs for a
        prolonged time
    Silicosis
    Poorly controlled diabetes mellitus
    Long-term hemodialysis
    Postgastrectomy
    Intestinal bypass surgery for obesity
    End-stage renal disease
Tuberculin reactors under age 35 years from Latin America, Asia, or Africa or from
    low-income groups
Tuberculin-positive residents of long-term care facilities (e.g., correctional institutions, nursing homes)
Tuberculin-positive staff of facilities in which many people could be exposed
Tuberculin-positive under age 35 years with no other risk factors (?)

---

* Increase ≥10 mm within a 2-year period for those under age 35 years; increase ≥15 mm for those age 35 years or older.
** Patient has never received a full course of antituberculous therapy.

after an initial tuberculin test. This diminished skin reactivity occurs more often in the elderly, and the repeated skin test can erroneously be interpreted as a new positive skin test reaction (conversion). Rather, the initial negative skin test reaction represents a false-negative result, and the result of the repeated test with an increase in size is positive but does not necessarily indicate a recent conversion.

The efficacy of INH is well documented in patients with a positive tuberculin skin test reaction and a fibrotic pulmonary lesion revealed by chest roentgenography. There are no studies supporting the efficacy of INH and the risk for disease in tuberculin reactors in the special clinical situations, and the recommendations are based on uncontrolled studies of tuberculosis in the various groups outlined (Table 66-1). Patients to be placed on either long-term prednisone or other cytotoxic drugs should undergo skin testing before starting the drugs to establish their tuberculin status before the immunosuppressive therapy.

Recommendations on the use of INH for immunosuppressed patients differ widely. Some authors advocate INH; others recommend deferring therapy because of the risk for hepatitis, such as that observed in renal transplant recipients. The duration of therapy for immunosuppressed patients is also unclear; some experts favor 1 year of therapy and others treatment for the duration of the immunosuppressed state. I favor using INH carefully for 1 year for the tuberculin-positive immunosuppressed patient. The greatest controversy concerns INH therapy in the tuberculin-positive adult (ages 21 to 35 years) with no other risk factors. Arguments on both sides of the issue have been clearly presented, and I favor chemoprophylaxis. An alternative approach to INH administration is careful observation of reactors and institution of therapy for active tuberculosis if it occurs. The benefits and risks of INH should be presented to the patient.

INH, the drug of choice for chemoprophylaxis, is given in a dose of 300 mg daily for adults and 10 mg/kg of body weight (up to 300 mg) in children. It is usually recommended for 6 to 12 months; however, 9 months of therapy is an acceptable duration for household contacts if the source case is being treated with a 9-month regimen. No more than a 1-month supply of INH should be given at any one time. In the recent trial of INH and placebo in Europe, patients randomly received 12, 24, or 52 weeks of treatment. There was a 93% reduction in tuberculosis for those with good compliance in the 52-week group. A 12-week treatment was too brief and eliminated fewer than one third of cases; 24 weeks of treatment eliminated 69% of the cases. INH for 1 year was particularly effective in patients with fibrotic lesions larger than 2 cm$^2$. There were more cases of hepatitis (than in controls) in patients being treated for 1 year, but the test population had a median age of 50 years. Nearly half the cases of hepatitis were observed during the initial 3 months of therapy. This study also demonstrated the importance of compliance for successful therapy. Rifampin (10 mg/kg of body weight, up to 600 mg) is recommended for 1 year for contacts who have presumably been infected by a source shedding INH-resistant bacilli, although this form of therapy has not been studied and is expensive. Twice-weekly INH treatment in a high dose (15 mg/kg of body weight) for 1 year may be tried if compliance is a problem.

The optimal preventive regimen for persons exposed to a source patient infected with multidrug-resistant *M. tuberculosis* is unknown. Susceptibility test results of the source-infecting strain may be helpful to guide therapy. If the infecting strain is less than 100% resistant to INH or rifampin, these drugs can be used. Potential alternative regimens include a combination of pyrazinamide plus ethambutol, or pyrazinamide plus either ofloxacin or ciprofloxacin. Clinical data are lacking on preventive therapy regimens that do not include INH, as this is the only drug approved for chemoprophylaxis. Shortening the duration of therapy with other drug combinations, as well as developing other regimens for prevention, should be a goal of future investigations. (N.M.G.)

## Bibliography

American Thoracic Society. Treatment of tuberculosis and tuberculosis infection in adults and children. *Am J Respir Crit Care Med* 1994;149:1359–1374.
    *Guidelines for screening and treatment. Persons with HIV infection should receive 12 months of INH preventive therapy. Children should be given 9 months of therapy.*
American Thoracic Society, American Academy of Pediatrics, Centers for Disease Control, Infectious Disease Society of America. Control of tuberculosis in the United States. *Am Rev Respir Dis* 1992;146:1623.
    *Indications for INH prophylaxis.*

Asch S, et al. Relationship of isoniazid resistance to human immunodeficiency virus infection in patients with tuberculosis. *Am J Respir Crit Care Med* 1996;153:1708–1710.
*INH-resistant tuberculosis was not more frequent in HIV-infected patients.*

Black M, et al. Isoniazid-associated hepatitis in 114 patients. *Gastroenterology* 1975; 69:289.
*A review of the cases of 114 patients with INH hepatitis, who had a 12% fatality rate. The clinical picture is indistinguishable from that of viral hepatitis.*

Byrd RB, Nelson R, Elliott RC. Toxic effects of isoniazid in tuberculosis chemoprophylaxis. *JAMA* 1979;241:1239.
*Ten percent of patients were unable to complete therapy with INH.*

Centers for Disease Control. Prevention and control of tuberculosis in facilities providing long-term care to the elderly: recommendations of the Advisory Committee for Elimination of Tuberculosis. *MMWR Morb Mortal Wkly Rep* 1990;39(RR10):7.
*A positive tuberculin skin test reaction is defined as an increase of 10 mm or more for a person under age 35 years or an increase of 15 mm or more for someone age 35 years or older.*

Centers for Disease Control. Management of persons exposed to multidrug-resistant tuberculosis. *MMWR Morb Mortal Wkly Rep* 1992;41(RR11):61.
*An approach to a tuberculin-positive contact suspected of having acquired infection with multidrug-resistant M. tuberculosis. Preventive therapy consists of pyrazinamide plus ethambutol, or pyrazinamide plus a fluoroquinolone.*

Centers for Disease Control. Prevention and treatment of tuberculosis among patients infected with human immunodeficiency virus: principles of therapy and revised recommendations. *MMWR* 1998;47 (No. RR-20):1–58.
*Describes use of a two month regimen of rifampin or rifabutin combined with pyrazinamide to prevent tuberculosis in patients with HIV infection.*

Colice GL. Decision analysis, public health policy, and isoniazid chemoprophylaxis for young adult tuberculin skin reactors. *Arch Intern Med* 1990;150:2517.
*Supports the use of INH for tuberculin-positive persons under age 35 years with normal chest roentgenographic findings and no other risk factors.*

Comstock GW, Baum C, Snider DE. Isoniazid prophylaxis among Alaskan Eskimos: a final report of the Bethel isoniazid studies. *Am Rev Respir Dis* 1979;119:827.
*Documents INH effectiveness in preventing tuberculosis.*

Comstock GW, Ferebee SH, Hammes LM. A controlled trial of community-wide isoniazid prophylaxis in Alaska. *Am Rev Respir Dis* 1967;95:935.
*Documents INH effectiveness in preventing tuberculosis.*

Curry FJ. Prophylactic effect of isoniazid in young tuberculin reactors. *N Engl J Med* 1967;277:562.
*Documents INH effectiveness in preventing tuberculosis.*

Dorken E, Grzybowski S, Enarson DA. Ten-year evaluation of a trial of chemoprophylaxis against tuberculosis in Frobisher Bay, Canada. *Tubercle* 1984;65:93.
*A regimen of INH plus ethambutol three times twice a week for 18 months was effective.*

Ferebee SH. Controlled chemoprophylaxis trials in tuberculosis. A general review. *Adv Tuber Res* 1970;17:28.
*Review of INH efficacy.*

Glassroth J, et al. Why tuberculosis is not prevented. *Am Rev Respir Dis* 1990; 141:1236.
*This report cites three reasons why tuberculosis is not prevented: (a) patients are not in the health care system until active tuberculosis occurs, (b) patients do not receive a tuberculin skin test or INH, or (c) patients fail to react to the skin test.*

Gordon FM, et al. A controlled trial of isoniazid in persons with anergy and human immunodeficiency virus infection who are at high risk for tuberculosis. *N Engl J Med* 1997;337:315–320.
*INH prophylaxis is not indicated for HIV-positive patients who are anergic unless they have been exposed to a patient with active tuberculosis.*

Halsey NA, et al. Randomised trial of isoniazid versus rifampicin and pyrazinamide for prevention of tuberculosis in HIV-1 infection. *Lancet* 1998;351:786–792.

*Twice-weekly isoniazid for 6 months or rifampin and pyrazinamide for 2 months were equally effective for chemoprophylaxis.*

Hawken MP, et al. Isoniazid preventive therapy for tuberculosis in HIV-1-infected adults: results of a randomized controlled trial. *AIDS* 1997;11:875–882.

*INH is not indicated for all HIV-infected persons.*

Hong Kong Chest Service, Tuberculosis Research Centre, Madras, British Medical Research Council. A double-blind, placebo-controlled clinical trial of three antituberculosis chemoprophylaxis regimens in patients with silicosis in Hong Kong. *Am Rev Respir Dis* 1992;145:36.

*At 5 years, the rate of active tuberculosis was halved in patients with silicosis receiving chemoprophylaxis with rifampin for 3 months, INH and rifampin for 3 months, or INH for 6 months, compared with those given placebo.*

Hsu KHK. Thirty years after isoniazid. *JAMA* 1984;251:1283.

*No control group. Effectiveness of INH prophylaxis was best demonstrated in children infected before age 4 years.*

International Union Against Tuberculosis Committee on Prophylaxis. Efficacy of various durations of isoniazid preventive therapy for tuberculosis: 5 years of follow-up in the IUAT trial. *Bull World Health Organ* 1982;60:555.

*A 24-week regimen of INH was effective.*

Israel HL, Gottlieb JE, Maddrey WC. Perspective: preventive isoniazid therapy and the liver. *Chest* 1992;101:1298.

*INH hepatic toxicity is reviewed, and three cases of fatal INH hepatitis are reported.*

Jordan TJ, Lewit EM, Reichman LB. Isoniazid preventive therapy for tuberculosis: decision analysis considering ethnicity and gender. *Am Rev Respir Dis* 1991;144:1357.

*Black women over age 50 years are at higher risk for INH hepatotoxicity.*

Jordan TJ, et al. Isoniazid as preventive therapy in HIV-infected intravenous drug abusers. *JAMA* 1991;265:2987.

*Analysis supports the use of INH for all HIV-seropositive patients with a history of IV drug use except tuberculin-negative black women who are not anergic.*

Livengood JR, et al. Isoniazid-resistant tuberculosis: a community outbreak and report of a rifampin prophylaxis failure. *JAMA* 1985;253:2847.

*Three options are available for the management of contacts of persons with known INH-resistant tuberculosis: (a) INH, (b) rifampin alone or in combination with INH, or (c) no antituberculous therapy and close observation of the patient for development of active disease. A possible case of rifampin prophylaxis failure is presented.*

Moreno S, et al. Isoniazid preventive therapy in human immunodeficiency virus-infected persons. *Arch Intern Med* 1997;157:1729–1734.

*INH prophylaxis in HIV-positive patients decreased the incidence of active tuberculosis and improved overall survival.*

Moulding TS, Redeker AG, Kanal GC. Twenty isoniazid-associated deaths in one state. *Am Rev Respir Dis* 1989;140:700.

*INH was used for prevention in 19 cases.*

Nazar-Stewart V, Nolan CM. Results of a directly observed intermittent isoniazid preventive therapy program in a shelter for homeless men. *Am Rev Respir Dis* 1992; 146:57.

*In a supervised program, INH could be given safely to the homeless in a dosage of 900 mg twice weekly.*

Passannante M, Gallagher CT, Reichman LB. Preventive therapy for multidrug-resistant tuberculosis, MDRTB: a Delphi survey. *Chest* 1994;106:431–434.

*No evidence that multidrug-resistant tuberculosis is more invasive than susceptible strains. Optimal therapy is unknown in this setting.*

Salpeter S. Fatal isoniazid-induced hepatitis: its risk during chemoprophylaxis. *West J Med* 1993;159:560–564.

*When liver function tests were monitored, the death rate from INH chemoprophylaxis for those over 35 years was 0.002% (1/43,334).*

Salpeter SR, et al. Monitored isoniazid prophylaxis for low-risk tuberculin reactors older than 35 years of age: a risk-benefit and cost effectiveness analysis. *Ann Intern Med* 1997;127:1051–1061.

*Based on cost decision analysis, INH is indicated for all adults with a positive PPD skin test reaction over 35 years of age if liver function tests are monitored.*

Snider DE Jr. Pyridoxine supplementation during isoniazid therapy. *Tubercle* 1980; 61:191.
*Useful in the elderly, alcoholics, and pregnant women to prevent peripheral neuropathy.*

Snider DE Jr, Caras GJ. Isoniazid-associated hepatitis deaths: a review of available information. *Am Rev Respir Dis* 1992;145:494.
*Deaths reviewed. Women may be at an increased risk for fatal INH-related hepatitis.*

Snider DE Jr, Caras GJ, Koplan JP. Preventive therapy with isoniazid: cost effectiveness of different durations of therapy. *JAMA* 1986;255:1579.
*According to a cost effectiveness analysis, a 6-month course of INH had an advantage over a 1-year regimen.*

Stead WW. Management of health care workers after inadvertent exposure to tuberculosis: a guide for the use of preventive therapy. *Ann Intern Med* 1995;122:906–912.
*In a heavily exposed health care worker, start INH even if the tuberculin skin test reaction is negative. If the skin test reaction is still negative at 3 months, discontinue INH.*

Stead WW, et al. Benefit-risk considerations in preventive treatment for tuberculosis in elderly persons. *Ann Intern Med* 1987;107:843.
*Among the elderly, INH hepatic toxicity developed in 4.4% of persons.*

Steiger Z, et al. Pulmonary tuberculosis after gastric resection. *Am J Surg* 1976; 131:668.
*Tuberculosis is likely to be reactivated following a gastrectomy in patients with chest roentgenographic evidence of inactive tuberculosis who have not been previously treated.*

Taylor WC, Aronson MD, Delbanco TL. Should young adults with a positive tuberculin test take isoniazid? *Ann Intern Med* 1981;94:808.
*Study does not support the use of INH for those under age 35 years with no other risk factors.*

Tsevat J, et al. Isoniazid for the tuberculin reactor: take it or leave it. *Am Rev Respir Dis* 1988;137:215.
*Based on decision analysis, this study suggests that INH prophylaxis provides minimal benefit to the person under age 35 years with a positive tuberculin test, normal chest roentgenographic findings, and no risk factors.*

Whalen CC, et al. A trial of three regimens to prevent tuberculosis in Ugandan adults infected with the human immunodeficiency virus. *N Engl J Med* 1997;337:801–808.
*A 6-month course of INH in PPD-positive, HIV-infected adults was effective in reducing the risk for active tuberculosis. Also effective in reducing the risk for tuberculosis were INH and rifampin for 3 months and INH, rifampin, and pyrazinamide for 3 months.*

## 67.  CHEMOTHERAPY OF TUBERCULOSIS

The potential to control tuberculosis has existed only since the late 1940s, when antituberculous medications became available. The impact of such medications became obvious quickly. Between 1932 and 1983, the number of new active cases declined from 96,500 to 23,500 per year, and mortality dropped from 71,000 to 1,980 per year. In 1986, however, the number of new cases increased by 2.6%. In 1991, 26,283 new cases were reported and were associated with direct health care expenditures estimated at $703 million. In 1997, 19,855 cases of tuberculosis were reported, representing a 7% decrease from what was seen the year before and a 26% decrease from what was noted in 1992—the peak year of the tuberculosis resurgence. Much of the increase seen since 1986 represents disease in persons simultaneously infected with HIV and tuberculosis. Outbreaks of multidrug-resistant tuberculosis have also occurred in this population and have spread to health care workers, resulting in significant morbidity and mortality. The problem has been compounded by the limited availability of streptomycin.

Through the 1970s, two-drug therapy administered for up to 2 years provided excellent results, with relapse rates predictably less than 5%. However, treatment of this length was associated with higher costs, increased side effects, and problems with compliance. During the past one to two decades, studies documented the efficacy and safety of shorter courses of chemotherapy using at least two effective agents. Treatment combining isoniazid (INH) and rifampin became commonplace. As an example, for sensitive organisms, daily therapy for 9 months with 300 mg of INH orally plus 600 mg of rifampin orally was associated with relapse rates of less than 3% and became a standard of care for uncomplicated pulmonary and extrapulmonary tuberculosis. However, the recent emergence of multidrug-resistant tuberculosis has required a reassessment of this issue.

In 1998, the FDA approved the first new antituberculous agent in almost 25 years. Rifapentine (Priftin; Hoechst Marion Roussel) functions as a long-active form of rifampin and has been approved for use in patients with tuberculosis but without HIV/AIDS. Doses may range from 600 mg/d to 300 mg twice weekly. Dosing with this drug can be as infrequent as once weekly, which, it is hoped, will decrease noncompliance. Preliminary data, however, suggest slightly higher relapse rates than are seen with rifampin. This new product is also likely to interact with protease inhibitors.

### Short-course Chemotherapy

Animal studies have demonstrated that INH plus a second bactericidal agent can rapidly cure murine TB. Other *in vitro* investigations have shown that tubercle bacilli can be killed only when dividing, and that organisms at different sites vary in their frequency of replication. Those that are dormant are most resistant to killing. *Mycobacterium tuberculosis* infection can be classified by the location of lesions as follows:

1. *Cavitary lesions: M. tuberculosis* replicates best at the high oxygen tensions found in body cavities. Numbers of bacteria approach $10^8$/g of tissue. Organisms in cavitary lesions are usually extracellular and in a neutral or alkaline pH. Streptomycin, INH, and rifampin are active against organisms at these sites and rapidly kill them.

2. *Closed caseous lesions* (organisms usually extracellular): Antituberculous drugs are less effective at these sites than within cavities. Organisms are metabolically less active and tend to number only $10^4$ to $10^5$/g of tissue. The pH remains neutral or slightly alkaline. Rifampin and INH are most effective at these locations.

3. *Within macrophages* (intracellular organisms): Organisms within macrophages have a low rate metabolic activity, may be intermittently dormant, and exist at an acid pH in numbers of $10^4$ to $10^5$/g of tissue. Those that are dormant are unresponsive to all medications. Although both INH and rifampin have modest activity within this acidic environment, pyrazinamide is most effective.

Patients infected with HIV are at increased risk for infections with *M. tuberculosis*. This pathogen is noted in 2% to 10% of patients with AIDS and often occurs in extrapulmonary locations. The likelihood of extrapulmonary disease increases with more advanced HIV infection. In recent studies of patients in whom tuberculosis has been newly diagnosed, up to 30% are simultaneously infected with HIV. Additionally, in patients with HIV infection, reactivation of latent infection is more likely, extrapulmonary disease is seen more often, and disease progresses more rapidly to active tuberculosis. The rate of development of active disease in patients with HIV is approximately 8% annually, compared with 10% in a lifetime for persons not infected with HIV. Fortunately, in the absence of multidrug-resistant tuberculosis, response to antituberculous therapy is similar to that seen in persons not infected with HIV.

### Multidrug-resistant Tuberculosis

Multidrug-resistant tuberculosis is being increasingly observed and is strongly associated with both HIV infection and increased mortality; fatality rates have approached 90% in some studies. The possibility of improved outcomes has been acknowledged in recent studies. These demonstrate that early identification of patients at risk and use of effective combination therapies can result in earlier bacteriologic conversion and prolonged survival. With appropriate management, survival of more than 1 year was seen in 59% of patients with multidrug-resistant tuberculosis. Factors that have been identified as increasing survival in patients with multidrug-resistant tuberculosis include initiation of treatment within 4 weeks of diagnosis, treatment with at least two effective agents for at least 2 consecutive weeks, and disease limited to the lungs. Appropriate treatment for at least 2 weeks consecutively is probably the most important of these. Multidrug resistance often extends beyond resistance to INH and rifampin. Consideration for multidrug-resistant tuberculosis is made on epidemiologic grounds, as most cases have occurred in closed populations within hospitals or prisons and in localized geographic areas, including Florida and New York. Health care workers exposed to actively infected persons have also become ill. Recent national data suggest that 7% to 8% of *M. tuberculosis* isolates are now INH-resistant, and that 1% to 2% of strains are multidrug-resistant. Forty-three states plus the District of Columbia reported strains of multidrug-resistant tuberculosis between 1993 and 1997. Other data from New York, an area with increased numbers of patients with AIDS, demonstrate that approximately 33% of isolates of *M. tuberculosis* are resistant to one drug and 19% are multiply resistant. Knowledge of applicable resistance patterns is mandatory to effect treatment.

Recommendations for empiric therapy of *M. tuberculosis* before the availability of sensitivities must take into account the HIV status of the patient and the likelihood of resistant organisms being present. Table 67-1 provides current recommendations for initial empiric therapy in HIV-negative patients. A four-drug regimen that usually consists of INH (300 mg daily), rifampin (600 mg daily), pyrazinamide (15 to 30 mg/kg daily, 2 g maximum), and ethambutol (15 mg/kg daily) or streptomycin (20 to 30 mg/kg daily, 1 g maximum) is generally recommended. A three-drug regimen that does not include ethambutol or streptomycin can be used if the likelihood of INH resistance is less than 4% in a community, and if there are no risk factors for multidrug-resistant tuberculosis. The same regimens can be used in patients who are HIV-positive; however, the length of therapy must be extended to at least 9 months, or 6 months beyond conversion of sputum cultures.

Fluoroquinolones have been studied in the treatment of tuberculosis and represent alternatives for some patients with multidrug-resistant tuberculosis. Both ciprofloxacin and ofloxacin possess significant antituberculous activity. However, INH plus rifampin plus ciprofloxacin (750 mg/d) was less effective than a traditional four-drug regimen in regard to time to sputum negativity and was associated with a higher relapse rate. Problems with efficacy of fluoroquinolones may be more noted in the HIV-infected population.

Directly observed therapy (DOT), generally twice or thrice weekly, is strongly advised for potentially noncompliant persons. Under DOT, the usual adult doses of drugs are as follows:

INH: 900 mg two to three times per week
Rifampin: 600 mg two to three times per week

Table 67-1. Initial empiric treatment of tuberculosis in HIV-negative patients

*Option 1*
In areas with documented rates of INH resistance of <4%, daily INH, RIF, and PZA for 8 wk, followed by 16 wk of INH plus RIF daily for 2–3 wk. If rates are > 4%, EMB or SM is added to the initial regimen until susceptibility to both INH and RIF is noted. Therapy is continued for at least 6 mo, and 3 mo beyond culture conversion.

*Option 2*
Administer INH, RIF, PZA, and either SM or EMB daily for 2 wk, followed by administration of the same drugs 2 times/wk (DOT) for an additional 6 wk, and (assuming organism sensitivity to both INH and RIF) subsequent administration of INH plus RIF 2 times/wk for an additional 16 wk (DOT).

*Option 3*
Treat by DOT 3 times/wk with INH, RIF, PZA, and EMB or SM for 6 mo.

INH, isoniazid; RIF, rifampin; PZA, pyrazinamide; EMB, ethambutol; SM, streptomycin; DOT, directly observed therapy.

Ethambutol: 2.5 g two to three times per week
Pyrazinamide: 3 to 4 g two to three times per week
Streptomycin: 1.0 to 1.5 g two to three times per week

DOT has been compared with the traditional treatment of tuberculosis. This investigation documented a decrease in relapse from 21% to 5.5%, and a decrease in primary and acquired drug resistance from 13% and 14% to 7% and 2%, respectively. The use of DOT should be expanded, and it may be cost effective for all populations.

The likelihood of adverse reactions to antituberculous medications is probably higher in HIV-infected patients, so these patients should be closely monitored. Additionally, other medications taken by patients with HIV infection (e.g., ketoconazole, fluconazole) may interact with antituberculous agents. For patients infected with susceptible organisms but incapable of tolerating both INH and rifampin, current recommendations are for at least 18 months of either INH or rifampin plus both ethambutol and pyrazinamide. Similar recommendations apply to patients infected with organisms resistant to either INH or rifampin.

When multidrug-resistant tuberculosis is considered, therapy should be initiated with four to six agents, one of which should be a quinolone. Isolates of *M. tuberculosis* should be tested against an expanded spectrum of antituberculous agents, including ciprofloxacin, ofloxacin, amikacin, and amoxicillin-clavulanate. The length of therapy is not defined but should probably be 18 to 24 months if multidrug-resistant tuberculosis is identified.

## Common Side Effects of Drugs Used in Short-course Chemotherapy

*Isoniazid*
Peripheral neuropathy and central nervous system events are rarely seen. Pyridoxine (vitamin $B_6$) deficiency, occurring especially in alcoholics, may provoke these problems. Prevention consists of daily administration of 50 to 100 mg of pyridoxine. Hepatitis is an uncommon but serious complication of INH administration. Incidence peaks at 2% to 3% for patients 50 years of age and may be enhanced by alcohol and rapid acetylation. Continued administration can lead to death. The problem is complex because transient and reversible elevations of hepatic enzymes develop in up to 20% of patients receiving INH. All persons taking INH should have a baseline measurement of hepatic function and should be informed of symptoms of hepatitis; use of INH should be discontinued if such symptoms arise. Persons over 35 years of age should be monitored regularly during therapy. Treatment should be discontinued if elevations three to five times normal are noted. Important drug interactions exist between INH and disulfiram and diphenylhydantoin; such interactions can result in psychosis or phenytoin toxicity.

*Rifampin*
Rifampin imparts an orange color to body secretions and may cause liver disease, especially in persons receiving INH. When used intermittently in doses above 600 mg/d, an influenza-like syndrome and thrombocytopenia may occur. Rifampin can induce hepatic enzymes that increase the metabolism of other drugs. Blood levels of birth control pills, warfarin, digoxin, and oral antidiabetic drugs are all decreased when rifampin is simultaneously administered. Ketoconazole, an agent often employed in patients with AIDS, may decrease rifampin absorption.

*Pyrazinamide*
Major clinical complications of this drug are hepatitis and arthralgia. The latter may result in severe but usually self-limited involvement of small and large joints. The cause of these complications is unclear, but it may be related to the hyperuricemia commonly noted in patients taking pyrazinamide. Therapy with salicylates is usually effective. Hepatitis can be observed in 1% to 4% of patients, but the use of pyrazinamide with INH does not appear to increase the risk. Hepatitis is dose-related and occurs less commonly with intermittent than with daily therapy. As with INH, hepatic enzymes may be transiently elevated, but this does not necessarily require discontinuation of therapy. (R.B.B.)

**Bibliography**

Ad Hoc Committee of the Scientific Assembly on Microbiology, Tuberculosis, and Pulmonary Infections. Treatment of tuberculosis and tuberculous infections in adults and children. *Clin Infect Dis* 1995;21:9–27.
*This publication (reprinted from* Am J Respir Crit Care Med *1994;149:1359–1374) reviews relevant data concerning drugs used in therapy, regimens, and monitoring of patients with tuberculosis. Specific measures for multidrug-resistant tuberculosis are given, and issues related to prophylaxis are addressed. An excellent source of information for most clinicians.*

Alangaden GJ, Lerner SA. The clinical use of fluoroquinolones for the treatment of mycobacterial diseases. *Clin Infect Dis* 1997;25:1213–1221.
*The authors review the rationale and clinical investigations regarding quinolones in the treatment of mycobacterial diseases. With regard to tuberculosis, ciprofloxacin and ofloxacin have been best studied, and both possess rapid bactericidal activity. In most instances, doses of ciprofloxacin or ofloxacin were 500 to 750 mg/d or 300 to 800 mg/d, respectively. Based on available data, the quinolones should not be considered front-line agents, but they can prove valuable in selected cases (especially multidrug-resistant tuberculosis) based on susceptibility studies. They do appear to be well tolerated when given for months at a time.*

Centers for Disease Control. Initial therapy for tuberculosis in the era of multidrug resistance. *MMWR Morb Mortal Wkly Rep* 1993;42:1–8.
*These recommendations of the Advisory Council for the Elimination of Tuberculosis take into account what is known about multidrug-resistant tuberculosis and the risks associated with HIV infection. A four-drug regimen is recommended as initial empiric therapy unless it is clear that the risk of INH resistance in a community is under 4%. Initial regimens should always employ at least three drugs.*

Centers for Disease Control. Tuberculosis morbidity—United States, 1997. *MMWR Morb Mortal Wkly Rep* 1998;47:253–257.
*Updated information is provided concerning the scope of the tuberculosis problem in the United States. Since 1992, the annual number of new cases of tuberculosis has declined. However, major geographic variations exist. Currently, fewer than 2% of* M. tuberculosis *isolates were multidrug-resistant, and 7% to 8% were INH-resistant. The editors attribute these encouraging trends to more thorough and rapid identification of patients with tuberculosis, and better and more complete treatment.*

Combs DL, O'Brien RJ, Geiter LJ. USPHS tuberculosis short-course chemotherapy trial 21: effectiveness, toxicity, and acceptability. The report of final results. *Ann Intern Med* 1990;112:397–406.
*This investigation represents a multicenter trial comparing 6 months of INH plus rifampin (pyrazinamide for first 8 weeks) with 9 months of INH plus rifampin. Patients receiving 6 months of treatment demonstrated quicker sputum conversions, better acceptance and completion of therapy, and similar rates of relapse. This study provides compelling evidence to use INH, rifampin, and pyrazinamide as standard therapy for pansensitive strains of* M. tuberculosis *for 6 months.*

Fischl MA, et al. An outbreak of tuberculosis caused by multiple-drug-resistant tubercle bacilli among patients with HIV infection. *Ann Intern Med* 1992;117:177–183.
*This investigation is a case-control study of patients with tuberculosis caused by either multidrug-resistant or sensitive strains. Patients with multidrug-resistant tuberculosis were more likely to be infected with HIV, to have had contact with HIV clinics, and to have received inhaled pentamidine. Many patients had had previous contact with patients harboring multidrug-resistant strains. The study documents potential nosocomial transmission.*

Goble M, et al. Treatment of 171 patients with pulmonary tuberculosis resistant to isoniazid and rifampin. *N Engl J Med* 1993;328:527–532.
*The authors describe their extensive experience with multidrug-resistant tuberculosis between 1973 and 1983, at which time most patients were probably not infected with HIV. Thirty-five percent failed to respond to multiple-drug regimens, and more than 50% ultimately relapsed. Deaths were noted in 37% of patients.*

Kennedy N, et al. Randomized controlled trial of a drug regimen that includes ciprofloxacin for the treatment of pulmonary tuberculosis. *Clin Infect Dis* 1996;22:827–833.

*This study, conducted in Tanzania, compared INH-rifampin-ciprofloxacin with standard four-drug treatment of pulmonary tuberculosis. The smears of all 168 patients who could be assessed were negative at 6-month follow-up, but the smears were slower to convert and the relapse rate was higher in those patients, both HIV-positive and HIV-negative, who received the quinolone-containing regimen. Also, INH-resistant strains developed in two patients in the quinolone arm of the study. It is known that several quinolones are bactericidal against M. tuberculosis, but the best dose and combination of other agents need to be defined better.*

Liu S, Shilkret KL, Finelli L. Initial drug regimens for the treatment of tuberculosis. *Chest* 1998;113:1446–1451.

*The authors reviewed the treatment regimens of 1,230 culture-positive patients residing in New Jersey to determine the adequacy of treatment based on Centers for Disease Control guidelines. Disturbingly, almost 40% of patients were initially placed on regimens with fewer than four effective drugs, despite the fact that almost all were in an area with substantial resistance. At least 6% to 7% of patients received fewer than two effective agents. However, outcome data were not presented. Treatment was much better at the hospital where tuberculosis experts were overtly available. The authors conclude that information about tuberculosis treatment needs to be disseminated better.*

Saloman N, et al. Predictors and outcome of multidrug-resistant tuberculosis. *Clin Infect Dis* 1995;21:1245–1252.

*The investigators identified 88 HIV-positive patients, 18 of whom had multidrug-resistant tuberculosis. Use of at least two agents effective in vitro resulted in enhanced 1-year survivorship and more rapid sputum conversion. The presence of multidrug-resistant tuberculosis did not predict poor outcome. This study reemphasizes the need for earlier and better identification of patients, use of multiple-drug regimens, and expanded susceptibility testing of patients at risk for multidrug resistance.*

Simone PM, Iseman MD. Drug-resistant tuberculosis: a deadly and growing danger. *J Respir Dis* 1992;13:960–971.

*This excellent review article summarizes the epidemiology and treatment of drug-resistant tuberculosis. The authors recommend continuation of treatment for at least 18 to 24 months after sputum conversion, although little data substantiate this. The article also provides short vignettes of first- and second-line antituberculous agents.*

Small PM, et al. Treatment of tuberculosis in patients with advanced human immunodeficiency virus infection. *N Engl J Med* 1991;324:289–294.

*Retrospective study of 132 patients in San Francisco with both tuberculosis and HIV infection. Tuberculosis was found to develop both before and after HIV diagnosis and was often extrapulmonary. Standard treatment regimens included INH plus rifampin (9 months) and INH plus rifampin with the addition of either ethambutol or pyrazinamide (6 months). Patients who adhered to the regimen did well. A single treatment failure occurred in a noncompliant person with multidrug-resistant tuberculosis. This investigation documents that standard therapy is effective for most patients with HIV infection and tuberculosis.*

Weis SE, et al. The effect of directly observed therapy on the rates of drug resistance and relapse in tuberculosis. *N Engl J Med* 1994;330:1179–1184.

*The authors conducted a retrospective study of patients treated for tuberculosis during two time frames, with DOT used in the latter in 90% of cases. Almost 1,000 patients comprised the study group. Despite the fact that many patients were substance abusers and homeless, use of DOT resulted in significantly fewer relapses and fewer numbers of resistant strains of M. tuberculosis. The authors conclude that DOT is cost effective, and that its use should be expanded in most populations.*

Wolinsky E. Statement of the Tuberculosis Committee of the Infectious Disease Society of America. *Clin Infect Dis* 1993;16: 627–628.

*This commentary reviews the rationale behind using at least three agents as initial therapy of tuberculosis and provides practical guidelines for the selection of agents when multidrug-resistant tuberculosis is suspected. The committee suggests that an injectable agent (amikacin, capreomycin, or kanamycin), a quinolone (ofloxacin or ciprofloxacin), pyrazinamide, and ethambutol be used. A fifth agent such as rifabutin can be added if tolerated.*

# XVIII. SELECTED LABORATORY PROCEDURES

# 68. LABORATORY REPORT OF A GRAM-NEGATIVE ROD IN THE BLOOD

When the microbiology laboratory reports that a blood culture is positive for a gram-negative bacillus, it must be assumed that the patient is bacteremic and a life-threatening infection is present. The history and physical examination will usually strongly suggest the source of infection. Specific identification of the gram-negative bacillus will also sometimes be helpful in identifying a primary infection.

## Etiologic Agents

Several studies have classified gram-negative bacteremia according to most common etiologic agent and most frequent source of infection. Kreger and associates, for example, reviewed 612 episodes of gram-negative bacteremia during a 10-year period. Table 68-1 shows the distribution of etiologic agents. *Escherichia coli* was the most common gram-negative rod causing bacteremia, being responsible for 31% of cases. Table 68-2 shows the sources of gram-negative bacteremia. Urinary tract infection is by far the most common source, with infection of the gastrointestinal and biliary tract second. The respiratory tract (i.e., bacteremic pneumonia) was the source in only 9% of cases, and skin and soft tissue in 6.5%.

The gram-negative organism most likely to cause bacteremia varies with several factors. If the bacteremia is acquired in the community, *E. coli* is the most common organism. Organisms such as *Pseudomonas aeruginosa* and *Serratia marcescens* are most likely to occur in the hospital. The longer the length of stay, the more likely it is that these relatively antimicrobial-resistant organisms will be found. The population studied will also affect the distribution of etiologic agents in gram-negative bacteremia. *P. aeruginosa* is more likely to occur in the neutropenic patient, whereas *E. coli* is by far the most common agent in the healthy young patient. Each hospital has its own profile of etiologic agents. Some organisms, such as *Acinetobacter* species, may be common in one hospital and unusual in another. The site of infection may also predict the etiologic agent. For example, *Proteus mirabilis* or *Providencia* species isolated from blood cultures suggest urinary tract infection. In bacteremic pneumonia, *Klebsiella pneumoniae* and *P. aeruginosa* are much more common than *Proteus* species, *Providencia,* or even *E. coli. Bacteroides* bacteremia suggests anaerobic infection of the colon or female genital tract, a liver abscess, or postoperative wound infection.

The pattern of gram-negative bacteremia has been changing with the introduction of new antimicrobials. For example, *Xanthomonas maltophilia* (formerly *Pseudomonas maltophilia*) infection has been increasing because of the aminoglycoside resistance of this organism. Isolates can be cultured from the hospital environment, and common-source outbreaks can occur. *Pseudomonas cepacia* has also caused an increasing incidence of bacteremia and outbreaks associated with hospital devices, such as a blood gas analyzer. *Pseudomonas fluorescens* has caused bacteremia in association with blood transfusion. An increasing number of *Pseudomonas* species have been implicated in bacteremia.

*Enterobacter* bacteremia has also been caused by contaminated blood products, but *Enterobacter* is reported to contaminate IV fluids more frequently. Compared with *K. pneumoniae* bacteremia, *Enterobacter* bacteremia appears to carry a higher mortality rate, is more often associated with surgery or infection of unknown source, and is more likely to be associated with polymicrobial bloodstream infection.

*Acinetobacter* species are causing more cases of nosocomial bacteremia, in part because of their relative resistance to third-generation cephalosporins. Bacteremia is frequently associated with an IV catheter or is secondary to pneumonia. The organism, on Gram's stain, frequently appears as a gram-negative coccus or diplococcus rather than as a rod.

A gram-negative bacillus on smear may represent bacteremia from a nonenteric gram-negative rod. For example, a group of slow-growing gram-negative bacilli, including *Haemophilus aphrophilus, Actinobacillus actinomycetemcomitans, Cardiobacterium hominis, Eikenella corrodens,* and *Kingella* species (HACEK group), can cause a picture of subacute bacterial endocarditis. These organisms are often difficult to grow,

Table 68-1.  Etiologic agents in gram-negative bacteremia

| Agent | Frequency (%) |
| --- | --- |
| *Escherichia coli* | 31 |
| *Klebsiella-Enterobacter-Serratia* | 22 |
| *Pseudomonas* species | 10 |
| *Proteus* and *Providencia* | 8 |
| *Bacteroides* | 7 |
| Other | 6 |
| Polymicrobial | 16 |

requiring prolonged incubation and subculturing to chocolate agar. *Haemophilus influenzae* can cause bacteremia secondary to pneumonia, otitis media, meningitis, or epiglottitis. These small, gram-negative coccobacilli can usually be distinguished from the larger enteric gram-negative rods on smear.

Dysgonic fermenter-2, now called *Capnocytophaga canimorsus,* is a slow-growing gram-negative bacillus that causes a zoonotic infection acquired through dog bites. It can cause fulminating bacteremia in splenectomized and alcoholic patients.

*Salmonella* bacteremia has become an increasing problem in patients with AIDS. Recurrent episodes of fever and chills and positive blood cultures are common. *Campylobacter* may also cause disease with bacteremia. *Shigella* species, rarely a cause of bacteremia, have been more commonly reported, particularly in AIDS patients.

*Flavobacterium* species, particularly *F. meningosepticum,* are nonmotile, catalase-positive, gram-negative bacilli that have become ubiquitous in some hospital environments. Hospital outbreaks of bacteremia can occur. The organism has an unusual sensitivity pattern, generally being sensitive to trimethoprim-sulfamethoxazole and vancomycin but resistant to aminoglycosides.

New genera and species of Enterobacteriaceae continue to emerge. In 1972, there were 11 genera and 26 species; in 1995, there were 28 genera and 115 species. Newer genera, which may cause episodes of urinary tract infection, wound infection, or bacteremia, include *Hafnia, Edwardsiella, Ewingella, Kluyvera,* and *Cedecea.* Many of these newer genera are particularly antibiotic-resistant.

### Clinical Approach
An internal medicine or infectious disease consultant will often be asked to assess a patient when the laboratory calls with the positive blood culture report. A history and physical examination should be directed at the most likely sources of infection (a urinary tract infection; gastrointestinal infection; pneumonia; skin, soft-tissue, or catheter infection). Urine Gram's stain and culture should be obtained. Chest roentgenography and sputum Gram's stain are necessary if pneumonia is suspected. A complete physical examination will include a pelvic examination in a woman in

Table 68-2.  Primary sources of gram-negative bacteremia

| Source | Frequency (%) |
| --- | --- |
| Urinary tract | 34.0 |
| Gastrointestinal tract | 14.0 |
| Respiratory tract | 9.0 |
| Skin | 6.5 |
| Biliary tract | 2.0 |
| Reproductive tract | 3.0 |
| Unknown | 30.0 |

whom no other definite source of infection can be defined. IV lines should be removed, and the patency of indwelling Foley catheters or nephrostomy tubes should be checked. Abdominal tenderness in the setting of gram-negative bacteremia will usually require a surgical consult and appropriate imaging examination.

Most patients reported to have gram-negative rods in a blood culture will require therapy with an antimicrobial that has a broad spectrum of gram-negative activity. In the case of a patient who appears well at the time of the report, blood cultures can be repeated while the patient is being closely observed. However, few blood cultures positive for gram-negative bacilli represent contamination. The great majority of such cases require rapid antimicrobial therapy. When infection caused by *H. influenzae*, endocarditis-causing organisms of the HACEK group, dysgonic fermenter-2, or anaerobes is suspected, a different approach to antimicrobial therapy will be required than in infection with the more common enteric gram-negative bacilli. (S.L.B.)

## Bibliography

Baltch AL, Griffin PE. *Pseudomonas aeruginosa* bacteremia: a clinical study of 75 patients. *Am J Med Sci* 1977;274:119.
   P. aeruginosa *bacteremia is nosocomial, arising from a urinary tract, respiratory tract, or intravascular focus of infection.*

Bisbe J, et al. *Pseudomonas aeruginosa* bacteremia: univariate and multivariate analyses of factors influencing the prognosis in 133 episodes. *Rev Infect Dis* 1988;10:629.
   Pseudomonas *bacteremia represented 25% of all cases of gram-negative bacteremia. Appropriate antimicrobial therapy is critical to survival.*

Bouza E, et al. *Enterobacter* bacteremia: an analysis of 50 episodes. *Arch Intern Med* 1985;145:1024.
   *Describes particular clinical characteristics of* Enterobacter *bacteremia.*

Bouza E, et al. *Serratia* bacteremia. *Diagn Microbiol Infect Dis* 1987;7:237.
   *Bacteremia caused by* S. marcescens *has become common in some institutions. Increasing resistance to gentamicin has developed.*

Crowe HM, Levitz RE. Invasive *Haemophilus influenzae* disease in adults. *Arch Intern Med* 1987;147:241.
   H. influenzae, *usually nontypable, caused bacteremia in 29 adults. Pneumonia was the most common source.*

DuPont HL, Spink WW. Infections due to gram-negative organisms: an analysis of 860 patients with bacteremia at the University of Minnesota Medical Center, 1958–1966. *Medicine (Baltimore)* 1969;48:307.
   *An analysis of the portal of entry in 655 adults with gram-negative bacteremia.*

Edmondson EB, Sanford JP. The *Klebsiella-Enterobacter (Aerobacter)-Serratia* group: a clinical and bacteriological evaluation. *Medicine (Baltimore)* 1967;46:323.
   *The lung is an important focus for* Klebsiella *bacteremia.*

Fainstein V, et al. *Haemophilus* species bacteremia in patients with cancer: a 13-year experience. *Arch Intern Med* 1989;149:1341.
   Haemophilus *bacteremia may occur in patients with cancer. Most isolates were nontypable.*

Flynn DM, Weinstein RA, Kabins SA. Infections with gram-negative bacilli in a cardiac surgery intensive care unit: the relative role of *Enterobacter*. *J Hosp Infect* 1988;11(Suppl A): 367.
   Enterobacter *is a particularly important cause of bacteremia in surgical patients.*

Freney J, et al. Postoperative infant septicemia caused by *Pseudomonas luteola* (CDC Group Ve-1) and *Pseudomonas oryzihabitans* (CDC Group Ve-2). *J Clin Microbiol* 1988;26:1241.
   *Several unusual* Pseudomonas *species have caused bacteremia—in this case, in an infant after open heart surgery.*

Glew RH, Moellering RC Jr, Kunz LJ. Infections with *Acinetobacter calcoaceticus* (*Herellea vaginicola*): clinical and laboratory studies. *Medicine (Baltimore)* 1977; 56:79.
   *The sources of bacteremia include intravascular cannulas and respiratory infections.*

Gregory WJ, McNabb PC. *Pseudomonas cepacia*. *Infect Control* 1986;7:281.
   *Reviews the epidemiology and microbiology of* P. cepacia.

Henderson DK, et al. Indolent epidemic of *Pseudomonas cepacia* bacteremia and pseudobacteremia in an intensive care unit traced to a contaminated blood gas analyzer. *Am J Med* 1988;84:75.
*P. cepacia is a cause of nosocomial bacteremia, often associated with contamination of hospital devices.*

Hicklin H, Verghese A, Alvarez S. Dysgonic fermenter-2 septicemia. *Rev Infect Dis* 1987;9:884.
*Dysgonic fermenter-2 causes bacteremia after dog bites, particularly in splenectomized and alcoholic patients.*

Isenberg HD, D'Amato RF. Enterobacteriaceae In: Gorbach SL, Bartlett JG, Blacklow NR, eds. *In Infectious Disease.* Philadelphia: WB Saunders, 1998.

Khabbaz RF, et al. *Pseudomonas fluorescens* bacteremia from blood transfusion. *Am J Med* 1984;76:62.
*P. fluorescens caused bacteremia after proliferating in refrigerated whole blood.*

Kreger BE, et al. Gram-negative bacteremia. III. Reassessment of etiology, epidemiology and ecology in 612 patients. *Am J Med* 1980;68:332.
*Definitive study on the clinical picture of gram-negative bacteremia, including etiologic agents and sources of infection.*

Levin DC, et al. Bacteremic *Haemophilus influenzae* pneumonia in adults: a report of 24 cases and a review of the literature. *Am J Med* 1977;62:219.
*A review of the clinical features of* H. influenzae *bacteremia.*

Lewis J, Fekety FR Jr. *Proteus* bacteremia. *Johns Hopkins Med J* 1969;124:151.
*The urinary tract and cutaneous wounds were the most common primary sites of infection.*

Mandell W, Neu HC. *Shigella* bacteremia in adults. *JAMA* 1986;255:3116.
*A case of* Shigella *bacteremia in a patient with AIDS.*

McCue JD. Improved mortality in gram-negative bacillary bacteremia. *Arch Intern Med* 1985;145:1212.
*Compares etiologic agents in community-acquired versus hospital-acquired gram-negative bacteremia.*

McGowan JE Jr. Changing etiology of nosocomial bacteremia and fungemia and other hospital-acquired infections. *Rev Infect Dis* 1985;7(Suppl 3):357.
*Describes changing trends between 1935 and 1983.*

Miller PJ, Wenzel RP. Etiologic organisms as independent predictors of death and morbidity associated with bloodstream infection. *J Infect Dis* 1987;156:471.
*Compares mortality rates and incidence of shock associated with various etiologic agents in gram-negative bacteremia.*

Morduchowicz G, et al. *Shigella* bacteremia in adults: a report of five cases and review of the literature. *Arch Intern Med* 1987;147:2034.
*Report of five cases of* Shigella *bacteremia. Patients were malnourished but did not have AIDS.*

Morrison AJ Jr, Hoffmann KK, Wenzel RP. Associated mortality and clinical characteristics of nosocomial *Pseudomonas maltophilia* in a university hospital. *J Clin Microbiol* 1986;24:52.
*P. maltophilia is becoming an increasingly common cause of nosocomial bacteremia. The organism is resistant to aminoglycosides but sensitive to trimethoprim-sulfamethoxazole.*

Myerowitz RL, Medeiros AA, O'Brien TF. Recent experience with bacillemia due to gram-negative organisms. *J Infect Dis* 1971;124:239.
*A blood culture that grows a gram-negative bacillus is virtually always significant.*

Ratner H. *Flavobacterium meningosepticum. Infect Control* 1984;5:237.
*This organism may cause hospital-acquired bacteremia. It has an unusual pattern of antimicrobial sensitivity.*

Smego RA Jr. Endemic nosocomial *Acinetobacter calcoaceticus* bacteremia. *Arch Intern Med* 1985;145:2174.
*A. calcoaceticus causes nosocomial bacteremia. The lungs and IV catheters are the most common primary sources.*

Young LS, et al. University of California/Davis Interdepartmental Conference on gram-negative septicemia. *Rev Infect Dis* 1991;13:666.
*Includes a good overview of empiric antimicrobial therapy.*

## 69. BLOOD CULTURE GROWING A GRAM-POSITIVE ROD

A report from the laboratory that a blood culture contains a gram-positive rod suggests that the organism is a diphtheroid or *Corynebacterium* species, *Clostridium* species, *Propionibacterium acnes, Listeria monocytogenes,* or *Bacillus* species. Other possibilities, although they are much less common, include *Rhodococcus equi, Erysipelothrix rhusiopathiae, Gardnerella vaginalis,* or *Lactobacillus* species. Some *Corynebacterium* species, *P. acnes,* and *Bacillus* species are part of the indigenous flora of the skin, and their isolation in a blood culture may represent nothing more than contamination. Other organisms, such as *Listeria* or *Clostridium,* may produce life-threatening disease, and their recovery from a blood culture may indicate the need for prompt therapy. A clinician who is assessing the importance of a blood culture positive for a gram-positive rod should consider the following factors:

1. *Does the patient have a single positive blood culture or multiple sets of positive blood cultures obtained during several days?* The finding of a single positive culture for a *Corynebacterium* species, *P. acnes,* or *Bacillus* species may represent nothing more than contamination. If the patient is febrile or has an implanted device, blood cultures should be repeated because, in selected clinical settings, these organisms can produce disease such as infective endocarditis. The patient with endocarditis will have multiple positive blood cultures because the bacteremia is generally continuous. In contrast, a single blood culture positive for an organism such as *Listeria* or, rarely, *Rhodococcus* or *Erysipelothrix* always indicates disease rather than contamination. Repeated blood cultures are indicated to determine if the patient has an illness associated with a sustained bacteremia. A single blood culture positive for a *Clostridium* species may be unimportant and secondary to a transient bacteremia, or it may reflect a life-threatening illness. Repeated blood cultures are indicated only if the patient is "ill." Often, a blood culture positive for *Clostridium* becomes evident after the patient has been sent home from the hospital. In this situation, antimicrobial therapy is usually unnecessary.

2. *Is the patient a normal or a compromised host?* Although any of the gram-positive rods can infect a normal host, *Listeria* has a predilection to produce infection in patients with impaired cellular immunity. Pregnant women and neonates are also susceptible to *Listeria. Rhodococcus* is also an intracellular pathogen that has a predilection for infecting the compromised host. *Corynebacterium jekeium* usually causes infection in neutropenic patients with central venous catheters.

3. *Does the patient have an implanted device, such as a cardiac valve prosthesis, arterial graft, ventriculoatrial shunt, or skeletal prosthesis?* Although *Staphylococcus epidermidis* is a major pathogen in patients with implanted devices, rarely *Corynebacterium* species, *P. acnes,* or a *Bacillus* species can cause an infection in this setting. The finding of multiple positive blood cultures for one of these organisms during several days suggests an infection of a prosthetic device regardless of how innocuous the organism is considered. If a patient has a single positive blood culture for a gram-positive rod and has an implanted device, obtain two to three sets of blood cultures within 24 hours. In a patient who is not receiving antimicrobials, this approach should detect the vast majority of cases of bacteremia. If the patient has an IV line and is febrile, the line should be changed and the tip cultured.

*Corynebacterium* species and *P. acnes* are the dominant organisms on the skin of adults. They are often called diphtheroids because they resemble, but do not include, *Corynebacterium diphtheriae.* Diphtheroids are aerobic gram-positive rods, do not form spores, and are not acid-fast. *P. acnes* organisms resemble diphtheroids and are anaerobic. The documentation of endocarditis caused by a diphtheroid may be difficult because the blood cultures may require prolonged incubation before demonstrating positivity, and *Corynebacterium* or *Propionibacterium* organisms frequently contaminate blood cultures. *Propionibacterium* is usually susceptible to penicillin, a cephalosporin, and the macrolides. Although it is an anaerobe, the organism is resistant to the imidazoles, such as metronidazole. Bacteremia caused by *Corynebacterium* species may be treated with a combination of penicillin with an aminoglycoside. If the patient is allergic to penicillin, vancomycin can be used.

*Listeria* is a β-hemolytic, aerobic, gram-positive rod that may be mistaken for a diphtheroid. In the laboratory, the organism has a characteristic tumbling motility. Both epidemic and sporadic disease occurs. Food-borne outbreaks were recognized in the 1980s, with coleslaw, milk, and cheese responsible for several outbreaks. *Listeria* has been isolated from uncooked beef, poultry, processed meats, and raw vegetables. It has been recommended that compromised hosts, pregnant women, and the elderly avoid soft cheeses, such as Mexican-style or feta cheese. Further, beef, pork, and poultry should be thoroughly cooked and raw vegetables well washed. Disease occurs mainly in pregnant women, neonates, and immunocompromised persons. Bacteremia and meningitis are the most common manifestations in nonpregnant persons. Focal infections such as endophthalmitis or a liver abscess are rare. In patients with meningitis, the cerebrospinal fluid glucose level is normal in more than 60% of patients, and the Gram's stain shows organisms in fewer than 40% of cases. In patients with bacteremia, gastrointestinal symptoms such as nausea, vomiting, and diarrhea may be prominent.

Ampicillin plus an aminoglycoside such as gentamicin is the therapy of choice in a patient without a history of penicillin allergy. If the patient is allergic to penicillin, then trimethoprim-sulfamethoxazole (TMP-SMX) or vancomycin can be selected. Cephalosporins should be avoided. Although controlled studies are lacking, patients with meningitis should be treated for 3 weeks to prevent relapse, and those with endocarditis should be treated for 4 weeks. The management of patients with infected synthetic grafts should consist of surgical resection in combination with 6 weeks of antimicrobial therapy.

Most *Bacillus* species isolated in the laboratory, except for *Bacillus anthracis,* are contaminants. The organism is an aerobic, gram-positive rod that forms spores. *Bacillus cereus* and *Bacillus subtilis* have been associated with post-traumatic endophthalmitis. Bacteremia generally occurs in the compromised patient with a central venous line. The IV catheter should be removed, and vancomycin plus an aminoglycoside should be administered. The organism is often resistant to penicillin and other β-lactam drugs, including the new cephalosporins. Clindamycin is an alternative drug in patients unable to tolerate vancomycin.

*R. equi* is a recently recognized human pathogen that can cause cavitary pulmonary disease and bacteremia in the compromised host. Although the optimal therapy is unknown, the organism is susceptible to vancomycin, erythromycin, clindamycin, or TMP-SMX. Most authors favor selecting two agents, with possible surgical drainage for an abscess. Prolonged therapy is usually required.

*Clostridium* species are anaerobic rods that are usually gram-positive. In clinical specimens, the organisms may appear to stain as gram-negative bacilli. Spore formation occurs but may not be present in clinical specimens. Clostridia are an interesting group of organisms in that a positive blood culture has been associated with life-threatening disease or an "insignificant transient bacteremia." *Clostridium perfringens* accounts for about 60% of blood culture isolates. An intraabdominal focus should be searched for in an ill patient with clostridial bacteremia. Some patients will have colon cancer. *Clostridium septicum* bacteremia is unusual; when present, it is often associated with an occult colon malignancy (about 40%). *C. septicum* bacteremia also occurs in patients with leukemia or in diabetic patients with infected foot ulcers. *C. perfringens* and *C. septicum* usually respond to penicillin or clindamycin. Approximately 25% of strains of *C. perfringens* are resistant to metronidazole. Rarely, a patient will have a blood culture positive for *Clostridium tertium*. Infection with *C. tertium* usually has a gastrointestinal source and often will respond without surgery to vancomycin or TMP-SMX. Interestingly, *C. tertium* is often resistant to clindamycin, penicillin, and metronidazole. (N.M.G.)

## Bibliography

Bodey GP, et al. Clostridial bacteremia in cancer patients: a 12-year experience. *Cancer* 1991;67:1928.
*Review. Fatality rate was 42%.*

Brook I, Frazier EH. Infections caused by *Propionibacterium* sp. *Rev Infect Dis* 1991;13:819.
*Usually causes bacteremia in the presence of a foreign body. Organism is commonly susceptible to penicillin and resistant to metronidazole.*

Brook I, Frazier EH. Significant recovery of nonsporulating anaerobic rods from clinical specimens. *Clin Infect Dis* 1993;16:476.
*Isolation of* Eubacterium *or* Lactobacillus *species from blood usually indicates contamination, but these organisms may rarely cause serious illness.*

Claeys G, et al. Endocarditis of native aortic and mitral valves due to *Corynebacterium accolens:* report of a case and application of phenotypic and genotypic techniques for identification. *J Clin Microbiol* 1996;34:1290–1292.
*A rare cause of endocarditis, which responded to penicillin.*

Cotton DJ, et al. Clinical features and therapeutic interventions in 17 cases of *Bacillus* bacteremia in an immunosuppressed patient population. *J Clin Microbiol* 1987; 25:672.
*Cure is unlikely without removal of the catheter.*

Dalton CB, et al. An outbreak of gastroenteritis and fever due to *Listeria monocytogenes* in milk. *N Engl J Med* 1997; 336:100–105.
*Gastroenteritis caused by contaminated milk.*

Donisi A, et al. *Rhodococcus equi* infection in HIV-infected patients. *AIDS* 1996; 10:359–362.
*R. equi is a rare cause of pulmonary infiltrates; infection is usually diagnosed by a positive blood culture (83%).*

Emmons W, Reichwein B, Winslow DL. *Rhodococcus equi* infection in the patient with AIDS: literature review and report of an unusual case. *Rev Infect Dis* 1991;13:91.
*A cause of a slowly progressive cavitary pneumonia.*

Funke G, et al. Clinical microbiology of Coryneform bacteria. *Clin Microbiol Rev* 1997;10:125–159.
*Comprehensive review of the various Coryneform bacteria.*

Gorbach SL, Thadepalli H. Isolation of *Clostridium* in human infections: evaluation of 114 cases. *J Infect Dis* 1975; 131 (Suppl):S81.
*Clostridial bacteremia may be clinically unimportant.*

Hof H, Nichterlein T, Kretschmar M. Management of listeriosis. *Clin Microbiol Rev* 1997;10:345–357.
*Ampicillin plus gentamicin remains the therapy of choice because the combination is bactericidal. TMP-SMX is an alternative in the penicillin-allergic patient.*

Husni RN, et al. *Lactobacillus* bacteremia and endocarditis: review of 45 cases. *Clin Infect Dis* 1997;25: 1048–1055.
*Lactobacilli occur as part of the normal gastrointestinal and genitourinary flora. Bacteremia is often (60%) polymicrobial in patients with underlying illnesses.*

Johnson WD, Kaye D. Serious infections caused by diphtheroids. *Ann N Y Acad Sci* 1970;174:568.
*Classic review. The majority of patients had endocarditis.*

Kaplan K, Weinstein L. Diphtheroid infections of man. *Ann Intern Med* 1969;70:919.
*Classic review. Penicillin is usually effective.*

Kudsk KA. Occult gastrointestinal malignancies producing metastatic *Clostridium septicum* infections in diabetic patients. *Surgery* 1992;112:765.
*In a patient with a soft-tissue infection caused by* C. septicum *in the absence of trauma, search for a gastrointestinal malignancy.*

Lasky JA, et al. *Rhodococcus equi* causing human pulmonary infection: review of 29 cases. *South Med J* 1991;84:1217.
*An uncommon pulmonary pathogen in the compromised host.*

Lombardi DP, Engleberg C. Anaerobic bacteremia: incidence, patient characteristics, and clinical significance. *Am J Med* 1992;92:53.
*The incidence of anaerobic bacteremia appears to be decreasing.*

Lorber B. Listeriosis. *Clin Infect Dis* 1997;24: 1–11.
*Review.*

Morris A, Guild I. Endocarditis due to *Corynebacterium pseudodiphtheriticum:* five case reports, review, and antibiotic susceptibilities of nine strains. *Rev Infect Dis* 1991;13:887.

*Penicillin plus an aminoglycoside should be effective.*

Myers G, et al. Clostridial septicemia in an urban hospital. *Surg Gynecol Obstet* 1992;174:291.

*Most patients had a gastrointestinal source, either a colonic neoplasm or mucosal translocation.*

Ognibene FP, et al. *Erysipelothrix rhusiopathiae* bacteremia presenting as septic shock. *Am J Med* 1985;78:861.

*A rare cause of bacteremia in fishermen and meat handlers.*

Patel RM et al. Lactobacillemia in liver transplant patients. *Clin Infect Dis* 1994; 18:207–212.

*A pathogen in compromised hosts. Penicillin is the drug of choice.*

Pinner RW, et al. Role of foods in sporadic listeriosis: II. Microbiologic and epidemiologic investigation. *JAMA* 1992;267:2046.

*Listeria was isolated from food in the refrigerators in 64% of infected patients. Ready-to-eat foods often grew serotype 4b, a disease-producing strain.*

Saxelin M, et al. Lactobacilli and bacteremia in southern Finland, 1989–1992. *Clin Infect Dis* 1996;22:564–566.

*Lactobacilli are found in dairy products and colonize the gastrointestinal tract. Despite their widespread occurrence, bacteremia is rare.*

Schuchat A, et al. Role of foods in sporadic listeriosis: I. Case-control study of dietary risk factors. *JAMA* 1992;267:2041.

*Patients were likely to have eaten soft cheese, sliced meats, cheese from a store delicatessen, or poultry products.*

Sliman R, Rehm S, Shlaes DM. Serious infections caused by *Bacillus* sp. *Medicine (Baltimore)* 1987;66:218.

*Underlying conditions included IV drug use, intravascular catheters, and malignancy.*

Speirs G, Warren RE, Rampling A. *Clostridium tertium* septicemia in patients with neutropenia. *J Infect Dis* 1988;158:1336.

*An uncommon cause of bacteremia in patients with a hematologic malignancy and granulocytopenia.*

Spera RV Jr, Kaplan MH, Allen SL. *Clostridium sordellii* bacteremia: case report and review. *Clin Infect Dis* 1992;15:950.

*An unusual cause of bacteremia.*

Spitzer PG, Hammer SM, Karchmer AW. Treatment of *Listeria monocytogenes* infection with trimethoprim-sulfamethoxazole: case report and review of the literature. *Rev Infect Dis* 1986;8:427.

*TMP-SMX is an alternative drug in the penicillin-allergic patient.*

## 70. STOOL FOR OVA AND PARASITES

Information obtained by history and physical examination may provide clues to parasitic infections of the gastrointestinal tract. Diarrhea, bloating, weight loss, or eosinophilia in the context of an appropriate epidemiologic history requires that a stool sample be examined for ova and parasites.

The number and frequency of fecal specimens to be collected varies with the diagnosis suspected. Because many pathogens are shed sporadically, it is generally advisable to inspect multiple specimens collected during several days. Many drugs and other substances can interfere with proper stool examination. Iron, bismuth, and mineral oil may interfere with stool examination for 1 week or more; barium and dyes, iodine preparations, and antimicrobials may cause difficulty for as long as several weeks. Fresh stool specimens are important to maximize the yield of trophozoites, such as *Entamoeba histolytica*. Prompt examination or fixation is particularly important for soft or watery specimens. Specimens that cannot be examined or fixed quickly should be refrigerated. Fecal specimens should not be incubated or frozen and thawed.

Fecal specimens should be collected in a wide-mouthed container or carton. Urine is harmful to some parasites and must not contaminate the specimen. Specimens should not be retrieved from toilet water because water is destructive to some eggs and protozoa. Purgation may increase the yield of some parasites, such as amebae, *Giardia*, and *Strongyloides*, and it should be considered when their presence is strongly suspected clinically but specimens have been negative.

The physician may want to screen the sample before submitting it to the laboratory. Macroscopic examination may reveal *Ascaris* or tapeworm proglottids. Wet mounts can be prepared with saline or iodine solution and examined for trophozoites, cysts, ova, or *Strongyloides* larvae. A fecal fleck is obtained with a wooden applicator stick. Flecks of mucus, pus, or blood will have a higher yield. The sample is mixed with a drop of saline solution and put on a microscope slide with cover slip. An iodine solution (1 g potassium iodide, 1.5 g iodine crystals to 100 mL of water) will stain protozoa and helminths.

The laboratory will usually perform three microscopic examinations, depending on the specimen submitted: a direct wet mount, a concentrated specimen wet mount, and permanent stain. Concentration techniques will vary depending on the parasite that is suspected. For example, a Baermann concentration method is used to detect *Strongyloides*. A Sheather sugar flotation method is recommended for concentration of *Cryptosporidium* cysts.

### Giardia lamblia

Cyst excretion in *Giardia* infection varies from one specimen to another and is observer-dependent. Only about 80% of infections are detected even when three daily specimens are studied. Cyst concentration techniques will improve overall yield. A recent study suggests that duodenal fluid obtained by aspiration is not superior to fecal specimens. Trophozoites can also be demonstrated in jejunal mucosal biopsy specimens. Immunologic methods to detect *Giardia* antigen in feces are under investigation and will likely provide additional sensitivity. A 65-kd *Giardia* antigen can be identified in feces by means of a counterimmunoelectrophoresis technique. DNA probes are also being developed.

### Entamoeba histolytica

Multiple stool specimens are necessary in the diagnosis of intestinal amebiasis. Specimens obtained by endoscopy with scraping of ulcers have a high yield. Biopsy material stained with paraaminosalicylic acid will demonstrate trophozoites. Wet preparations can identify amebae with their linear motility. Permanent stains with trichrome or iron hematoxylin are used to identify *E. histolytica* by nuclear morphology and ingestion of RBCs. Concentration methods are superior to direct stool examination for detection of cysts. Results of an indirect hemagglutination serum test are positive in active intestinal infection.

Stool examination is useful in the diagnosis of cestode infections. Eggs or proglottids of *Taenia* species are demonstrated with concentration methods and thick smears. A perianal swab or adhesive tape method detects 90% of cases. These thick smears are diagnostic in more than 95% of patients with infection. Specific detection of *Taenia* eggs by DNA hybridization studies has recently been reported.

The thick-smear technique is also the procedure of choice to detect *Schistosoma* eggs. Rectal biopsy may be necessary in some patients. When biopsy is performed, tissue should be crushed and examined with low-power microscopy.

### Strongyloides

Concentration techniques such as formalin-ethylacetate and zinc sulfate flotation lack sensitivity in diagnosis of infection with this nematode. Multiple stool samples and long periods of inspection are often inadequate to ensure diagnosis. The Baermann technique uses the hydrothermotropism of the larva to improve sensitivity. In one study of 736 patients, the Baermann technique found 243 positive cases, compared with 55 cases when a concentration method was used. An agar-plate method has recently been devised. In this method, nematodes are suspected by the burrows in agar that they leave behind. The larvae themselves are viewed with a dissecting microscope. This method appears to be more sensitive than the Baermann technique.

Serodiagnostic studies in which antigens derived from filariform larvae are used have a sensitivity greater than 80% and should be performed when the disease is suspected but cannot be confirmed by stool analysis. After treatment, titers fall or become negative altogether.

Hookworm infection is usually easily diagnosed by finding the typical oval eggs on direct stool smear. Concentration methods are helpful for mild infections. *Ascaris* infection also is relatively easy to diagnose by direct smear. Adult worms at times will be seen by barium studies or cholangiography.

Antibody and antigen capture assays in dipstick dot enzyme-linked immunosorbent assay format are now being developed for the detection of *Strongyloides* in feces. These systems utilize parasite antigens that do not cross-react and can therefore identify organisms even in multiple infections.

## Other Organisms

*Cryptosporidium* infection is diagnosed by finding cysts in stool or biopsy material. Modified acid-fast stain will demonstrate the organism. Yeasts, similar in shape and size, will not stain with acid-fast stain. A direct immunofluorescence antibody stain based on a murine monoclonal antibody to the cyst cell wall should improve sensitivity. An enzyme-linked immunosorbent assay method has also been used to detect anticryptosporidial immunoglobulin in serum.

*Isospora belli,* also a cause of diarrhea in AIDS patients, will stain with acid-fast stain but is larger and ellipsoid in shape compared with *Cryptosporidium.* (S.L.B.)

## Bibliography

Arakaki T, et al. A new method to detect *Strongyloides stercoralis* from human stool. *Jpn J Trop Med Hyg* 1988;16:11.
*The agar-plate method is probably the most sensitive approach to the diagnosis of* Strongyloides *infection.*

Arakaki T, et al. Efficacy of agar-plate culture in detection of *Strongyloides stercoralis* infection. *J Parasitol* 1990;76:425.
Strongyloides *furrows could be distinguished from those of Necator, which were thicker.*

Berk SL, et al. Clinical and epidemiologic features of strongyloidiasis: a prospective study in rural Tennessee. *Arch Intern Med* 1987;147:1257.
*Repeated stool samples and use of the ether extraction method did not improve* Strongyloides *detection (only 2 of 512 repeated specimens were positive).*

Blumencranz H, et al. The role of endoscopy in suspected amebiasis. *Am J Gastroenterol* 1983;78:15.
*Endoscopy may be diagnostic in amebiasis. When results of stool studies are negative, it may also detect concomitant disease, such as inflammatory bowel disease.*

Butcher PD, Clark C, Farthing MJG. *Giardia lamblia* cloned genomic DNA probes: uses in faecal diagnosis and genetic analysis of clinical isolates. *Gut* 1988;29:A722.
Giardia *species can be detected by DNA probe.*

Craft JC, Nelson JD. Diagnosis of giardiasis by counterimmunoelectrophoresis of feces. *J Infect Dis* 1982;145:499.
*A countercurrent immunoelectrophoresis test for* Giardia *fecal antigen was as sensitive as combined examination of feces and duodenal fluid.*

Flisser A, et al. Specific detection of *Taenia saginata* eggs by DNA hybridization. *Lancet* 1988;2:1429.
*DNA probe has been used to distinguish* Taenia solium *from* T. saginata.

Genta RM. Global prevalence of strongyloidiasis: critical review with epidemiologic insights into the prevention of disseminated disease. *Rev Infect Dis* 1989;11:755.
*Excellent review of laboratory diagnosis of strongyloidiasis.*

Goka AKJ, et al. Diagnosis of *Strongyloides* and hookworm infections: comparison of faecal and duodenal fluid microscopy. *Trans R Soc Trop Med Hyg* 1990;84:829.
*Fecal microscopy was insensitive in the diagnosis of* Strongyloides *and hookworm infection. Examination of duodenal fluid improved diagnosis.*

Hruska JF. Gastrointestinal and intra-abdominal infection. In: Reese RE, Betts RF, eds. *A practical approach to infectious diseases,* 3rd ed. Boston: Little, Brown, 1991.
*Excellent review of the diagnosis and treatment of gastrointestinal parasites.*

Kamath KR, Murugasu R. A comparative study of four methods for detecting *Giardia lamblia* in children with diarrheal disease and malabsorption. *Gastroenterology* 1974;66:16.
*Mucosal impression smears and biopsy gave the highest yield of positive test results. Duodenal aspiration was more commonly positive than stool examination.*

Koga K, et al. An evaluation of the agar-plate method for the detection of *Strongyloides stercoralis* in northern Thailand. *J Trop Med Hyg* 1990;93:183.
*The agar-plate method was most sensitive. A few cases were missed by this method. A smear was required to distinguish* Strongyloides *from hookworm.*

Lima JP, Delgado PG. Diagnosis of strongyloidiasis: importance of Baermann's method. *Am J Dig Dis* 1961;6:899.
*Baermann's method, which is based on the thermohydrotropism of* Strongyloides, *was more sensitive than concentration methods.*

Madanagopalan N, et al. A correlative study of duodenal aspirate and faeces examination in giardiasis, before and after treatment with metronidazole. *Curr Med Res Opin* 1975;3:99.
*Duodenal aspiration and stool examination supplement the diagnostic yield in* Giardia *infection.*

Pelletier LL Jr. Chronic strongyloidiasis in World War II Far East ex-prisoners of war. *Am J Trop Med Hyg* 1984;33:55.
*Five hours of microscopy per case resulted in a 90% rate of detection of positive cases.*

Rosenthal P, Liebman WM. Comparative study of stool examinations, duodenal aspiration, and pediatric Entero-Test for giardiasis in children. *J Pediatr* 1980;96:278.
*Entero-Test was an efficient, safe method for diagnosis of giardiasis in children.*

Rosoff JD, Stibbs HH. Isolation and identification of a *Giardia lamblia*-specific stool antigen (GSA 65) useful in coprodiagnosis of giardiasis. *J Clin Microbiol* 1986; 23:905.
*A Giardia lamblia-specific antigen was demonstrated in 36 of 40 infected patients. Antigen is detected by countercurrent immunoelectrophoresis with rabbit monospecific antiserum.*

Siddiqui AA, et al. *Strongyloides stercoralis:* identification of antigens in natural human infections from endemic areas of the United States. *Parasitol Res* 1997; 83:655.
*Describes eight immunodominant antigens found in immunoprecipitates of infected patients. These antigens may be targets for immunodiagnosis by testing of stool samples.*

Smith JW, Bartlett MS. Diagnostic parasitology: introduction and methods. In: Balows A, ed. *Manual of clinical microbiology,* 5th ed. Washington, DC: American Society for Microbiology, 1991.
*An excellent overview of stool examination. Describes wet-mount concentration procedures and permanent stains.*

Thornton SA, et al. Comparison of methods for identification of *Giardia lamblia. Am J Clin Pathol* 1983;80:858.
*Trichrome was the superior stain for cysts and trophozoite in giardiasis.*

Ungar BLP, et al. Enzyme-linked immunosorbent assay for the detection of *Giardia lamblia* in fecal specimens. *J Infect Dis* 1984;149:90.
*An enzyme-linked immunosorbent assay is sensitive and specific for detection of G. lamblia in human feces. Stools became negative after successful treatment.*

# 71. ANTIMICROBIAL SUSCEPTIBILITY TESTS

Under ideal circumstances, the use of antimicrobials would follow a logical sequence of events in which a pathogen is isolated from a clinical specimen, *in vitro* antimicrobial susceptibility tests are performed, and, based on the results of the laboratory tests, the patient is administered an agent that exhibits inhibitory activity against the offending microbe. In practice, however, etiologic agents frequently are not recovered from patients with an infectious syndrome, and empiric antimicrobial therapy is usually necessary. Nevertheless, in many circumstances, the clinical microbiology laboratory does play an important role in assisting the physician in selecting antimicrobial therapy.

Antimicrobial susceptibility testing is indicated for microbes that are isolated from appropriately collected clinical specimens and that have unpredictable drug susceptibility patterns. For example, susceptibility assays would be appropriate for a *Staphylococcus aureus* recovered from the blood of a febrile drug user or for a *Pseudomonas aeruginosa* isolated from the sputum of a patient with pneumonia acquired in an ICU. On the other hand, testing is not required for pathogens that are predictably susceptible to antimicrobials of choice; for example, *in vitro* tests are not necessary for group A streptococci, as the bacterium remains susceptible to penicillin and erythromycin. With recent changes in the susceptibility of some common human bacterial pathogens, especially *Streptococcus pneumoniae* and *Enterococcus* species, *in vitro* testing that was previously not necessary is now often required. Because of technical and other difficulties, the need to perform susceptibility tests on anaerobic bacteria must be determined on a case-by-case basis. Finally, because of the requirement for special techniques, antimycobacterial susceptibility testing is usually performed at a regional laboratory, and antifungal and antiviral assays at a research facility.

In most hospitals, the microbiologist, infectious disease physician, and pharmacist contribute to the decision concerning which of the many available antimicrobials are to be used in the susceptibility assays. For example, all third-generation cephalosporins are very active *in vitro* against *Escherichia coli* and other Enterobacteriaceae, and these drugs have been shown to be effective in clinical trials; nevertheless, an institution may elect to have just one or two of these drugs on the formulary and so the laboratory will test (or report results) for the formulary agents only. Similarly, although a number of cephalosporins demonstrate *in vitro* activity against methicillin-resistant *S. aureus,* clinical observations indicate that this class of drug is not effective in treating patients infected with the microbe; accordingly, the laboratory will not determine the susceptibility of methicillin-resistant *S. aureus* to cephalosporins. In short, the clinician should not expect to find results for every antimicrobial on susceptibility test reports.

### Disk Diffusion Testing

Introduced in the 1960s, the disk diffusion test or Kerby-Bauer method is an important technique for evaluating the ability of an antimicrobial to inhibit the growth of a bacterium. Disk susceptibility testing is based on the principle that there exists an inverse linear relationship between the concentration of drug necessary to prevent bacterial proliferation and the zone or area of growth inhibition around an antimicrobial-impregnated disk; thus, the smaller the concentration of drug required to prevent growth, the larger the zone of inhibition. In the procedure, an agar plate (e.g., Mueller-Hinton medium) is streaked with a standardized bacterial inoculum containing approximately $1 \times 10^8$ colony-forming units (CFU), and as many as 12 paper disks containing a standard quantity of antimicrobial are dropped onto the plate, which is then incubated at 35°C for 16 to 18 hours. The diameter of the area around each disk that is free from visible bacterial growth is measured to the nearest millimeter. The zones of growth inhibition are compared with reference values, and the results are reported as "susceptible," "intermediately susceptible," or "resistant" to each agent tested; of note, a computer program is available that can provide a "calculated minimum inhibitory concentration (MIC)" based on the zone size. The disk technique is an inexpensive, rapid, reproducible, and relatively simple means of evaluating antimicrobial susceptibility; however, standardized procedures must be followed. In addition, the disk diffusion test can be employed only for microbes that grow rapidly on artificial media; thus, this technique is not reliable for evaluating the susceptibility of anaerobic and other fastidious bacteria.

### Antibiotic Gradient Diffusion Testing

A relatively new method for assessing susceptibility, the E test uses a plastic strip that is coated with a continuous antimicrobial gradient on one side and has an MIC scale printed on the other. The strip is placed on an agar plate inoculated with the bacterium of interest; following incubation, the intersection of the strip with the edge of the elliptic zone of inhibition is identified, and the MIC is read from the scale. In comparative studies, data from the E test have correlated very well with the results of broth or agar dilution susceptibility assays. The E test has greatly facilitated the ability of microbiology laboratories to determine MICs for fastidious microbes, especially *S. pneumoniae*. On the other hand, the costs of the E test strips are substantial, and the expense of the assay has limited its use.

### β-Lactamase Assays
Although they are not susceptibility tests, assays that detect the presence of β-lactamase represent an essential component of the microbiologic evaluation of some common bacteria, especially *Haemophilus influenzae* and *Neisseria gonorrhoeae*. β-Lactamases are enzymes capable of hydrolyzing the β-lactam ring of penicillins (penicillinases) or cephalosporins (cephalosporinases), thereby inactivating the drugs. Once a pathogen has been isolated from a clinical specimen, β-lactamase production can be detected rapidly by a number of methods, such as the chromogenic cephalosporin assay. The results of screening for β-lactamase are often available 12 to 24 hours before the results of *in vitro* susceptibility tests are known. Production of β-lactamase by *H. influenzae* indicates that the pathogen is resistant to ampicillin and amoxicillin.

### Dilution Susceptibility Tests
To determine the actual concentration of an antimicrobial required to inhibit bacterial growth, dilution tests must be performed. Broth (or agar) containing twofold dilutions of a drug (usual range of concentrations, 0.125 to 128.0 µg/mL) is inoculated with a standardized bacterial inoculum ($5 \times 10^5$ CFU/mL), and the cultures are incubated at 35°C for 18 to 24 hours. The lowest concentration of drug that prevents visible growth of the bacterium is the MIC, which is expressed in micrograms per milliliter (µg/mL). In general, an organism is considered to be susceptible when the achievable peak serum concentration is twofold to fourfold greater than the measured MIC. Tests that assess the MIC require strict attention to detail because a variety of technical factors (e.g., size of the bacterial inoculum, concentration of cations in the medium) can influence outcome. To ensure a uniformity in the methodology and interpretation of MIC and other susceptibility tests, most microbiology facilities use the National Committee for Clinical Laboratory Standards (NCCLS).

Broth microdilution tests represent the most prevalent susceptibility assays; agar dilution testing, in which twofold dilutions of an antimicrobial are incorporated into the growth medium (e.g., Mueller-Hinton agar), remains primarily a research tool. The wide use of the broth microdilution assays results from the commercial availability of 96-well microtiter plates containing up to 12 antimicrobials and the automated systems that inoculate and read the plates and that report MIC values for each of the drugs tested. Broth microdilution tests are also useful in evaluating the antimicrobial susceptibility of fastidious bacteria, including anaerobic microbes. Obviously, the testing of an increasing number of antimicrobials against the many microbes isolated daily in a busy clinical microbiology laboratory has been facilitated by the introduction of automated broth microdilution systems. Of note, although these microdilution systems provide MIC data, the results are often reported to clinicians in terms of "susceptible," "moderately susceptible," or "resistant." Finally, antifungal susceptibility is currently performed by means of a broth macrodilution assay.

On occasion, the lowest concentration of antimicrobial required to kill a bacterium must be measured; this value is referred to as the minimum bactericidal concentration (MBC) or minimum lethal concentration (MLC). To determine the MBC, a broth dilution system is employed. Tubes containing a broth medium, a standard bacterial inoculum, and varying concentrations of an antimicrobial are incubated for 18 to 20 hours. Aliquots of broth from tubes with no visible growth (the first of which corresponds to the MIC) are subcultured onto agar medium containing no drugs. Expressed in micrograms per milliliter, the MBC is the concentration of antimicrobial that kills at least 99.9% of the original bacterial inoculum. The MBC determination is a time-consuming test, and fortunately it is not often indicated. In general, an MBC determination should be reserved for patients who have infections in which host defenses do not contribute to cure (e.g., endocarditis) and who are failing to respond to apparently appropriate antimicrobial therapy (e.g., MIC of drug against offending pathogen is low).

Measuring the MBC might reveal tolerance, the phenomenon in which normally microbicidal drugs, such as penicillins and cephalosporins, inhibit the growth of a bacterium but do not kill it. Tolerance has been defined on the basis of the ratio of MBC to MIC, and it is said to be present when MBC/MIC is greater than 16 or 32. Usually associated with *S. aureus,* tolerance should be suspected in the patient with endocarditis who fails to respond to ostensibly adequate antimicrobial therapy.

### Serum Bactericidal Test

The serum bactericidal test is an assay that quantifies the killing ability of serum from an antimicrobial-treated patient. In this assay, serum is obtained immediately before (trough) or soon after (peak) the administration of an antimicrobial. Twofold dilutions of the serum are made with culture medium (Mueller-Hinton broth with pooled human serum), and the mixtures are inoculated with the patient's bacterial isolate. The serum bactericidal titer is defined as the highest dilution at which more than 99% of the bacterial inoculum is killed. The serum bactericidal test has been used to monitor antimicrobial therapy in patients with infectious endocarditis. The test has also been used in granulocytopenic or immunosuppressed patients who have gram-negative bacteremia and in patients whose therapy has been changed from the parenteral to the oral route, including children with acute osteomyelitis and IV drug users with endocarditis. In general, a peak titer of 1:8 or 1:16 or more is considered desirable. Because its precise role remains uncertain, the test should be reserved for selected adults with bacterial endocarditis or other life-threatening infections that fail to respond to therapy.

### Combination Antimicrobial Therapy

Patients who are critically ill with gram-negative pneumonia or other serious infections are often administered a number of antimicrobials, each of which possesses *in vitro* activity against the offending pathogen. A combination of drugs can produce a bactericidal effect that is equal to, greater than, or less than the sum of the activities of the individual agents; these effects are referred to as indifference, synergism, or antagonism, respectively.

Therapy with predictably synergistic antimicrobial combinations represents an attractive method of treating normal or immunosuppressed patients with serious infections caused by pathogens that are difficult to eradicate. In general, the combination of an aminoglycoside with a β-lactam drug will produce synergy against most aerobic gram-negative bacilli; thus, for the patient with a severe pneumonia caused by *P. aeruginosa, Serratia marcescens,* or *Enterobacter* species, the combination of an aminoglycoside with a third-generation cephalosporin, a ureidopenicillin (e.g., ticarcillin), or a monobactam (e.g., aztreonam) has appeal. However, therapy with synergistic combinations has proved to offer a significant advantage over treatment with a single drug or with nonsynergistic pairings in few infections; of note, enterococcal endocarditis is one disease in which the administration of a synergistic combination (penicillin plus gentamicin) is essential for cure. It must be emphasized that predicting which drug combinations will exert synergistic killing in an individual patient can be difficult, and some drug combinations can be antagonistic. *In vitro* assays (the two-dimensional broth dilution method and the time-kill curve method) have been developed to quantify the bactericidal activity of combinations of antimicrobials. These tests are technically difficult and labor-intensive, and they should be considered only in selected circumstances.

### Antiviral Susceptibility Testing

During the past two decades, a number of antiviral medications have been introduced into clinical practice; obviously, the AIDS pandemic has accelerated the widespread use of agents with activity against herpes simplex virus, varicella-zoster virus, cytomegalovirus, and, of course, HIV. Not surprisingly, treatment failures have occurred, and interest in the *in vitro* susceptibility testing of important viral pathogens has developed. Although not generally available, these assays have the potential to detect resistance and permit the selection of more effective therapy. In the most common clinical circumstance, a change in susceptibility to the antiviral agent is inferred when the expected outcome is not achieved. For example, a rising "viral load" of HIV-1 as determined by a quantitative molecular assay (polymerase chain reaction) suggests the evolution of resistance to the antiretroviral agents the patient is receiving; conversely, a declining viral load indicates susceptibility.

Antiviral susceptibility tests are characterized as genotypic or phenotypic assays. Genotypic assays allow the detection, by polymerase chain reaction amplification, of viral genes that are known to confer resistance; these remain primarily research tools. Phenotypic assays are somewhat similar to the common bacterial susceptibility tests noted earlier. Cell cultures containing various concentrations of the antiviral drug are infected with a standard inoculum of the virus. Following incubation, the activity of the drug is assessed by quantifying phenomena such as decrease in virus yield, inhibition of cytopathic effect, or reduction in the elaboration of viral products. Results are expressed as the drug concentration that produces a 50% inhibition ($IC_{50}$). Phenotypic assays are commonly employed to assess the susceptibility of herpes simplex virus, varicella-zoster virus, HIV-1, and others. Many factors can influence the outcome of these tests, and the results do not invariably correlate with the clinical response to an agent.

## Summary

Although the results of susceptibility assays are valuable in guiding antimicrobial therapy, they do not guarantee a response to treatment, and they cannot predict outcome. Host factors and the nature of the infection play critical roles in determining whether a patient will respond to antiinfective agents. For example, the patient with an abscess or an obstructed biliary tract may fail to respond to antimicrobial therapy, regardless of the results of *in vitro* susceptibility tests. By extension, surgical intervention to drain an abscess or to relieve an obstruction may be more important than potent antimicrobials in improving the likelihood of a favorable outcome. To strengthen the chances of a response, adequate dosages of the antimicrobial must be administered, and to achieve this goal, the clinician may need to review the pharmacokinetics of the agents being considered for use and to monitor serum drug levels during therapy. (A.L.E.)

## Bibliography

Brook I. Inoculum effect. *Rev Infect Dis* 1989;11:361.
  *For some antimicrobials, especially β-lactam drugs, an increase in the size of the bacterial inoculum produces a substantial elevation in the MIC. This article provides a detailed review of the problem and its clinical relevance.*
Gutmann L, et al. Synergism and antagonism in double β-lactam antibiotic combinations. *Am J Med* 1986;80 (Suppl 5C):21.
  *In this extensive review, the authors report that most combinations of the β-lactam antimicrobials, such as the ureidopenicillins (e.g., piperacillin), third-generation cephalosporins (e.g., ceftazidime), and monobactams (e.g., aztreonam), produce an indifferent effect, and they caution that antagonism can occur when β-lactam drugs are combined.*
Jorgensen JH. Laboratory issues in the detection and reporting of antimicrobial resistance. *Infect Dis Clin North Am* 1997;11:785.
  *A contemporay review of the methodology and limitations of* in vitro *testing in the detection of antimicrobial resistance.*
Washington JA. In vitro testing of antimicrobial drugs. *Infect Dis Clin North Am* 1989;3:375.
  *A thorough review of the indications, methodology, and limitations of* in vitro *testing. The importance of technical and biologic variables in the performance of bactericidal tests and in the detection of tolerance is noted.*
Weinstein MP, et al. Multicenter collaborative evaluation of a standardized serum bactericidal test as a prognostic indicator in infective endocarditis. *Am J Med* 1985;78:262.

*Employing a standard method to evaluate the serum bactericidal activity in patients with endocarditis, the investigators found that peak titers of 1:64 or more and trough titers of 1:32 or more were associated with a bacteriologic cure in all patients.*

Weinstein MP, et al. Multicenter collaborative evaluation of a standardized serum bactericidal test as a predictor of therapeutic efficacy in acute and chronic osteomyelitis. *Am J Med* 1987;83:218.

*Based on data from 48 patients with infections of bone, the authors conclude that for patients with acute osteomyelitis, serum bactericidal titers of 1:2 or greater should be maintained at all times; for patients with chronic osteomyelitis, titers of 1:4 or greater should be achieved.*

Wolfson JS, Swartz MW. Serum bactericidal activity as a monitor of antibiotic therapy. *N Engl J Med* 1985;312:968.

*A thorough review of this controversial assay that emphasizes the paucity of clinical data concerning efficacy.*

## 72. SPECIAL TESTS OF ANTIMICROBIAL ACTIVITY IN INFECTIOUS DISEASES

The optimal management of a bacterial infection requires the isolation and identification of a causative pathogen from a body site and demonstration of its susceptibility to antimicrobial agents by standard microbiologic testing. This methodology takes into account achievable serum levels of the antimicrobials and compares them with the amount of an agent determined to be necessary to inhibit the growth of the isolate. Generally, organisms are considered susceptible to antimicrobials when the antimicrobial concentration in serum is two to ten times greater than the amount needed for inhibition of growth. It has not been demonstrated that higher "therapeutic indices" improve clinical outcome. Selection of an antimicrobial is based on degree of activity, safety, cost, host factors, and pharmacokinetic considerations. The microbiologic systems that are commercially available work well for rapidly growing aerobic pathogens but have limitations for those that are more fastidious. In practice, decision making may be complicated by the inability to perform adequate susceptibility testing (e.g., anaerobes and other fastidious organisms), the need to employ an antimicrobial agent not available on the panels of automated systems, or the need to treat infection outside the bloodstream, where the concentration of antimicrobial may be substantially different (higher or lower) from the usual serum levels.

On occasion, more sophisticated antimicrobial testing procedures need to be employed. Those available in many clinical laboratories include measurement of antimicrobial blood levels, serum bactericidal testing (SBT), and the determination of minimum inhibitory concentration (MIC) of an antimicrobial. In general, these studies are not routinely indicated because they are labor-intensive and do not add to the efficacy of treatment; however, knowledge of their indications, benefits, and limitations can help the clinician manage antimicrobials in selected situations.

### Antimicrobial Levels

This test is used when the clinician wants to know the concentration of a specific agent in serum (or rarely other body fluids or tissues). Results are given in micrograms per milliliter ($\mu g/mL$) or micrograms per gram ($\mu g/g$). The peak level may be compared with the MIC of the organism to help determine "antibiotic efficacy" and toxicity; the trough level is used to guide additional dosing and also to help prevent toxicity. Knowledge of such levels is useful for antimicrobials with therapeutic serum levels close to those associated with toxicity and with pharmacokinetics that may be difficult to predict. In practice, serum levels are most useful for the management of aminoglycosides (especially gentamicin and tobramycin) and perhaps vancomycin. Determination of levels of aminoglycosides and vancomycin is especially useful in patients with rapidly changing renal function. Additionally, numerous other factors, including weight, hematocrit, and body temperature, may confound serum levels of aminoglycosides.

The value of measuring peak levels for aminoglycosides has been recently challenged with the documentation of efficacy and safety of once-daily dosing of aminoglycosides (see Chapter 75). With once-daily dosing, peak levels above 20 µg/mL are generally attained without enhanced toxicity. Thus, measurement of peak levels is rarely indicated. Alternatively, renal and auditory toxicity may occur when trough levels are above 2 µg/mL; these should be measured after the second or third daily dose. Current assay technology allows values to be returned expeditiously. For patients with significantly impaired or rapidly changing renal function, serum levels should be ordered more frequently, so that dosing can be individualized.

Use of serum levels to monitor vancomycin is controversial but still very common. As an example, a large university hospital performed more than 6,500 assays in a year, and estimates are that on a national basis more than 5 million tests are performed annually. This agent is less toxic than aminoglycosides and has a higher therapeutic index. In fact, whether vancomycin is associated with ototoxicity and nephrotoxicity at all is largely unknown! Recent reviews demonstrate a lack of correlation between serum levels of vancomycin and either toxicity or clinical success. With this in mind, most investigators consider that measurement of blood levels is generally not indicated. Situations in which they might be employed include the following: (a) patients with rapidly changing renal function, where use of nomograms is burdensome; (b) those receiving aminoglycosides (in which case potentially toxic synergy may occur); (c) patients receiving supernormal dosages; and (d) those on hemodialysis dialysis with high-flux dialysis membranes.

Determination of levels of antimicrobial in tissues and fluids other than blood is generally employed for investigational use but may occasionally be of clinical benefit. As an example, many antimicrobials are concentrated in urine and may have clinical efficacy therein despite apparent resistance by standard testing (which is based on serum levels). In unusual circumstances, a clinician might wish to document high urine concentrations of a selected antimicrobial and compare that value with the MIC for the organism. Alternatively, for abscesses that cannot be totally extirpated, documentation of significant levels of antimicrobial within the abscess fluid may confirm for the physician that the agent and dosage are correct.

### Serum Bactericidal Test

The SBT was developed in 1912 and modified by Schlichter in 1947. In practice, the Schlicter test is an inhibitory rather than a bactericidal test. The SBT attempts to answer the physiologic question of what dilution of a patient's serum (with accompanying antimicrobials, antibodies, and other inhibitory factors) is capable of killing the organisms causing infection in that person. Results are provided as a dilution of the patient's serum (e.g., 1:4, 1:16) at which the tested organism is killed. The higher the dilution, the more active the serum. In this test, dilutions of the patient's serum are prepared with liquid media with or without the addition of pooled human serum and are inoculated with the offending organism. After overnight growth, tubes demonstrating no visible growth (the one with the lowest dilution is the serum inhibitory concentration) are incubated on agar. The SBT result is then defined as the highest serum dilution at which more than 99.9% of the inoculum is killed. In theory, this test should be a useful gauge of antimicrobial treatment because it takes into account the susceptibility of the offending pathogen, the activity of the antimicrobial in conjunction with other inhibitory factors within human serum, and the pharmacokinetics of the product(s). Additionally, it can be performed in patients who simultaneously receive multiple antimicrobial agents. Major problems include lack of interlaboratory standardization, controversy over the importance of peak versus trough SBT results, and what defines optimal results for different infections.

The SBT is most commonly employed to gauge response in infective endocarditis, infections of bone or joint, and infections in neutropenic patients, when bactericidal (as opposed to bacteriostatic) activity may be necessary for a satisfactory clinical outcome. In addition, the SBT has been employed to guide the changeover from parenteral to oral therapy, often in bacterial endocarditis or osteomyelitis. In these situations, it provides the physician with the knowledge that the antimicrobial, in a physiologic setting, is capable of killing the offending pathogen. The use of this test, however, remains controversial, and several authorities feel that its value has not yet been proved.

With regard to infective endocarditis, recent studies suggest that dilutions obtained within 1 hour of antimicrobial administration of more than 1:64 and trough values of more than 1:32 are associated with bacteriologic cures, whereas clinical and microbiologic failures cannot be predicted by SBT determinations. There is no information to support the concept that extremely high dilutions (e.g., >1:1,024) are clinically more effective than lower favorable ones. Similar data are available for osteomyelitis and for selected infections in the neutropenic patient. In my opinion, the SBT should be employed infrequently. It may be indicated for selected cases of infective endocarditis, hematogenous osteomyelitis, and bacteremia in neutropenic patients when infection is caused by unusual pathogens, an unusual drug regimen is employed, or patient response has been unsatisfactory despite apparent adequacy of therapy. In these instances, an adequate SBT result, typically above 1:8 at peak, demonstrates that antimicrobial activity is satisfactory, and adverse clinical or bacteriologic experiences probably do not mean that the antimicrobial employed is ineffective.

### Determinations of Minimal Inhibitory and Bactericidal Concentrations

Determinations of MIC and minimum bactericidal concentration (MBC) are laboratory tests that evaluate the minimum concentration of an antimicrobial required to inhibit or kill an organism *in vitro*. The MIC, when compared with achievable serum levels of an antimicrobial, determines whether the organism is susceptible or resistant. For instance, if an organism has an MIC of 4 µg/mL but achievable serum concentrations of a given agent are only 2 µg/mL, the organism is likely to be resistant. This information is now incorporated into virtually all automated antimicrobial susceptibility systems, and results for any antimicrobial agent versus the offending pathogen are either noted in the standard microbiology report or are available on request from laboratory personnel.

The MBC is determined by incubating on agar those tubes demonstrating no visible growth from the MIC determination. The MBC is an antimicrobial concentration that kills more than 99.9% of the original inoculum. This test is extremely time-consuming for laboratory personnel and is currently of little clinical value. For selected patients in whom knowledge about antimicrobial killing may be of value (e.g., immunocompromised patients with unresponsive, overwhelming bacteremia or with infective endocarditis), the SBT is more physiologic. (R.B.B.)

### Bibliography

Cantu TG, Yamanaka-Yuen NA, Lietman PS. Serum vancomycin concentrations: reappraisal of their clinical value. *Clin Infect Dis* 1994;18:533–543.
*After performing a literature review on the subject, the authors concluded that measurement of serum concentrations of vancomycin are generally not indicated. It is not even clear whether the product is associated with ototoxicity or nephrotoxicity when it is employed as monotherapy. For determination of drug levels to be useful, certain criteria must be met: (a) Drug concentrations must be correlated with toxicity/efficacy; (b) there must be variations between patients with regard to pharmacokinetics; (c) efficacy or toxicity of drug must be either difficult to measure or substantially delayed in onset; and (d) a sensitive assay must exist. In the case of vancomycin, the first two criteria are not met.*

Fernandez de Gatta MD, et al. Cost effectiveness analysis of serum vancomycin concentration monitoring in patients with hematologic malignancies. *Clin Pharmacol Ther* 1996;60:332–340.
*This was a prospective, randomized investigation of 70 febrile, immunocompromised patients receiving vancomycin. One group received active pharmacologic intervention—monitoring of vancomycin serum concentrations and adjustment of vancomycin dose—while the other arm acted as a control. Patients who received active intervention fared no better regarding clinical response but had significantly less nephrotoxicity and lower hospital costs. However, this finding may not conflict with*

*recommendations against routine testing, as many of these patients might have been receiving other agents that could have caused cumulative / synergistic toxicity.*

Follin SL, et al. Falsely elevated serum vancomycin concentrations in hemodialysis patients. *Am J Kidney Dis* 1996;27:67–74.

*Maintenance hemodialysis patients may have significantly overestimated serum vancomycin levels if the tests are performed with the fluorescence polarization immunoassay (FPIA). This widely employed method may result in false determinations of further vancomycin dosing regimens. The authors suggest use of an alternative enzyme multiplied immunoassay technique (EMIT) method.*

Jordan GW, Kawachi MM. Analysis of serum bactericidal activity in endocarditis, osteomyelitis, and other bacterial infections. *Medicine (Baltimore)* 1981;60:49–61.

*This retrospective review of a 5-year clinical experience with SBT in the management of a variety of infections concludes that (a) SBT is a useful indicator of antimicrobial efficacy in infective endocarditis; (b) for infections caused by susceptible bacteria, antimicrobial combinations offer no advantage over monotherapy; (c) SBT was useful when second-line antimicrobials were indicated; (d) SBT was useful in adjusting dosages in complex cases; and (e) SBT determinations may be useful in the management of endocarditis caused by "tolerant" staphylococci.*

Moellering RC Jr. Editorial: monitoring serum vancomycin levels: climbing the mountain because it is there? *Clin Infect Dis* 1994;18:544–546.

*An editorial response to the Cantu article. Dr. Moellering is in general agreement with the conclusions, but feels that four indications for vancomycin monitoring might exist, as mentioned in the text of this chapter.*

Mulhern JG, et al. Trough serum vancomycin levels predict the relapse of gram-positive peritonitis in peritoneal dialysis patients. *Am J Kidney Dis* 1995;25:611–615.

*Thirty-one episodes of gram-positive peritonitis in patients on chronic ambulatory peritoneal dialysis were assessed to discover risks for relapse. All patients received four weekly doses of vancomycin, with the last two adjusted to maintain a trough level greater than 12 μ/mL. Relapse was seen only in those who failed to maintain a mean 4-week concentration at this level.*

Washington JA II. The role of the microbiology laboratory in the diagnosis and antimicrobial treatment of infective endocarditis. *Mayo Clin Proc* 1982;57:22–32.

*This overview of the SBT and the MBC test describes the techniques and limitations involved in both. It also reviews the history of the use of the SBT in infective endocarditis and describes the differences in several published reports in regard to how the SBT was employed.*

Weinstein MP, et al. Multicenter collaborative evaluation of a standardized serum bactericidal test as a prognostic indicator of infective endocarditis. *Am J Med* 1985;78:262–268.

*Employing standardized methodology for SBT, this investigation demonstrated the statistical relevance of peak SBT levels above 1:64 and trough SBT levels above 1:32 as a prediction of bacteriologic cure in cases of infective endocarditis. Trough levels above 1:8 correlated with bacteriologic cure. However, the SBT result failed to predict bacteriologic failure or clinical outcome.*

Wolfson JS, Swartz MN. Serum bactericidal activity as a monitor of antibiotic therapy. *N Engl J Med* 1985;312:968–975.

*This excellent overview of the rationale, technique, and advantages and disadvantages of the SBT concludes that far more data are necessary to determine its efficacy in monitoring infections.*

# XIX. ANTIMICROBIAL, ANTIVIRAL, ANTIPARASITIC, AND ANTIFUNGAL AGENTS

# 73. PRINCIPLES OF ANTIMICROBIAL THERAPY

There are at least five basic principles on which successful antimicrobial therapy must be based. These principles require knowledge of an antimicrobial's spectrum of activity, distribution and pharmacokinetics, toxicity, synergy and antagonism with other antimicrobials, and cost.

## Principle 1: Spectrum of Activity

This principle is relevant to choosing an antimicrobial directed against a specific pathogen. First, the physician must determine the particular pathogen that is causing infection. Once the agent has been identified, an antimicrobial with particular activity against the organism causing disease can be chosen.

Identification of the most likely bacterium causing an infection is based on history, physical examination, epidemiology, and Gram's stain and culture of appropriate body fluids. For example, in a patient with pneumonia, several aspects of the history might be important. Whether the pneumonia is community-acquired or hospital-acquired will provide a clue to the likely etiologic agent. Another clue to the identity of the organism causing pneumonia might be a patient history that includes having a sick parakeet, as psittacosis presents in a nonspecific manner. A history of a single shaking chill suggests to some the likelihood of a pneumococcal infection. Sputum that is foul-smelling or has a fecal odor suggests an anaerobic component to the pneumonia. Physical examination, in addition to suggesting the focus of infection, may also be important in determining an etiologic agent. In a patient with cellulitis, for example, erysipelas seen on physical examination suggests group A β-hemolytic streptococcal infection. In a patient with gram-negative bacteremia, a black fluid-filled lesion suggesting ecthyma gangrenosum makes the diagnosis of *Pseudomonas* bacteremia most likely.

An increasing number of rapid laboratory tests are available for early, specific diagnosis; however, for bacterial infections, Gram's stain of the infected material is still extremely important in defining optimal antimicrobial therapy. In a patient with bacterial pneumonia, sputum Gram's stain is essential for optimal management. A patient who presents with empyema requires thoracentesis and Gram's stain of pleural fluid before antimicrobial therapy can be determined.

Once the physical examination and laboratory results, including Gram's stain, have been assessed, the physician makes the best possible determination about the likely bacterial pathogens causing infection. An antimicrobial with optimal activity against these pathogens must then be chosen. Narrow-spectrum antibiotics are preferred to prevent the emergence of resistance; however, the choice of narrow- versus broad-spectrum therapy will depend on the severity of illness, clinical clues to etiology, and issues of local hospital epidemiology.

## Principle 2: Volume of Distribution and Pharmacokinetics

An antimicrobial may have excellent activity against a particular bacterium, but treatment will not be successful unless it reaches the site of infection in adequate concentrations. For example, aminoglycosides alone are not usually chosen for gram-negative pneumonia because of concern about concentrations of aminoglycosides in bronchial washings. Nor would a first-generation cephalosporin be used for pneumococcal meningitis. Although the cephalosporin would have excellent activity against the pneumococcus, it does not enter the cerebrospinal fluid in adequate concentrations to be effective. Hence, in choosing an antimicrobial, it is necessary to know the specific pharmacokinetics of each and what antimicrobials can be expected to reach therapeutic levels in various body fluids.

## Principle 3: Antimicrobial Toxicity

The benefits of an antimicrobial must outweigh the risks. To make this assessment, the clinician must appreciate the side effects of each agent that is used and must then assess the benefits versus the risks of the drug in question. For example, in an elderly patient with *Klebsiella pneumoniae* pneumonia, a combination of cephalosporin and aminoglycoside may be chosen. This combination may have some nephrotoxic side effects (and the combination of cephalosporin and aminoglycoside likely causes increased nephrotoxicity compared with aminoglycoside alone), but in the case of a life-threatening infection such as *K. pneumoniae* pneumonia, this combination of anti-microbials would be the therapy of choice for many clinicians. In contrast, a patient presenting with cystitis and found to have *K. pneumoniae* in the urine would be treated with a very different regimen, one with a less toxic profile.

The toxicity of an antimicrobial must be assessed in regard to the specific patient. The likelihood of toxicity from an aminoglycoside is greater in an elderly patient with underlying renal disease than in a young adult. A patient who has had an episode of anaphylaxis to penicillin should not be treated with a cephalosporin.

### Principle 4: Issues of Synergy and Antagonism

When one antimicrobial enhances the other with more than just an additive effect, the interaction is called synergy. When an antimicrobial interferes with the activity of a second one, the effect is called antagonism. A bacteriostatic antimicrobial, for example, frequently slows the killing rate of a bactericidal antimicrobial.

Several examples of *in vitro* synergism have been shown to be important in the clinical setting. For example, the newer penicillins in combination with aminoglycosides are synergistic for *Pseudomonas aeruginosa*. In neutropenic patients with *Pseudomonas* bacteremia, the combination of a newer penicillin and an aminoglycoside is generally considered to be a combination of choice because of this synergistic relationship. There have also been some examples of clinical antagonism. For example, an early study on pneumococcal meningitis showed that the combination of penicillin and tetracycline was much less successful than penicillin alone in the treatment of this disease.

The use of more than one antimicrobial has become increasingly common in therapy, so the clinician must understand the potential synergistic and antagonistic relationships involved in combination antimicrobial therapy.

### Principle 5: Cost of Antimicrobials and Antimicrobial Administration

In life-threatening infections, cost will not play a major role in choosing antimicrobial therapy; however, for mild infections such as cystitis or for antimicrobial prophylaxis, regimens may vary 10-fold in cost. Therefore, the clinician must have some understanding of the cost of various antimicrobials.

### Other Issues in Selection

For some infections, bactericidal antimicrobials are mandatory. For example, in endocarditis, treatment with a bacteriostatic drug such as erythromycin has a higher failure rate than treatment with a bactericidal drug such as penicillin. In this infection, a high level of inhibition is insufficient; for cure, adequate "killing" must be achieved. In some types of bacterial meningitis, a bactericidal drug is also recommended. For example, in gram-negative bacillary meningitis, a third-generation cephalosporin is preferred to chloramphenicol.

For some infections, the ability of antimicrobials to penetrate phagocytes may be necessary for cure. *Legionella pneumophila,* for example, can survive within phagocytic cells. Erythromycin, rifampin, and ciprofloxacin may penetrate alveolar macrophages and be curative in this infection. Some β-lactamase-stable cephalosporins have good *in vitro* activity against *Legionella* but are ineffective in treatment.

Because antimicrobials are often given intermittently, the ability of the offending agents to multiply between doses can present an important problem. Many antimicrobials produce an inhibitory effect on bacteria for a number of hours after exposure. With gram-positive cocci, this post-antimicrobial effect is similar for all antimicrobial agents. However, for gram-negative bacilli, some antimicrobials, such as aminoglycosides and ciprofloxacin, have a post-antimicrobial effect, whereas others, such as cephalosporins, may not. The clinical relevance of this phenomenon needs further evaluation. (S.L.B.)

### Bibliography
Allan UD Jr. Antibiotic combinations. *Med Clin North Am* 1987;71:1079.
  *Advantages and disadvantages of combination antimicrobial therapy.*

Bryan CS. Strategies to improve antibiotic use. *Infect Dis Clin North Am* 1989;3:723.
*Strategies for effective selection of antimicrobials.*

Gleckman RA. Antibiotic use in the elderly: a selective review. *Infect Dis Clin North Am* 1989;3:507.
*Describes antimicrobial-related adverse events and drug interaction problems with antimicrobials. These tend to be more serious in elderly patients.*

Gross PA. The potential for clinical guidelines to impact appropriate antimicrobial agent use. *Infect Dis Clin North Am* 1997;11:803.
*Practice guidelines will become more important in antibiotic selection. These guidelines will require selection of narrow-spectrum antibiotics, when possible, with lowest possible toxicity.*

Hessen MT, Kaye D. Principles of selection and use of antibacterial agents. *Infect Dis Clin North Am* 1995;9:531.
*Includes basic principles of pharmacodynamics, monitoring of therapy, and reasons for treatment failure.*

Hughes WT, et al. 1997 Guidelines for the use of antimicrobial agents in neutropenic patients with unexplained fever. *Clin Infect Dis* 1997;25:551.
*Evidence-based guidelines for the selection of antibiotics for patients with neutropenia.*

Kirst HA, Sides GD. New directions for macrolide antibiotics: pharmacokinetics and clinical efficacy. *Antimicrob Agents Chemother* 1989;33:1419.
*The new macrolide antimicrobials may provide an advantage based on their tissue penetration properties.*

Levison ME, Bush LM. Pharmacodynamics of antimicrobial agents: bactericidal and post-antibiotic effects. *Infect Dis Clin North Am* 1989;3:415.
*Emphasizes the importance of drug concentration at the site of infection and the clinical relevance of post-antimicrobial effects.*

The Medical Letter. The choice of antibacterial drugs. *Med Lett Drugs Ther* 1996;38:25.
*Lists drugs of choice for common pathogens. Good consensus evaluation of value of new antimicrobial agents.*

Moellering RC. Principles of antiinfective therapy. In: Mandell GL, Douglas RG Jr, Bennett JE, eds. *Principles and practice of infectious diseases.* New York: Churchill Livingstone, 1990.
*Excellent discussion of general principles of antimicrobial therapy.*

Neu HC. General concepts on the chemotherapy of infectious diseases. *Med Clin North Am* 1987;71:1051.
*Includes a discussion of bactericidal versus bacteriostatic drugs and intracellular versus extracellular location of bacteria, plus a brief description of the mechanism of action of each drug.*

Rahal JJ Jr. Antibiotic combinations: the clinical relevance of synergy and antagonism. *Medicine (Baltimore)* 1978;57:179.
*Reviews the relationship between in vitro testing and the clinical relevance of antimicrobial combinations.*

Shlaes DM, et al. Society of Healthcare Epidemiology of America and Infectious Disease Society of America Joint Commission on the Prevention of Antimicrobial Resistance: guidelines for the prevention of antimicrobial resistance in hospitals. *Clin Infect Dis* 1997;25:584.
*Antibiotic selection must take into account prevention of the emergence of resistance. Narrow-spectrum antibiotics are preferred, but their selection will depend on local hospital epidemiology.*

Symposium on antimicrobial agents. *Mayo Clin Proc* 1987;62:788.
*Reviews general principles of antimicrobial therapy as well as major categories of antimicrobial agents. Excellent summary.*

Winston DU, et al. β-Lactam antibiotic therapy in febrile, granulocytopenic patients. *Ann Intern Med* 1991;115:849.
*Discusses double β-lactam therapy. Basic principles of antimicrobial therapy are used to evaluate treatment.*

Yoshikawa TT. Antimicrobial therapy for the elderly patient. *J Am Geriatr Soc* 1990; 38:1353.

*Describes the principles of antimicrobial therapy as they apply to elderly patients and includes important issues of pharmacokinetic differences related to aging.*
Young LS. Empirical antimicrobial therapy in the neutropenic host. *N Engl J Med* 1986;315:580.
*Reviews evidence for synergy in the treatment of* Pseudomonas *infection.*

## 74. CHOOSING A CEPHALOSPORIN

In 1979, there were 10 cephalosporins available for use in the United States. Since then, the number has increased to about 30. Choosing from among these many similarly named antimicrobials has become a challenge for even the most knowledgeable internist.

The cephalosporins are synthetic or semisynthetic derivatives of products produced by the fungus *Cephalosporium acremonium.* The original compound, cephalosporin C, is closely related to penicillin in both structure and mechanism of action. The initial cephalosporins were recognized for their bactericidal activity against both gram-positive cocci and gram-negative bacilli, as well as their good safety profile. Cephalosporins have been developed during the past 10 years with increased intrinsic antibacterial activity and modified pharmacokinetic properties, so that drugs with a longer half-life and greater oral absorbability are available.

The conceptual organization of cephalosporins as first-, second-, or third-generation remains useful (Table 74-1). First-generation cephalosporins are similar, whereas third-generation cephalosporins must be appreciated for their unique differences.

First-generation cephalosporins remain active against most aerobic gram-positive cocci. They are resistant to hydrolysis by the penicillinase produced by *Staphylococcus aureus.* First-generation cephalosporins have been used extensively in staphylococcal infections with good success. They are not active against methicillin-resistant staphylococci. In the hospital setting, they are often used as second-line antimicrobials against staphylococci because oxacillin and nafcillin have a narrower spectrum and therefore are usually preferred for methicillin-sensitive organisms. In patients who have manifest allergy to penicillin, first-generation cephalosporins are drugs of choice for methicillin-sensitive staphylococcal infections. They are generally regarded as safer than clindamycin or vancomycin. In patients who have had anaphylactic reactions to penicillin, cephalosporins are not used.

First-generation cephalosporins are also widely used for streptococcal infection, excluding infections caused by enterococci. They are particularly useful to treat streptococcal cellulitis and pneumococcal pneumonia in patients who have had a rash in reaction to penicillin. First-generation cephalosporins are not preferred drugs for endocarditis caused by *viridans* streptococci. Because they penetrate the blood–brain barrier poorly, they cannot be used in pneumococcal meningitis.

Many strains of gram-negative bacilli, particularly *Escherichia coli, Klebsiella pneumoniae,* and *Proteus mirabilis,* are sensitive to first-generation cephalosporins. When *in vitro* susceptibility tests are available and demonstrate susceptibility, first-generation cephalosporins are generally good choices against these agents because they are less expensive and induce less resistance than the second- and third-generation cephalosporins. The first-generation cephalosporins cannot be used as empiric therapy for life-threatening gram-negative bacillary infection because many of these bacilli (*Pseudomonas* and *Serratia* species in particular) are resistant. First-generation cephalosporins also cannot be used for infections caused by *Haemophilus influenzae* or for anaerobic infection.

The first-generation cephalosporins cephalothin, cephapirin, and cephradine can be considered interchangeable, and the same Kirby-Bauer disk is used to test susceptibility for all of them. Cefazolin has a longer half-life, and higher serum concentrations are obtained with IM injection. First-generation cephalosporins are still recommended for many types of IM injection and surgical prophylaxis; however, agents with better

Table 74-1. Classification of cephalosporins

**First-generation cephalosporins**
Cephalothin (Keflin)
Cephapirin (Cefadyl)
Cephradine (Velosef)
Cefazolin (Ancef, Kefzol)
*Oral*
Cephalexin (Keflex)
Cefadroxil (Duricef)

**Second-generation cephalosporins and carbacephems**
Activity *Haemophilus influenzae*
  Cefamandole (Mandol)
  Cefuroxime (Zinacef)
  Cefonicid (Monocid)
Activity *Bacteroides fragilis*
  Cefoxitin (Mefoxin)
  Cefotetan (Cefotan)
  Cefmetazole
*Oral*
Cefaclor (Ceclor)
Cefdinir (Omnicef)
Cefuroxime axetil (Ceftin)
Cefprozil (Cefzil)
Loracarbef (Lorabid)

**Third-generation cephalosporins**
Moxalactam (Moxam)
Cefotaxime (Claforan)
Ceftizoxime (Cefizox)
Ceftiaxone (Rocephin)
Cefoperazone (Cefobid)
Antipseudomonal
  Ceftazidime (Fortaz)
  Cefepime
*Oral*
Cefixime (Suprax)
Cefpodoxime (Vantin)

anaerobic activity are recommended for colorectal surgical prophylaxis. These drugs cannot be used for meningitis, as they do not penetrate inflamed meninges.

Second-generation cephalosporins are generally somewhat less active than first-generation cephalosporins against gram-positive cocci but have a broader spectrum against gram-negative bacilli, such as *Enterobacter* species, *Citrobacter,* and *Morganella*. More importantly, some provide excellent activity against *H. influenzae,* and others have added activity against anaerobic bacteria, particularly *Bacteroides fragilis.* The second-generation cephalosporins cefamandole, cefuroxime, and cefonicid and the oral drugs cefaclor, cefuroxime axetil, loracarbef, cefdinir, and cefprozil have become the antimicrobials of choice to treat infection with *H. influenzae,* both β-lactamase-positive and β-lactamase-negative strains. Other second-generation cephalosporins, such as cefoxitin, cefotetan, and cefmetazole, have little *H. influenzae* activity but are useful for mixed anaerobic and gram-negative bacillary infection.

The third-generation cephalosporins have the widest spectrum of gram-negative activity. Most have activity against both *H. influenzae* and anaerobes, although differences exist among individual members of the group. Ceftazidime has excellent activity against *Pseudomonas aeruginosa* and is one of the drugs of choice for infection with this organism. Other third-generation agents, such as cefoperazone, have moderate activity against *Pseudomonas*. Third-generation cephalosporins generally have lost activity against gram-positive cocci. Third-generation cephalosporins have been used to treat meningitis caused by *H. influenzae, Neisseria meningitidis, Streptococcus pneumoniae,* and many gram-negative bacilli. Treatment failure has recently been reported for pneumococcal meningitis caused by penicillin-resistant strains. Moxalactam, rarely used because of its tendency to cause gastrointestinal bleeding, was the third-generation cephalosporin of choice for anaerobic infection. Ceftizoxime has been considered a good anaerobic agent by some investigators.

In addition to the etiologic agent and spectrum of activity of the drug, the choice of a cephalosporin may depend on its side-effect profile. The major adverse reaction to all cephalosporins is hypersensitivity or allergic reactions. All can cause a drug fever, eosinophilia, and diarrhea. Gastrointestinal bleeding has occurred with all cephalosporins but is more common in those with a methylthiotetrazole ring at the R2 position. Such cephalosporins include moxalactam, cefoperazone, cefamandole, and cefotetan. These same cephalosporins can cause a disulfiram-like reaction in patients who have been drinking alcohol. Flushing, tachycardia, nausea, and vomiting are manifestations of this syndrome. Cephalosporins do not cause nephrotoxicity in themselves but may increase the likelihood of aminoglycoside nephrotoxicity when a cephalosporin and aminoglycoside are used together.

Cefixime, cefpodoxime proxetil, and cefetamet pivoxil are oral third-generation cephalosporins that have an additional spectrum of activity against gram-negative bacilli, but not *Pseudomonas*. They are generally less likely to be used for gram-negative bacillary infection than are quinolones. Cefpodoxime has better antistaphylococcal activity than the others, but none should be drugs of choice for gram-positive infection.

Cefepime is one of the newest cephalopsorins and has been considered by some to be a fourth-generation agent. Cefepime targets multiple penicillin-binding proteins and is resistant to many β-lactamases. The antibiotic covers many strains of *Pseudomonas* while maintaining activity against gram-positive cocci, including *S. aureus*.

The following considerations are important in choosing the right cephalosporin:

1. The first-generation cephalosporins such as cephalothin and cefazolin are good second-line drugs for staphylococcal (not methicillin-resistant *S. aureus*) or streptococcal infection. They can be used in patients with penicillin-induced rash but not in patients who have experienced anaphylaxis. They are useful in gram-negative bacillary infections when susceptibility tests show the organism to be sensitive.

2. Second-generation cephalosporins with *H. influenzae* activity (cefamandole, cefuroxime, cefonicid, cefaclor) are among the drugs of choice for lower respiratory infection. These antimicrobials are active against *S. pneumoniae, H. influenzae,* and *Moraxella catarrhalis,* the common respiratory pathogens in acute tracheobronchitis and community-acquired pneumonia.

3. Cefoxitin and cefotetan are second-generation cephalosporins with good anaerobic activity against *Bacteroides fragilis*. They cover some but not all gram-negative bacilli. For hospital-acquired gram-negative infection, broader-spectrum gram-negative coverage (to include *P. aeruginosa*) is necessary.

4. The third-generation cephalosporin ceftazidime is an excellent antipseudomonal agent with or without addition of an aminoglycoside. The other third-generation cephalosporins are generally not recommended for *Pseudomonas* infection.

5. Third-generation cephalosporins have become the drugs of choice for gram-negative meningitis. They are also valuable in treating infection caused by resistant gram-negative bacilli, for which aminoglycosides might formerly have been necessary.

6. Ceftriaxone, the third-generation cephalosporin with the longest half-life, is commonly used to treat serious infections at home. The drug can be administered by a visiting nurse once or twice per day.

7. Ceftizoxime and cefotaxime, the third-generation cephalosporins with names that sound the most alike, actually are the most alike. They maintain coverage of gram-positive cocci better than do other third-generation cephalosporins but provide little *Pseudomonas* coverage. Some believe that ceftizoxime is a drug of choice for anaerobic infection. Moxalactam, which has the best *in vitro* activity against anaerobes, is no longer recommended because it causes gastrointestinal bleeding. (S.L.B.)

## Bibliography

Cherubin CE, et al. Penetration of newer cephalosporins into cerebrospinal fluid. *Rev Infect Dis* 1989;11:526.
  *Compares cerebrospinal fluid concentrations of second- and third-generation cephalosporins. The most clinical data are available for cefotaxime.*
Ehmann WC. Cephalosporin-induced hemolysis: a case report and review of the literature. *Am J Hematol* 1992;40:121.
  *Review of 13 cases of cephalosporin-induced hemolytic anemia.*
Ennis DM, Cobb CG. The newer cephalosporins. *Infect Dis Clin North Am* 1995;9:687.
  *Describes structure, side effects, and activity of the newer second- and third-generation oral cepalosporins.*
Finland M, Kaye D, Turck M. Clinical symposium on cefazolin. *J Infect Dis* 1973; 128:S312.
  *Includes 22 articles on the spectrum, pharmacology, uses, and adverse effects of a long-acting first-generation cephalosporin.*
Fong IW, Tompkins KB. Review of *Pseudomonas aeruginosa* meningitis with special emphasis on treatment with ceftazidime. *Rev Infect Dis* 1985;7:604.
  *Ceftazidime has been successful in the treatment of* Pseudomonas *meningitis, making intraventricular aminoglycoside therapy rarely necessary.*
Goldberg DM. The cephalosporins. *Med Clin North Am* 1987;71:1113.
  *Review article on cephalosporins, with more than 100 references.*
Gorbach SL. The role of cephalosporins in surgical prophylaxis. *J Antimicrob Chemother* 1989;23(Suppl D):61.
  *For colorectal surgery, the choice of a cephalosporin should be based in part on its anaerobic activity.*
Gustaferro CA, Steckelberg JM. Cephalosporin antimicrobial agents and related compounds. *Mayo Clin Proc* 1991;66:1064.
  *Bacterial resistance has developed to cephalosporins with respect to β-lactamase production, alterations in binding proteins, and modifications of the cell wall.*
John CC. Treatment failure with the use of a third-generation cephalosporin for penicillin-resistant pneumococcal meningitis. Case report and review. *Clin Infect Dis* 1994;18:188.
  *Describes treatment failures of third-generation cephalosporins with minimum inhibitory concentrations greater than 2 µg/mL against pneumococci. Vancomycin is likely the drug of choice for these strains.*
Kaiser AB. Overview of cephalosporin prophylaxis. *Am J Surg* 1988;155(5A):52.
  *Comprehensive review of cephalosporin prophylaxis in surgery that also stresses the difficulty in making definitive choices for prophylaxis.*
Landesman SH, et al. Past and current roles for cephalosporin antibiotics in treatment of meningitis: emphasis on use in gram-negative bacillary meningitis. *Am J Med* 1981;71:693.
  *Describes role of cephalosporins in meningitis.*
Meideros AA. Nosocomial outbreaks of multiresistant bacteria: extended-spectrum β-lactamases have arrived in North America. *Ann Intern Med* 1993;119:428.
  *Reports on a nosocomial outbreak of Klebsiella infection resistant to third-generation cephalosporins.*
Neu HC. Cephalosporin antibiotics: molecules that respond to different needs. *Am J Surg* 1988;155(5A):1.
  *The presence of a methoxyl group at C7 of the cephalosporin nucleus confers activity against many anaerobes.*
Neu HC, Prince AS. Interaction between moxalactam and alcohol. *Lancet* 1980;1:1422.
  *Description of Antabuse-like reaction with moxalactam and alcohol.*
Quenzer RW. A perspective of cephalosporins in pneumonia. *Chest* 1987;92:3.
  *Describes an approach to cephalosporin therapy in patients with pneumonia.*
Rankin GO, Sutherland CH. Nephrotoxicity of aminoglycosides and cephalosporins in combination. *Adverse Drug React Acute Poisoning Rev* 1989;8:73.
  *A review of cephalosporin potentiation of aminoglycoside nephrotoxicity.*
Rouse MS, et al. Animal models as predictors of outcome of therapy with broad-spectrum cephalosporins. *J Antimicrob Chemother* 1992;29(Suppl A):39.

*Suggests that animal models of endocarditis and meningitis may be most useful in assessing cephalosporin efficacy.*

Sanders CC. Cefepime. The next generation? *Clin Infect Dis* 1993;17:369.
*Cefepime has activity against many strains of* Pseudomonas *and also maintains good coverage of many gram-positive cocci. Hence, it is a broad-spectrum antipseudomonal antibiotic.*

Sattler FR, Weitekamp MR, Ballard JO. Potential for bleeding with new β-lactam antibiotics. *Ann Intern Med* 1986;105:924.
*Moxalactam is no longer recommended because of its propensity to cause gastrointestinal bleeding.*

Scully BE, Neu HC. Clinical efficacy of ceftazidime: treatment of serious infection caused by multiresistant *Pseudomonas* and other gram-negative bacteria. *Arch Intern Med* 1984;144:57.
*A proven role for ceftazidime in serious* Pseudomonas *infection.*

Thoburn R, Johnson JE, Cluff LE. Studies on the epidemiology of adverse drug reactions. IV. The relationship of cephalothin and penicillin allergy. *J Am Med* 1966; 198:111.
*A history of penicillin allergy or a positive skin test reaction with these drugs was a predisposing factor to cephalothin reactions.*

Thompson RL. Cephalosporin, carbapenem, and monobactam antibiotics. *Mayo Clin Proc* 1987;62:821.
*Part of the Mayo Clinic symposium on antimicrobials. Includes good summary of spectrum of activity and details on adverse reactions.*

Weinstein L, Kaplan K. The cephalosporins: microbiological, chemical, and pharmacological properties and use in chemotherapy of infection. *Ann Intern Med* 1970;72:729.
*Discussion of first-generation cephalosporins.*

Wiedemann B. Selection of β-lactamase producers during cephalosporin and penicillin therapy. *Scand J Infect Dis* 1986;49 (Suppl):100.
*Discusses the selection of cephalosporins with respect to their impact on β-lactamase production.*

## 75. SINGLE DAILY DOSING OF AMINOGLYCOSIDES

The aminoglycosides are a group of structurally related antibiotics that kill bacteria by inhibiting protein synthesis. They share similar pharmacokinetic profiles, and their structure does not allow easy penetration into cells. Aminoglycosides are excreted primarily by the kidney, and they are active mainly against gram-negative bacteria. These compounds have been available for approximately 50 years. During that time, they have waxed and waned in favor based on the availability of other, similar products, presumed toxicity, and questions of efficacy in some clinical instances. By the early 1990s, some clinicians questioned whether these products would survive, as numerous other agents with similar spectra of activity and enhanced safety records emerged. However, during the past several years in the United States, gentamicin, tobramycin, and amikacin have acquired renewed importance, in part because of new information about dosing that renders them safer and probably more effective than previously. Potential parenteral uses of these aminoglycosides include (a) empiric therapy of presumed gram-negative infections, (b) therapy of proven gram-negative infections caused by organisms not treatable by alternative agents, (c) therapy against selected gram-positive pathogens in combination with penicillins or vancomycin for synergy, (d) empiric therapy of the febrile granulocytopenic patient, and (e) management of selected mycobacterial infections.

Parenterally administered aminoglycosides historically have been considered difficult to use in seriously ill patients because of their narrow toxic-therapeutic ratio. This was based on the premise that toxicity was in part related to peak concentrations of the product. For gentamicin and tobramycin, toxic levels have historically been considered to be greater than 12 μg/mL (peak) or greater than 2 μg/mL (trough). Clinical variables such as weight, renal function, hemoglobin, temperature, obesity, and "metabolic state" influence aminoglycoside levels. Nomograms attempting to predict dosing generally were unsuccessful, and several studies exist that demonstrate the problem of obtaining therapeutic levels early in the course of severe illness. Lack of such levels was associated with adverse outcomes, especially in critically ill patients.

The toxic effects of aminoglycosides include ototoxicity, nephrotoxicity, and neuromuscular blockade. Classic investigations of the ototoxicity and nephrotoxicity of these products concluded that ototoxicity (either auditory or vestibular) occurs in up to 5% of patients, is difficult to monitor, and is often irreversible. The mechanism of toxicity appears to be related to uptake and accumulation by cochlear or vestibular cells. The time of contact between affected cells and antibiotic seems to be important. Nephrotoxicity (generally defined by relatively minor changes in serum creatinine values) has been seen in up to 25% of patients, appears more commonly with gentamicin than with tobramycin, and is generally minor clinically and often reversible. However, some investigations have indicated a prolonged hospitalization, and occasional patients have required dialysis. The mechanism of toxicity is related to the reabsorption of the drug in the lumen of the renal tubule. Animal data suggest that this process can become saturated and thus does not continue beyond a specific level. Neuromuscular blockade is rarely noted and is associated with rapid administration of the drug. Thus, difficulties with both therapeutic efficacy and toxicity are major reasons why aminoglycosides appear to have been used sparingly in recent years.

The rationale for once-daily dosing of aminoglycosides is based on the fact that bacterial killing with these agents is related to drug concentration; progressively increased bactericidal activity is demonstrated by concentrations up to 10 to 12 times the minimum inhibitory concentration (MIC) for an organism. Because *Pseudomonas aeruginosa* is the most resistant organism likely to be treated, and because the MIC of gentamicin for this organism is 2 μg/mL, peak levels of gentamicin above 20 μm/mL should be sought. Aminoglycosides also have a prolonged post-antibiotic effect, which indicates that killing continues after serum levels have fallen below the MIC for an organism. This is in contrast to what is noted with β-lactam antibiotics; with these agents, killing is time-dependent, and post-antibiotic effects are less pronounced. These aminoglycoside "virtues" make it likely that dosing regimens that produced higher peak levels more rapidly would be more clinically effective so long as toxicity was not augmented. More rapid killing could also decrease the emergence of resistance. Furthermore, single-dose aminoglycosides are less likely to result in toxicity because when they are given in a large single dose, contact with the agent is limited.

A number of studies have been conducted, primarily in immunocompetent patients, to compare the safety and efficacy of daily dosing with traditional dosing of aminoglycosides. In an investigation of approximately 2,200 patients, nephrotoxicity developed in fewer than 2% of patients, and ototoxicity was observed in about 0.1%. In two thirds of patients with vestibular dysfunction, the dysfunction resolved. Two metaanalyses have been completed. Data indicate that single daily dosing in patients with normal renal function is associated with decreased nephrotoxicity and equal ototoxicity in comparison with traditional dosing regimens. In one metaanalysis, nephrotoxicity (defined as an increase in serum creatinine of 50%) was reduced from 7.5% to 5.5% ($p = .05$). Another metaanalysis demonstrated no significant differences in therapeutic outcome or toxicity, but indicated that ease of administration, reductions in nursing and other professional time, and apparent equivalency of outcomes implied that single daily dosing is advantageous. No studies have concluded that once-daily dosing of aminoglycosides results in unfavorable outcomes.

Most investigations of once-daily aminoglycosides have been conducted in patients with normal renal function and illnesses that are not life-threatening. Use in febrile neutropenic patients and in those with critical illness needs to be studied further. However, it is the opinion of the author that the principles on which once-daily dosing is predicated should allow it to be used in these circumstances as well.

Aminoglycosides are also employed for their synergistic activity in selected streptococcal infections. Once-daily regimens are adequate for the management of *viridans* streptococcal endocarditis, but they should not be used for enterococcal endocarditis.

Table 75-1.  Situations in which once-daily aminoglycosides are not indicated

Dialysis
Severe burns
Pregnancy
Enterococcal endocarditis
Quadriplegia
Bilateral amputation
Ascites

Other clinical situations in which once-daily dosing is currently not indicated include severe burns, pregnancy, and dialysis. Table 75-1 summarizes the clinical conditions in which once-daily dosing is not appropriate.

When once-daily aminoglycoside dosing is utilized, the initial dose should be at least the total daily dose. Data generated at Hartford Hospital suggest that a 7-mg dose of gentamicin or tobramycin per kilogram be employed. The initial dose of amikacin would be 15 mg/kg. These doses provide optimal peak levels against *P. aeruginosa,* the target organism in most cases. Dose adjustments might be necessary depending on the $MIC_{90}$ values for target organisms at other institutions. Such dosing routinely results in peak antibiotic concentrations above 20 μg/mL (gentamicin and tobramycin), which is approximately 10 times the MIC. The need for aminoglycoside monitoring is controversial. No antibiotic levels have to be obtained initially if patients are less than 60 years of age, have normal values of serum creatinine, are neither quadriplegics nor amputees, and are not receiving other potential nephrotoxic agents. Repeated doses are then administered at 24-hour intervals. However, all patients should have serum creatinine values regularly monitored, and patients who receive aminoglycosides for longer than 5 days require determination of a trough aminoglycoside level; this should be done thereafter at weekly intervals. This result should be below 2 μg/mL. For patients at higher risk, trough levels are monitored after the third dose. Once-daily aminoglycoside dosing is also appropriate for patients with renal dysfunction. The dosing interval is based on creatinine clearance (Cockcroft-Gault equation). The dosing interval is 24 hours (creatinine clearance >60 mL/min), 36 hours (clearance 40 to 60 mL/min), or 48 hours (clearance 20 to 40 mL/min).

Economic data demonstrate that once-daily aminoglycoside dosing can conserve hospital resources and save money. One study showed a net saving of $128,000 based on decreased nephrotoxicity and lower administration and preparation costs. (R.B.B.)

## Bibliography

Ambrose PG, Owens RC Jr, Quintiliani R. The aminoglycosides: rationale and guidelines for once-daily dosing. *Contemp Intern Med* 1997;9:9–13.
  *This article provides an excellent overview of the principles and practices of once-daily aminoglycoside dosing. It stresses the need to individualize dosing by hospital, based on likely target organisms, and provides data for dose modification in patients with renal dysfunction.*
Barza M, et al. Single or multiple daily doses of aminoglycosides: a metaanalysis. *BMJ* 1996;312:338–345.
  *A second metaanalysis performed by different investigators demonstrates a tendency toward enhanced clinical outcomes with once-daily aminoglycoside dosing, and a clear advantage in regard to prevention of nephrotoxicity.*
Edson RS, Terrell CL. The aminoglycosides. *Mayo Clin Proc* 1991;66:1158–1164.
  *Excellent and succinct overview of the structure, mode of action, mechanisms of resistance,* in vitro *activity, and clinical uses of the aminoglycosides.*
Hatala R, Dinh T, Cook DJ. Once-daily aminoglycoside dosing in immunocompetent adults: a metaanalysis. *Ann Intern Med* 1996;124:717–725.
  *In a metaanalysis of 13 investigations of aminoglycoside dosing that met the criteria of the authors, no differences could be detected in bacteriologic cure as an outcome variable. Once-daily dosing trended toward decreased mortality and lessened toxicity.*

Lietman PS, Smith CR. Aminoglycoside nephrotoxicity in humans. *Rev Infect Dis* 1983;5 (Suppl 2):S284–S293.

*Reviews the pathophysiology, incidence, and risk factors of aminoglycoside-induced nephrotoxicity in humans. Studies employed multiple doses daily. Investigators describe comparative differences among the aminoglycosides, based on their previous investigations, and point out that serious nephrotoxicity is uncommon. Issues related to toxicity include dosage, agent, concomitant agents, and personal factors.*

McCormack JP, Jewesson PJ. A critical reevaluation of the "therapeutic range" of aminoglycosides. *Clin Infect Dis* 1992;14:320–329.

*A thorough review of the aminoglycoside literature that assesses several issues: (a) relationship between peak serum levels and outcome, (b) relationship between minimum serum level and outcome, (c) whether monitoring of levels improves treatment outcome, (d) relationship between serum levels and toxicity, and (e) relationship between monitoring of serum levels and decreased toxicity. The critical literature review fails to answer most of these questions, but suggestions for aminoglycoside use and monitoring are provided.*

Prins JM, et al. Once versus thrice daily gentamicin in patients with serious infections. *Lancet* 1993;341:335–339.

*The authors conducted a randomized trial of once-daily (4 mg/kg per day) versus thrice-daily (1.3 mg/kg every 8 hours) dosing in patients hospitalized with a variety of serious infections. Patients with neutropenia or severe renal dysfunction were excluded. Efficacy was equivalent in the two groups, whereas nephrotoxicity was 5% (once-daily dosing) versus 24% (thrice-daily dosing). No differences were noted in ototoxicity. The authors concluded that once-daily dosing for this population was as effective and less nephrotoxic than the standard treatment regimen.*

## 76. ANTIMICROBIAL-ASSOCIATED COLITIS

Gastrointestinal side effects frequently complicate antimicrobial therapy. Of the adverse effects, diarrhea and an occasionally lethal pseudomembranous colitis have been the subject of numerous reports. Pseudomembranous colitis occurred in the pre-antimicrobial era, usually as a complication of an abdominal operation.

In 1977, based on studies in a hamster model, it was reported that clindamycin-associated colitis was caused by a toxin-producing organism, *Clostridium difficile*. Most cases of antimicrobial-associated diarrhea can be classified as *C. difficile*-associated or idiopathic. The role of other pathogens, such as *Candida albicans*, as a cause of antimicrobial-associated, *C. difficile*-negative disease requires more evidence.

Nearly all patients with *C. difficile* disease report use of an antimicrobial within the prior 6 weeks. Almost all antimicrobials have been implicated in cases of *C. difficile* disease; those most commonly involved are the cephalosporins, ampicillin or amoxicillin, and clindamycin. Most cases (total numbers) are associated with cephalosporin use, although the incidence rates are probably highest following clindamycin. Rarely, some antineoplastic drugs have been involved, such as fluorouracil and methotrexate. *C. difficile* should be considered as a cause of both community-acquired and nosocomial diarrhea; this organism is the most frequent cause of nosocomial diarrhea. In the hospital setting, numerous outbreaks of diarrhea as well as sporadic cases have been associated with *C. difficile*. The organism has been recovered from the hands of hospital personnel, and transmission via the hands appears to be an important mode of spread from patient to patient. In one study, use of vinyl gloves was associated with a fivefold decline in the incidence of *C. difficile* diarrhea.

*C. difficile* is an anaerobic gram-positive rod. Disease is localized to the colon. Pseudomembranes consisting of fibrin, mucus, epithelial cells, and leukocytes may be present adhering to the underlying mucosa. Only 3% of healthy adults will be culture-positive for *C. difficile*, in contrast to colonization rates of 50% in newborns. Colitis results from toxin production by the organism. Pathogenesis appears to involve four factors: (a) alteration in the intestinal flora secondary to antimicrobial therapy, (b) presence of *C. difficile,* usually from an exogenous source but sometimes in the patient's endogenous flora, (c) presence of an organism capable of producing toxins A and B, and (d) age-related susceptibility (the illness is uncommon in children, and the elderly are at an increased risk).

The spectrum of disease ranges from asymptomatic to life-threatening. The typical patient notes profuse watery diarrhea with abdominal pain 4 to 9 days after starting to take an antimicrobial. Diarrhea may begin after the antimicrobial has been discontinued. Fever and leukocytosis are often present. Fever and abdominal pain may occur without diarrhea. Fecal leukocytes are present in about half the patients, and the stool guaiac test result may be positive. A leukemoid reaction and hypoalbuminemia may occur. If the disease is untreated, complications include toxic megacolon, colonic perforation, and shock. The death rate may be 10% in elderly debilitated patients.

The diagnosis depends on demonstrating disease by endoscopy and/or *C. difficile* toxin by specific assay. Sigmoidoscopy is adequate in 67% of cases, but in about 33% of cases, disease involves only the right side of the colon. Computed tomography may suggest the diagnosis, demonstrating a characteristic thickening of the colon. A barium enema is best avoided because of the possibility of colonic perforation. Diagnosis is usually established by demonstrating the presence of toxin B by tissue culture assay. Endoscopy may be helpful when the result of the toxin assay for *C. difficile* is negative. Results of tissue culture assays for *C. difficile* toxin are positive in 95% to 100% of patients with antimicrobial-associated pseudomembranous colitis, 15% to 25% of patients with antimicrobial-associated diarrhea without confirmed pseudomembranous colitis, 2% to 8% of patients with antimicrobial exposure without diarrhea, and none of healthy adults. False-negatives occur in about 10% of patients. Stool culture for *C. difficile* is available but is used mainly for epidemiologic studies. Other available tests include a latex particle agglutination test, enzyme immunoassays, polymerase chain reaction, and a dot immunobinding assay. The latex agglutination test lacks the sensitivity (60%) of the tissue culture assay but has a specificity of 96%. One enzyme immunoassay had a sensitivity of 85%, in comparison with 94% for the tissue culture assay. The specificity of the enzyme immunoassay was excellent (98%). Further data are needed to define the role of the dot immunobinding assay and polymerase chain reaction in the diagnosis.

Therapy for antimicrobial-associated colitis consists of stopping the implicated antimicrobial and providing supportive care. If an antimicrobial is still needed to treat the underlying infection, an agent should be selected that is infrequently associated with this disease, such as a quinolone or an aminoglycoside. Although data are lacking, avoid use of a cephalosporin, ampicillin, or clindamycin. Oral vancomycin (125 mg four times daily) or metronidazole (500 mg thrice daily) should be selected for patients with severe disease. Some patients with mild-to-moderate disease will respond if the implicated antimicrobial is discontinued and supportive therapy with fluids is provided. An advantage of metronidazole is its low cost. Treatment should be given usually for 7 to 10 days. Antidiarrheal agents must be avoided because they promote toxin retention in the colon. Corticosteroids are not indicated. Patients who are unable to take oral vancomycin should receive it by nasogastric tube. For patients who cannot take oral medications, parenteral metronidazole should be given along with oral vancomycin via a nasogastric tube or by a long tube. More data are needed on the optimal management of patients who cannot take oral medications. Most patients respond to oral vancomycin with defervescence within 24 hours and a reduction in diarrhea and abdominal cramps within 4 to 5 days. Response is poorer in patients with a toxic megacolon or other causes of an ileus.

Approximately 20% of patients will relapse within 4 weeks of completing therapy. Most relapses occur within 3 to 10 days after discontinuation of therapy. The frequency of relapse is the same whether vancomycin or metronidazole is used as initial therapy. Relapse does not depend on the duration of treatment, and repeated toxin assays are not indicated. Treatment of patients who relapse with oral vancomycin or metronidazole is usually effective. Bartlett has suggested two regimens for patients who have multiple relapses: (a) vancomycin plus rifampin for 10 to 14 days, or

(b) vancomycin or metronidazole orally for 10 to 14 days followed by a 3-week course of cholestyramine, or cholestyramine plus lactobacilli, or vancomycin orally every other day. Other methods to restore the normal colon flora include administration of *Saccharomyces boulardii* orally for 1 month or of *Lactobacillus* preparations. (N.M.G.)

## Bibliography

Bartlett JG. The 10 most common questions about *Clostridium difficile*-associated diarrhea/colitis. *Infect Dis Clin Pract* 1992;1:254.
*Answers to questions regarding* C. difficile *issues.*

Bartlett JG. *Clostridium difficile* infection: pathophysiology and diagnosis. *Semin Gastrointest Dis* 1997;8:12–21.
*A review of diagnostic tests for the detection of* C. difficile *toxins. Latex particle agglutination lacks sensitivity, and enzyme-linked immunosorbent assays and dot immunoblot assays may have a role in rapid diagnosis.*

Bartlett JG, et al. Antibiotic-associated pseudomembranous colitis due to toxin-producing clostridia. *N Engl J Med* 1978;298:531.
*A toxin-producing clostridial species* (C. difficile) *resistant to clindamycin is the likely cause of antimicrobial-associated pseudomembranous colitis.*

Climo MW, et al. Hospital-wide restriction of clindamycin: effect on the incidence of *Clostridium difficile*-associated diarrhea and cost. *Ann Intern Med* 1998;128:989–995.
*Use of other antibiotics with anaerobic activity, such as cefotetan, ticarcillin-clavulanate, and imipenem-cilastatin, and a decreased use of clindamycin were associated with a decreased incidence of* C. difficile *diarrhea.*

DiPersio JR, et al. Development of a rapid enzyme immunoassay for *Clostridium difficile* toxin A and its use in the diagnosis of *C. difficile*-associated disease. *J Clin Microbiol* 1991;29:2724.
*A direct enzyme immunoassay test for* C. difficile *toxin A had a sensitivity of 85% and specificity of 98%. Results were available in 2.5 hours, compared with 24 to 48 hours for the tissue culture assay for toxin.*

Do AN, et al. Risk factors for early recurrent *Clostridium difficile*-associated diarrhea. *Clin Infect Dis* 1998;26:954–959.
*Relapse is more common than reinfection. Risk factors for relapse include a history of renal insufficiency and leukocytosis (cell count* $\geq 15,000/mm^3$*).*

Fekety R. Guidelines for the diagnosis and management of *Clostridium difficile*-associated diarrhea and colitis. *Am J Gastroenterol* 1997;92:739–750.
*Review. Unnecessary use of antibiotics should be avoided within the first 2 months after treatment of an episode of* C. difficile *infection.*

Fekety R, et al. Recurrent *Clostridium difficile* diarrhea: characteristics of and risk factors for patients enrolled in a prospective, randomized, double-blinded trial. *Clin Infect Dis* 1997;24:324–333.
*Factors associated with recurrent* C. difficile *disease included (a) onset of initial disease in the spring, (b) prior episodes of* C. difficile *disease, (c) use of antibiotics for another infection during or shortly after the* C. difficile *episode, (d) female sex, and (e) certain strains of* C. difficile.

Fishman EK, et al. Pseudomembranous colitis: CT evaluation of 26 cases. *Radiology* 1991;180:57.
*The computed tomographic findings are nonspecific and demonstrate an increase in bowel wall thickness with the "accordion sign."*

George RH, Symonds JM, Dimock F. Identification of *Clostridium difficile* as a cause of pseudomembranous colitis. *Br Med J* 1978;1:695.
C. difficile *was isolated from the stools of patients with pseudomembranous colitis.*

Gerding DN, et al. *Infect Control Hosp Epidemiol* 1995;16:459–477.
*A review of the diagnosis, epidemiology, infection control, and treatment of* C. difficile *disease. Testing stools of asymptomatic patients for* C. difficile, *including testing for cure, is not indicated.*

Ho M, et al. Increased incidence of *Clostridium difficile*-associated diarrhea following decreased restriction of antibiotic use. *Clin Infect Dis* 1996;23(Suppl 1):S102–S106.
C. difficile *disease increased after broad-spectrum antibiotics were removed from formulary restriction status.*

Hutin Y, Casin I, Lesprit P, et al. Prevalence of and risk factors for *Clostridium difficile* colonization at admission to an infectious diseases ward. *Clin Infect Dis* 1997; 920–924.
*Clostridium difficile was detected in the stool of 13% of patients on admission and was usually related to use of antibiotics in the prior month.*
Jacobs J, et al. *Eur J Clin Microbiol Infect Dis* 1996;15:561–566.
*In hospitalized patients with fewer than six stools per day, the prevalence of* C. difficile *is low (3%); in patients with more than six stools per day, the yield is 27%.*
Johnson S, Gerding DN. *Clostridium difficile*-associated diarrhea. *Clin Infect Dis* 1998;26:1027–1036.
*Review. The pathogenesis of* C. difficile *colitis involves exogenous acquisition of the organism and antibiotic exposure.*
Johnson S, et al. Prospective, controlled study of vinyl glove use to interrupt *Clostridium difficile* nosocomial transmission. *Am J Med* 1990;88:137.
*Hand carriage of* C. difficile *by hospital personnel is an important means of spread of this organism. The use of vinyl gloves can reduce the incidence of disease.*
Johnson S, et al. Treatment of asymptomatic *Clostridium difficile* carriers (fecal excretors) with vancomycin or metronidazole. *Ann Intern Med* 1992;117:297.
*Asymptomatic excretion of* C. difficile *should not be treated.*
Katz DA, Lynch ME, Littenberg B. Clinical prediction rules to optimize cytotoxin testing for *Clostridium difficile* in hospitalized patients with diarrhea. *Am J Med* 1996;100:487–495.
*Patients without a history of antibiotic use within the past month and without either diarrhea (at least three watery stools) or abdominal pain are unlikely to have a positive result on* C. difficile *toxin assay.*
Keighly MRB, et al. Randomized controlled trial of vancomycin for pseudomembranous colitis and postoperative diarrhea. *Br Med J* 1978;2:1667.
*Oral vancomycin (125 mg every 6 hours) was effective for pseudomembranous colitis caused by toxigenic strains of* C. difficile.
Kelly CP, LaMont JT. *Clostridium difficile* infection. *Annu Rev Med* 1998;49:375–390.
*Review. Response usually occurs within 3 days after start of therapy.*
Kreutzer EW, Milligan FD. Treatment of antibiotic-associated pseudomembranous colitis with cholestyramine resin. *Johns Hopkins Med J* 1978;143:67.
*Cholestyramine (4 g thrice daily), an anion-binding resin that may bind the toxin, was effective in 12 patients with pseudomembranous colitis.*
Lemann F, et al. Arbitrary primed PCR rules out *Clostridium difficile* cross-infection among patients in a haematology unit. *J Hosp Infect* 1997;35:107–115.
*Polymerase chain reaction can be helpful to type strains in the evaluation of an outbreak.*
Manabe YC, et al. *Clostridium difficile* colitis: an efficient clinical approach to diagnosis. *Ann Intern Med* 1995;123:835–840.
*Predictors of a positive* C. difficile *toxin assay included a positive fecal leukocyte test, semiformed stool, use of a cephalosporin, and onset of diarrhea 6 days after start of antibiotic therapy.*
McFarland LV, et al. Nosocomial acquisition of *Clostridium difficile* infection. *N Engl J Med* 1989;320:204.
*Fifty-nine percent of health care workers had a positive hand culture for* C. difficile *after contact with an infected patient.*
Renshaw AA, Stelling JM, Doolittle MH. The lack of value of repeated *Clostridium difficile* cytotoxicity assays. *Arch Pathol Lab Med* 1996:120:49–52.
*In only 1% of cases was a repeated* C. difficile *toxin assay useful if performed within a 7-day period.*
Rifkin GD, et al. Antibiotic-induced colitis: implication of a toxin neutralized by *Clostridium sordellii* antitoxin. *Lancet* 1977;2:1103.
*A clostridial toxin was isolated from two patients with pseudomembranous colitis. Oral vancomycin (500 mg every 6 hours) was given for 10 days, with resolution of the illness.*
Salcedo J, et al. Intravenous immunoglobulin therapy for severe *Clostridium difficile* colitis. *Gut* 1997;41:366–370.
*IV immunoglobulin may have a role in patients with* C. difficile *colitis who fail standard antibiotic therapy.*

Stanley RJ, Melson GL, Tedesco FJ. The spectrum of radiographic findings in anti-
biotic-related pseudomembranous colitis. *Radiology* 1974;111:519.
*Plaquelike mucosal lesions on barium enema are highly suggestive.*
Tedesco FJ, Barton RW, Alpers DH. Clindamycin-associated colitis: a prospective
study. *Ann Intern Med* 1974;81:429.
*The authors noted a 21% incidence of diarrhea and a 10% incidence of pseudomem-
branous colitis in patients receiving clindamycin.*

# 77. PERIOPERATIVE ANTIMICROBIAL PROPHYLAXIS

Infections following surgical procedures are a major cause of morbidity and occasional
mortality. Currently, postoperative wound infections represent up to 24% of all nosocomial infections, prolong hospital stay by 7 to 14 days, and cost in excess of $1 billion
annually. Another way of viewing such data is that 2% to 3% of all surgical procedures
are complicated by infection, resulting in more than 3,000 deaths annually. The majority of postoperative wounds harbor bacteria in low counts. The role of antibiotics is to
reduce the likelihood of bacterial proliferation. These agents have been demonstrated
to decrease the likelihood of infection following selected types of surgery; however,
their indiscriminate use may result in emergence of resistant pathogens, increased
costs, adverse reactions, and a false sense of security.

Asepsis and good surgical technique still remain cornerstones in the prevention of
wound infection. The cleanliness of the operating room environment, adequacy of preoperative skin preparation, judicious shaving, level of activity in the operating room,
and duration of both preoperative hospitalization and surgical procedure are other
potential factors. Patient factors such as poor nutrition, diabetes mellitus, old age,
remote foci of infection, and lack of immunologic integrity can contribute greatly to the
risk for wound infection. As an example, the presence of a remote focus of infection
may increase the risk of postoperative infection fourfold.

## Classification of Surgical Procedures

Surgical procedures have historically been classified as clean (class 1), clean/contam-
inated (class 2), contaminated (class 3), and dirty/infected (class 4). Table 77-1 defines
and gives examples of procedures within each class. In general, a major break in asepsis moves a procedure into the next higher class. Such a classification of procedures
has been useful to help define anticipated postoperative infection rates. Clean operations are generally associated with infection rates below 2%. Clean/contaminated procedures performed without prophylaxis have historically been associated with wound
infection rates higher than 8%, and often much higher. Factors within class 1 and
2 procedures that are associated with a higher likelihood of infection include abdominal surgery, surgery lasting more than 2 hours, and the presence of more than three
underlying diseases. The other classes are associated with infection rates above 30%;
in these situations, the administration of antimicrobial agents should be considered
therapeutic. Factored into this classification should be categorization based on three
independent factors established by the Centers for Disease Control and Prevention as
important in the likelihood of postoperative wound infection. These are as follows:
American Society of Anesthesiology (ASA) score of at least 3, duration of surgery
beyond a given length of time for each surgical procedure, and class 3 or 4 surgery.
Based on these criteria (scores of 0 to 3), the risk for infection increases from less than
2% to 13%. Thus, a patient with multiple comorbidities (ASA class 3 or greater) for
whom prolonged surgery is anticipated may benefit from antibiotic prophylaxis even
if undergoing class 1 surgery.

Parenteral antimicrobials have been used for perioperative prophylaxis for several
decades; however, only since the early 1980s have well-designed and controlled studies been performed that document efficacy in selected situations. Factors to be con-

Table 77-1. Classification of surgical procedures

| Class | Definition | Examples |
|---|---|---|
| 1. **Clean** | Nontraumatic, un-infected procedure without surgical procedural breaks; no entry into gastrointestinal, respiratory, or genitourinary tracts. | Thyroidectomy, laminectomy, herniorrhaphy, breast surgery |
| 2. **Clean/contaminated** | Entry into gastrointestinal, respiratory, or genitourinary tracts under controlled conditions without unusual contamination. Wounds may be mechanically drained. | Appendectomy, hysterectomy, elective colorectal surgery, most elective biliary tract procedures |
| 3/4. **Contaminated/dirty** | Surgery with overt spillage of gastrointestinal contents, open traumatic wounds, entry into infected biliary, gastrointestinal, or genitourinary tracts. | Perforated diverticulitis, ruptured appendix, drainage of intra-abdominal abscess, repair of open compound fracture |

sidered in prophylaxis include timing, duration, choice of agent, type of surgical procedure, and cost.

Animal studies performed by Burke in 1961 and subsequently corroborated by human investigations demonstrate the importance of the timing of the initial dose. Antimicrobial agents administered postoperatively (i.e., after contamination has occurred) or more than 2 hours preoperatively give no greater protection than placebo. Most experts now recommend that therapy be initiated 30 minutes before skin incision so that adequate tissue levels have been achieved when tissues are incised. This can be conveniently performed by anesthesiology within the operating suite during other surgical preparations. Levels should be maintained throughout the procedure, but prolonging them beyond this has not been proved necessary; it may increase costs, encourage the emergence of resistant organisms, and increase adverse reactions without decreasing morbidity. Recent studies show the benefit of single-dose perioperative antimicrobial prophylaxis for many surgical procedures, including biliary tract and vaginal hysterectomy. No well-performed investigations have demonstrated enhanced efficacy with multiple-dose regimens.

The agent chosen for prophylaxis should be safe and effective against most anticipated pathogens. To utilize agents most effectively, clinicians must know about the likely postoperative pathogens in their institution. Of especial importance are data regarding the risk for infection with methicillin-resistant *Staphylococcus aureus* or methicillin-resistant *Staphylococcus epidermidis,* as a risk for these pathogens requires increased prophylactic use of vancomycin (with the attendant risks for immediate complications and potential for emergence of vancomycin-resistant *Enterococcus faecium*). The pharmacokinetic properties of the agent employed should allow availability throughout the procedure. Cefazolin, the agent most commonly used, can be given as a single preoperative 1-g dose for procedures lasting under 4 hours. For prolonged procedures, a second dose may be given at about 4 hours. Alternatively, some experts recommend use of an agent with an extended half-life (e.g., cefotetan, ceftriaxone) when surgery is anticipated to extend beyond this length of time. Some authorities also recommend that antimicrobials used for treatment of established infections not be routinely used for prophylaxis.

The role of prophylaxis for clean surgical procedures is controversial. With most of these, infection rates are low, and large numbers of patients would have to receive antimicrobials to prevent small numbers of infections. However, when large numbers of patients have been studied, benefits have been shown for several apparently low-risk procedures (e.g., herniorrhaphy), and patients undergoing some types of breast surgery. Patients with implantation of hardware or grafts and cardiac surgery patients should receive prophylaxis. Additional clean procedures in which prophylaxis should be employed include those lasting more than 4 hours, procedures in patients with distant foci of infection, and procedures in insulin-dependent diabetics. In the presence of these risks, infection rates approach 8%—approximately 300% more than in patients undergoing similar procedures without such risks.

Clean/contaminated surgical procedures benefit the most from antimicrobial prophylaxis, and in general perioperative prophylaxis represents a standard of care. Risks for infection from selected procedures may decline from above 15% to well below 8%.

## Specific Procedures
### Biliary Tract Surgery
Cholelithiasis is associated with the presence of bacteria in bile in more than 50% of patients. The organisms most commonly identified are *Escherichia coli, Klebsiella* and *Proteus* species, and *Enterococcus faecalis*. Risk factors for postoperative infection are age over 70 years, cholelithiasis, jaundice, and positive bile cultures. In general, agents active against the common gram-negative enteric bacteria have proved effective. These include trimethoprim-sulfamethoxazole and cefazolin. For high-risk patients, 1 g of cefazolin is recommended. Trimethoprim-sulfamethoxazole is a reasonable alternative.

### Colorectal Surgery
Antimicrobial prophylaxis should always be used for this surgery. Patients given oral antimicrobials as well as cleansing enemas had decreased rates of postoperative wound infection when compared with controls given only vigorous purgation; however, recent limitations on length of preoperative stay may impede the ability to perform satisfactory bowel cleansing. Oral neomycin plus erythromycin decreased wound infection rates from 43% to 9% in comparison studies. Similar results have been achieved with metronidazole and doxycycline. A standardized regimen for oral prophylaxis is given in Table 77-2.

The value of additional parenteral antimicrobials remains controversial. One study demonstrated that cefoxitin decreased infection rates from 18.3% to 6.6%. Many clinicians now add either a single preoperative dose of cefotetan or cefoxitin to a bowel preparation including nonabsorbable antimicrobials.

When emergency colorectal operations must be performed on an unprepared bowel, the likelihood of fecal soilage is great. In this event, parenteral antimicrobial prophylaxis should be initiated. Cefoxitin or cefotetan are reasonable choices. Follow-up treatment depends on surgical findings. Gross spillage necessitates continuing antimicrobials for therapeutic reasons, but if no evidence of bowel perforation is noted, these agents can be discontinued.

### Obstetric and Gynecologic Surgery
Patients undergoing vaginal hysterectomy benefit most from parenteral antimicrobial prophylaxis. Surgical wound infection rates decline from between 20% and 40% to between 4% and 8%. Cefazolin has been the most frequently studied antimicrobial and is considered the agent of choice. Other agents with proven effectiveness are ampicillin and cefoxitin. Single-dose prophylaxis is sufficient.

Data for abdominal hysterectomy and cesarean section are less conclusive. For the former, antimicrobials as diverse as cefazolin and metronidazole have demonstrated statistically significant decreases in pelvic and wound infections. However, mechanical methods, such as closed suction drainage, may be equally effective. Patients under-

Table 77-2. Bowel preparation for elective colorectal operations

| | |
|---|---|
| Two days before surgery | Low-residue or liquid diet<br>Magnesium citrate (30 mL of 50% solution) at 10 a.m., 2 p.m., and 6 p.m.<br>Fleet Enema in evening until clear |
| One day before surgery | Clear liquid diet<br>Magnesium citrate ×2, or whole-gut lavage with polyethylene glycol electrolyte solution, 1L/h × 2–4 h until clear (before use of oral antibiotics)<br>Neomycin-erythromycin, 1 g each at 1 p.m., 2 p.m., and 11 p.m. |
| Day of surgery | Operate early a.m.<br>Appropriate parenteral antibiotic (generally cefoxitin or cefotetan) 30 min before initiation of surgery |

Adapted from Nichols RL. Prophylaxis for surgical infections. In: Gorbach SL, Bartlett JG, Blacklow NR, eds. *Infectious diseases,* 2nd ed. Philadelphia: WB Saunders, 1988: 470–480.

going cesarean sections should be given prophylaxis if the procedures are unscheduled or associated with prolonged rupture of membranes. The timing of prophylaxis in cesarean sections remains controversial. Some clinicians administer the drug after cord clamping to reduce the possibility of antimicrobial transfer to the neonate.

Cost-benefit analyses of the use of cefazolin in both vaginal and abdominal hysterectomies demonstrate the importance of antimicrobial prophylaxis in both of these procedures. Costs were reduced by $1,777 and $716, respectively, and for vaginal and abdominal procedures, wound infection rates declined from 21.4% to 2.3% and from 21.1% to 14.1%, respectively. The authors report that savings would be substantially higher if more expensive drugs or prolonged prophylaxis had been utilized. A single IV dose of 1 g of cefazolin, therefore, appears to be a prudent choice for antimicrobial prophylaxis in most obstetric and gynecologic operations. (R.B.B.)

### Bibliography

Classen DC, et al. The timing of prophylactic administration of antibiotics and the risk of surgical-wound infection. *N Engl J Med* 1992;326:281–286.
*Approximately 2,800 patients were prospectively monitored to determine the relationship of postoperative wound infection to the timing of antimicrobial prophylaxis. Rates of infection were statistically higher when prophylaxis was initiated either more than 2 hours preoperatively or postoperatively. The authors could not differentiate between groups that were given a first dose just before surgery or intraoperatively. This large clinical study confirms many animal data.*
Cruse PJE, Foord R. The epidemiology of wound infections: a 10-year prospective study of 62,939 wounds. *Surg Clin North Am* 1980;60:27–40.
*The authors prospectively followed more than 60,000 surgical wounds during a 10-year period. The survey included telephone follow-up with patients at 28 days. There was a direct relationship between surgical wound class and risk for postoperative infection. The rate for clean procedures was 1.5%, and for class 4 procedures, 40%. Infection prolonged hospital stay by an average of 10 days. The authors conclude that wound infections can be decreased by such factors as shortened hospital stay, preoperative hexachlorophene shower, minimal shaving, excellent surgical technique, and expeditious surgery.*
DiPiro JT, et al. Single-dose systemic antibiotic prophylaxis of surgical wound infections. *Am J Surg* 1986;152:552–559.
*The authors critically evaluate the available literature on single-dose antimicrobial prophylaxis in surgery. Data are broken out by type of study and surgical procedure.*

*Approximately 40 studies were identified, and in no instance was single-dose prophylaxis demonstrated to be inferior to a multiple-dose regimen.*

Haley RW, et al. Identifying patients at high risk of surgical wound infection. *Am J Epidemiol* 1985;121:206–215.

*Information concerning more than 59,000 surgical patients was analyzed to establish risks for postoperative infections. Factors associated with postoperative infection included abdominal operation, surgical procedure longer than 2 hours, class 3 or 4 surgery, and diagnosis of more than three underlying conditions. Addition of factors other than surgical class identified at least twice as many infections.*

Hirschmann JV, Inui TS. Antimicrobial prophylaxis: a critique of recent trials. *Rev Infect Dis* 1980;2:1–23.

*Although somewhat dated and not limited to prophylaxis in surgery, this excellent article critically assesses published literature concerning antimicrobial prophylaxis. It depicts problems in study design that accompany many investigations and reviews data based on individual types of surgical procedures. It is one of the first reviews that demonstrate the value of short-course (often single-dose) prophylaxis.*

Kaiser AB. Antimicrobial prophylaxis in surgery. *N Engl J Med* 1986;315:1129–1137.

*This review article presents historical data and criteria for study design and assessment and recommendations for antimicrobial prophylaxis by type of surgery in tabular form.*

Martin CE, the French Study Group on Antimicrobial Prophylaxis in Surgery, the French Society of Anesthesia and Intensive Care. Antimicrobial prophylaxis in surgery: general concepts and clinical guidelines. *Infect Control Hosp Epidemiol* 1994;15:463–471.

*The authors review basic principles of antibiotic prophylaxis in surgery and present recommendations for numerous specific procedures. They spend much time describing the ideal antibiotic, which of course does not exist.*

The Medical Letter. Antimicrobial prophylaxis in surgery. *Med Lett Drugs Ther* 1997; 39:97–102.

*The latest in a series of recommendations from this group of experts seeking to update us on the most recent recommendations. They continue to conclude that cefazolin remains the agent of choice for most procedures. Cefoxitin or cefotetan is sensible for colorectal or appendiceal procedures. Routine vancomycin use should be discouraged. Recommendations for numerous procedures are provided.*

Nichols RL. Prophylaxis for surgical infections. In: Gorbach SL, Bartlett JG, Blacklow NR, eds. *Infectious diseases*, 2nd ed. Philadelphia: WB Saunders, 1998:470–480.

*Dr. Nichols presents an excellent overview of the rationale, indications, and antibiotic choices for perioperative prophylaxis. Cephalosporins remain the mainstay of antibiotic prophylaxis, unless resistance issues in particular hospitals or specific operations are recognized.*

Nichols RL, et al. Current practices of preoperative bowel preparation among North American colorectal surgeons. *Clin Infect Dis* 1997;24:609–619.

*The authors sent questionnaires to more than 800 colorectal surgeons and received responses from 58%. All utilized some form of mechanical bowel preparation. Almost 90% also utilized antibiotics (the majority both oral and parenteral). The most common regimen was a combination of oral neomycin plus either metronidazole or erythromycin plus a parenteral antibiotic.*

Platt R, et al. Perioperative antibiotic prophylaxis for herniorrhaphy and breast surgery. *N Engl J Med* 1990;322:153–160.

*This important investigation validates the concept that patients with "clean" surgery, unassociated with implants or other major risks, may benefit from antimicrobial prophylaxis. In this study, ceforanide was employed versus placebo in more than 1,200 patients undergoing herniorrhaphy or breast surgery. For both surgical procedures, postoperative wound infection was less likely to develop in patients who received antimicrobial prophylaxis. It remains uncertain whether all patients undergoing clean surgical procedures would benefit similarly.*

Shapiro M, et al. Risk factors for infection at the operative site after abdominal or vaginal hysterectomy. *N Engl J Med* 1982;307:1661–1666.

*Three hundred women undergoing vaginal hysterectomy and 1,125 women undergoing abdominal hysterectomy were prospectively followed to determine factors associated with postoperative surgical wound infections. Longer duration of surgery, young age, lack of antimicrobial prophylaxis, and abdominal approach were associated with infection. The effect of antimicrobial prophylaxis diminished significantly with prolonged surgery, being unmeasurable after 3 hours. This is one of the few studies demonstrating the importance of antimicrobial availability throughout the surgical procedure, which has important implications for other forms of surgery.*

Ulualp K, Condon RE. Antibiotic prophylaxis for scheduled operative procedures. *Infect Dis Clin North Am* 1992;6:613–625.

*A contemporary review that includes information on normal flora of various body areas and antimicrobial pharmacokinetics. Recommends specific antimicrobials for various types of procedures.*

## 78. ANTIFUNGAL CHEMOTHERAPY

Fungi are an important cause of human infection. Some, such as *Histoplasma capsulatum* and *Coccidioides immitis,* are indigenous to selected geographic areas and are unlikely to be contracted by persons who do not live or travel there. Others, including *Candida* species and *Cryptococcus neoformans,* are more universally distributed and are seen primarily in patients with selected forms of immunosuppression or exposure to broad-spectrum antibiotics. Patients with HIV/AIDS are especially predisposed to infection by these fungi, with various clinical presentations. Numerous antifungal agents have been approved, and Table 78-1 provides typical dosages for many of them. However, data on efficacy, safety, and dosing, as well as on the necessary length of treatment, are much less well established than for most antibacterial agents. Reports of carefully controlled, prospective, and blinded studies are few, and problems regarding the use of most of the antifungals are complicated further by a lack of standards for susceptibility testing and blood level determinations.

### Classes of Antifungal Drugs

Antifungal agents can be grouped into several classes. The *polyenes,* which include amphotericin B, nystatin, and candicidin, are characterized by the presence of a hydrophilic region and four to seven double bonds. None is absorbed well after oral administration, and all are considered to be relatively toxic when parenterally administered. Additionally, all are poorly soluble in aqueous solvents. The mechanism of action, probably through binding to fungal ergosterol (a component of the fungal cell wall), allows for the formation of channels within the fungal cell membrane, with a resultant loss of vital elements. Lack of binding characterizes the occasionally resistant organism, such as *Candida lusitaniae.*

The *azoles* (imidazoles and triazoles) include miconazole, terconazole, fluconazole ketoconazole, and econazole. Imidazoles differ from triazoles by having two (rather than three) nitrogen atoms in the five-member azole ring. The triazole configuration increases tissue penetration, prolongs half-life, and enhances efficacy while decreasing toxicity. Unlike polyenes, which are active primarily against systemic mycoses, azoles are also effective against dermatophytes. The mechanism of action is through inhibition of intracellular cytochrome P-450, which is required for demethylation of the ergosterol precursor lanosterol and is generally fungistatic.

### Specific Drugs

*Amphotericin B*

Amphotericin B is the standard treatment for disseminated fungal infections, against which all other agents and combinations are judged. It is active against virtually all pathogenic fungi, although occasional resistance and tolerance are encountered. Pharmacokinetically, the drug is poorly absorbed after oral administration, and it must be given intravenously for systemic infections. Its lack of absorption has made ampho-

Table 78-1. Dosages of commonly employed antifungal agents

| Agent | Dosage |
|-------|--------|
| *Intravenous* | |
| Amphotericin B deoxycholate | 0.3–1.5 mg/kg per day |
| Liposomal amphotericin B | 3–5 mg/kg |
| Miconazole | 600–800 mg q8h |
| Fluconazole | 200–800 mg first dose, then 100–400 mg q24h |
| *Oral* | |
| Flucytosine | 150 mg/kg per day (four divided doses) |
| Fluconazole | 100–200 mg/d |
| Ketoconazole | 200 mg/d |
| Itraconazole (capsules) | 200–400 mg/d |
| Itraconazole (liquid) | 100 mg bid |
| Amphotericin B (liquid) | 100–500 qid |
| Griseofulvin | 500 mg qd or bid |

tericin B a useful component for bowel decontamination or treatment of candidal overgrowth syndromes in selected clinical situations. After parenteral administration, less than 5% is recovered in urine, and only 40% can be found in serum and other fluids. The remainder is presumably absorbed by cell membranes and is then slowly released during prolonged periods. The drug can be detected for more than 8 weeks after commonly employed dosages. Blood levels of amphotericin B are typically below 2 μg/mL, an amount barely greater than the minimum inhibitory concentrations required for many of the fungi treated with this compound. The drug penetrates poorly into body fluids other than serum, and cerebrospinal fluid levels have been demonstrated to be only about 2% to 3% of simultaneous serum levels. Nevertheless, occasional cures of central nervous system infections, such as cryptococcal meningitis, have been effected with this drug.

The solubility of amphotericin B is poor, and it is marketed with deoxycholate to ensure colloidal dispersion. It must be reconstituted with sterile water and then added to 5% dextrose in water (5% D/W) in an amount sufficient to provide a final concentration of 0.1 mg/mL. This formulation cannot be mixed with other solutions, and other compounds should not be admixed. It is no longer necessary to cover the bottle with a paper bag during administration. A 22-mm filter causes partial retention of the agent and should be avoided.

Amphotericin B is administered in doses of 0.5 to 0.7 mg/kg per day. Doses of 1.0 to 1.5 mg/kg per day have been employed for disseminated aspergillosis and meningeal fungal infections. Larger doses are associated with enhanced toxicity without increased efficacy. Normally, a test dose of 1 mg in 50 to 200 mL of 5% D/W is given over 1 to 2 hours to prevent possible anaphylaxis. If the agent is tolerated, the dose is increased to up to 0.5 mg/kg per day, usually administered in 500 mL of 5% D/W over 4 to 6 hours. In most cases, the maximum daily dose is 50 mg. Generally, dose escalation is at a rate of 0.1 to 0.3 mg/kg per day, although this can be increased for severe disease. Generally, dosage modification for renal dysfunction is not needed. Although anecdotal reports of successful infusions lasting fewer than 4 to 6 hours have been published, occasionally severe adverse reactions, including cardiac arrest, have occurred with more rapid administration. Alternatively, the drug may be administered on alternate days with double the usual daily dose. This is especially useful for outpatients. The length of treatment depends on the disease. Under many circumstances, it may be necessary to render therapy for several months. Amphotericin B may be utilized in selected cases of mucosal disease and has been employed widely for patients with HIV/AIDS-related stomatitis and esophagitis. Dosage in these situations is generally 0.3 to 0.5 mg/kg, with total doses as low as 200 to 300 mg. Although most cases of this disease are now treated with oral antifungals, selected cases may still require this form of management. In unusual circumstances, amphotericin B can be administered by alternative routes. As an example, selected cases of *C. immitis* meningitis may benefit from intrathecal therapy. Intraarticular regimens of less than 15 mg per dose have been employed for selected fungal arthritides.

Adverse reactions to amphotericin B are common and may be severe. This compound is considered to be a rather toxic agent and should be administered by persons comfortable with its use. Chills, fever, and hypotension may be encountered, especially early in therapy. Such problems usually subside as medication is continued. Concurrent administration of hydrocortisone within the bottle may be beneficial. Premedication with 1 g of acetaminophen or salicylic acid, 30 to 45 minutes before infusion of amphotericin, is also useful. Nephrotoxicity is the most significant side effect of this agent and occurs in up to 80% of cases. Elevations of serum creatinine to 2 to 3 mg/dL are routinely noted and may necessitate intermittent discontinuation of the drug. There is often evidence of tubular disease, and proximal renal tubular acidosis may be observed. Renal vasoconstriction and abnormalities of glomerular filtration may also be important. Maintenance of adequate fluid and sodium loading may prove protective. Significant decreases in serum potassium may also be observed with amphotericin B. Profound hypokalemia may occur when amphotericin B is given with other drugs that may also cause this effect.

Anemia is routinely observed and is thought to be secondary to either bone marrow suppression or inhibition of erythropoietin production. Thrombocytopenia or neutropenia rarely occurs, and aplastic anemia has not been reported. Adult respiratory distress syndrome has been reported when amphotericin B is used with granulocyte transfusion. The etiology may be related to lysis of aggregates of transfused granulocytes that are trapped in the pulmonary parenchyma.

An oral suspension of amphotericin B (100 mg/mL) has recently become available, with use primarily targeted at HIV/AIDS patients. The recommended dose is 1 to 5 mL (100 to 500 mg) four times daily for a minimum of 2 weeks.

Several forms of liposomal amphotericin B have recently been approved by the FDA and appear to be associated with decreased nephrotoxicity and an increased capacity for dosing to at least 5 mg/kg. Table 78-2 summarizes comparative data. No one is distinctly better than the others, but any one may be the therapy of choice for invasive infections with *Aspergillus* species; use for other fungal infections is uncertain. All have the capacity to cause acute severe reactions, similar to those seen with amphotericin B, and should be administered with a test dose and dose escalation. Fortunately, many of the patients who receive the liposomal preparations will already have had experience of amphotericin B and are less likely to have acute adverse reactions. The liposomal preparations have also been recommended for use in patients with nephrotoxicity from amphotericin B. Expense precludes their routine use, and it is uncertain whether they are beneficial for most fungal infections.

*Flucytosine*

Flucytosine is a fluorinated pyrimidine related to fluorouracil; it is useful for selected candidal and cryptococcal infections. Its mechanism of action is incompletely understood but is probably related to its conversion to fluorouracil within the fungal cell. It is well absorbed from the gastrointestinal tract and penetrates into most tissues. Most of the compound is excreted in active form in the urine, with levels averaging 200 to 500 μm/mL. Peak serum values are only 70 to 80 mg/mL. Renal insufficiency (as may be seen with concurrent use of amphotericin B) may result in potentially toxic levels of flucytosine unless the dosage is regulated. The usual dosage of this drug is 150 mg/kg per day in four divided doses. The compound is supplied in either 250-mg or 500-mg tablets.

Flucytosine is relatively safe and usually well tolerated. Bone marrow depression may occur in the presence of renal dysfunction. The cause of this depression is not completely known but appears to be related to the metabolism of the parent compound to 5-fluorouracil. Suppression rarely occurs when blood levels of flucytosine are below 100 mg/mL. The presence of renal impairment necessitates dosage reduction. One method is to give a dose (37.5 mg/kg) at varying intervals depending on creatinine

Table 78-2. Liposomal amphotericin B preparations

| | Trade name | | |
| --- | --- | --- | --- |
| | Abelcet | Amphotec | AmBisome |
| FDA-approved indications* | Invasive fungal infections refractory to amphotericin B. | Invasive aspergillosis in patients intolerant of full-dose amphotericin B. | Empiric treatment of possible fungal infection in febrile neutropenics. *Aspergillus, Candida,* or *Cryptococcus* infection in patients who cannot tolerate amphotericin B. |
| Approval date (U.S.) | 1995 | 1996 | 1997 |
| Daily cost** | $693.32 (5 mg/kg daily) | $480 (4 mg/kg daily) | $1,099 (5 mg/kg daily) |

* Amphotericin B indications: progressive/invasive fungal infections including cryptococcosis, North American blastomycosis, systemic candidiasis, coccidioidomycosis, histoplasmosis, sporotrichosis, aspergillosis, mucormycosis, and several others that are less common.
** Amphotericin B daily cost (1 mg/kg daily): $33.20.

clearance (e.g., every 6 hours at more than 40 mL/min, every 12 hours at 20 to 40 mL/min, and every 24 hours at 10 to 20 mL/min). No nomogram is satisfactory for the anuric patient; however, blood levels can be measured by high-pressure liquid or gas chromatography. Flucytosine is cleared by hemodialysis or peritoneal dialysis, and a single dose of 37.5 mg/kg is recommended after each treatment. Bone marrow depression develops in about 5% of patients who receive this drug, typically anemia or neutropenia. Nausea, diarrhea, and vomiting are occasionally seen but are infrequently severe and rarely necessitate discontinuation of therapy.

The use of flucytosine as monotherapy is indicated only in selected patients with candiduria, in whom rapid achievement of high levels may preclude emergence of resistance. It is most frequently employed in combination with amphotericin B for serious cryptococcal infections. For cryptococcal meningitis in the HIV-negative patient, use of the two agents reduces the dose of amphotericin B (from 0.6 to 0.3 mg/kg) and the duration of therapy (from 10 to 6 weeks). In the presence of HIV infection, cryptococcal meningitis is not curable, and the addition of flucytosine may intensify anemia and other adverse reactions. However, some authorities recommend its use for the first 2 weeks of treatment. In a recent study of flucytosine plus fluconazole (vs. fluconazole alone) in AIDS patients with cryptococcal meningitis, survivorship was enhanced at 2 months (32% vs. 12%) and headache was decreased at 1 month in those who received the combination. Other data suggest that the combination may also be useful for the therapy of serious candidal infections. Flucytosine is not effective against infections caused by species of *Aspergillus* or *Mucor.*

*Ketoconazole*
Ketoconazole is an oral preparation active *in vitro* against *Candida, Coccidioides, Blastomyces, Histoplasma,* and most dermatophytes. The usual daily dose is 200 to 400 mg. Ketoconazole is extensively metabolized, and the dosage need not be altered in renal failure. Levels in the cerebrospinal fluid and urine are low, and the drug

should not be considered for use in infections at these sites. Orally administered keto-conazole requires gastric acid for absorption, and this product must be given with food. In achlorhydric patients, administration with 8 oz of orange juice, cola, or ginger ale will improve absorption.

Ketoconazole has been successfully used to treat candidal infections involving mucous membranes, including esophagitis. It is inferior to fluconazole for esophageal candidiasis in AIDS patients, but its early use may prove initially less expensive. Outcomes in the treatment of thrush in patients with HIV infection are similar for the two agents. Ketoconazole has also been reported useful in the management of coccidioidomycosis, histoplasmosis, cryptococcal infection (nonmeningeal), sporotrichosis, and blastomycosis. Chronic relapsing forms of coccidioidomycosis and paracoccidioidomycosis appear to be stabilized with low doses of this agent given for up to 1 year. One study has documented the efficacy and limited toxicity of high doses (up to 1,200 mg/d) in the management of fungal infections of the central nervous system.

Side effects of ketoconazole are minor, although hepatitis may occur and should be considered in patients on long-term, high-dose therapy. At least one fatal case of hepatitis caused by this drug has been reported, in a patient who was receiving only 200 mg/d for 2 months. Additionally, it may depress synthesis of both testosterone and corticosteroids, which may result in oligospermia, gynecomastia, and abnormalities of menstruation. These side effects are associated more with high daily doses than with prolonged therapy and are reversible on discontinuation of the drug.

Drug interactions are an important consideration with the use of ketoconazole. Agents that should be given with caution at the same time as ketoconazole include (but are not limited to) histamine$_2$ antagonists, rifampin, terfenadine, cisapride, didanosine, protease inhibitors, and cyclosporine.

*Fluconazole*
Fluconazole is available in both oral and IV formulations. *In vitro* activity occurs against species of *Candida, C. neoformans, H. capsulatum, C. immitis,* and *Blastomyces* species. Activity against *Aspergillus* and *Mucor* is limited. Unlike ketoconazole, it is well absorbed orally and is not affected by gastric acidity. It distributes well to tissues, and levels within inflamed meninges are 60% to 80% of those in serum. Clinically, fluconazole in doses of 100 mg daily has been successfully used for oropharyngeal and esophageal candidiasis. It is more effective than clotrimazole troches for the former and at least as effective as ketoconazole. A study employing a daily 100-mg dose of fluconazole in AIDS patients demonstrated its superiority (endoscopically and clinically) over ketoconazole (200 mg daily) for therapy of *Candida* esophagitis.

Oral fluconazole at a dosage of 200 mg/d is the agent of choice to maintain suppression of cryptococcal meningitis in AIDS patients after initial therapy with amphotericin B. If amphotericin B cannot be utilized for primary treatment, 400 mg of fluconazole per day for 8 weeks (followed by 200 mg/d for suppression) may be employed.

IV fluconazole is an important agent for the management of invasive candidal infections in seriously ill patients. Its ease of administration and excellent safety profile make it an appealing alternative to amphotericin B for disseminated candidal infections. At dosages of 400 to 800 mg/d, it appears to be as effective as amphotericin B for invasive candidiasis in critically ill patients who are not neutropenic. However, some species of *Candida* are inherently resistant to fluconazole, so epidemiologic information regarding individual hospitals is vital. A loading dose that is double the daily dose should be administered to reach steady state promptly. Amphotericin B remains the agent of choice for *Candida* endophthalmitis.

Fluconazole inhibits cytochrome P-450 hepatic enzymes. Drug interactions resulting in higher levels of warfarin (Coumadin), cyclosporine, and hydantoin, among others, have been observed. Life-threatening cardiac arrhthymias may result from the combined use of fluconazole with terfenadine or cisapride.

*Itraconazole*
Itraconazole, available as capsules or as an oral suspension, is a triazole with potent *in vitro* activity against *Candida, Cryptococcus, Aspergillus, Mucor,* and others. The oral solution has been approved for oral and esophageal candidiasis. The dosage is 100

to 200 mg/d; the solution should be vigorously swished for several seconds and swallowed. Strains of *Candida* resistant to fluconazole may remain sensitive to this agent. Adverse effects are generally minor, although a case of fatal hepatitis has been reported. Itraconazole capsules require gastric acid for absorption and should be taken with food. Acid beverages enhance absorption (see earlier section on ketoconazole). The oral solution (10 mg/mL, 150-mL bottle) has enhanced bioavailability in fasting situations. Generally, patients should not take oral solution and capsules simultaneously.

The recommended doses of itraconazole range from 100 mg/d (superficial infections) to 200 mg/d (deep-seated systemic infections). Doses of up to 400 mg daily can be employed for recalcitrant infections. The length of therapy ranges from 3 days (vaginal candidiasis) to many months.

Itraconazole appears well tolerated in patients with HIV infection and has been successfully employed both therapeutically and suppressively for cryptococcal meningitis. Similarly, it appears to be a well-tolerated and effective agent for histoplasmosis in patients with AIDS and may become the agent of choice for this disease.

*Clotrimazole*
Clotrimazole is a topical product useful in treating infections caused by both dermatophytes and *Candida albicans*. It is available as a 1% ointment, a topical solution, a lozenge, and 100- and 500-mg vaginal tablets. Because of its broad spectrum of activity, it is often employed when a specific organism has not been identified. A controlled clinical trial has demonstrated the effectiveness of clotrimazole lozenges given five times daily to treat chronic oral candidiasis; however, efficacy is less than that seen with fluconazole or ketoconazole.

*Griseofulvin*
Griseofulvin is an oral agent that is active only against dermatophytes. Therefore, an accurate diagnosis is necessary before treatment is begun. Griseofulvin is supplied as 125-mg, 250-mg, and 500-mg capsules or tablets, and peak blood levels of about 1 mg/mL are reached. The usual dosage for adults is 500 mg twice daily, and therapy should be continued for more than 4 weeks even if the infection clears before that time. For stubborn nail infections, therapy should be anticipated to last more than 3 months.

Side effects are minor and consist primarily of nausea, which may be noted in up to 15% of patients. Occasionally, neuritis and mild confusion can be noted. Hematologic and hepatic dysfunction occur rarely. Adverse drug interactions with warfarin can be seen.

*Miscellaneous Agents*
Terbinafine, a well-absorbed oral antifungal, is used in the United States primarily for the management of dermatophytes associated with onychomycosis. When administered at a dosage of 250 mg/d for fingernail or toenail onychomycosis (6 weeks or 12 weeks, respectively), it is at least as effective as griseofulvin.

Supersaturated potassium iodide is employed for the management of lymphocutaneous sporotrichosis. The drug is given orally, and treatment is initiated with a dose of 5 drops mixed in a liquid three times daily. The dose is increased by up to 4 drops per day to a maximum of 120 drops per day. If treatment is continued for several months, supersaturated potassium iodide is effective and may preclude the need for harsher regimens. Toxicity is manifested by gastrointestinal upset or increased lacrimation or salivation. An acneiform rash may be noted at any stage of therapy and is generally not considered a reason to discontinue treatment. (R.B.B.)

## Bibliography
Anaissie EJ, et al. Fluconazole versus amphotericin B in the treatment of hematogenous candidiasis: a matched cohort study. *Am J Med* 1996;101:170–176.
*Patients with cancer and hematogenous candidiasis were matched for underlying conditions. Forty-five patients received each agent. Rates of survival and clinical response were no different, but drug-related adverse reactions were significantly higher in those who received amphotericin B (67% vs. 9%). This investigation could not identify different candidal species as being associated with outcome. The authors*

*conclude that fluconazole is a satisfactory alternative to amphotericin B for hematoge-*
*nous candidiasis and is less toxic. Several other studies have reached the same con-*
*clusion. However, it must be remembered that certain azole-resistant* Candida *species*
*do not respond to fluconazole, and this caveat must be a factor in the choice of anti-*
*fungals for severe infections.*

Bennett JE, et al. A comparison of amphotericin B alone and combined with flucytosine in the treatment of cryptococcal meningitis. *N Engl J Med* 1979;301:126–131.
*Multicenter study of 50 patients with cryptococcal meningitis in the pre-AIDS era.*
*Demonstrates that the addition of flucytosine to amphotericin B allows a reduction*
*in the course of therapy from 10 to 6 weeks and a decrease in amphotericin B dosage*
*from 0.6 to 0.3 mg/kg per day. Combination therapy resulted in greater cure rates,*
*fewer relapses, and more rapid sterilization of cerebrospinal fluid.*

Bozette SA, et al. A placebo-controlled trial of maintenance therapy with fluconazole
after treatment of cryptococcal meningitis in AIDS. *N Engl J Med* 1991;324:580–584.
*In patients with AIDS, fluconazole was an effective suppressant of cryptococcal*
*meningitis versus placebo (3% vs. 37% relapse) following initial successful therapy*
*with amphotericin B. The dosage of fluconazole was 100 to 200 mg daily and was*
*well tolerated.*

Como JA, Dismukes WE. Oral azole drugs as systemic antifungal therapy. *N Engl J*
*Med* 1994;330:263–273.
*The authors provide an excellent review of the chemistry, mechanisms of action,*
*pharmacology, drug interactions, and uses of the oral azole antifungals. The section*
*on drug interactions is particularly useful. Although fluconazole and itraconazole*
*have potential roles in the treatment of systemic candidiasis, their efficacy, particu-*
*larly in neutropenic patients, requires further study.*

Grant SM, Clissold SP. Fluconazole: a review of its pharmacodynamic and pharmacokinetic properties and therapeutic potential in superficial and systemic mycoses.
*Drugs* 1990;39:877–916.
*Excellent single-source reference on the properties of this antifungal agent. Deals pri-*
*marily with the oral preparation and reviews published data concerning its clinical*
*applications.*

Kauffman CA. Role of azoles in antifungal therapy. *Clin Infect Dis* 1996;22(Suppl
2):S148–S153.
*A succicnt review of the subject that does not stress infections in HIV/AIDS. Seventy-*
*two articles are cited, and problems related to the emergence of azole resistance are*
*mentioned.*

Laine L, et al. Fluconazole compared with ketoconazole for the treatment of *Candida*
esophagitis in AIDS. *Ann Intern Med* 1992;117:655–660.
*Randomized trial of two agents that demonstrates more rapid clinical and endo-*
*scopic improvement in patients treated with fluconazole (90% vs. 50%). Patients*
*treated with ketoconazole often improved clinically but not endoscopically. Suggested*
*reasons for differences in outcome include better absorption of fluconazole and*
*enhanced in vitro activity against* Candida *species.*

Larsen RA. Azoles and AIDS. *J Infect Dis* 1990;162:727–730.
*This commentary continues to recommend amphotericin B as the primary therapy*
*for cryptococcal meningitis in AIDS, but describes fluconazole as a satisfactory agent*
*for suppression following successful initial therapy. The author points out the value*
*of fluconazole and itraconazole in selected AIDS patients with histoplasmosis and*
*significant candidal infections.*

Mayanja-Kizza H, et al. Combination therapy with fluconazole and flucytosine for
cryptococcal meningitis in Ugandan patients with AIDS. *Clin Infect Dis* 1998;
26:1362–1366.
*The authors performed a randomized trial on 58 AIDS patients with cryptococcal*
*meningitis who received either fluconazole (200 mg/d orally for 2 months) or flu-*
*conazole plus flucytosine (150 mg/kg per day in three divided doses for the first*
*2 weeks). All patients then received 200 mg of fluconazole thrice weekly for an addi-*
*tional 4 months. The death rate within the study period was substantially decreased*
*in patients who received the combination, and the severity of headache similarly*
*decreased significantly in this group. There appeared not to be a correlation between*

*clinical outcome and results of the in vitro susceptibility tests performed on 32 isolates. This combination of antifungals needs to be better studied, and the doses may need to be increased to obtain maximal benefits. The regimens were well tolerated.*

The Medical Letter. Systemic fungal infections. *Med Lett Drugs Ther* 1996;38:9–12.

*A concise overview of products available for the management of deep fungal infections. It contains no information on the lipsomal amphotericin B preparations. A chart of indications and doses is provided.*

Pathak A, Pien FD, Carvalho L. Amphotericin B use in a community hospital, with special emphasis on side effects. *Clin Infect Dis* 1998;26:334–338.

*A retrospective review of 102 patients who received amphotericin B deoxycholate during an approximate 3-year period was conducted. A major outcome was that the vast majority of patients tolerated the product well! Most could be treated without premedication. The major value of this investigation is to emphasize the relative safety of the cheapest and best-studied of the amphotericin B products. The liposomal preparations should be reserved for a very small subset of patients who require high doses, or in whom significant renal failure from amphotericin B clearly develops.*

Singh RM, Perdue BE. Amphotericin B: a class review. *Formulary* 1998;33:424–447.

*An excellent overview comparing the available formulations of amphotericin. Three lipsomal forms have been approved by the FDA. All are substantially more expensive than amphotericin B deoxycholate, and it remains uncertain how much better they are clinically. It is very difficult to detect important differences among the three liposomal forms. One of them should probably be used to treat invasive disease associated with Aspergillus infection. Although these forms are marketed as having advantages in patients with renal dysfunction associated with amphotericin B deoxycholate, the author has not found this problem to be significant when the original formulation is used carefully. All forms may be associated with acute toxicities and should be administered with a loading dose followed by dose escalation.*

Walsh TJ, et al. Amphotericin B lipid complex for invasive fungal infections: analysis of safety and efficacy in 556 cases. *Clin Infect Dis* 1998;26:1383–1396.

*Patients who clinically failed therapy with amphotericin B or who had renal failure (drug-induced or before treatment) or acute amphotericin B toxicity were enrolled to receive amphotericin B lipid complex. Most patients were infected with either Aspergillus or Candida. Approximately 60% demonstrated a clinical response, including 40% with Aspergillus. Renal function improved in those who entered the study with renal failure. The authors correctly conclude that amphotericin B lipid complex is indicated for selected conditions.*

## 79. NEW ORAL ANTIMICROBIALS

Interest in oral antibiotics has been renewed, and a number of factors have contributed to this. Various "negative" features are associated with infusion of an antibiotic (discomfort, restriction, phlebitis, bacteremia, excess fluid administration, and cost), and the new oral antimicrobial agents offer excellent absorption. The "pressure" to provide cost effective treatment has influenced clinicians to reconsider their practice patterns, and physicians have recently observed that oral antibiotic treatment (either initially or as a follow-up to IV infusion) is effective management for patients with such infections as chronic osteomyelitis, pyelonephritis, and community-acquired pneumonia, disorders previously considered indications for exclusively parenteral treatment.

This chapter explores specific themes that relate to the new oral antibiotics. Why does a need exist to develop new antibiotics? What factors must be considered when an oral antibiotic is selected? What have we learned concerning patient compliance? What are the clinically meaningful differences between the newer FDA-approved compounds, and what are their advantages and/or limitations? An effort will be made to examine critically the following newer compounds: cephalosporins, loracarbef, macrolides/azalide, fluoroquinolones, and fosfomycin tromethamine.

New antimicrobial agents need to be developed for several reasons: drug allergy, untoward events attributed to available compounds, the potential for drug-drug interactions, the discovery of new pathogens, limited present therapeutic options, and bacterial resistance. During the last few years, researchers have identified numerous novel infectious organisms, including hepatitis G virus, *Chlamydia*-like microorganism Z, *Legionella*-like amebal pathogens (LLAPs), *Ehrlichia* species, and *Bartonella* species. In addition, there are serious concerns worldwide about the emerging antimicrobial resistance of numerous bacteria, including *Streptococcus pneumoniae, Enterococcus* species, gram-negative bacilli, and *Mycobacterium tuberculosis.* Recently, quinolone-resistant *Escherichia coli,* gonococci, and *Campylobacter,* multidrug-resistant *Salmonella typhimurium,* and methicillin-resistant *Staphylococcus aureus* with reduced vancomycin susceptibility have all been recognized.

Some of the most important features of an oral drug that influence the selection process include efficacy, track record of safety, potential for drug-drug interactions, compliance concerns, safety during pregnancy, and cost. Although numerous studies have evaluated additional features of antibiotics, such as protein binding, post-antibiotic effect, and bactericidal-bacteriostatic status, it has been difficult to relate these characteristics to the therapeutic efficacy of each compound in the clinical arena.

A frequent observation is the failure of patients to comply with an oral medication regimen. Numerous patients do not follow the medication schedule, do not complete the course of therapy, or inform their physician that they have not taken the medication as recommended. Researchers have consistently demonstrated that patient compliance is enhanced when oral antibiotics are prescribed to be taken no more frequently than twice a day. Each of the new compounds reviewed in this article (cephalosporins, loracarbef, macrolides, azalide, fluoroquinolones, and fosfomycin tromethamine) achieves this goal.

### Cephalosporins

Three new cephalosporin compounds have been approved by the FDA for clinical administration. These drugs are cefprozil (Cefzil), cefpodoxime (Vantin), and ceftibuten (Cedax). They are indicated for the treatment of otitis media, streptococcal pharyngitis/tonsillitis, and exacerbation of chronic bronchitis by susceptible strains of bacteria.

Cefprozil, prescribed as 500 mg taken twice daily, is also approved for the management of acute maxillary sinusitis. Ceftibuten is prescribed as 400 mg taken once a day or as 200 mg taken twice daily. Cefpodoxime is prescribed as 200 mg taken twice daily and is FDA-approved for the management of gonococcal urethritis and community-acquired pneumonia caused by susceptible strains of *S. pneumoniae* and *Haemophilus influenzae.* Cefpodoxime rivals cefixime as an effective single-dose therapy for the patient with uncomplicated cervicitis or urethritis caused by *Neisseria gonorrhoeae.* The most common untoward event attributed to these safe compounds is diarrhea. These three cephalosporins do not, however, appear to add any unique feature or advantage to the present antibiotic arsenal and cannot be recommended as initial treatment of any established infection. They should not be prescribed for the patient who has experienced an immediate or accelerated hypersensitivity reaction to a member of the penicillin or cephalosporin family of drugs.

FDA approval has recently been given to a new, extended-spectrum oral cephalosporin, cefdinir, a compound that inhibits the growth of three bacterial respiratory pathogens: *S. pneumoniae, H. influenzae,* and *Moraxella (Branhamella) catarrhalis.* Cefdinir is a safe, effective treatment for patients with acute community-acquired sinusitis, exacerbation of chronic bronchitis, and community-acquired pneumonia. The most common untoward event attributed to this compound is diarrhea.

### Carbacephem

Loracarbef (Lorabid), technically a carbacephem, is a β-lactam antibiotic that resembles a cephalosporin and has a spectrum of activity similar to that of cefaclor and cefuroxime. Loracarbef is FDA-approved for the treatment of otitis media, sinusitis, exacerbation of chronic bronchitis, community-acquired pneumonia, streptococcal pharyngitis/tonsillitis, skin infections, and uncomplicated urinary tract infections caused by susceptible pathogens.

The compound, which is prescribed as 200 mg taken twice daily, is a safe agent. The major untoward events produced by loracarbef are headache and diarrhea. This drug is not indicated for the penicillin-allergic patient, and it is not appropriate therapy for the patient with pneumonia caused by *Legionella* species, *Mycoplasma pneumoniae,* or *Chlamydia pneumoniae.*

Loracarbef is an expensive compound that is comparable in therapeutic efficacy to traditional agents, and thus it does not appear to be the preferred treatment for any established infection.

### Macrolides/Azalide

The new macrolides (clarithromycin, dirithromycin) and azalide (azithromycin) offer a therapeutic advance in comparison with erythromycin. The newer compounds require less frequent dosing, are better tolerated, and have expanded indications. They are, however, considerably more expensive.

Dirithromycin (Dynabac) is taken once a day, but because this macrolide does not inhibit the growth of *H. influenzae,* its empiric administration to patients with an exacerbation of chronic bronchitis or community-acquired pneumonia is severely restricted.

Clarithromycin (Biaxin) and azithromycin (Zithromax) are FDA-approved for the treatment of streptococcal pharyngitis/tonsillitis (disorders for which penicillin is the drug of choice), acute exacerbation of chronic bronchitis, community-acquired pneumonia, and uncomplicated skin infections caused by susceptible pathogens. In addition, each of these compounds is appropriate prophylaxis for disseminated infection with *Mycobacterium avium* complex in the severely immunocompromised, HIV-infected patient.

Azithromycin is also an effective treatment for patients with *Chlamydia trachomatis*-related urethritis/cervicitis, genital ulcer disease caused by *Haemophilus ducreyi,* and moderate or severe shigellosis caused by multidrug-resistant *Shigella* strains. Azithromycin should not be taken with food. Azithromycin has two particularly desirable features. Treatment durations, compared with those of traditional drug courses, can be abbreviated, and this compound, unlike clarithromycin and erythromycin, does not appear to have a potential for drug-drug interaction. Of interest, because of the possibility of a role of *C. pneumoniae* in the pathogenesis of coronary artery disease, azithromycin is being evaluated to determine its ability to interfere with the development of coronary artery disease.

In contrast to azithromycin, clarithromycin can be ingested with food, and it has been approved to treat acute maxillary sinusitis and, in conjunction with additional agents, disseminated *M. avium* complex infection in AIDS patients and peptic ulcer disease caused by *Helicobacter pylori.* Clarithromycin appears to be the preferred compound to treat patients with cutaneous, disseminated *Mycobacterium chelonei* infections. Unfortunately, however, clarithromycin has the potential to precipitate drug-drug interactions when it is coadministered with cisapride, digoxin, carbamezepine, ergotamine, theophylline, terfenadine, astemizole, cyclosporine, felodipine, warfarin, and buspirone.

### Fluoroquinolones

The fluoroquinolones have held a great appeal for clinicians for various reasons: These compounds have a broad spectrum of activity, are bactericidal, are administered infrequently, can be prescribed to penicillin-allergic patients, are safe, rarely cause antimicrobial-related *C. difficile* pseudomembranous colitis, and constitute effective treatment for a wide range of infections.

Prime indications for treatment with fluoroquinolones include chronic bacterial prostatitis, complicated urinary tract infection, bacterial enterocolitis, and gram-negative osteomyelitis. Additional unique indications for the use of fluoroquinolones include the prevention of spontaneous bacterial peritonitis and the treatment of an acute infectious exacerbation superimposed on cystic fibrosis. In combination with additional antibiotics, fluoroquinolones have been prescribed to treat selected outpatients with pelvic inflammatory disease or with solid tumors complicated by fever and neutropenia. The fluoroquinolones have also been widely used as therapy for patients with respiratory tract infections and urinary tract infections.

Four new fluoroquinolones have recently been marketed: sparfloxacin (Zagam), levofloxacin (Levaquin), grepafloxacin (Raxar), and trovafloxacin (Trovan). Sparfloxacin has been approved by the FDA for the management of community-acquired pneumonia and exacerbation of chronic bronchitis. Levofloxacin is FDA-approved for these indications and also for the treatment of acute maxillary sinusitis, skin infections, and urinary tract infections. Each of these compounds is prescribed to be taken once a day, does not interact with theophylline (in contrast to some other fluoroquinolones), and possesses activity against some penicillin-resistant S. pneumoniae. In addition, both compounds inhibit the growth of "traditional" bacterial respiratory pathogens, as well as the growth of what are occasionally referred to as "atypical" pathogens—namely, Legionella species, C. pneumoniae, and M. pneumoniae.

Certain features of these two new fluoroquinolones distinguish them further. Levofloxacin is available for IV as well as oral administration. Sparfloxacin has the potential to produce severe and protracted phototoxicity, and this compound can increase the risk for arrhythmias, such as torsade de pointes, when prescribed with selected antiarrhythmic agents. It would thus appear that levofloxacin is the preferred agent, particularly when patients receive disopyramide, amiodarone, quinidine, procainamide, sotalol, and bepridil. Sparfloxacin should not be used in patients with known $QT_c$ prolongation or in patients receiving $QT_c$-prolonging drugs. Levofloxacin dosage requires adjustment in patients with renal compromise.

Grepafloxicin has a spectrum of activity similar to that of the other quinolones, but it does display enhanced activity, in comparison with ciprofloxacin, against S. pneumoniae. Grepafloxacin is administered once a day and is an effective treatment for patients with lower respiratory tract infections caused by traditional respiratory pathogens and in patients with gonococcal/chlamydial urethritis and cervicitis. The most common untoward event produced by this medication is nausea. Grepafloxacin is contraindicated for patients who have hepatic failure, in whom the $QT_c$ interval is prolonged, or who are receiving $QT_c$-prolonging drugs.

Trovafloxacin (Trovan), another fluoroquinolone, is available as both an IV and an oral preparation. Compared with ciprofloxacin, trovafloxacin exhibits enhanced in vitro activity against staphylococci, streptococci, penicillin-resistant S. pneumoniae, Bacteroides, Clostridium, and C. trachomatis. This compound has been noted to be an effective treatment for upper and lower respiratory tract infections and uncomplicated urinary tract infections caused by traditional bacterial pathogens, and for genital infections caused by N. gonorrhoeae and C. trachomatis. The main untoward event produced by this drug is dizziness. Because trovafloxacin can produce dizziness, it is probably contraindicated for people who must operate heavy machinery, drive a car, or engage in activities that require mental alertness and coordination. A desirable feature of the drug is that its absorption is not altered by concomitant food intake or concurrent enteral feeding. Furthermore, dose reduction is not required in cases of renal insufficiency, and drug interactions do not occur when the drug is given concomitantly with cimetidine, theophylline, digoxin, warfarin, or cyclosporine. Finally, photoxicity rarely occurs.

### Fosfomycin Tromethamine

Fosfomycin tromethamine (Monuril) is a phosphoric acid bactericidal single-dose agent designed for the management of women with acute symptomatic bacterial cystitis caused by E. coli. The favorable features of this compound include excellent compliance, safety (transient adverse events, mild diarrhea), and lack of cross-sensitization with other antibacterials. This agent produces clinical and microbiologic responses that are comparable with those achieved by standard, traditional, single- or multiple-dose treatments. The compound has been given a category B pregnancy status. Fosfomycin is prescribed as a single, 3-g dose of dissolved granules, to be taken without regard to food.

A number of concerns are relevant to fosfomycin tromethamine. It is an expensive treatment, and the agent cannot be coadministered with metoclopramide, as this gastrointestinal motility agent reduces the urinary concentration of fosfomycin tromethamine.

Perhaps the major disadvantage of fosfomycin tromethamine, however, is the fact that it does not inhibit the growth of Staphylococcus saprophyticus. This is important because numerous studies have identified *S. saprophyticus* as the second most common cause of acute, symptomatic bacterial cystitis in young women.

### Conclusion

The newer antimicrobial agents should be reserved for judiciously selected indications. There is no compelling reason to prescribe these newer compounds to patients with streptococcal pharyngitis, acute maxillary sinusitis, acute bronchitis, an exacerbation of chronic bronchitis, or bacterial cystitis. Many time-honored, safe, effective, and less expensive drugs are available to manage patients with these infections. Excessive and inappropriate use of the newer agents will result in exorbitantly expensive medicine and foster the emergence of drug-resistant pathogens. (R.A.G.)

### Bibliography

Ernst ME, Ernst EJ, Klepser ME. Levofloxacin and trovafloxacin: the next generation of fluoroquinolones? *Am J Health Syst Pharm* 1997;54:2569–2584.
*A review of two new fluoroquinolones.*

Gelfand M, Johnson R. Single-dose fosfomycin tromethamine: evaluation in the treatment of uncomplicated lower urinary tract infection. *Adv Therapy* 1997;14:49–63.
*A review of a single-dose treatment for acute bacterial cystitis.*

Gleckman RA, Borrego F. Adverse reactions to antibiotics. *Postgrad Med* 1997;101: 97–108.
*Potential for drug-drug interactions and antimicrobial-related side effects influence the choice of drug therapy.*

Goa KL, Bryson HM, Markham A. Sparfloxacin: a review of its antibacterial activity, pharmacokinetc properties, clinical efficacy, and tolerability in lower respiratory tract infections. *Drugs* 1997;53:700–725.
*A detailed review of the fluoroquinolone sparfloxacin.*

Gwaltney JM Jr, et al. Comparative effectiveness and safety of cefdinir and amoxicillin-clavulanate in the treatment of acute community-acquired bacterial sinusitis. *Antimicrob Agents Chemother* 1997;41:1517–1520.
*Cefdinir is an effective treatment for patients with acute maxillary sinusitis, but the compound is often associated with diarrhea.*

Haria M, Lamb HM. Trovafloxacin. *Drugs* 1997;54:435–445.
*A review of the fluoroquinolone trovafloxacin.*

Joshi N, Milfred D. The use and misuse of new antibiotics: a perspective. *Arch Intern Med* 1995;155:569–577.
*Administration of new compounds should be restricted to specific indications.*

Sclar DA, Tartaglione TA, Fine M. Overview of issues related to medical compliance with implications for the outpatient management of infectious diseases. *Infect Agents Dis* 1994;3:266–273.
*There is a direct relationship between frequency of dose and compliance.*

Wagstaff AJ, Balfour JA. Grepafloxacin. *Drugs* 1997;53:817–824.
*A review of the new fluoroquinolone grepafloxacin.*

## 80. ANTIBIOTIC FAILURE

When clinicians prescribe an antibiotic to a patient with an established infection, it is expected that the patient will recover. This course of events is particularly anticipated when the host is immunocompetent. It is well recognized, however, that some immunocompromised patients, such as profoundly and persistently leukopenic leukemic patients with an invasive fungal infection, often succumb to their infection *despite* appropriate antimicrobial chemotherapy.

Failure to respond to antimicrobial treatment is frequently manifested by persistent fever, lack of clinical improvement, and clinical deterioration and/or persistent or worsening laboratory or radiographic abnormalities. The seasoned clinician appreciates, however, that fever can be a manifestation of a noninfectious process, such as an adverse event caused by a drug, chemical thrombophlebitis at an infusion site, deep-venous thrombosis, pulmonary embolism, pulmonary aspiration of gastric contents, neoplasm, or an immunologic disorder. The antimicrobial agents most frequently associated with drug-induced fever include sulfonamides, β-lactam antibiotics, and amphotericin B. Drug fever is usually not accompanied by rash or eosinophilia, and it customarily subsides within 72 hours of discontinuation of the medication.

Resolution of a bacterial infection depends largely on three factors: host defenses, nature of the pathogen, and characteristics of the antimicrobial administered. Failure of resolution of the infection should encourage the clinician to search for factors that would compromise the host, enhance bacterial pathogenicity, or reduce the effectiveness of the prescribed antibiotic.

### Host Factors

When a patient is not responding to the designated antibiotic, it is extremely tempting to administer alternative antimicrobial agents with an extended spectrum of inhibitory activity. On occasion, this approach is valid, particularly for a patient who is seriously ill. In general, however, it is preferable for the clinician to consider any host-related features that could be contributing to persistent infection, and to reassess the diagnostic possibilities.

If an infection does not respond to antibiotic treatment alone, the patient should be evaluated for the presence of obstruction, necrotic tissue, hematoma, abscess, or a prosthetic device and, if necessary, corrective action taken. Additional concerns relating to the host that need to be considered are compliance with medication and the presence of an infection in a protected ("privileged") site. Infections in protected sites, which require treatment with antimicrobials having unique penetration properties, include meningitis, endocarditis, chronic bacterial prostatitis, and endophthalmitis.

An important consideration, when the patient appears not to be responding to antibiotic therapy, is the accuracy of the diagnosis. Gout, thrombophlebitis, and Lyme disease can resemble a traditional bacterial cellulitis; Charcot's joint often simulates osteomyelitis; and pulmonary infarction, lung cancer, adult respiratory distress syndrome (ARDS), and aspiration of gastric contents can imitate bacterial pneumonia.

### Organism

The lack of a clinical response can suggest features unique to the offending pathogen. Resistance to the antibiotic prescribed, the presence of multiple organisms (abdominal and pelvic infections as well as infections involving the feet of diabetic patients are typically polymicrobic), and the need to administer combination treatment should be considered when infection persists despite what appears to be appropriate antibiotic treatment.

Results of susceptibility reports generated by automated systems can be false, and this can result in misleading identification of heterogeneous methicillin sodium-resistant staphylococci and β-lactamase-resistant Enterobacteriaceae. It is beneficial to explore this possibility with the microbiology technologist.

Selected infections, including tuberculosis, endocarditis caused by *viridans* streptococci and enterococci, brucellosis, disseminated *Mycobacterium avium* complex infection, and life-threatening infection caused by *Pseudomonas aeruginosa,* require combination antibiotic therapy for clinical resolution to be achieved.

### Drug

Assuming the antimicrobial possesses an appropriate spectrum of activity to curtail the growth of an infectious organism, what additional factors relevant to the ability of a drug to influence the outcome of an infection must be considered? Three specific features of the antimicrobial certainly can contribute to therapeutic efficacy.

Bactericidal compounds are preferred for patients with bacterial endocarditis or gram-negative bacillary meningitis. Bactericidal agents are also indicated when life-threatening infections develop in granulocytopenic hosts.

Table 80-1. Failure to respond to antibiotic therapy

| | Condition being treated | | | |
|---|---|---|---|---|
| | Acute maxillary sinusitis | Exacerbation of chronic bronchitis | Community-acquired pneumonia |
| Compliance | X | X | X |
| Inappropriate antibiotic (resistant or unusual organism) | X | X | X* |
| Incorrect diagnosis | Allergic fungal sinusitis Dental sepsis Acute invasive fungal sinusitis | Pneumonia, CHF, neoplasm | CHF, neoplasm, pulmonary embolism, BOOP, Wegener's granulomatosis |
| Immunocompromised state | HIV infection Diabetes mellitus Leukemia | HIV infection | HIV infection Profound leukopenia |
| Complication requiring attention | Facilitate drainage | Excessive bronchospasm and secretions | Obstructive neoplasm Empyema |

CHF, congestive heart failure; BOOP, bronchiolitis obliterans-organizing pneumonia.
* Tuberculosis, fungal infection, legionellosis, nocardiosis, actinomycosis, *Pneumocystis carinii* pneumonia.

When a β-lactim antibiotic is prescribed, it is best to maintain blood and tissue concentrations above the minimal inhibitory concentration (MIC) for the organism causing infection throughout the entire dosing interval. Lower doses or longer dosing intervals, sometimes used to save money, raise the risk for treatment failure. Alternatively, aminoglycoside antibiotics exhibit concentration-dependent killing of organisms and are probably best administered once a day.

Drug-drug interaction has the potential to diminish antimicrobial efficacy. The ingestion of food impairs the bioavailability of azithromycin, and milk products diminish the absorption of the tetracyclines. The coadministration of antacids, iron, didanosine, and multivitamins that contain zinc decreases absorption of the tetracyclines and fluoroquinolones. In addition, the bioavailability of fluoroquinolones is impaired by ingestion of sucralfate.

Table 80-1 lists some considerations that the clinician might ponder when a patient appears not to be responding to antibiotic treatment of acute maxillary sinusitis, exacerbation of chronic bronchitis, or community-acquired pneumonia.

When a patient is persistently febrile (longer than 96 hours) after antibiotic treatment has been initiated to manage pyelonephritis, concerns should focus on a drug-resistant uropathogen, obstructive uropathy, intrarenal or perinephric abscess, an adverse drug reaction, diabetes mellitus compromising the host, or xanthogranulomatous pyelonephritis. (R.A.G.)

## Bibliography

Bartlett JG, et al. Community-acquired pneumonia in adults: guidelines for management. *Clin Infect Dis* 1998;26:811–838.
*Reviews why patients fail to respond to the antibiotic treatment of community-acquired pneumonia and provides an assessment of a nonresponding patient.*

Borrego F, Gleckman R. Preventing antibiotic treatment failure. *Contemp Intern Med* 1996;8:9–15.
*An approach for evaluating patients whose infection fails to respond to antibiotics.*

Cunha BA. Differentiating pneumonitis and pneumonia in your SLE patient. *J Crit Illness* 1997;12:779–783.
*In a patient with systemic lupus erythematosus, pneumonitis, as a complication of the systemic disorder, can resemble infectious pneumonia.*

Cunha BA, Ortega AM. Antibiotic failure. *Med Clin North Am* 1995;79:663–671.
*A review of the causes of antibiotic failure.*

Feinsilver SH, Fein AM, Niederman MS. Nonresolving, slowly resolving, and recurrent pneumonia. In: Niederman MS, Sarois GA, Glassroth J, eds. *Respiratory infections: a scientific basis for management.* Philadelphia: WB Saunders, 1994:277–290.
*Outlines the diagnostic and therapeutic approach for the patient with pneumonia in whom the infection is not resolving.*

Genovese MC. Fever, rash, and arthritis in a woman with silicone gel breast implants. *West J Med* 1997;167:149–158.
*Difficulty of differentiating a connective tissue disease (systemic inflammatory illness) from an infectious or neoplastic process.*

Melby MJ, et al. Acute adrenal insufficiency mimicking septic shock: a case report. *Pharmacotherapy* 1988;8:69–71.
*Acute adrenal insufficiency can resemble septic shock.*

Mulligan MJ, Cobbs CG. Bacteriostatic versus bactericidal activity. *Infect Dis Clin North Am* 1989;3:389–398.
*Outlines those conditions in which bactericidal activity appears necessary for successful antibiotic treatment.*

Schattner A. Quinidine hypersensitivity simulating sepsis. *Am J Med* 1998;104: 488–490.
*Adverse drug reaction can resemble an infectious disease.*

Wallace JM. Mimics of infectious pneumonia in persons infected with human immunodeficiency virus. In: Niederman MS, Saros GA, Glassroth J, eds. *Respiratory infections: a scientific basis for management.* Philadelphia: WB Saunders, 1994:217–223.
*Malignant and infiltrative disorders in the HIV-infected patient that resemble infectious pneumonia.*

## 81. WHO REALLY NEEDS PARENTERAL ANTIBIOTICS?

Although much has been written concerning the indications, abuses, and recommended dosing regimens of antibiotics for many diseases, far less is known about the most appropriate route of administration for these agents. Historically, clinicians in the United States acquired the notion that hospitalized patients should receive antibiotics parenterally, whereas those at home could be treated with oral antibiotic agents. This was no doubt based on a sense of differing degrees of illness between hospitalized and ambulatory patients. This feeling is not shared universally, and clinicians in other parts of the world employ oral antibiotics more regularly to treat hospitalized patients. This concept of the use of parenteral antibiotics in hospitalized patients has been nurtured by external forces that include insurers, community services, and governmental regulatory agencies. As an example, until the past decade, there was no generally available infrastructure for the administration of parenteral antibiotics outside the setting of acute care. Similarly, insurers did not ordinarily provide compensation to patients for the purchase of antibiotics, and the costs associated with the purchase and administration of parenteral antibiotics in the community would have been prohibitive.

During the past decade, as the result of various changes, the decision regarding when to use parenteral or oral agents has become less clearly defined. Table 81-1 summarizes many of these issues. Managed care has forced health care providers to reconsider the costs of treatment, including those associated with administration of antibiotics. Parenteral antibiotics administered in the hospital are expensive, and the adverse effects of both high-dose parenteral agents and the administration paraphernalia have been well publicized. In essence, clinicians have been challenged to demonstrate the superiority of more expensive therapies.

In the mid-1980s, the concept of outpatient parenteral antibiotic therapy was addressed in earnest, and numerous investigations now document the safety, efficacy, and cost effectiveness of this modality of care. Most urban and suburban areas are now equipped with an infrastructure to deliver outpatient parenteral antibiotic therapy in the home, infusion center, or physician's office. During this time, substantial progress has been made in the development of oral antibiotic agents. Numerous drugs now exist that can be given once or twice daily, have excellent bioavailability, "cover" likely pathogens for many infections, are well tolerated, and can be obtained at a reasonable price. Indeed, the cost of the most expensive oral antibiotic is less than 3% of that associated with parenteral antibiotics given in the acute care setting. Several investigators have now documented the safety and efficacy of oral antibiotic therapy for diseases historically treated parenterally. Examples include selected cases of osteomyelitis, pyelonephritis, septic arthritis, and infective endocarditis. The discussion that follows attempts to put these issues in perspective, define populations that can reasonably be treated with oral antibiotics, and realistically address the question of who really needs parenteral antibiotics.

### Bioavailability and Pharmacodynamic Issues of Oral Antibiotics

Several antibiotics are well absorbed after oral administration, and serum levels are obtained that are similar to those following parenteral therapy. Metronidazole, doxycycline, many quinolones, rifampin, trimethoprim-sulfamethoxazole, and chloramphenicol are examples. Thus, provided the patient has a functional gastrointestinal tract, there are few reasons to administer these agents parenterally. Additionally, one or a combination of them can provide coverage for many infections. Drug and food interactions are a concern with selected oral antibiotics. The absorption of quinolones and tetracycline may be inhibited by divalent cations. Others, including penicillin G and the early form of azithromycin, must be given without food, whereas selected antimicrobials such as itraconazole and ketoconazole require the presence of food (gastric acid) for adequate absorption. These issues become critical when antiretroviral agents are considered (see Chapter 90).

Many β-lactam antibiotics and clindamycin represent examples of agents for which oral and parenteral dosing regimens are substantially different. As an example, the

Table 81-1. Changing face of antibiotic treatment

1. External forces (government, insurers) requiring "cost effectiveness" and cost cutting with preservation of clinical outcomes
2. Availability of newer oral antibiotics with excellent bioavailability and daily or twice-daily dosing
3. Studies demonstrating efficacy of oral antibiotic therapy for conditions historically treated parenterally
4. Recognition of significant unique adverse effects associated with parenteral use of antibiotics

dose of nafcillin or oxacillin for serious staphylococcal infections may be 8 to 12 g/d, whereas the usual dose of dicloxacillin rarely exceeds 2 g/d. Presumably, this is because of likely gastrointestinal adverse reactions associated with higher oral doses. Because the efficacy of β-lactams is based on the length of time the minimum inhibitory concentration for the organism is exceeded (time-dependent killing), oral and parenteral products could be anticipated to have different clinical outcomes. This is a reason why hospitalized patients treated with β-lactam antibiotics for severe infections generally are treated parenterally.

## Availability of Oral Products
A number of important antimicrobial agents cannot be administered orally for systemic infections. Examples include amphotericin B, vancomycin, aminoglycosides, and foscarnet. Amphotericin B has historically been considered the gold standard for serious systemic fungal infection; aminoglycosides were important agents for significant gram-negative infections, and vancomycin remains the standard of care for infections associated with methicillin-resistant *Staphylococcus aureus,* systemic infections caused by *Staphylococcus epidermidis,* and many other severe, gram-positive infections in patients with histories of immediate β-lactam allergy.

## Host Factors to Consider in the Choice of Oral or Parenteral Antibiotics
The host factors to consider in the decision to use oral antibiotics are summarized in Table 81-2. Compliance with an oral regimen administered outside the hospital requires (a) ability to purchase the agent, (b) understanding of how to take it, and (c) ability to cope with adverse reactions. The writing of the script does not guarantee the intake of the product. Numerous examples of patients unable to afford an oral agent exist, and the prescribing physician needs to ascertain the patient's ability to pay. Compliance has been simplified with the recent availability of products requiring dosing once (or twice) daily. Several investigations demonstrate that products requiring three to four doses per day are less likely to be taken regularly (and so could result in poor outcomes). Adverse reactions range from life-threatening to annoying. The patient must understand that certain adverse reactions are possible and do not mandate drug discontinuation.

Gastrointestinal function must be sufficient to allow drug absorption. Patients with severe nausea, vomiting, or diarrhea are not candidates for initial oral antibiotic ther-

Table 81-2. Host factors to consider in use of oral antibiotics

1. Ability to absorb antibiotic
2. Drug-drug or drug-food interaction
3. Compliance with oral antibiotic regimen
    Ability to pay
    Ability to understand regimen and potential adverse reactions
4. Allergy potential
5. End-organ function and ability to metabolize and excrete product

apy. Achlorhydria may aid in the absorption of selected agents and be deleterious for others.

Allergy may preclude the use of selected products. However, it is the opinion of the author that its importance is overemphasized and often results in the use of expensive, less effective agents. Immediate reactions to penicillin occur in fewer than one in 10,000 patients. Maculopapular rash, probably the most common manifestation of allergy, is generally not associated with defined mechanisms of true allergy and often will not recur with repeated dosing of the offending product. The clinician must question the patient about the type of allergy and consider whether the adverse reaction truly represents an allergic problem.

Age and end-organ function are of occasional importance. The quinolones are contraindicated in persons less than 18 years old and should be used in persons less than this age only in highly specific circumstances and with the consent of the patient. Tetracyclines should not be given to young children, typically until all the secondary teeth are in place. Tetracyclines and quinolones are contraindicated in pregnancy, and sulfa preparations should be administered with care, especially late in the third trimester. Patients with neurologic disturbances may be at risk for complications with the use of selected quinolones, and patients with severe renal failure may need dosage adjustments with many oral antibiotics.

### Antibiotic Susceptibility Profiles

Antibiotics now exist that provide *in vitro* activity against most pathogens. The availability of newer quinolones (sparfloxacin, grepafloxacin, levofloxacin, and trovafloxacin) has provided the clinician with a class of product that has excellent *in vitro* activity against most enteric gram-negative bacilli and many gram-positive cocci (including many strains of *S. aureus* and penicillin-resistant *Streptococcus pneumoniae*), and reasonable activity against *Pseudomonas aeruginosa*. Trovafloxacin is the first of the available quinolones to have excellent anaerobic activity. Thus, for many infections in appropriate hosts, the oral quinolones may be considered for treatment of infections historically treated parenterally.

Metronidazole is an oral agent with excellent bioavailability and is active against the majority of anaerobes associated with human infection. It is also the agent of choice for *Clostridium difficile* diarrhea. Trimethoprim-sulfamethoxazole has good activity against many strains of *S. aureus* and many enteric gram-negative bacilli. It is also an agent of choice for *Pneumocystis carinii* pneumonia and is well-studied as an oral agent to treat mild-to-moderate infection with this pathogen. Rifampin has broad-spectrum antibacterial activity, but it is now associated with the problem of rapid emergence of resistance when employed as monotherapy. *In vitro,* it is one of the most active agents against *S. aureus* and has been clinically utilized successfully (in conjunction with a second antistaphylococcal agent) against this pathogen. Chloramphenicol is active against many gram-positive, enteric gram-negative, and anaerobic bacteria. It also is active against rickettsiae. It is well absorbed, associated with few adverse reactions, and inexpensive in most parts of the world. Bone marrow aplasia is a life-threatening but rare complication that has precluded its use in the United States for most indications. However, studies assessing the risk of this agent against the risks of alternative parenteral antibiotic therapy (e.g., IV line sepsis) have not been performed.

### Oral Agents for Severe Infections

Studies that have been performed during the past decade indicate the value of oral antibiotic therapy for numerous conditions historically treated parenterally. Several examples are presented. The combination of ciprofloxacin plus rifampin has been successfully employed in patients with uncomplicated right-sided endocarditis associated with *S. aureus*. This condition has also been successfully treated with trimethoprim-sulfamethoxazole, and outcomes in patients with methicillin-resistant *S. aureus* infection were slightly better than with vancomycin. Oral antistaphylococcal agents now represent the therapy of choice for uncomplicated staphylococcal osteomyelitis and septic arthritis in children. In most instances, the dose is several times higher than usual, and the serum bactericidal test is used to help assess the optimal dose. In adults, a quinolone plus rifampin usually results in satisfactory serum bactericidal levels. A recent study of ciprofloxacin plus rifampin in the management of infected orthopedic prostheses demonstrated that patients who received this combination (plus appropriate early debridement) were all cured after 3 to 6 months of oral treatment. The quinolones have revolutionized the management of acute pyelonephritis, and in patients otherwise fit to be treated outside the hospital, they now represent the treatment of choice (in the absence of pregnancy and other contraindications).

Step-down from parenteral to oral therapy has received increasing recognition as a method to decrease the length of parenteral treatment and hasten discharge from the hospital. This has been best studied with community-acquired pneumonia, for which numerous studies have now demonstrated the safety and efficacy of this approach. In many instances, patients with community-acquired pneumonia can be placed on oral antibiotics after 2 to 3 days in the hospital and discharged on the same day. Criteria for the switch to oral antibiotics include (a) a functional gastrointestinal tract, (b) improving clinical and laboratory parameters, and (c) being afebrile for two consecutive 8-hour intervals.

## Conclusions

The availability of newer oral products plus the publication of several important investigations now demonstrate the adequacy of oral antibiotic therapy for many conditions historically treated parenterally. Parenteral administration of antibiotics should be reserved for highly selected patients in the following situations: (a) No oral antibiotic is available, (b) the patient's gastrointestinal function will not support absorption of an oral antibiotic, (c) drug-food or drug-drug interactions are present that preclude the use of an oral antibiotic, (d) severe sepsis is present and high concentrations of antibiotic must be attained rapidly (often at a sequestered focus, such as a heart valve or the meninges). Clinicians, insurers, and patients must understand that oral antibiotic therapy does not represent poor treatment, and that in many circumstances it is equally effective, less expensive, and potentially safer than parenteral antibiotic therapy. (R.B.B.)

## Bibliography

Gentry LO, Rodriguez GG. Oral ciprofloxacin compared with parenteral antibiotics in the treatment of osteomyelitis. *Antimicrob Agents Chemother* 1990;34:40–43.
   *A prospective, randomized trial of ciprofloxacin versus standard parenteral antibiotic therapy was conducted for adults with biopsy-proven osteomyelitis. Success rates were approximately 75% in both groups. Adverse effects were more common in patients treated parenterally. Most failures were noted in patients with polymicrobial infections involving P. aeruginosa. For many patients with osteomyelitis, oral quinolone therapy is a rational alternative to parenteral antibiotics.*
Greenberg RN. Overview of patient compliance with medication dosing: a literature review. *Clin Ther* 1984;6:592–596.
   *In studies of compliance with antibiotic dosing, once- and twice-daily regimens were associated with substantially better compliance than regimens that required dosing three or four times daily. With regimens that required dosing more frequently than twice daily, compliance dropped to less than 50%, and this was not related to social class, income, or occupation. The current availability of numerous products that can be taken once or twice daily makes oral antibiotic treatment far more appealing than previously.*
Heldman AW, et al. Oral antibiotic treatment of right-sided staphylococcal endocarditis in injection drug users: prospective randomized comparison with parenteral therapy. *Am J Med* 1996;101:68–76.
   *Ciprofloxacin plus rifampin was compared with either oxacillin or vancomycin to treat febrile drug users hospitalized with suspected right-sided infective endocarditis. Treatment failures and drug toxicity were more common among those treated parenterally. For selected patients with endocarditis, a totally oral antibiotic regimen appears reasonable.*
MacGregor RR, Graziani AL. Oral administration of antibiotics: a rational alternative to the parenteral route. *Clin Infect Dis* 1997;24;457–467.

*Many of the issues that have led to the reassessment of the role of oral antibiotics are summarized, pharmacokinetic data are presented for several oral agents, and various studies that justify oral antibiotic treatment for many infections historically treated parenterally are reviewed. The authors make a good case for the expanded use of oral antibiotics, and they ask for the input of physicians to foster the ongoing study of older oral antibiotics, for which industrial sponsorship is unlikely.*

Zimmerli W, et al. Role of rifampin for treatment of orthopedic implant-related staphylococcal infections. *JAMA* 1998;279:1537–1541.

*The authors conducted a randomized trial of ciprofloxacin with and without rifampin for orthopedic implant-related staphylococcal infections. Patients were treated orally after an initial 2-week course of parenteral antibiotics. Initial debridement of infected materials was carried out, but the implant was left in place. All isolates were susceptible to both ciprofloxacin and rifampin. Patients who completed a 3- to 6-month course of ciprofloxacin plus rifampin were cured without removal of the implant. The rate of cure was substantially lower among those who received only ciprofloxacin (100% vs. 58%). This investigation is the most recent one demonstrating a role for the oral treatment of a condition that has historically been treated parenterally. The antibiotics used were highly bioavailable, well tolerated, and given no more than twice daily.*

# XX. AIDS

# 82. ACQUISITION AND TRANSMISSION OF HIV

Infection associated with HIV has been recognized for almost two decades, and morbidity and mortality have taken enormous tolls worldwide. The best estimates are that a total of about 42 million persons throughout the world have acquired HIV since inception of the epidemic, of whom about 12 million have died. Estimates for selected AIDS data, which demonstrate the profound impact of this disease on the global population, are shown in Table 82-1. Unfortunately, despite the availability of life-prolonging medications, up to 60 million cases will have developed by the millennium. Two thirds of all cases have occurred in sub-Saharan Africa. Almost 25% of those who have died have been children. Estimates are that 8 million children have become orphans on account of this disease. Table 82-2 summarizes international data by region.

In the United States, the first 50,000 cases were reported between 1981 and 1987. The second 50,000 cases were reported by 1989, and by the beginning of 1998, a total of 641,000 cases of AIDS had been reported to the Centers for Disease Control and Prevention. Current estimates are that up to 900,000 persons are HIV-positive. Blacks (40%), Caucasians (38%), and Hispanics (19%) are most notably involved. Dramatic changes have occurred among selected groups at risk for HIV. Currently, 84% of cases have occurred in men, 15% in women, and about 1% in children. However, between 1985 and 1996, the percentage of AIDS cases in women increased from 7% to 20%, mostly associated with heterosexual sex or IV drug use. AIDS among heterosexuals increased from 5% (1988) to 18% (1995). In male subjects, homosexuality (48%), IV drug use (20%), or both (7%) are the most prominent associations; acquisition through heterosexual sex accounts for 5% of cases. Similar data for women demonstrate IV drug use (8%) and heterosexual sex (10%) to be the most frequent associations. Among hospitalized patients, seroprevalence ranges from 0.2% to 14.2%.

Among persons ages 18 to 22, approximately 33,000 are HIV-positive. Homosexual contact was the most common mode of spread among white men of this age, whereas heterosexual contact was most common among women. This is especially noted within minorities. In 1996, about 7,500 persons above age 50 were reported with AIDS. Of these, 12% were above age 65. Homosexuality and an absence of acknowledged risk factors were most common in persons above age 50. In this group, persons had a higher risk for death within 1 month of an AIDS diagnosis, and the diagnosis of an AIDS-defining opportunistic infection was more common in this group.

Globally, major disparities in mortality from AIDS are being recognized between developing countries and the United States. This is mostly related to the availability of antiretroviral medications. Data from the United States demonstrate that HIV-related deaths declined in 1996 by 23% in comparison with deaths in 1995. This was noted among all risk groups and in all geographic regions. Similarly, 1996 data demonstrate substantial decreases in the diagnosis of AIDS-related opportunistic infections. During that year, about 57,000 opportunistic infections were diagnosed, representing a decline of 6% from the previous year.

The rate of progression to AIDS following seroconversion can be gauged from the baseline CD4-cell count and viral load (HIV RNA). This information has been generated from a cohort of male homosexuals, and it is uncertain how to extrapolate it to others. Data have been provided in chart form (Table 82-3). As an example, the risk for AIDS within 3 years in persons with CD4-cell counts above 750 and HIV RNA below 500 is nil, and it rises to only 3.6% after 9 years. Alternatively, for patients with baseline CD4-cell counts above 750 but with viral loads above 3,000, the risk for AIDS rises to 3% at 3 years and 40% at 9 years. Up to 11% of patients infected with HIV demonstrate prolonged survivorship. Such persons demonstrate ongoing viral replication, and virus can regularly be cultured from their lymph nodes. Characteristics of patients with long-term survival include low viral load, noncytopathogenicity of HIV strains, absence of enhancing antibodies, a cytokine response characterized by elevated amounts of interleukin-2 (the $T_H1$ response), and an enhanced CD8-cell response. Thus, a combination of decreased viral virulence and enhanced immune response probably contributes to prolonged survival in this subset.

Table 82-1. Global HIV/AIDS estimates, 1997

| Category | Number |
|---|---|
| New cases, adults, 1997 | 5,200,000 |
| New cases, women, 1997 | 2,100,000 |
| Total adults with HIV/AIDS | 29,400,000 |
| Total women with HIV/AIDS | 12,200,000 |
| AIDS deaths, adults, 1997 | 1,800,000 |
| AIDS deaths, women, 1997 | 800,000 |
| Total AIDS deaths, adults | 9,000,000 |
| Total AIDS deaths, women | 3,900,000 |
| Total AIDS orphans | 8,200,000 |

Health care workers comprise an important subset at risk for HIV infection because of their potential exposure to HIV-infected body fluids, most notably blood. The risk for seroconversion following exposure to HIV-infected blood is approximately 0.3%. The risk after mucous membrane exposure is about 0.09%. HIV seroconversion after skin exposure has occurred; the risk is thought to be less than that following exposure to mucous membranes. Seroconversion occurs at a mean of 46 days following exposure; in 95%, seroconversion occurs within 6 months. In most persons (81%), primary HIV syndrome develops within 1 month after seroconversion. Through June 1997, 52 health care workers with documented HIV seroconversion following occupational exposure had been reported. Most of these exposures were to blood and were percutaneous. Enhanced risks for seroconversion include deep injury, exposure into a vein or artery, or visible contamination. Currently, the benefit of assessing risk by measurement of viral load from the source is unknown.

Antiretroviral therapy is indicated for health care workers following possible actual HIV exposure. Medications should be initiated as soon as feasible, preferably within hours. However, treatment begun after many days should still be considered in the setting of high risk, as it may favorably affect the acute retroviral syndrome. The basic regimen is zidovudine (AZT) 300 mg and 3 lamivudine (3TC) 150 mg both twice daily. For health care workers with more severe exposures (e.g., large-bore needle, deep puncture), the addition of either 750 mg of nelfinavir thrice daily or 800 mg of indinavir every 8 hours is indicated. Therapy is continued for 4 weeks. Exposed health care workers should be checked for seroconversion at 6 weeks and then at 3, 6, and 12 months.

Studies of HIV in pregnancy provide excellent documentation of the feasibility of preventing the spread of disease by antiretroviral therapy. Aids Clinical Trials Group (ACTG) 076, a federally funded investigation, demonstrated a decline in spread of HIV to the newborn from approximately 24% to 8% (i.e., a 70% reduction) with the use of zidovudine during pregnancy, the peripartum period, and the first 6 weeks of life. This regimen may be initiated in the naive patient after 10 to 12 weeks of gestation. The recommendations for additional agents are inconclusive, and administration should be based on stage of disease, medications risks, and other relevant factors.

Table 82-2. International epidemiology of HIV/AIDS

| Region | HIV/AIDS (No.) | HIV prevalence (%) |
|---|---|---|
| Africa | 21,000,000 | 7.4 |
| Asia | 6,000,000 | 10–50 |
| Europe | 700,000 | 0.23 |
| Australia | 12,000 | 0.11 |
| Americas | 2,400,000 | 0.5–2.0 |
| United States | 650,000–900,000 | 0.5 |

Table 82-3. Risk for development of AIDS

| CD4 count | HIV RNA | 3 y | 6 y | 9 y |
|---|---|---|---|---|
| <350 | <1,500 | N/A | N/A | N/A |
| | 1,501–7,000 | 0 | 19 | 31 |
| | 7,001–20,000 | 8 | 42 | 66 |
| | 20,001–55,000 | 40 | 73 | 86 |
| | >55,000 | 73 | 93 | 96 |
| 351–500 | <1,500 | N/A | N/A | N/A |
| | 1,501–7,000 | 4 | 22 | 47 |
| | 7,001–20,000 | 6 | 40 | 60 |
| | 20,001–55,000 | 15 | 57 | 79 |
| | >55,000 | 48 | 78 | 94 |
| >500 | <1,500 | 1 | 5 | 11 |
| | 1,501–7,000 | 2 | 15 | 33 |
| | 7,001–20,000 | 7 | 26 | 50 |
| | 20,001–55,000 | 15 | 48 | 71 |
| | >55,000 | 33 | 67 | 76 |

N/A, not available.

For patients with known HIV infection who are on therapy and become pregnant, medications should generally be continued. (R.B.B.)

### Bibliography

Centers for Disease Control and Prevention. Update: trends in AIDS incidence—United States, 1996. *MMWR Morb Mortal Wkly Rep* 1997;46:861–867.
*Recent data concerning the incidence of AIDS in the United States. The information demonstrates decreases in AIDS-related opportunistic infections and deaths in comparison with data from 1995. This in turn reflects the positive impact of antiretroviral and antiopportunistic medications. Unfortunately, such trends are not seen worldwide.*
Centers for Disease Control and Prevention. Public Health Service guidelines for the management of health-care worker exposures to HIV and recommendations for postexposure prophylaxis *MMWR Morb Mortal Wkly Rep* 1998;(RR7):1–35.
*An excellent in-depth review of the problems and recommendations for management. All issues—identification, treatment, and counseling—are addressed. The authors stress the need for rapid initiation of antiretroviral treatment when indicated, and this requires the availability of appropriate facilities within the health care system.*
Centers for Disease Control and Prevention. Public Health Service Task Force recommendations for the use of antiretroviral drugs in pregnant women infected with HIV-1 for maternal health and for reducing perinatal HIV-1 transmission in the United States. *MMWR Morb Mortal Wkly Rep* 1998;47(RR2):1–30.
*This document provides the most recent recommendations for the management of HIV in pregnancy. At least zidovudine is indicated, and for patients who have been on antiretroviral therapy and then become pregnant, medications should generally be continued. These recommendations should be available to and followed by all health care workers dealing with pregnant women.*
Janssen RS, et al. HIV infection among patients in U.S. acute-care hospitals. *N Engl J Med* 1992;327:445–452.
*A multiple-hospital survey based on anonymous blood samples from 20 hospitals in 15 U.S. cities. Almost 5% of 195,829 specimens were HIV-positive. Seroprevalence rates were 0.2% to 14.2%. Most patients were hospitalized for non–HIV-related reasons. The authors estimate that 225,000 patients with HIV infection were hospitalized in 1990 in the United States, and they recommend voluntary HIV testing for persons ages 15 to 54 in hospitals with more than one newly diagnosed AIDS case per 1,000 discharges annually.*

Marcus R, CDC Cooperative Needlestick Surveillance Group. Surveillance of health care workers exposed to blood from patients infected with the human immunodeficiency virus. *N Engl J Med* 1988;319:1118–1123.

*Approximately 1,200 health care workers with blood exposures, more than 60% of them nurses, were followed. Most exposures resulted from needlestick injuries, and about a third were potentially preventable. The seroprevalence rate was 0.4%.*

Pantaleo G, et al. Studies in subjects with long-term, nonprogressive human immunodeficiency virus infection. *N Engl J Med* 1995;332:209–216.

*This and a companion article provide insights regarding a small subset of HIV-infected patients who are nonprogressors. Such persons continue to demonstrate viral replication, albeit with low viral loads. Lymph nodes and general immune function remain intact. The virus appears to be attenuated.*

Rosenberg PS, Biggar RJ. Trends in HIV incidence among young adults in the United States. *JAMA* 1998;279:1894–1899.

*Estimates are that about 33,000 persons ages 18 to 22 are HIV-positive. Male acquisition is primarily homosexual, whereas female acquisition is primarily heterosexual. The latter is increasing, and the former is decreasing.*

Vlahov D, et al. Prognostic indicators for AIDS and infectious death in HIV-infected injection drug users. *JAMA* 1998;279:35–40.

*The authors studied a cohort of more than 500 HIV-infected drug users for up to 8 years. As has been previously noted for male homosexuals, there was a direct correlation between baseline CD4-cell count, HIV RNA, and progression to AIDS-defining disease or infectious death. Of the two parameters, HIV RNA showed the more direct correlation. Simple assessments can be used to gauge the prognosis in IV drug users and male homosexuals.*

## 83. PRIMARY HIV INFECTION (HIV-MONONUCLEOSIS SYNDROME)

The clinical spectrum of the acute retroviral syndrome of primary HIV-1 infection is the result of the initial penetration and widespread dissemination of the HIV virus. The illness is often referred to as an HIV-mononucleosis or glandular feverlike disorder. Table 83-1 lists some of the protean signs and symptoms manifested during primary HIV infection. The acute clinical response to HIV-2 infection is similar to the clinical illness associated with primary HIV-1 infection. Some of the distinguishing features of primary HIV infection are an exanthem (macular or maculopapular oval or rounded lesions) with a predilection for the upper thorax, face, and forehead and oral-genital-anal ulcers. The most common manifestations include fever, fatigue, pharyngitis, myalgias, and headache. When symptoms and signs do develop (estimated to occur in 50% to 70% of infected patients), they appear after an incubation period of 11 days to 6 weeks. Clinical manifestations usually resolve spontaneously within 1 to 4 weeks (average duration, 25 days), although resolution occasionally requires more than 40 days. On occasion, concomitant AIDS-defining disorders develop, such as *Pneumocystis carinii* pneumonia, miliary tuberculosis, tuberculous meningitis, candidal esophagitis, cytomegalovirus (CMV) pneumonitis, CMV colitis, CMV encephalitis, ocular cryptococcosis, and prolonged cryptosporidiosis, so that when a symptom complex is unusual in severity and/or duration for primary HIV infection, the possible presence of a coexistent, treatable infecting agent needs to be considered. Rarely, it is difficult to determine if the patient has acute primary HIV infection with severe immunosuppression or advanced AIDS with the inability to demonstrate antibody.

Lymphadenopathy occurs commonly, appearing in the second week of illness, and most often involves the axillary, occipital, and cervical nodes. The adenopathy persists following the acute illness, but the size of affected nodes tends to decrease with time.

Laboratory findings include (initially) a reduction of total lymphocyte and T-cell subset counts, followed (by the beginning of the second week) by an increase in the concentration of CD8 cells and an inversion of the ratio of CD4 to CD8 cells. These latter

Table 83-1. Abnormal signs and symptoms described
in patients with primary HIV infection

| Systemic | Mucocutaneous |
|---|---|
| Fever | Ulcers (gingiva, buccal mucosa, |
| Sweats | anus, penis) |
| Malaise | Oral candidiasis |
| Weight loss | Conjunctivitis |
| Arthralgia | Enanthem of palate |
| Myalgia | **Dermatologic** |
| **Hematologic** | Macular rash |
| Generalized lymphadenopathy | Alopecia |
| Splenomegaly | **Neuropsychiatric** |
| **Digestive** | Depression |
| Sore throat | Irritability |
| Pharyngitis (with/without exudate) | Headache |
| Anorexia | Stiff neck |
| Vomiting | Photophobia |
| Nausea | Encephalopathy |
| Diarrhea | Myelopathy |
| Retrosternal pain | Neuropathy |
| Odynophagia | Guillain-Barré syndrome |
| Esophageal ulcers | **Respiratory** |
| Candidal esophagitis | Cough (nonproductive) |

findings can be accompanied by thrombocytopenia and, less commonly, atypical lymphocytes. Virus has been recovered from seminal fluid, peripheral blood (mononuclear cells and plasma), cerebrospinal fluid (often with a lymphocytic elevation), and bone marrow.

A number of studies have noted an association between specific features of symptomatic primary HIV infection, such as persistent fever and neurologic manifestations (encephalitis, meningitis, neuritis), peak plasma levels of HIV-1 RNA (determined more than 120 days after onset of disease), and accelerated progression of disease to AIDS and death.

The traditional screening test, the enzyme-linked immunosorbent assay (ELISA), may not detect antibodies to HIV for 1 to 2 months or even longer after development of disease, and rarely, the lack of antibody formation persists well beyond the expected "window" period. The diagnosis of primary HIV infection during the period of high viral replication in the absence of detectable antibody ("window of infectivity" period) has been established by the detection of p24 antigen. However, the detection of HIV RNA in plasma is a more sensitive test than the detection of p24 antigen, and this test can detect primary infection 3 to 5 days earlier. Culture of HIV from peripheral blood mononuclear cells is also a more sensitive test than detection of p24 antigen.

The diverse manifestations of primary HIV infection can resemble those of numerous other conditions, including drug reaction, Epstein-Barr virus (EBV) infection, influenza, CMV infection, rubella, parvovirus infection, hepatitis B, syphilis, toxoplasmosis, Lyme disease, leptospirosis, "aseptic" meningitis, and herpes encephalitis. The presence of a skin rash (rare in EBV infection unless the patient has received an antimicrobial), mucocutaneous ulcers, diarrhea, and cough suggest primary HIV infection rather than EBV infection. Pharyngeal exudate, lymphadenopathy, atypical lymphocytes, and abnormal levels of liver enzymes are noted in both these viral infections.

When patients manifest signs and symptoms compatible with acute HIV infection, a quantitative determination of viral load should be performed. If this "early" laboratory test demonstrates evidence of HIV (which should be confirmed in 6 weeks with the ELISA and Western blot antibody tests because false-positive HIVRNA tests have been reported), patients should be counseled regarding their disease. Patients must also be informed about the spread of HIV and the need to notify persons for whom they may have been a source of high-risk exposure (vaginal, rectal, oral-genital sex; sharing of needles, syringes) and be made aware of the various treatment options (no therapy; referral to a specialist at an AIDS center; monotherapy or combination antiretroviral treatments).

Zidovudine monotherapy during acute primary infection has resulted in increased CD4-cell counts and reduced development of "minor" opportunistic infections (oral candidiasis, oral hairy leukoplakia, herpes zoster). However, because patients with primary infection may harbor zidovudine-resistant strains of HIV, because acute curtailment of viral production helps the immune system to clear virus (resulting in a lower viral "set point"), and because combination treatments have the capacity to exert a potent antiviral effect (reduce virus in peripheral blood, peripheral lymph nodes, and gastrointestinal lymphoid tissue), some experts recommend that patients receive triple therapy with compounds that affect different parts of the viral life cycle. Certainly, therapy (consisting of two nucleoside analog reverse transcriptase inhibitors plus a protease inhibitor) should be recommended to patients with plasma RNA concentrations greater than 5,000 copies per milliliter regardless of the CD4-cell count. Patients must be counseled regarding their willingness to commit themselves to this costly, complex, and potentially toxic regimen. For those patients who cannot tolerate or comply with the three-drug regimen containing a protease inhibitor, the recommended alternative treatment consists of two nucleoside analog reverse transcriptase inhibitors and one non-nucleoside reverse transcriptase inhibitor (nevirapine, delavirdine or efavirenz). The drugs should be prescribed for at least 6 months (perhaps indefinitely) and be initiated simultaneously, *not* in sequence. Unfortunately, however, there is a paucity of clinical trial data to guide the clinician. (R.A.G.)

## Bibliography

Berger DS, et al. Acute primary human immunodeficiency virus type 1 infection in a patient with concomitant cytomegalovirus encephalitis. *Clin Infect Dis* 1996;23:66–70.
*Primary HIV infection can occur with a coexistent opportunistic infection that normally develops in a patient with profound immunosuppression (AIDS).*

Boufassa F, et al. Influence of neurologic manifestations of primary human immunodeficiency virus infection on disease progression. *J Infect Dis* 1995;171:1190–1195.
*Neurologic manifestations of primary HIV infection are associated with an accelerated progression of disease.*

Centers for Disease Control. Persistent lack of detectable HIV-1 antibody in a person with HIV infection—Utah 1995. *MMWR Morb Mortal Wkly Rep* 1996;45:181–185.
*A patient with confirmed HIV infection in whom results of enzyme immunoassays for HIV antibody were persistently negative beyond the expected "window period."*

Kahn JO, Walker BD. Acute human immunodeficiency virus type 1 infection. *N Engl J Med* 1998;339:33–39.
*A contemporary assessment of primary HIV infection.*

Kinloch-Delöes S, et al. A controlled trial of zidovudine in primary human immunodeficiency virus infection. *N Engl J Med* 1995;333:408–413.
*Antiretroviral therapy administered during primary infection may improve the subsequent clinical course and increase the CD4-cell count.*

Lafeuillade A, et al. Effects of a combination of zidovudine, didanosine, and lamivudine on primary human immunodeficiency virus type 1 infection. *J Infect Dis* 1997; 175:1051–1055.
*Triple-drug therapy has a potent antiviral effect during primary HIV-1 infection.*

Lapins J, et al. Mucocutaneous manifestations in 22 consecutive cases of primary HIV-1 infection. *Br J Dermatol* 1996;134:257–261.
*A review of the mucocutaneous manifestations of primary HIV-1 infection.*

Nui MT, et al., DATRI 002 Study Group. Zidovudine treatment in patients with primary (acute) human immunodeficiency virus type 1 infection: a randomized, doubleblind, placebo-controlled trial. *J Infect Dis* 1998;178:80–91.
*An example of clinical studies designed to assess the merits of drug treatment of primary HIV.*

Quinn TC. Acute primary HIV infection. *JAMA* 1997;278:58–62.
*A review of the clinical spectrum, diagnosis, and treatment.*

Schacker T, et al. Clinical and epidemiologic features of primary HIV infection. *Ann Intern Med* 1996;125:257–264.
*Detection of HIV RNA in plasma is more sensitive than p24 antigenemia to test for HIV seroconversion.*

Schacker TW, et al. Biological and virologic characteristics of primary HIV infection. *Ann Intern Med* 1998;128:613–620.
*Peak plasma HIV-1 RNA levels in the first 120 days were not predictive of disease progression.*

Vanhems P, et al. Acute human immunodeficiency virus type 1 disease as a mononucleosis-like illness: is the diagnosis too restrictive? *Clin Infect Dis* 1997;24:965–970.
*The mean duration of primary HIV infection is 25 days, and the most common abnormalities are fever, lethargy, rash, myalgia, and headache.*

Vanhems P, et al. Severity and prognosis of acute human immunodeficiency virus type 1 illness: a dose-response relationship. *Clin Infect Dis* 1998;26:323–329.
*Clinical expression of disease correlates with rate of progress.*

Veugelers PJ, et al. Incidence and prognostic significance of symptomatic primary human immunodeficiency virus type 1 infection in homosexual men. *J Infect Dis* 1997;176:112–117.
*Fever is associated with faster disease progression.*

## 84. TREATMENT OF *PNEUMOCYSTIS CARINII* PNEUMONIA IN AIDS

The CD4 lymphocyte plays a central role in protection against respiratory tract infections. Alveolar macrophages, natural killer cells, and B lymphocytes depend on adequate numbers and function of CD4 cells. As the CD4-cell count inevitably falls in patients with HIV infection, the ability of the lung defense mechanisms to protect against infection decreases. Pathogens such as *Pneumocystis carinii* and *Mycobacterium tuberculosis*, often residing in the host for years, overwhelm defense mechanisms as the CD4 count falls below a critical level. Although the pathogens against which an intact system of cell-mediated immunity is required are most problematic, humoral defenses are also impaired, and bacterial infections such as bacterial pneumonia are also more common and serious in AIDS patients.

Of all the respiratory infections seen in patients with AIDS, none is more common than *Pneumocystis carinii* pneumonia (PCP). Despite the decrease in frequency of this disease secondary to antibiotic prophylaxis, PCP remains an important cause of death in the United States. Patients are at risk for this infection once the CD4-cell count falls below 200/μL. The clinical symptoms are usually more insidious than would be seen with bacterial pneumonia. Low-grade fever with shortness of breath or exercise intolerance is frequent. Cough is present but usually nonproductive. The process is frequently associated with weight loss, fatigue, and a general decline in well-being during several weeks. Diffuse crackles may be heard on chest auscultation, but often the physical examination is not helpful. The disease is usually confined to the lungs, but in some cases, after pentamidine aerosol prophylaxis, disseminated infection can occur.

Chest roentgenography reveals a diffuse interstitial process, often affecting all portions of the lung field equally. However, variations in the characteristic picture are becoming more frequently reported. Chest roentgenographic patterns of consolidation, nodular lesions, pneumatoceles, and spontaneous pneumothoraces are all well described. Hilar adenopathy and pleural effusions are uncommon and should suggest another or a concomitant process. Initially, the chest roentgenographic findings may be normal with diffusely abnormal findings on gallium scan. Measurement of arterial blood gases is necessary to assess the need for supplementary oxygen but is not helpful in determining the specific cause of a pulmonary infection.

Survival of an acute episode is correlated with the extent of abnormalities on chest x-ray films and the alveolar-arterial oxygen gradient. Long-term survival is correlated with the degree of interstitial edema noted on transbronchial biopsy and a low alveolar-arterial oxygen gradient at the time of diagnosis. Persistence of cysts after 3 weeks of therapy also is a poor prognostic sign.

The recommended approach to the diagnosis of PCP is as follows: When clinical data and chest x-ray findings suggest PCP, induce sputum for examination of cysts and trophozoites. The patient's mouth is cleaned to avoid extraneous debris. Sputum is induced by inhalation of 3% saline solution through an ultrasonic nebulizer. The specimen is processed by trained personnel. The specimen is digested, centrifuged, and stained with Giemsa stain, silver methenamine, or toluidine blue. Direct immunofluorescent assays are being used at some institutions. The sensitivity of sputum examination is somewhere between 50% and 90%. Sensitivity is lower in patients who have been receiving aerosolized pentamidine.

Because a negative test result does not rule out PCP, bronchoscopy is the next procedure of choice, both to increase sensitivity and to search for other potential respiratory pathogens. Both bronchoalveolar lavage (BAL) and transbronchial biopsy are sensitive to detect *Pneumocystis carinii* and most other respiratory pathogens in AIDS. Broaddus et al. found that both procedures had similar sensitivities of 86% to 87%. Transbronchial biopsy was somewhat more sensitive than BAL for the diagnosis of PCP (97% vs. 86%). Most centers are now using BAL alone and consider biopsy with repeated bronchoscopy when the diagnosis remains elusive after the first procedure. Open lung biopsy is now considered an infrequent last resort and must be approached in the light of overall benefits versus risk and impact on prognosis.

Many clinicians are treating PCP empirically, especially when mild, although generally this is not formally recommended. In one study, 43 of 45 patients would have been given a correct diagnosis of PCP by clinical criteria alone. However, three patients would have been given an incorrect diagnosis and treated inappropriately. Not all studies report the same success with empiric treatment. In another study, only 57% of AIDS patients treated for PCP actually had the infection.

Table 84-1 lists the potential regimens for the treatment of PCP. Treatment depends on the degree of illness, which is often categorized as mild, moderate, or severe (Pao$_2$ <70 mm Hg). In patients who are not acutely ill, outpatient therapy with oral drug regimens can be initiated with careful follow-up. Trimethoprim-sulfamethoxazole (TMP-SMX) remains the drug of choice for all cases of PCP, regardless of severity. For mild or moderate disease, two double-strength tablets of TMP-SMX four times per day (15 to 20 mg/kg) remains the regimen of choice. TMP-SMX is also the regimen of choice

Table 84-1. Treatment regimens for *Pneumocystis carinii* pneumonia

**Mild-to-moderate disease (patient not acutely ill, Po$_2$ > 70 mm Hg)**
A. TMP-SMX 2 tablets DS PO tid for 21 d
B. Dapsone 100 mg PO qd *plus* TMP 100 mg PO tid for 21 d
C. Ataquone 750 mg PO tid for 21 d
D. Clindamycin 600 mg PO tid plus primaquine 30 mg PO daily

**Moderate-to-severe disease (Po$_2$ <70 mm Hg)**
A. TMP-SMX (TMP 20 mg/kg per day; SMX 100 mg/kg per day) q6h for 21 d
B. Pentamidine isethionate 4 mg/kg per day IV for 21 d
C. Clindamycin 900 mg IV q8h *plus* primaquine 30 mg PO qd
D. Trimetrexate 45 mg/m$^2$ IV daily plus leucovorin 20 mg/m$^2$ PO or IV for course of therapy, extended 3 d after completion of trimetrexate

In addition to A, B, C, or D:

Prednisone 40 mg PO bid for 5 d

*then*

Prednisone 40 mg PO qd for 5 d

*then*

Prednisone 20 mg PO qd for 11 d

TMP-SMX, trimethoprim-sulfamethoxazole; DS, = double strength.

for severe disease, in which case it is given parenterally, usually for 10 to 14 days. Monitoring of sulfa levels to maintain them between 100 and 150 > µg/mL has been recommended to reduce toxicity, especially in the setting of renal insufficiency. Some toxicity can be expected with TMP-SMX regimens in more than half of all patients, although most adverse reactions are not life-threatening. Adverse reactions such as fever, rash, neutropenia, and thrombocytopenia usually develop after about 1 week. They are much more likely to occur in AIDS patients than in other immunosuppressed patients. Folic or folinic acid plays no role in preventing hematologic toxicity and is not recommended.

Dapsone plus TMP may be as effective as TMP-SMX and at least as well tolerated. A randomized San Francisco General Hospital study found that either regimen was more than 90% effective for mild-to-moderate disease. Side effects include rash, neutropenia, nausea and vomiting, and hemolytic anemia, often in association with glucose-6-phosphate dehydrogenase deficiency.

Clindamycin plus primaquine has been used for mild-to-moderate disease, with 600 mg of clindamycin taken orally three times daily and 30 mg of primaquine taken orally each day. For severe disease, 900 mg of clindamycin is given intravenously every 8 hours, with the oral dose of primaquine remaining the same. In one randomized study from Canada, TMP-SMX was compared with clindamycin-primaquine. No differences in outcome, rate of relapse, survival, or adverse effects were noted. Hemolytic anemia in association with glucose-6-phosphate dehydrogenase deficiency is also a concern with primaquine.

Atovaquone is a hydroxynaphthoquinone that inhibits protozoal mitochondrial electron transport and pyrimidine biosynthesis. It is approved only for treatment of mild-to-moderate disease ($PaO_2$ >60 mm Hg). The drug is generally well tolerated but is only half as effective (20% to 31% failure rate) as TMP-SMX. Adverse reactions include rash, fever, nausea and vomiting, and abnormal levels of liver enzymes. The drug is variably absorbed and should be avoided if a patient has diarrhea and other gastrointestinal problems. Serum levels of 15 µ/mL or greater correlate with a favorable response.

As noted, when a patient is acutely ill or hypoxic with PCP, TMP-SMX administered intravenously (TMP, 20 mg/kg per day; SMX, 100 mg/kg per day) is still the regimen of choice. If toxicity develops, IV pentamidine isethionate can be used (4 mg/kg per day over 1 to 2 hours) for 21 days. Dosage adjustment is required when the glomerular filtration rate is below 50 mL/min. IV pentamidine is about as effective as IV TMP-SMX for severe disease. Pancreatitis, azotemia, leukopenia, hyperglycemia, or hypoglycemia can all develop and make drug cessation necessary. Pentamidine-induced cardiac toxicity has been reported, including *torsades de pointes* and other forms of ventricular tachycardia. Delivery of the drug to the lung via aerosolization has been used in the treatment of mild disease but has been associated with a high rate of relapse and treatment failure.

Trimetrexate is a quinazoline analog of methotrexate that has been approved for moderate-to-severe disease in patients who have not responded to TMP-SMX. Leucovorin is given concomitantly to avoid the complications of myelosuppression. In a randomized study of patients with moderate-to-severe disease, TMP-SMX was more effective than trimetrexate-leucovorin. Mortality rates were twice as high with trimetrexate and relapses were more common. The drug is probably best reserved for those in whom both TMP-SMX and pentamidine are contraindicated or who have failed to respond to these preferred drugs.

A number of clinical trials have supported the use of corticosteroids in moderate-to-severe disease. Corticosteroids moderate the intense inflammatory reaction that can occur in response to protozoal killing early in the course of treatment. Based on the results of five randomized trials, a panel of experts from the National Institutes of Health recommended the adjunctive use of corticosteroids within 24 to 72 hours for patients above the age of 13 who had severe disease (defined as $PaO_2$ <70 mm Hg or $PaO_2 - PaO_2$ >35 mm Hg). Table 84-2 summarizes the recommendations for steroid use. In those with the most severe disease, corticosteroids will decrease mortality from about 40% to 20%. The potential to exacerbate certain concomitant disease, such as tuberculosis, must be recognized. However, in one study the incidence of tuberculosis was not found to be increased by the use of corticosteroids as empiric therapy of PCP.

Table 84-2. Corticosteroid use in *Pneumocystis carinii* pneumonia

**Indication**
For patients with documented PCP who are acutely ill, with PaO$_2$ <70 mm Hg
**Dosage**
Prednisone 40 mg bid for 5 d
Prednisone 40 mg qd for 5 d
Prednisone 20 mg qd for 11 d
Give first dose of prednisone 30 min before TMP-SMX.*
Begin as soon as possible, within 72 h of therapy.
**Other**
Do not continue unless PCP is documented.
Be alert for exacerbation of any concomitant disease.

PCP, *Pneumocystis carinii* pneumonia; TMP-SMX, trimethoprim-sulfamethoxazole.
* See Table 84-1 for dose.

Disseminated, deep-seated fungal infection has been reported in some patients treated empirically with corticosteroids. All patients with severe disease should be hospitalized and treated with supplemental oxygen. Noninvasive ventilatory support by means of continuous positive airway pressure has been useful in buying time and avoiding mechanical ventilation. When intubation and mechanical ventilation are being considered, the prognosis, overall HIV history, and patient preferences must all be taken into account. Patients who require mechanical ventilation for respiratory failure secondary to PCP generally have a poor prognosis. (S.L.B.)

### Bibliography

Bozzette SA, et al. A controlled trial of early adjunctive treatment with corticosteroids for *Pneumocystis carinii* pneumonia in the acquired immunodeficiency syndrome. *N Engl J Med* 1990;323:1451.
*Early corticosteroid treatment reduced risks for respiratory failure and death in PCP. There were few adverse effects.*
Brenner M, et al. Prognostic factors and life expectancy of patients with acquired immunodeficiency syndrome and *Pneumocystis carinii* pneumonia. *Am Rev Respir Dis* 1987;136:1199.
*Patients in whom PCP was diagnosed before 1985 had more advanced disease at the time of diagnosis and a worse prognosis. The extent of disease on chest x-ray films and the alveolar-arterial gradient could be correlated with prognosis.*
Broaddus C, et al. Bronchoalveolar lavage and transbronchial biopsy for the diagnosis of pulmonary infections in the acquired immunodeficiency syndrome. *Ann Intern Med* 1985;102:747.
*This study compared BAL with transbronchial biopsy for the diagnosis of pulmonary infection in AIDS. Both were sensitive for* Pneumocystis carinii *infection. The sensitivity for* Pneumocystis carinii *infection when they were used together was 100%.*
Brooks KR, et al. Acute respiratory failure due to *Pneumocystis carinii* pneumonia. *Crit Care Clin* 1993;9:31.
*Management of PCP in AIDS is discussed with respect to ventilatory support and critical care.*
Fallon J, Masur H. Infectious complications of HIV: *Pneumocystis carinii* and other protozoa. In: Fallon J, Masur H, eds. *AIDS: etiology, diagnosis, treatment and prevention.* Philadelphia: JB Lippincott Co, 1992.
*Good, succinct review of PCP.*
Gagnon S, et al. Corticosteroids as adjunctive therapy for severe *Pneumocystis carinii* pneumonia in the acquired immunodeficiency syndrome. *N Engl J Med* 1990;323:1444.
*Also shows that early adjunctive corticosteroid therapy improves survival and prevents respiratory failure in PCP.*

Golden JA, et al. Bronchoalveolar lavage as the exclusive diagnostic modality for *Pneumocystis carinii* pneumonia: a prospective study among patients with acquired immunodeficiency syndrome. *Chest* 1986;90:18.
*BAL detected PCP in 36 of 37 patients, making lung biopsy of little value in this disease.*

Hughes WT, et al. Comparison of atovaquone (566C80) with trimethoprim-sulfamethoxazole to treat *Pneumocystis carinii* pneumonia in patients with AIDS. *N Engl J Med* 1993;328:1521.
*Atovaquone had a lower rate of efficacy but also a lower rate of treatment-limiting adverse effects, making it an option in mild disease when patients cannot be treated with TMP-SMX.*

Jones BE, et al. Tuberculosis in patients with HIV infection who receive corticosteroids for presumed *Pneumocystis carinii* pneumonia. *Am J Respir Crit Care Med* 1994; 149:1686.
*The incidence of active tuberculosis was not increased in patients with HIV infection who were treated with corticosteroids for PCP.*

Kovacs JA, et al. Diagnosis of *Pneumocystis carinii* pneumonia: improved detection in sputum with use of monoclonal antibodies. *N Engl J Med* 1988;318:589.
*Examination of induced sputum was a sensitive test in the diagnosis of PCP. Immunofluorescent stain had a 92% sensitivity; Giemsa DifQuik was 76% sensitive.*

Levine SJ. *Pneumocystis carinii*. *Clin Chest Med* 1997;17:665.
*This article reviews in great detail the clinical manifestations, prognostic markers, and treatment options for PCP.*

Miller RF, Mitchell DM. AIDS and the lung: update 1995. *Thorax* 1995;50:191.
*Concise review article on PCP that includes molecular biology and details of treatment options.*

Miller RF, et al. Empirical treatment without bronchoscopy for *Pneumocystis carinii* pneumonia in the acquired immunodeficiency syndrome. *Thorax* 1989;44:559.
*Describes the experience with an empiric approach to treatment in comparison with the use of bronchoscopy for diagnosis.*

Montaner JSG, et al. Corticosteroids prevent early deterioration in patients with moderately severe *Pneumocystis carinii* pneumonia and the acquired immunodeficiency syndrome (AIDS). *Ann Intern Med* 1990;113:14.
*Oral corticosteroids prevented early deterioration in AIDS patients who were moderately ill in this prospective, randomized, double-blind, placebo-controlled study.*

Murray JF, et al. NHLBI Workshop summary. Pulmonary complications of the acquired immunodeficiency syndrome: an update. *Am Rev Respir Dis* 1987;135:504.
*An overall approach to the evaluation of AIDS patients with pulmonary infection is presented in this report from the National Heart, Lung, and Blood Institute Workshop.*

National Institutes of Health. Special report: consensus statement on the use of corticosteroids as adjunctive therapy for *Pneumocystis* pneumonia in the acquired immunodeficiency syndrome. *N Engl J Med* 1990;323:1500.
*Excellent review of steroid trials in PCP. Includes a National Institutes of Health consensus statement recommending an oral tapering regimen of corticosteroids for patients with documented, moderate-to-severe PCP.*

Phair J, et al. The risk of *Pneumocystis carinii* pneumonia among men infected with human immunodeficiency virus type 1. *N Engl J Med* 1990;322:161.
*PCP is unlikely to occur in a patient who has a CD4 count above 200/mm³. Prophylaxis should be reserved for patients with a CD4-cell count below this level.*

Pitchenik AE, et al. Sputum examination for the diagnosis of *Pneumocystis carinii* pneumonia in the acquired immunodeficiency syndrome. *Am Rev Respir Dis* 1986; 133:226.
*Results of sputum examination were positive in 55% of patients. Examination of induced sputum is recommended as a first step in the diagnosis of PCP.*

Safrin S, et al. A double-blind, randomized comparison of oral trimethoprim-sulfamethoxazole, dapsone-trimethoprim, and clindamycin-primaquine for treatment of mild-to-moderate *Pneumocystis carinii* pneumonia in patients with AIDS. *Ann Intern Med* 1996;124:792.

*One third of patients were unable to tolerate an oral TMP-SMX regimen. Describes the alternative oral regimens for mild-to-moderate disease.*

Sattler FR, et al. Trimetrexate with leucovorin versus trimethoprim-sulfamethoxazole for moderate to severe episodes of *Pneumocystis carinii* pneumonia in patients with AIDS. *J Infect Dis* 1994;170:165.

*Failure rare, relapses and mortality rates higher in the trimetrexate group. Trimetrexate-leucovorin can be used to treat PCP in patients who have failed TMP-SMX and pentamidine or who have contraindications to these regimens.*

Smith D, Gazzard B. Treatment and prophylaxis of *Pneumocystis carinii* pneumonia in AIDS patients. *Drugs* 1991;42:628.

*Good description of treatment options in PCP, particularly with regard to toxicity profile.*

Toma E, et al. Clindamycin-primaquine versus trimethoprim-sulfamethoxazole as primary therapy for *Pneumocystis carinii* pneumonia in AIDS: a randomized, double-blind pilot trial. *Clin Infect Dis* 1993;17:178.

*There were no differences in outcome, survival, or relapse between these regimens. Therapy-limiting adverse reactions occurred in 18% of patients receiving clindamycin-primaquine. Patients should be screened for deficiency of glucose-6-phosphate dehydrogenase before receiving this regimen.*

Wachter RM, Luce JM, Hopewell PC. Critical care of patients with AIDS. *JAMA* 1992; 267:541.

*Discusses medical and ethical issues involved in the management of respiratory failure in AIDS patients.*

## 85. TUBERCULOSIS AND SYPHILIS IN THE AIDS ERA

Since 1986, syphilis and tuberculosis have reemerged as significant health care problems, in part related to the AIDS epidemic. Between 1986 and 1990, what was considered an epidemic of syphilis was noted in the United States. During this time, rates were approximately 12 to 21 cases per 100,000 population per year. Since that time, rates of primary plus secondary syphilis have declined by about 84%, and nationally are at 3.2 cases per 100,000 population. This is attributed to better management and control strategies for both syphilis and HIV/AIDS. Similar recent declines have been noted for tuberculosis. In 1995, approximately 22,800 cases of tuberculosis were reported to the Centers for Disease Control, representing three consecutive years of decline. By 1997, reported cases had further declined to 19,855 (7.4 cases per 100,000 population). This represents a 26% decline since 1992. For cases reported with susceptibilities, 7.6% of isolates were resistant to isoniazid (INH), and 1.3% were multiply drug-resistant. Unfortunately, HIV status was reported only in about 50% of patients with tuberculosis, and the range of coinfection by state was nil to 48%. The simultaneous presence of HIV with either tuberculosis or syphilis is of major concern because of the differences in clinical presentation and the potential for altered responses to therapy.

### Tuberculosis

Although pulmonary and extrapulmonary tuberculosis were described early in the AIDS epidemic, the full impact of this mycobacterial infection has been recognized only within the past several years. Between 1984 and 1991, there were approximately 39,000 more cases of tuberculosis than had been anticipated. By 1991, the number of new cases rose to approximately 26,280, an increase of 2.3% over the previous year, with most cases geographically linked to regions associated with HIV infection. Subsequently, numbers have declined to fewer than 20,000 cases per year. A recent prospective investigation of more than 1,100 HIV-infected persons without AIDS-defining diagnoses demonstrated that tuberculosis developed in 31 of them (16 with pulmonary tuberculosis only, seven with only extrapulmonary disease, and eight simultaneously infected with pulmonary and extrapulmonary tuberculosis) during a median follow-up period of 53 months. These numbers, representing 0.7 cases per 100 patient-years, were related to geographic area and the magnitude of initial results of purified protein derivative testing. The risk for development of tuberculosis was eight-fold higher in persons with tuberculin test reactions larger than 5 mm than for those with smaller measurements. Negative results on skin testing for mumps were also statistically associated with the development of tuberculosis. Of eligible patients, only 55% received prophylactic INH, and only 59% of these completed 6 months of prophylaxis.

Studies of the prevalence of HIV among patients with proven or suspected tuberculosis demonstrate rates of up to 46%, with many urban centers reporting rates in excess of 10%. Alternatively, an average of 3.8% of patients with AIDS also appear on tuberculosis registries (range, 0 to 10%). This correlation is apparent mostly in IV drug users and selected minorities.

The pathogenesis of tuberculosis in patients with HIV infection involves either reactivation of previously latent disease or new acquisition of *Mycobacterium tuberculosis,* most commonly by droplet inhalation. Both modes are probably exacerbated by concomitant HIV infection because of its impact on cell-mediated immunity, especially as related to the decline in numbers of CD4 cells and macrophage and monocyte dysfunction.

*Clinical Presentation and Diagnosis*
Tuberculosis may present at any time in the course of HIV/AIDS and is therefore one of the few AIDS-defining opportunistic infections associated with CD4-cell counts greater than 200/μL. Thus, many patients may present to tuberculosis clinics and physicians' offices before being given a diagnosis of HIV infection. Pulmonary involvement is seen in approximately 75% of patients and may present as it does in persons who are not infected with HIV. This is especially true in patients with higher CD4-cell counts. Alternatively, patients may present with atypical disease, which includes disease affecting primarily the lower lobes, dissemination, hilar adenopathy, and extrapulmonary involvement. Several studies now demonstrate a marked increase in extrapulmonary tuberculosis in patients coinfected with HIV; extrapulmonary may coexist with pulmonary involvement. Common extrapulmonary manifestations include lymphadenitis, dissemination (miliary), meningitis, and focal disease at other anatomic locations. A recent investigation of HIV and tuberculosis demonstrated that HIV-positive patients were more likely to have extrapulmonary tuberculosis, but smears for acid-fast bacilli in patients with pulmonary tuberculosis were positive more frequently among the cohort without HIV seropositivity. Other opportunistic infections, such as *Pneumocystis carinii* pneumonia, cytomegalovirus pneumonia, and fungal infections, need to be considered and may not be distinguishable on clinical or radiographic grounds. Tuberculous lymphadenitis may involve nodes about the neck and affect those of the hilum and mediastinum. The clinical presentation is usually that of fever and tender lymphadenopathy. Lymph node aspiration demonstrates acid-fast bacilli in more than 67% of cases. When disease involves the lung, the diagnosis is based on a high index of suspicion plus positive results on acid-fast smear and culture of sputum. Alternatively, screening of asymptomatic HIV-positive patients by chest roentgenography is not warranted.

Skin testing can provide important clues but does not prove the presence of active infection. Results of skin testing follow the degree of immunosuppression resulting from HIV infection. Tuberculin reactivity is thought to be maintained throughout early HIV infection. Overall, about 40% of patients with HIV infection and tuberculosis react positively to intermediate-strength purified protein derivative (Mantoux test). Current recommendations are to consider a 5-mm induration as a positive result in patients with HIV, and (unless specifically contraindicated) all tuberculin-positive patients should receive INH prophylaxis. Debate continues regarding the value of controls and the determination of anergy. The most clinical experience has been acquired with mumps and *Candida* antigens as controls; however, it has not been routinely demonstrated that anergy to these is associated with increased risks for the development of tuberculosis. Most recent guidelines from the Centers for Disease Control no longer recommend the routine use of controls in tuberculin testing.

The diagnosis of active tuberculosis requires either identification of the organism or a clinical or radiographic response to specific therapy. The best data demonstrate that smears will be positive in 30% to 80% (expectorated sputa) and 30% to 75% (bronchoscopy) of cases with pulmonary involvement. The likelihood of recovery of organisms is higher in patients with higher CD4-cell counts. For disease outside the lungs, a high index of suspicion is necessary so that appropriate smears and cultures can be obtained. When lysis-centrifugation techniques are used, blood cultures for *M. tuberculosis* are positive in up to 40% of cases and should be obtained when dissemination is considered.

Chest x-ray findings are generally abnormal in patients with pulmonary tuberculosis but may be normal in those with strictly endobronchial disease. "Usual" changes, such as involvement of the upper lobes with or without cavitation and effusion, are often noted, but atypical presentations, such as infiltrates in lower lobes, miliary patterns, and mediastinal adenopathy, are also regularly seen. No features should be considered pathognomonic of tuberculosis, and virtually all have important differential diagnoses.

### Treatment

The therapy of *M. tuberculosis* infection has been complicated by the recent emergence in some geographic areas of primary drug resistance to front-line medications such as INH and rifampin. At least 12 such outbreaks have been reported since 1990, and they often involve the development of new infection rather than reactivation. Although to date most cases have occurred in inner-city or prison populations, there is little reason to think that highly resistant strains will not emerge in other venues. This problem has been complicated by recent difficulties in obtaining streptomycin. In the absence of this drug, medications employed in the treatment of tuberculosis in patients with HIV are similar to those in other populations. Most data suggest that patients respond well, and treatment failures or relapses are noted in fewer than 5% of cases. However, most investigators treat patients for more prolonged periods. Table 85-1 summarizes treatment recommendations.

Standard therapy for sensitive organisms should include INH, rifampin, and pyrazinamide for 2 months, followed by INH plus rifampin for either an additional 7 months or 6 months after culture negativity (whichever is longer). Patients with proven or presumed multiply resistant organisms (generally at least to both INH and rifampin) need to be treated with multiple-drug regimens, often containing third-line or investigational agents (e.g., ciprofloxacin, ofloxacin, and amikacin). Mortality rates in these outbreaks have been in excess of 75%, often within 4 months of diagnosis. Of the quinolones, ofloxacin and ciprofloxacin have been best studied. They should not be employed as first-line agents, but rather in conjunction with other agents when the use of INH and rifampin is impossible. Susceptibility testing to these agents should be performed. Com-

Table 85-1. Therapy of tuberculosis in the HIV-positive patient

| Category | Agents (dose per day) | Duration |
|---|---|---|
| Empiric, INH resistance >4% | INH 300 mg<br>Rifampin 600 mg<br>Pyrazinamide 20–30 mg/kg<br>Ethambutol 15 mg/kg | 6 mo* |
| Empiric, INH resistance <4% | Same as above, without ethambutol | 6 mo |
| INH-resistant TB | Four-drug regimen, as above, but delete INH in favor of pyrazinamide A for full 6 months | 6 mo |
| Multiple-drug resistance | Regimen with at least two, and preferably three, effective agents | Up to 24 mo |

INH, isoniazid.
*adjust regimen after two months, based on results of susceptibility testing; treat 6 months after culture is negative.

pliant patients who tolerate complex regimens can be expected to do better. In one published study, the response rate was better than 50% when patients took medicines for at least 2 consecutive weeks within a month of diagnosis. The optimal length of treatment has not been determined but is at least 12 months following culture negativity. Therapy for at least 18 months is recommended if neither INH nor rifampin can be used because of intolerance.

Tuberculin skin testing should be employed in all HIV-positive patients, and chemoprophylaxis should be offered to all HIV-positive patients with positive (>5 mm) tuberculin test results who do not demonstrate active tuberculosis. Selected anergic patients felt to be at high risk for infection may also be offered prophylaxis. Several options now exist. The standard is INH for 12 months. Alternatives are summarized in Table 85-2. Thus, 2-month regimens with rifampin and pyrazinamide offer the alternative of more pills for shorter periods, but without significantly enhanced toxicity. Issues of drug interactions must be addressed. Although some authorities recommend prophylaxis indefinitely, there are no data to support duration in excess of 12 months. All HIV-positive persons exposed to tuberculosis should receive prophylaxis, regardless of skin test reactivity. Prophylactic formulations for persons exposed to multidrug-resistant tuberculosis are experimental but could involve rifampin alone (resistance to INH only) or combinations of ciprofloxacin or ofloxacin plus pyrazinamide (resistance to multiple drugs).

Recommendations for the prevention of transmission of tuberculosis in health care settings have been published. These stress the need to employ multifactorial methods: early identification and treatment of patients, prevention of spread of droplet nuclei into the air by use of source-control methodology, reduction of air contamination, decontamination of equipment, and surveillance.

## Syphilis

The incidence of syphilis has risen during the past several years; this is in large part related to HIV infection. In 1990, more than 50,000 cases of syphilis were reported, an increase of approximately 75% from 1985. Most cases were transmitted heterosexually. Since this time, rates have fallen considerably, in part because of better methods of detection and management of both HIV infection and syphilis. Interactions between HIV infection and syphilis are well described. These include an enhanced likelihood of HIV transmission in patients with primary syphilis, altered serologic responses, more rapid progression of primary syphilis to neurosyphilis, and potential for delayed response to therapy.

That primary syphilis (and other ulcerative genital lesions) is associated with increased transmission of HIV has been well established. Several investigations in Africa and the United States document increased rates of HIV positivity in persons treated for syphilis or having a history of genital ulcers. The reasons for this association include the disruption of epithelial barriers in ulcers (thus facilitating HIV transmission) and the availability of large numbers of activated T lymphocytes at the base of genital lesions, which may expedite entry of HIV into the immune system.

Table 85-2. Regimens for tuberculosis prevention

| Regimen | Dose | Duration | Other issues |
|---|---|---|---|
| INH | 300 mg qd | 12 mo | Standard regimen |
| INH | 900 mg twice weekly, direct observation | 12 mo | Higher likelihood of compliance |
| Rifampin plus pyrazinamide | 600 mg plus 15–20 mg/kg daily | 2 mo | Drug interactions; shortest regimen, no increase adverse reactions |
| Rifampin plus pyrazinamide | 600 mg plus 50 mg/kg twice weekly, direct observation | 2 mo | See above |

A modification of serologic response to syphilis in persons infected with HIV has been documented but is the exception rather than the rule. Selected patients may demonstrate marked fluctuations in titers. However, in most instances, both reaginic tests [Venereal Disease Research Laboratory (VDRL), rapid plasma reagin (RPR)] and specific treponemal tests [fluorescent treponemal antibody absorption (FTA-ABS), microhemagglutination specific for *Treponema pallidum* (MHA-Tp)] should be used in the same manner as in non–HIV-infected populations. The diagnosis of neurosyphilis requires a combination of techniques that includes interpretation of cerebrospinal fluid (CSF) VDRL test results and chemical and cellular results of lumbar puncture. The serologic response to therapy may also be altered in patients who are HIV-positive. Response may be delayed, and a higher percentage of persons may become nonreactive on specific treponemal testing.

Clinical syphilis is clearly modified in patients with HIV. Although no data exist that document more severe primary disease, accelerated progression to neurosyphilis has been noted. Up to 1.5% of patients with AIDS have neurosyphilis. Other studies have noted that 44% of persons with neurosyphilis had AIDS, despite appropriate therapy for early disease.

Neurosyphilis in the AIDS era has changed. Most cases now appear to represent early neurosyphilis, with an average age of onset below 40. Primary manifestations of meningitis, meningovascular disease, and uveitis are noted. Late neurosyphilis manifested as tabes dorsalis or paresis occurs less commonly. The most common manifestations of early neurosyphilis are meningitis, cranial nerve palsies, and meningovascular disease. The cranial nerves most affected include the ophthalmic and auditory nerves. At least 95% of persons have abnormal CSF findings that are nondiagnostic but include elevated protein, pleocytosis, and hypoglycorrhachia. Cell counts range from 40 to 400/mm³, often with a lymphocyte predominance. Virtually all patients with neurosyphilis demonstrate CSF cell counts of more than 5/mm³. CSF protein levels are generally below 500 mg/dL but may occasionally be higher. Interpretation is complicated by other illnesses, including HIV infection, that can cause similar central nervous system abnormalities.

The treatment of primary and secondary syphilis in patients with HIV infection is similar to that in non–HIV-infected patients. IM injection of 2.4 g of benzathine penicillin is recommended. Some experts would treat with three doses, each a week apart. VDRL studies should be repeated at 6 and 12 months, and a fourfold reduction in titer is expected at 6 months. For patients who fail to respond, CSF examination and (if CSF unremarkable) repeated treatment for 3 weeks is recommended. The need for routine lumbar puncture in HIV-infected patients with syphilis is uncertain. It should

Table 85-3. Therapy of syphilis in HIV-infected patients

| Classification | Penicillin regimen | Dose | Alternative agent | Dose |
|---|---|---|---|---|
| Primary/ secondary | Benzathine | 2.4 million U IM once | Doxycycline | 100 mg PO bid for 14 d |
| Early latent | Benzathine | 2.4 million U IM once | Unknown | Unknown |
| Late latent or unknown duration | Benzathine | 2.4 million U IM weekly × 3 | Unknown | Unknown |
| Neurosyphilis | Aqueous penicillin G | 18–24 million U IV × 10–14 d | Procaine penicillin | 2.4 million U IM daily plus probenicid 500 mg PO qid, both for 10–14 d |

be performed diagnostically in all persons with neurologic findings or complaints, both to define the length of parenteral therapy and to monitor response. Patients with advanced syphilis (late latent syphilis or neurosyphilis) of the central nervous system are preferably treated parenterally for 10 to 14 days with 18 to 24 million units of IV aqueous penicillin G, given daily in four to six divided doses. The treatment of patients with early neurosyphilis is associated with high cure rates. Table 85-3 summarizes the recommendations for treatment of syphilis in HIV-infected persons. Few data exist to recommend agents other than penicillin for neurosyphilis or latent syphilis. Recent investigations have documented a disturbingly high failure rate (23%) with IV ceftriaxone administered in doses of up to 2 g daily. Under all circumstances, vigilant follow-up is indicated to define failure or relapse. (R.B.B.)

## Bibliography

Ad Hoc Committee of the Scientific Assembly on Microbiology, Tuberculosis, and Pulmonary Infections. Treatment of tuberculosis and tuberculosis infection in adults and children. *Clin Infect Dis* 1995;21:9–27.

*An excellent summary of available data and recommendations for the management of tuberculosis in the United States. Medications employed in management are discussed, along with proposed regimens. The value of directly observed therapy is reinforced.*

Alpert PL, et al. A prospective study of tuberculosis and human immunodeficiency virus infection: clinical manifestations and factors associated with survival. *Clin Infect Dis* 1997;24:661–668.

*More than 100 HIV-positive patients with tuberculosis were identified, prospectively followed, and compared with an HIV-negative cadre. Those who were HIV-positive were more likely to have extrapulmonary tuberculosis and were less likely to have sputum smears positive for acid-fast bacilli. Improved survivorship was correlated with rapid initiation of treatment and less severe HIV disease.*

Barnes PF, et al. Tuberculosis in patients with human immunodeficiency virus infection. *N Engl J Med* 1991;324:1644–1650.

*Excellent overview of epidemiology, clinical features, diagnosis, and management of tuberculosis in patients with HIV infection. Provides therapeutic strategies based on the likelihood of drug resistance and ways to distinguish presumptively* M. tuberculosis *from* Mycobacterium avium *complex.*

Busillo CP, et al. Multidrug-resistant *Mycobacterium tuberculosis* in patients with human immunodeficiency virus infection. *Chest* 1992;102:797–801.

*This investigation demonstrates that since 1990, approximately one third of patients with tuberculosis have harbored multidrug-resistant strains. Resistance is defined as resistance to INH plus at least one other first-line agent. Often, resistance was noted to at least three agents. Approximately 75% of patients died despite therapy with at least four drugs. Optimal therapy is unknown.*

Centers for Disease Control and Prevention. Tuberculosis morbidity—United States, 1997. *MMWR Morb Mortal Wkly Rep* 1998;47:253–257.

*Excellent recent data are provided that demonstrate the continued decline in rates of active tuberculosis in the United States. Most of this decline is attributable to cases in persons born in the United States. Rates among immigrants have actually increased slightly. Of isolates for which susceptibility data are available, about 8% demonstrate resistance to INH, and 1.3% are multidrug-resistant. Furthermore, cases of multidrug-resistant tuberculosis appear to be decreasing.*

Centers for Disease Control and Prevention. 1998 Guidelines for treatment of sexually transmitted diseases. *MMWR Morb Mortal Wkly Rep* 1998;47(RR1):28–49.

*An extremely contemporary review of guidelines for the management of syphilis, with especial reference to HIV/AIDS. Best single source of recommendations for the management of syphilis. Provides information for treatment that includes tables for penicillin desensitization.*

Centers for Disease Control and Prevention. Primary and secondary syphilis—United States, 1997. *MMWR Morb Mortal Wkly Rep* 1998;47:493–497.

*This article provides recent data on the epidemiology of primary and secondary syphilis. During the past several years, the incidence has declined by up to 84%. Rates remain higher for blacks and are highest in the South.*

Chaisson RE, et al. Tuberculosis in patients with the acquired immunodeficiency syndrome: clinical features, response to therapy, and survival. *Am Rev Respir Dis* 1987;136:570–574.
*This vintage investigation documents the interaction between tuberculosis and HIV infection, demonstrating the frequency of extrapulmonary disease and the fact tuberculosis may antedate the diagnosis of HIV. A good clinical response to therapy was generally noted.*

Flood JM, et al. Neurosyphilis during the AIDS epidemic, San Francisco, 1985–1992. *J Infect Dis* 1998;177:931–940.
*The authors review their experience with 117 patients who had neurosyphilis, of whom approximately 65% were HIV-infected. Most were young and presented with early neurosyphilis. High VDRL titers were often noted. Treatment of this cadre was generally curative.*

Hook EW III, Marra CM. Acquired syphilis in adults. *N Engl J Med* 1992;326:1060–1069.
*Provides excellent demographic data on the impact of HIV on the prevalence of syphilis and insights into the natural history of syphilis and the impact of HIV. Points out difficulties in defining "cure" and the need for further information regarding optimal treatment.*

Hopewell PC. Impact of human immunodeficiency virus infection on the epidemiology, clinical features, and control of tuberculosis. *Clin Infect Dis* 1992;15:540–547.
*Provides timely data on epidemiology, clinical features, and pathogenesis of tuberculosis in the setting of HIV. Defines reasonable management strategies and describes important drug interactions. Redefines the need for relevant procedures of infection control to limit the spread of tuberculosis, including disease caused by multidrug-resistant strains.*

Musher DM, Hamill RJ, Gaughn RE. Effect of human immunodeficiency virus (HIV) infection on the course of syphilis and on the response to treatment. *Ann Intern Med* 1990;113:872–881.
*This article represents an exhaustive review of the English literature dealing with syphilis before and after the introduction of penicillin, and provides excellent insights into the natural history of the disease. Also extensively reviews data on the impact of HIV on syphilis and provides strategies for management.*

## 86. HIV-1 AND INFECTIONS OF THE CENTRAL NERVOUS SYSTEM

Neurologic disorders are common in persons infected with the human immunodeficiency virus type 1 (HIV-1). Indeed, at autopsy, 70% to 80% of patients with AIDS have pathologic findings in the central nervous system (CNS), including infections, neoplasms, and degenerative conditions of uncertain etiology, such as vacuolar myelopathy; furthermore, diseases within the CNS have become major immediate causes of death in patients with AIDS.

The high prevalence and variety of diseases affecting the CNS is a consequence of the direct involvement of the brain by HIV-1 as well as the profound immunosuppression that occurs as the systemic retroviral illness progresses. Because the spectrum of problems involving the CNS is broad and because many of these conditions respond to specific therapies, the evaluation of the HIV-1–infected patient with neurologic symptoms or signs must be systematic, expeditious, and thorough. This chapter focuses on the prevalent infectious syndromes that involve the meninges and brain. Although the common CNS syndromes are discussed as distinct clinical entities, it must be emphasized that the patient with advanced HIV-1 disease can present with multiple disorders; for example, patients with AIDS can experience cryptococcal meningitis and cerebral toxoplasmosis concurrently.

### Meningitis
A neurotropic retrovirus, HIV-1 appears to invade the CNS during the primary infection. The virus has been isolated from the cerebrospinal fluid (CSF) of adults with acute

HIV-1 infection and from those with AIDS, and HIV-1 RNA has been detected by polymerase chain reaction (PCR) in the CSF of most patients at all stages of the disease. In addition, HIV-1 has been detected in a number of CNS cell populations, including endothelial cells, macrophages, and microglial cells. Finally, HIV-1 DNA has been found in the brains of about 50% of patients with asymptomatic infection and 100% of patients with AIDS.

Patients with acute HIV-1 infection can present with fever, malaise, myalgias, arthralgias, headache, and photophobia; on occasion, an acute encephalopathy dominates the clinical picture. The CSF abnormalities in patients with acute HIV-1 infection include a lymphocytic pleocytosis (<200 cells per cubic millimeter) and an elevated protein concentration. Thus, the possibility of HIV-1 infection should be considered in the adult who has aseptic meningitis and risk factors for infection with the virus (a history of IV drug use, homosexuality, or heterosexual promiscuity). In the patient with aseptic meningitis and risk factors, PCR or another assay to detect HIV-1 RNA in serum should be performed, and HIV-1 serologies should be obtained 1 and 3 months following the episode to detect seroconversion. The symptoms in patients with acute HIV-1 meningitis usually resolve within 4 weeks. Of note, some patients can experience a chronic meningitis syndrome, apparently caused by HIV-1.

Many patients with latent-stage (asymptomatic) HIV-1 infection have abnormal CSF profiles, typically a lymphocytic pleocytosis (<30 cells per cubic millimeter) and a high protein level (>60 mg/dL); these CSF abnormalities may or may not be accompanied by clinical evidence of meningitis. The CSF of patients with AIDS is characterized by an elevated protein level but no pleocytosis. Because of the high prevalence of abnormal spinal fluid findings in this patient population, the results of the CSF analysis must be interpreted with caution in patients who have an enigmatic neurologic process.

Patients with HIV-1 infection are at risk to experience meningitis caused by a variety of microbes, and reports of infection with bacteria (*Streptococcus pneumoniae, Listeria monocytogenes*), spirochetes (*Treponema pallidum*), mycobacteria (*Mycobacterium tuberculosis, Mycobacterium avium-intracellulare*), and fungi (*Cryptococcus neoformans, Histoplasma capsulatum, Coccidioides immitis*) have appeared in the medical literature. In addition, lymphomatous meningitis can develop in these patients as a complication of a systemic lymphoma. Accordingly, the appropriate microbiologic, serologic, or cytologic tests should be performed in the HIV-infected patient with an acute or chronic meningitis syndrome and epidemiologic, clinical, or laboratory evidence of one of these conditions. Of note, PCR of the CSF for the detection of *M. tuberculosis* DNA appears to be a very rapid, sensitive, and specific assay for establishing a diagnosis of tuberculous meningitis.

Although uncommonly, HIV-1–infected patients can present with acute syphilitic meningitis or meningovascular syphilis, a dramatic manifestation of neurosyphilis. In addition, these patients are at risk to experience asymptomatic neurosyphilis. Because the spinal fluid Venereal Disease Research Laboratory (VDRL) test in the setting of HIV-1 infection can be nonreactive, the possibility of neurosyphilis should be considered in the patient with positive peripheral blood serologies [VDRL, rapid plasma reagin (RPR)] and compatible cellular and biochemical CSF findings; for example, in one report of 11 patients with oligosymptomatic or asymptomatic neurosyphilis, the CSF VDRL assay was determined to be 100% specific but only 33% sensitive. In any case, *T. pallidum* can be recovered from the CSF in 20% to 25% of adults with primary or secondary syphilis, and so the potential for relapse within the CNS exists in penicillin-treated, HIV-positive patients. Finally, the utility of *T. pallidum* DNA PCR in the CSF remains under investigation.

*C. neoformans,* a fungus found in bird excreta and soil throughout the United States, is the most common cause of nonviral meningitis in patients infected with HIV-1. Before the widespread use of fluconazole, cryptococcal meningitis was reported in about 10% of patients infected with AIDS; the prevalence appears substantially lower at present. Often the initial manifestation of the underlying retroviral disease, cryptococcal meningitis is usually seen in HIV-1–infected patients whose CD4-cell counts are below 100/mm$^3$. The illness presents as a subacute or chronic meningitis syndrome with fever, lethargy, nausea, headache, and nonfocal findings on neurologic examination; papilledema can be present. Results of computed tomography (CT) and magnetic resonance imaging (MRI) are usually normal. The CSF findings are variable, but a pleocytosis, a depressed glucose concentration (hypoglycorrhachia), and an elevated protein level are characteristic; however, in patients with advanced retroviral disease, the spinal fluid cell count, glucose level, and protein level can all be normal. Fortunately, cryptococcal antigen is detectable in the CSF and serum in more than 90% of patients, typically at high titer (>1:1,024). Spinal fluid cultures will reveal the presence of the fungus in virtually all patients, and blood cultures will be positive in 50% to 60% of cases. Higher-dose amphotericin B (0.7 mg/kg per day) with or without flucytosine (100 mg/kg per day) appears to be the treatment of choice for the initial 2 weeks of therapy; fluconazole or itraconazole can be utilized for consolidation therapy. However, some authorities recommend that fluconazole alone be employed as initial therapy in patients with mild disease. Liposomal amphotericin B has also been shown to be effective as initial therapy for crytococcal meningitis, and the use of the agent might be considered in patients who cannot tolerate amphotericin B. In any case, primary therapy for cryptococcal meningitis should be continued until the CSF cultures are sterile. Of note, because of defects in the mechanisms through which the polysaccharide is eliminated, cryptococcal antigen can remain detectable for extended periods of time.

Because relapse occurs in 40% to 60% of treated patients, lifelong suppressive therapy (secondary prophylaxis) is required, and fluconazole (200 mg orally per day) should be used for this purpose. Finally, low-dose fluconazole (200 mg orally thrice weekly) represents effective primary prophylaxis for the infection, and the antifungal should be given to patients with AIDS whose CD4-cell counts are below 100/mm$^3$.

### Space-occupying Lesions in the Brain

HIV-1–infected patients frequently present with abnormal findings on the neurologic examination and parenchymal lesions revealed by CT of the brain. Although a number of diseases can result in space-occupying lesions in the brain, the most common entities are toxoplasmosis and lymphoma. Pyogenic brain abscesses, cryptococcomas, tuberculomas, Kaposi's sarcoma, and even cytomegalovirus (CMV) infection are rare causes of intracerebral masses in these patients.

A protozoan pathogen, *Toxoplasma gondii* is capable of causing single or multiple cerebral abscesses. The disease usually results from the reactivation of viable organisms encysted in extraneural sites during the primary infection. The risk for cerebral disease approaches 10% among persons with HIV-1 infection who have serologic evidence of prior infection with *T. gondii;* indeed, toxoplasmosis is the most common cause of intraparenchymal brain lesions in HIV-1–infected patients. The problem is usually seen in persons with CD4-cell counts below 100/mm$^3$.

Most patients with cerebral toxoplasmosis present with focal neurologic problems, such as aphasia, hemiparesis, and complete hemiplegia, that evolve during 1 to 2 weeks; headache, fever, seizures, and changes in mental status also occur. In other patients, toxoplasmosis can present as an acute confusional state, with or without focal findings; these patients can have a diffuse necrotizing encephalitis rather than focal lesions. CT with contrast material will demonstrate single or multiple enhancing lesions in virtually all patients; the lesions are most commonly seen in the region of the basal ganglia or at the junction of the gray and white matter in the cerebral hemispheres. Although the test is not often required, MRI can detect lesions not visualized by CT; with MRI, multiple abscesses will be detected in more than 80% of patients. *Toxoplasma* serologies are positive in more than 95% of patients with CNS infection. Because the CSF changes are nondiagnostic, the standard analysis of CSF has been considered rarely helpful in the management of these patients; however, PCR of the CSF to detect *T. gondii* DNA may prove to be a very useful assay. In any case, because the intracranial pressure of patients with intracerebral mass lesions can be increased, a lumbar puncture in this setting does carry a risk for herniation.

Primary lymphoma of the CNS, which has been associated with the Epstein-Barr virus, is the lesion most frequently confused with toxoplasmosis. Although rare in the general population, the disease occurs in about 5% of patients with AIDS; most persons with the malignancy have a CD4-cell count below 50/mm$^3$. In contrast to patients with toxoplasmosis, those with CNS lymphoma tend to present without focal neurologic signs but with a slowly evolving encephalopathy that is characterized by apathy and an altered mental status; nevertheless, the overlap in the clinical manifestations of the two diseases is great. Unfortunately, the anatomic location and CT appearance of toxoplasmosis and lymphoma are similar. Equally important, in up to 40% of patients, the malignancy is multicentric, and so the presence of more than one ring-enhancing lesion on CT does not exclude the possibility of a lymphoma; furthermore, 60% to 70% of patients with primary CNS lymphoma will have positive serologic tests for *T. gondii*. Of note, in recent investigations, PCR for Epstein-Barr virus DNA in CSF appears to be a very sensitive method for identifying patients with primary CNS lymphoma, and single-photon emission computed tomography (SPECT) with thallium 201 has been reported as a novel method for accurately distinguishing toxoplasmosis from lymphoma.

The approach to the HIV-1–infected patient with a space-occupying brain lesion varies from institution to institution; however, for the AIDS patient with multiple ring-enhancing lesions, empiric antitoxoplasmal therapy is usually given and the clinical response to treatment is monitored. Most patients with cerebral toxoplasmosis demonstrate an improvement in their systemic or neurologic symptoms within 2 weeks and a radiologic response within 3 weeks; of note, abnormalities on CT can persist for up to 6 months. The usual therapy is a combination of pyrimethamine (200 mg by mouth on the first day and then 75 to 100 mg daily), sulfadiazine (1 to 1.5 g orally every 6 hours), and folinic acid (10 to 15 mg daily) given for 4 to 6 weeks; clindamycin (600 mg by vein or by mouth every 6 hours) can be used in patients intolerant of sulfadiazine. When given with pyrimethamine and folinic acid, azithromycin, clarithromycin, and dapsone are among the other agents that have been shown to be effective in the therapy of CNS toxoplasmosis. A stereotactic or open brain biopsy is reserved for patients with single lesions that suggest lymphoma and for patients who fail to respond to antitoxoplasmal therapy within 7 to 14 days.

The outlook for patients with cerebral toxoplasmosis tends to be good, and many survive for extended periods of time. In contrast, the prognosis for patients with primary CNS lymphoma is poor; most succumb within 2 to 4 months. Finally, because the discontinuation of antitoxoplasmal therapy results in a recrudescence of the infection in up to 50% of treated patients, long-term (lifelong) suppressive therapy is indicated; pyrimethamine (25 to 50 mg daily) and folinic acid (5 to 10 mg daily) plus sulfadiazine (0.5 to 1.0 g four times daily) or clindamycin (300 mg four times daily) should be given.

## Encephalopathy

Patients infected with HIV-1 can present with changes in mental status because of meningitis or cerebral mass lesions. These patients can also experience a deterioration in cognitive function caused by intercurrent conditions, including viral encephalitis (CMV, herpes simplex virus, herpes zoster virus, human herpesvirus 6) and metabolic encephalopathy (hypoxemia, drugs). Of note, PCR of the CSF for CMV DNA appears to be a rapid and sensitive technique for establishing a diagnosis of CMV encephalitis or ventriculoencephalitis, and PCR of the CSF has been employed to monitor the response of AIDS patients with CMV disease to antiviral (ganciclovir) therapy.

HIV-infected persons are also at risk for the development of progressive multifocal leukoencephalopathy (PML), which is caused by the reactivation of papovaviruses, usually Jamestown Canyon (JC) virus, and is characterized by personality changes, an altered mental status, aphasia, ataxia, and hemiparesis; occasionally, new-onset seizures are the first manifestation of PML. CT in patients with PML characteristically reveals hypodense, nonenhancing lesions confined to the white matter. Traditionally, a brain biopsy has been required for definitive diagnosis; however, PCR of the CSF for JC virus DNA appears to be a very promising assay. Unfortunately, most patients with PML die within a few months of diagnosis. The most common cause of a deterioration in cognitive function in patients infected with HIV-1, however, is the AIDS dementia complex.

Also referred to as AIDS-related dementia and AIDS encephalopathy, the AIDS dementia complex is characterized by a progressive impairment in cognitive function that is accompanied by behavioral changes and motor abnormalities. Not common in HIV-1–infected persons who are asymptomatic and constitutionally well, the prevalence of the AIDS dementia complex increases with advanced degrees of immunosuppression; the risk for the disorder also rises with age and appears to be greatest in patients with AIDS who are more than 50 years of age. Depending on the criteria used, the disorder has been detected in 25% to 90% of all patients with AIDS. Early in the course, patients with the AIDS dementia complex experience impairments in cognitive function, such as forgetfulness and an inability to concentrate, and personality changes, including apathy, withdrawal, and depression. As the condition progresses, often during a period of months, the cognitive function deteriorates, and the behavioral and motor abnormalities become more prominent; leg weakness, a loss of balance, and clumsiness of the arms and hands are common complaints. Late in the course, ataxia, psychiatric disturbances, mutism, paraplegia, incontinence, and myoclonus occur. Intercurrent illness can accentuate the neurologic findings at any stage. CT reveals cortical atrophy in about 75% of patients with the AIDS dementia complex; the CSF and electroencephalogram findings are usually abnormal, but the changes are not diagnostic of the condition. Most patients succumb within a few months following the onset of severe dementia.

The AIDS dementia complex results from infection of the CNS by HIV-1. The histopathology of the brains of many patients is compatible with a diffuse viral infection, suggesting a direct insult by HIV-1; however, the brains of other patients indicate that immune and other indirect mechanisms of injury contribute prominently to the neuropathology. Apoptosis, which is induced by soluble factors, including cytokines (e.g., tumor necrosis factor-$\alpha$), that are produced by neighboring and uninfected cells, is one important mechanism of neuronal injury. Of note, the magnitude of cytokine production appears to be related to the extent of viral replication. Thus, it is not surprising that clinical investigations have shown that the severity of AIDS dementia complex parallels CSF levels of HIV-1 RNA. A number of other potential mechanisms of neuronal damage have been suggested; these include neurotoxicity by quinolinic acid released by HIV-infected macrophages and cellular injury by HIV-specific cytotoxic T cells. In any case, the severity of the dementia reflects the extent of the pathologic changes in the brain.

Because the CNS changes are attributable to infection with HIV-1, clinicians have been hopeful that antiretroviral therapy would prove useful in the prevention and therapy of the AIDS dementia complex, and initial reports have in general indicated a benefit of antiretroviral drugs. In particular, long-term therappy with zidovudine prevents the onset of neurocognitive defects in patients with symptomatic HIV-1 disease or AIDS, and the medication improves neurocognitive functions, such as memory and attention, in HIV-1–infected patients with AIDS dementia complex; these benefits appear to be sustained for at least months. Didanosine also appears to be effective. The impact of combination antiretroviral therapy (e.g., reverse transcriptase inhibitors plus protease inhibitors) on the incidence and clinical course of AIDS dementia complex remains to be determined. (A.L.E.)

## Bibliography

Anaissie E, et al. Central nervous system histoplasmosis. *Am J Med* 1988;84:215.
*The manifestations of CNS histoplasmosis in patients with AIDS include meningitis, multiple brain abscesses, or a single, large, space-occupying lesion.*

Appleman ME, et al. Cerebrospinal fluid abnormalities in patients without AIDS who are seropositive for the human immunodeficiency virus. *J Infect Dis* 1988;158:193.
*The authors report that 38.6% of 114 asymptomatic persons infected with HIV-1 had abnormal findings in the CSF.*

d'Arminio MA, et al. A comparison of brain biopsy and CSF-PCR in the diagnosis of CNS lesions in AIDS patients. *J Neurol* 1997;244:35.
*The detection of JC virus DNA, CMV DNA, Epstein-Barr virus DNA, or T. gondii DNA by PCR of CSF represents a promising method for establishing etiologic diagnoses in AIDS patients with intracranial lesions.*

Arribas JR, et al. Level of cytomegalovirus (CMV) DNA in cerebrospinal fluid of subjects with AIDS and CMV infection of the central nervous system. *J Infect Dis* 1995;172:527.
*The authors conclude that PCR of CSF for CMV DNA is more useful than clinical and neuroradiologic tests to document CMV infection of the CNS and that the levels of CSF DNA correlate with the severity of infection.*

Berger JR, et al. Progressive multifocal leukoencephalopathy associated with human immunodeficiency virus. *Ann Intern Med* 1987;107:78.

*Detailed descriptions of the clinical features and radiologic findings of progressive multifocal leukoencephalopathy are provided by the authors, who present 16 patients and review 12 previously reported cases.*

Brouwers P, et al. Effect of combination therapy with zidovudine and didanosine on neuropsychological functioning in patients with symptomatic HIV disease: a comparison of simultaneous and alternating regimens. *AIDS* 1997;11:59.

*In this small, nonblinded study, zidovudine and didanosine were both effective in improving memory and attention in patients with AIDS dementia.*

Carrigan DR, Harrington D, Knox KK. Subacute leukoencephalitis caused by CNS infection with human herpesvirus 6 manifesting as acute multiple sclerosis. *Neurology* 1996;47:145.

*Human herpesvirus 6 has been added to the list of viral agents that can produce diffuse or multifocal demyelination in the CNS of adults with AIDS.*

Chuck SL, Sande MA. Infections with *Cryptococcus neoformans* in the acquired immunodeficiency syndrome. *N Engl J Med* 1989;321:794.

*After a retrospective review of the records of 106 patients with cryptococcal meningitis, the authors concluded that the addition of flucytosine to amphotericin B neither enhances survival nor prevents relapse; in addition, they noted that flucytosine had to be discontinued in 53% of the patients because of leukopenia or thrombocytopenia.*

Cinque P, et al. Diagnosis and clinical management of neurological disorders caused by cytomegalovirus in AIDS patients. *J Neurovirol* 1998;4:129.

*The central and peripheral nervous system disorders caused by CMV in patients infected with HIV are reviewed, and the role of PCR of the CSF in the diagnosis and management of the diseases is discussed.*

Dannemann B, et al. Treatment of toxoplasmal encephalitis in patients with AIDS: a randomized trial comparing pyrimethamine plus clindamycin to pyrimethamine plus sulfadiazine. *Ann Intern Med* 1992;116:33.

*In this study of 59 patients with cerebral toxoplasmosis, the clinical response to therapy and survival were comparable with pyrimethamine (a loading dose of 200 mg orally followed by 75 mg daily) plus sulfadiazine [100 mg/kg body weight (up to 8 g/d) given orally in four divided doses per day] and pyrimethamine plus clindamycin (1,200 mg given intravenously every 6 hours for 3 weeks followed by 300 mg orally every 6 hours).*

Dismukes WE. Cryptococcal meningitis in patients with AIDS. *J Infect Dis* 1988; 157:624.

*The author provides a detailed review of the clinical manifestations and laboratory findings of the disease in patients infected with HIV-1.*

Epstein LG, Gendelman HE. Human immunodeficiency virus type 1 infection of the nervous system: pathogenic mechanisms. *Ann Neurol* 1993;33:429.

*The authors review the mechanisms through which HIV-1 produces disease in the CNS, emphasizing the role that retrovirus-infected macrophages play in initiating neurotoxicity.*

Gabuzda DH, Hirsch MS. Neurologic manifestations of infection with human immunodeficiency virus. *Ann Intern Med* 1987;107:383.

*Aseptic meningitis, subacute encephalitis, and the other neurologic syndromes attributable to HIV-1 infection are reviewed.*

Gorman JM, et al. The effect of zidovudine on neuropsychiatric measures in HIV-infected men. *Am J Psychiatry* 1993;150:505.

*In a prospective, 6-month study of 50 HIV-infected men, a significant improvement in neuropsychiatric parameters was not detected in subjects receiving zidovudine.*

Grant I, et al. Evidence for early central nervous system involvement in the acquired immunodeficiency syndrome (AIDS) and other human immunodeficiency virus (HIV) infections. *Ann Intern Med* 1987;197:828.

*Employing extensive neuropsychologic testing, the authors detected abnormalities in 53% of patients with asymptomatic HIV-1 infection, 47% of patients with AIDS-related complex, and 87% of patients with AIDS.*

Grant IH, et al. *Toxoplasma gondii* serology in HIV-infected patients: the development of central nervous system toxoplasmosis in AIDS. *AIDS* 1990;4:519.
*The authors detected antibody to* T. gondii *in 32% of 411 patients, and they observed that symptomatic CNS infection developed in 24% of the patients with antitoxoplasmal antibodies.*

Hollander H. Cerebrospinal fluid normalities and abnormalities in individuals infected with human immunodeficiency virus. *J Infect Dis* 1988;158:855.
*The CSF changes that occur at each stage of infection with HIV-1 are reviewed in detail.*

Holton PD, et al. Prevalence of neurosyphilis in human immunodeficiency virus-infected patients with latent syphilis. *Am J Med* 1992;93:9.
*In this study of HIV-1–infected patients with latent syphilis, the investigators found that 9% also had asymptomatic neurosyphilis. The authors conclude that HIV-1–infected persons who have positive results on serum testing for syphilis (VDRL, RPR) should undergo a lumbar puncture to detect evidence of asymptomatic neurosyphilis.*

Holtzman DM, Kaku DA, So YT. New-onset seizures associated with human immunodeficiency virus infection: causation and clinical features in 100 cases. *Am J Med* 1989;87:173.
*The authors found that although toxoplasmosis and HIV encephalopathy were the most frequently identified causes of recent-onset seizures, the spectrum of infectious and noninfectious causes was broad.*

van der Horst CM, et al. Treatment of cryptococcal meningitis associated with the acquired immunodeficiency syndrome. *N Engl J Med* 1997;337:15–21.
*In this double-blind, multicenter trial, patients given a higher dose of amphotericin B plus flucytosine for the initial 2 weeks of therapy demonstrated a higher CSF sterilization rate and a lower mortality rate at 2 weeks than did patients treated with amphotericin B alone; however, the overall case-fatality rates at 10 weeks were similar. Subsequent consolidation therapy was of comparable efficacy with fluconazole or itraconazole.*

Johns DR, Tierney M, Felsenstein D. Alteration in the natural history of neurosyphilis by concurrent infection with the human immunodeficiency virus. *N Engl J Med* 1987;316:1569.
*In this report of four HIV-1–infected men with neurosyphilis, the authors note that such patients can present with a variety of clinical illnesses, including acute syphilitic meningitis and meningovascular syphilis. The authors also emphasize that neurosyphilis can evolve in HIV-1–infected persons who have received conventional antimicrobial therapy for early-stage syphilis.*

Jurado R, Carpenter SL, Rimland D. Case report: trimethoprim-sulfamethoxazole–induced meningitis in patients with HIV infection. *Am J Med Sci* 1996;312:27.
*A reminder that medications, including trimethoprimsulfamethoxazole, can lead to an aseptic meningitis syndrome.*

Kalayjian RC, et al. Cytomegalovirus ventriculoencephalitis in AIDS: a syndrome with distinct clinical and pathologic features. *Medicine (Baltimore)* 1993;72:67.
*The authors describe the unique clinical, CSF, and pathologic findings of this terminal complication of AIDS.*

Katz DA, Berger JR, Duncan RC. Neurosyphilis: a comparative study of the effects of infection with human immunodeficiency virus. *Arch Neurol* 1993;50:243.
*In this retrospective review of 46 patients hospitalized with neurosyphilis, the investigators found that the HIV-1–infected group more frequently presented with signs of secondary syphilis and symptomatic meningitis; in addition, a higher WBC count and a lower glucose concentration were usually observed in the CSF of patients with an underlying retroviral infection.*

Leenders AC, et al. Liposomal amphotericin B (AmBisome) compared with amphotericin B, both followed by oral fluconazole in the treatment of AIDS-associated cryptococcal meningitis. *AIDS* 1997;11:1463.
*In a study of 28 patients, liposomal amphotericin B (4 mg/kg per day) was found to be less nephrotoxic, have equal clinical efficacy, and produce a more rapid sterilization of the CSF than amphotericin B alone (0.7 mg/kg per day).*

Luft BJ, Remington JS. Toxoplasmic encephalitis in AIDS. *Clin Infect Dis* 1992;15:211.
*The authors provide an in-depth review of the problem and an algorithm useful in the management of patients with space-occupying brain lesions.*

Luft BJ, et al. Toxoplasmic encephalitis in patients with the acquired immunodeficiency syndrome. *N Engl J Med* 1993;329:995.
*In a study of 49 patients with suspected CNS toxoplasmosis treated empirically with oral clindamycin (600 mg four times daily) and pyrimethamine (75 mg daily), the authors found that 86% of the patients who responded improved neurologically within 7 days. The investigators also concluded that patients with a presumptive diagnosis of toxoplasmosis who experience an early neurologic deterioration or fail to respond after 10 to 14 days of therapy should be considered candidates for brain biopsy.*

Malessa R, et al. Oligosymptomatic neurosyphilis with false-negative CSF-VDRL in HIV-infected individuals. *Eur J Med Res* 1996;1:299.
*Using clinical criteria and the response to antibiotic therapy for neurosyphilis, the authors conclude that the CSF VDRL test was only 33% sensitive in detecting infection with* T. pallidum *among the 11 HIV-infected patients studied.*

Malone JL, et al. Syphilis and neurosyphilis in a human immunodeficiency virus type 1-seropositive population: evidence for frequent serologic relapse after therapy. *Am J Med* 1995;99:55–63.
*Patients with reactive CSF VDRL assays are among those at high risk to experience relapses or treatment failures; these patients require prolonged monitoring and occasionally multiple courses of therapy.*

Melton ST, Kirkwood CK, Ghaemi SN. Pharmacotherapy of HIV dementia. *Ann Pharmacol* 1997;31:457.
*A comprehensive review of the AIDS dementia complex, with emphasis on the beneficial effects of zidovudine on the incidence and course of the disorder.*

Moulignier A, et al. AIDS-associated cytomegalovirus infection mimicking central nervous system tumors: a diagnostic challenge. *Clin Infect Dis* 1996;22:626.
*The authors report their findings in three patients with AIDS whose clinical and neuroradiologic findings initially suggested neoplasm but in whom brain biopsy confirmed a diagnosis of focal infection caused by CMV.*

Murray-Pulsifer K. Two central nervous system infectious diseases in a patient with AIDS. *J Fam Pract* 1993;36:660.
*The author describes a patient with AIDS and concurrent cryptococcal meningitis and toxoplasmal encephalitis.*

Powderly WG, et al. A controlled trial of fluconazole or amphotericin B to prevent relapse of cryptococcal meningitis in patients with the acquired immunodeficiency syndrome. *N Engl J Med* 1992;326:793.
*In a prospective randomized trial that compared fluconazole (200 mg daily given orally) with amphotericin B (1 mg/kg body weight given weekly intravenously), the investigators found that the relapse rate for symptomatic cryptococcal meningitis was 2% among patients assigned to fluconazole versus 18% among patients administered amphotericin B. In addition, bacteremias and serious drug-related toxicities were more common in the amphotericin B-treated group.*

Price RW, Brew BJ. The AIDS dementia complex. *J Infect Dis* 1988;158:1079.
*The clinical manifestations and pathophysiology of the condition are reviewed, and a detailed scheme for the clinical staging of the disorder is presented.*

Qureshi AI, et al. Human immunodeficiency virus and stroke in young patients. *Arch Neurol* 1997;54:1150.
*Infection with HIV is associated with an increased risk for stroke and cerebral infarction in young patients.*

Rolfs RT, et al. A randomized trial of enhanced therapy for early syphilis in patients with and without human immunodeficiency virus unfection. *N Engl J Med* 1997; 337:307.
*The addition of a 10-day course of oral amoxicillin plus probenecid did not improve the efficacy of benzathine penicillin G alone in the therapy of primary or secondary syphilis in HIV-infected patients; clinically defined failure rates were uncommon in both HIV-infected and non–HIV-infected patients.*

Schmitt FA, et al. Neuropsychological outcome of zidovudine (AZT) treatment of patients with AIDS and AIDS-related complex. *N Engl J Med* 1988;319:1573.
*Cognitive abnormalities attributable to the AIDS dementia complex may be decreased with the use of zidovudine.*

Sidtis JJ, et al. Stable neurological function in subjects treated with 2'3'-dideoxyinosine. *J Neurovirol* 1997;3:233.
*Didanosine (dideoxyinosine, DDI) may have a benefit in the prevention and therapy of AIDS dementia complex similar to that of zidovudine.*

Snider WD, et al. Neurological complications of acquired immune deficiency syndrome: analysis of 50 patients. *Ann Neurol* 1983;14:403.
*In this early report, the authors found that toxoplasmosis, progressive multifocal leukoencephalopathy, cryptococcal meningitis, subacute encephalitis (AIDS dementia complex), and lymphoma represented the most common CNS complications of infection with HIV-1.*

Tagliati M, et al. Cerebellar degeneration with human immunodeficiency virus infection. *Neurology* 1998;50:244.
*The authors describe 10 HIV-infected patients with isolated cerebellar degeneration of unknown cause.*

White M, et al. Cryptococcal meningitis in patients with AIDS and patients with neoplastic disease. *J Infect Dis* 1992;165:960.
*In this retrospective analysis of 41 cases of cryptococcal meningitis in patients with underlying neoplastic disease or AIDS, the investigators found that the patients with AIDS had a higher serum cryptococcal antigen titer, a lower CSF WBC count, a better response to therapy, and a longer overall survival.*

Yechoor VK, et al. Tuberculous meningitis among adults with and without HIV infection. Experience in an urban public hospital. *Arch Intern Med* 1997;156:1710.
*In this retrospective review of 31 adult patients with tuberculous meningitis, the authors concluded that although the incidence of the infection is higher among HIV-infected patients, the presenting clinical, laboratory, and radiographic features are similar in HIV-infected and non–HIV-infected patients; further, the response to therapy appears to be comparable in patients with and without an underlying retroviral disease.*

Zuger A, et al. Cryptococcal disease in patients with the acquired immunodeficiency syndrome. *Ann Intern Med* 1986;104:234.
*The authors present a summary of the clinical manifestations and response to treatment in 34 patients with the infection, and they emphasize the importance of long-term suppressive therapy in preventing relapse.*

---

## 87. DISSEMINATED *MYCOBACTERIUM AVIUM* COMPLEX INFECTION

Before the AIDS era, disease caused by *Mycobacterium avium* and *Mycobacterium intracellulare* was relatively rare. Infection occurred in patients who presented with chronic, slowly progressive, cavitary pulmonary disease. Disseminated disease was even rarer (<100 cases reported) and was seen in those with underlying defects in cellular immunity. Since the beginning of the AIDS epidemic, *Mycobacterium avium-intracellulare* complex (MAC) infection has been seen in 23% of patients infected with HIV. This percentage reflects underdiagnosis, as MAC disease has been noted at autopsy in more than 50% of patients with HIV disease.

The organism has been recovered from soil, water, air, and animals such as poultry. The portal of entry of the organism is likely the gastrointestinal or respiratory tract. Because the organism is ubiquitous, methods to prevent its acquisition are not likely to be found. The major risk factor predisposing patients to infection is a low CD4-cell count. Disseminated MAC infection occurs with CD4-lymphocyte counts below 100/mm$^3$. Evidence suggests that MAC disease results from primary acquisition rather than reactivation. When dissemination occurs, the main sites affected are the blood, bone marrow, liver, spleen, and lymph nodes; however, the organism has been recovered from almost every site in the body. Pathologically, the tissue reveals massive numbers of acid-fast bacilli ($10^{10}$ colony-forming units per gram) with a minimal inflammatory response or evidence of tissue destruction. Granulomas, if present, are poorly formed. Phagocytosis of the organisms occurs, but there appears to be little macrophage-mediated killing.

Most laboratories are unable to distinguish *M. avium* from *M. intracellulare* and report the isolates as MAC. However, nucleic acid probes show that the majority of isolates infecting AIDS patients are *M. avium*. There are also nucleic acid probes for *Mycobacterium tuberculosis* complex, which consists of *M. tuberculosis, Mycobacterium bovis, Mycobacterium africanum,* and *Mycobacterium microti.* Unlike *M. tuberculosis,* which is niacin-positive, MAC is niacin-negative. When the BACTEC system is used, the growth of isolates of the *M. tuberculosis* complex are inhibited by a compound, *p*-nitro-a-acetylamino-b-hydroxypropiophenone (NAP), in contrast to isolates of MAC, which are not inhibited by its presence. Mycobacteria can be recovered from blood cultures by using a lysis-centrifugation system (Isolator) or the radiometric blood culture system (BACTEC). With the BACTEC system, the time to culture positivity is usually 5 to 30 days, depending on the magnitude of the bacteremia. The number of colony-forming units of mycobacteria in the blood usually ranges between $10^1$ and $10^4$/mL, whereas in tissue, up to $10^{10}$/g have been noted.

Disseminated MAC infection should be suspected in any HIV patient with a CD4-cell count below 100/mm³ and systemic symptoms of fever, malaise, and weight loss. Anemia is present, and an increased need for blood transfusions is reported. In one study, disseminated MAC infection (31.9%) was the most frequent cause of fever of unknown origin, followed by *M. tuberculosis* infection (26.2%) and *Pneumocystis carinii* infection (9.5%). Chronic diarrhea and abdominal pain occur when organisms invade the colon. Chronic malabsorption has been described, with pathologic changes in the small intestine resembling those of Whipple's disease. Extrahepatic biliary obstruction secondary to periportal lymphadenopathy also occurs. The lungs can be involved, but the symptoms are usually not prominent. On physical examination, hepatosplenomegaly is often present. Abdominal computed tomography in patients with MAC infection shows lymphadenopathy (86%), hepatic (45%) and splenic (23%) enlargement, and diffuse thickening of the jejunal wall (18%).

The diagnosis of disseminated MAC infection depends on detecting the organism by culture of blood, bone marrow, or any other sterile body site. The diagnosis may also be established by obtaining a culture from the liver, spleen, or a lymph node. Positive cultures of sputum and stool may indicate disseminated disease or reflect colonization. Similarly, a smear of sputum, bronchial washings, or stool that is positive for acid-fast bacilli may indicate disseminated disease or colonization. In patients with disseminated disease, two blood cultures will detect 70% to 98% of cases. Occasionally, a buffy coat smear for acid-fast bacilli will be positive for mycobacteria. In a patient with pulmonary disease, a smear that is positive for acid-fast bacilli is more likely to represent *M. tuberculosis* than MAC. In patients with unexplained fever, a liver or bone marrow biopsy may yield a diagnosis more rapidly than a blood culture by demonstrating acid-fast bacilli on smear (Table 87-1).

The median survival of untreated patients with MAC infection was 4 months, compared with 11 months for matched controls. In another study of the natural history of MAC infection, severe anemia and death were associated with disseminated MAC infection.

Therapy of MAC infection is difficult because the organisms are resistant to the first-line agents: isoniazid, rifampin, pyrazinamide, and streptomycin. Drugs capable of inhibiting the organisms include rifabutin, ethambutol, clarithromycin, ciprofloxacin, ofloxacin, azithromycin, and amikacin. Various combinations of these drugs have been used, including regimens containing three or four drugs. To date, the preferred regimen consists of 500 mg of clarithromycin given orally twice daily plus 15 mg of ethambutol per kilogram once daily with or without 300 mg of rifabutin once daily or 500 to 750 mg of ciprofloxacin twice daily. Azithromycin can be given as 500 mg once daily instead of clarithromycin. Also, amikacin can be added to the two- or three-drug regimen in a dose of 10 to 15 mg/kg per day given intramuscularly in two divided doses. A dose of clarithromycin greater than 1 g daily has been associated with increased mor-

Table 87-1.  Interpretation of positive test results
for *Mycobacterium avium-intracellulare* complex

| Result | Interpretation |
| --- | --- |
| Positive stool AFB smear or culture | Colonization versus disseminated infection |
| Positive sputum AFB smear or culture | Colonization versus disseminated infection |
| Positive blood culture | Disseminated infection |
| Positive lymph node, liver, or bone marrow AFB smear or culture | Disseminated infection |

AFB, acid-fast bacilli.

tality. Rifabutin was more effective in a higher dose (600 mg/d) than in a lower dose (300 mg/d), but the higher dose was associated with the development of reversible uveitis in half the patients. Clofazimine is no longer recommended, as it has been associated with increased mortality. Aspirin or nonsteroidal antiinflammatory drugs can be administered for relief of symptoms. Survival after a diagnosis of MAC infection has increased from 4.5 months without therapy to about 9 months with the macrolide combination therapy. To prevent recurrences, the drugs used for initial therapy should be given as lifelong therapy.

In untreated patients, MAC bacteremia occurred in nearly 20% of patients with CD4-cell counts below 50/mm$^3$ and in only 6% of those with an initial CD4-cell count above 100/mm$^3$. Chemoprophylaxis for MAC infection is now strongly recommended as a standard of care. Before initiation of prophylaxis, patients should be assessed with a tuberculin skin test, chest roentgenography, and one blood culture to exclude active disease caused by *M. tuberculosis* or MAC.

Azithromycin (1,200 mg given orally once weekly) or clarithromycin (500 mg given orally twice daily) is preferred for chemoprophylaxis. Rifabutin (300 mg orally once daily) can be given as an alternative agent. Either macrolide is superior to rifabutin. In a study, the combination of azithromycin plus rifabutin was superior to either agent alone, but adverse effects, compliance issues, and possible drug interactions limit the use of both drugs together for chemoprophylaxis. One issue is the development of macrolide-resistant isolates in patients taking azithromycin or clarithromycin for prophylaxis. This has not been a serious problem with the use of macrolides because prophylaxis failures are rare. I prefer using azithromycin once weekly for prophylaxis. (N.M.G.)

### Bibliography
American Thoracic Society. Diagnosis and treatment of disease caused by nontuberculous mycobacteria. *Am Rev Respir Dis* 1990;142:940.
*Review.*
Amsden GW, Peloquin CA, Berning SE. The role of advanced-generation macrolides in the prophylaxis and treatment of *Mycobacterium avium* complex (MAC) infections. *Drugs* 1997;54: 69–80.
*Review of therapy and prophylaxis of MAC disease.*
Benator DA, Gordin FM. Nontuberculous mycobacteria in patients with human immunodeficiency virus infection. *Semin Resp Infect* 1996;11:285–300.
*Review.*
Brown BA, et al. Relationship of adverse events to serum drug levels in patients receiving high-dose azithromycin for mycobacterial lung disease. *Clin Infect Dis* 1997;24:958–964.
*Reversible hearing loss and gastrointestinal symptoms occurred frequently in elderly patients given a 600-mg daily dose.*

Chaisson RE, Moore RD, Richman DD. Incidence and natural history of *Mycobacterium avium* complex infections in patients with advanced human immunodeficiency virus disease treated with zidovudine. *Am Rev Respir Dis* 1992;146:285.
*Anemia and death are a consequence of MAC infection.*

Freedberg KA, Cohen CJ, Barber TW. Prophylaxis for disseminated *Mycobacterium avium* complex (MAC) infection in patients with AIDS: a cost effectiveness analysis. *J Acquir Immune Defic Syndr Hum Retrovirol* 1997;15:275–282.
*According to a cost effectiveness model, azithromycin represents the best value when started in patients with a CD4-cell count below 25/mm³.*

Griffith DE, et al. Azithromycin activity against *Mycobacterium avium* complex lung disease in patients who were not infected with human immunodeficiency virus. *Clin Infect Dis* 1996;23:983–989.
*A 600-mg daily dose of azithromycin was associated with a high frequency of gastrointestinal upset and hearing loss; these were not seen with a lower dose (300 mg) of the drug.*

Grinsztejn B, et al. Mycobacteremia in patients with the acquired immunodeficiency syndrome. *Arch Intern Med* 1997;157: 2359–2363.
*In patients with AIDS, a blood culture was useful to detect both* M. tuberculosis *and* MAC.

Gyure KA, et al. Symptomatic *Mycobacterium avium* complex infection of the central nervous system. *Arch Pathol Lab Med* 1995;119:836–839.
*A rare cause of central nervous system infection.*

Hawkins CC, et al. *Mycobacterium avium* complex infection in patients with acquired immunodeficiency syndrome. *Ann Intern Med* 1986;105:184.
*A positive stool culture and smear for acid-fast bacilli correlated with the presence of organisms in the blood.*

Heifets L. Susceptibility testing of *Mycobacterium avium* complex isolates. *Antimicrob Agents Chemother* 1996;40: 1759–1767.
*The most effective drugs for MAC based on minimum inhibitory concentrations include clarithromycin or azithromycin plus ethambutol and rifabutin. Isoniazid and pyrazinamide are inactive.*

Horsburgh CR Jr. *Mycobacterium avium* complex infection in the acquired immunodeficiency syndrome. *N Engl J Med* 1991;324:1332.
*Review.*

Horsburgh CR Jr, et al. Survival of patients with acquired immune deficiency syndrome and disseminated *Mycobacterium avium* complex infection with and without antimycobacterial chemotherapy. *Am Rev Respir Dis* 1991;144:557.
*Untreated patients with disseminated MAC infection had a median survival of 4 months.*

Jacobson MA, et al. Randomized, placebo-controlled trial of rifampin, ethambutol, and ciprofloxacin for AIDS patients with disseminated *Mycobacterium avium* complex infection. *J Infect Dis* 1993;168:112.
*Rifampin, ethambutol, and ciprofloxacin were associated with gastrointestinal side effects in 75% of patients.*

Kilby MJ, et al. The yield of bone marrow biopsy and culture compared with blood culture in the evaluation of HIV-infected patients for mycobacterial and fungal infections. *Am J Med* 1998;104:123–128.
*A single blood culture for MAC will usually establish the diagnosis, and only infrequently (17%) will a bone marrow culture contribute to the diagnosis.*

Modilevsky T, Sattler FR, Barnes PF. Mycobacterial disease in patients with human immunodeficiency virus infection. *Arch Intern Med* 1989;149:2201.
*In patients with MAC infection, blood cultures were positive in 96% of patients, whereas the yield from sputum smear was only 16%. This study also compared clinical findings and diagnostic yield in patients with* M. tuberculosis *infection versus findings in those with MAC infection.*

Nightingale SD, et al. Two controlled trials of rifabutin prophylaxis against *Mycobacterium avium* complex infection in AIDS. *N Engl J Med* 1993;329:828.
*MAC bacteremia developed in about 8% of patients receiving prophylactic rifabutin, and in 18% of those in the placebo group. However, no statistically significant difference in survival was noted between the two groups.*

Oldfield EC III, et al. Once-weekly azithromycin therapy for prevention of *Mycobacterium avium* complex infection in patients with AIDS: a randomized, double-blind, placebo-controlled multicenter trial. *Clin Infect Dis* 1998;26:611–619.

*Azithromycin (1,200 mg once weekly) is safe and effective in preventing disseminated MAC infection in patients with CD4-cell counts below 100/mm³.*

Phair JP, Young LS. Clinical challenges of *Mycobacterium avium. Am J Med* 1997; 102:1–55.

*Symposium devoted to epidemiology and prophylaxis (azithromycin) of MAC infection.*

Prego V, et al. Comparative yield of blood culture for fungi and mycobacteria, liver biopsy, and bone marrow biopsy in the diagnosis of fever of undetermined origin in human immunodeficiency virus-infected patients. *Arch Intern Med* 1990;150:333.

*In a small study, liver biopsy revealed acid-fast bacilli in a higher percentage of cases than did bone marrow biopsy (75% vs. 25%).*

Radin DR. Intraabdominal *Mycobacterium tuberculosis* vs. *Mycobacterium avium-intracellulare* infections in patients with AIDS: distinction based on CT findings. *AJR Am J Roentgenol* 1991;156:487.

*Radiographic differences are illustrated.*

Rastogi N, et al. Spectrum of activity of levofloxacin against nontuberculous mycobacteria and its activity against the *Mycobacterium avium* complex in combination with ethambutol, rifampin, roxithromycin, amikacin, and clofazimine. *Antimicrob Agents Chemother* 1996;40:2483–2487.

*Levofloxacin may be used as part of combination therapy for MAC infection.*

Salzman SH, et al. The role of bronchoscopy in the diagnosis of pulmonary tuberculosis in patients at risk for HIV infection. *Chest* 1992;102:143.

*Unlike bronchoscopy in* M. tuberculosis *infection, bronchoscopy was rarely helpful in the diagnosis of MAC infection. Transbronchial biopsy had a higher yield than bronchoalveolar lavage in patients with* M. tuberculosis *infection.*

Shafran SD, et al. A comparison of two regimens for the treatment of *Mycobacterium avium* complex bacteremia in AIDS: rifabutin, ethambutol, and clarithromycin versus rifampin, ethambutol, clofazimine, and ciprofloxacin. *N Engl J Med* 1996;335:377–383.

*Addition of clofazimine was associated with an increased mortality rate.*

USPHS/IDSA Prevention of Opportunistic Infections Working Group. Preface to the 1997 USPHS/IDSA guidelines for the prevention of opportunistic infections in persons infected with human immunodeficiency virus. *Clin Infect Dis* 1997;25 (Suppl 3):S299–S335.

*Guidelines to prevent opportunistic infections.*

Wallace RJ Jr, et al. Clarithromycin regimens for pulmonary *Mycobacterium avium* complex. The first 50 patients. *Am J Respir Crit Care Med* 1996;153:1766–1772.

*In HIV-negative patients with pulmonary disease caused by MAC, a regimen of clarithromycin, ethambutol, and rifampin or rifabutin plus an initial 2-month course of streptomycin was usually successful.*

Yajko DM, et al. High predictive value of the acid-fast smear for *Mycobacterium tuberculosis* despite the high prevalence of *Mycobacterium avium* complex in respiratory specimens. *Clin Infect Dis* 1994;19:334–336.

*An expectorated sputum specimen that is positive for acid-fast bacilli is more likely to grow* M. tuberculosis *than MAC on culture.*

---

## 88. FEVER AND FEVER OF UNKNOWN ORIGIN IN THE HIV-INFECTED PATIENT

---

It has been estimated that approximately 650,000 to 900,000 Americans are infected with HIV. These persons are predominantly young and middle-aged adults. When they have an early morning oral temperature above 99°F, or above 100°F at any time of the day, they are considered febrile. When they have fever for more than 4 weeks without an obvious cause, their condition can be defined as fever of unknown origin (FUO).

When an HIV-infected patient manifests fever, certain general concepts can guide the clinician: Infection is the most common cause; an untoward drug reaction may explain the fever; when the CD4-cell count is below 200/mm³, the clinician should resist the temptation to attribute the fever to the HIV infection itself; prophylactic trimetho-prim-sulfamethoxazole (TMP-SMX) reduces, but does not eliminate, the possibility of *Pneumocystis carinii* pneumonia (PCP) and invasive toxoplasmosis; fever can be the exclusive presentation of PCP, toxoplasmosis, invasive cryptococcal disease, tubercu-losis, or lymphoma; for the IV drug addict with HIV infection, most fevers are caused by bacterial infections (pneumonia, soft-tissue infections, bacteremia, endocarditis, septic arthritis, osteomyelitis, tuberculosis); fever combined with autoimmune phe-nomena can resemble a vasculitis (systemic lupus erythematosus); fever can be caused by a neoplasm (particularly lymphoma), a disorder unrelated to the HIV infection, or two disorders (two infections or infection plus neoplasm) occurring simultaneously. Of note is the fact that although the presence of fever can signify a serious infection, fever may not be the focus of the patient's concern.

Fever is the most common sign of primary HIV infection, and it has a median dura-tion of 14 days. Some researches have noted that a fever lasting 1 week or longer has been associated with a higher risk for AIDS and death. When fever develops in an HIV-infected patient with a CD4-cell count above 200/mm³, diagnostic considerations would include traditional bacterial infections (on occasion PCP also), alcohol-related disorders (hepatitis, pancreatis, tuberculosis), HIV-related diseases [lymphoma, sinusitis, symp-tomatic B (formerly considered AIDS-related complex and consisting of fever, lethargy, night sweats, weight loss, diarrhea, adenopathy, and splenomegaly)], disorders un-related to HIV, and side effects from alternative medications (such as the febrile hepati-tis syndrome precipitated by jin bu huan).

It is essential that the physician assessing a febrile, HIV-infected patient with a CD4-cell count above 200/mm³ perform a careful and thorough examination, document that the patient has HIV infection (exclude factitious HIV infection), and, if no obvi-ous clues to the source of the fever are revealed by the medical history and physical examination, arrange for a CBC count, blood cultures, evaluation of liver enzymes, and chest roentgenography. However, it is important to appreciate that chest roentgeno-graphic findings may be "negative" in a patient who has PCP or tuberculosis. Analy-sis of induced sputum with stains and cultures can be invaluable to establish the diagnosis of PCP or pulmonary tuberculosis, and if the patient is febrile and coughing and the chest roentgenographic findings are "negative," bronchoalveolar lavage should be considered.

Patients who appear "toxic," have a WBC count below 500/mm³, or inject illicit drugs are candidates for hospitalization and empiric infusion of an antibiotic. Neutropenia is a risk factor for bacteremia in the HIV-infected patient, and the possibility of endo-carditis cannot be excluded in the febrile IV drug abuser. For febrile HIV-infected patients who are not candidates for hospital admission, outpatient management should consist of the following: Obtain the patient's current telephone number and mailing address; maintain daily communication; provide the patient with a means to contact the clinician and/or "cover" 24 hours a day; recommend no antipyretic; have the patient record temperatures morning, afternoon, and evening; and schedule return visits to review the diagnostic test results and reassess the patient. If the patient remains febrile without adequate explanation, consider further evaluation (laboratory, radiographic).

For the patient with a CD4-cell count below 200/mm³, the initial diagnostic work-up is similar to that described above. In addition, there must be a concern for the opportunis-tic and unusual infections [such as PCP, *Mycobacterium avium* complex (MAC) infection, tuberculosis, invasive histoplasmosis, toxoplasmosis, cryptococcosis, *Helicobacter cinaedi* infection, bartonellosis] and neoplasms (non-Hodgkin's lymphoma) that characterize the advanced immunocompromised state known as AIDS, as well as drug-induced fever. Some researchers suggest that persistent fever does not correlate with cytomegalovirus (CMV) viremia or systemic CMV infection. Febrile patients with AIDS are not candidates for a diagnostic evaluation when they require hospice care, have advanced dementia, or have advanced systemic neoplasms recalcitrant to chemotherapy. Febrile AIDS patients who present a particular diagnostic challenge include the following: patients with tuber-culosis or PCP who have either no respiratory symptoms or normal chest roentgenographic findings; those with central nervous system toxoplasmosis in the absence of neurologic manifestations; patients with symptoms of invasive MAC infection weeks to months before detection of the organism on blood cultures; patients with disseminated histoplasmosis and no pulmonary symptoms or chest roentgenographic abnormalities; and patients receiving numerous medications, any one of which has the potential to cause fever. The list of medications capable of producing drug-related fever is extensive and includes such compounds as antimicrobials (TMP-SMX, clindamycin, amphotericin B, dapsone, β-lactams, pentamidine), antivirals (zidovudine, stavudine, interferon alfa, ganciclovir, protease inhibitors), antimycobacterials (isoniazid, rifampin), hematopoietic growth factors, antineoplastic agents (bleomycin, methotrexate), antiepileptics (phenytoin, carbamezipine), and thalidomide.

Numerous investigations have identified rather charateristic CD4-cell counts for specific opportunistic infections (PCP, <200/μL; toxoplasmosis, <100/μL; histoplasmosis, <100/μL; MAC infection, <50/μL; and CMV infection, <50/μL); however, there are well-documented exceptions to this general rule, and it has been observed that in patients who have received treatments that include a protease inhibitor, the CD4-cell count may increase to above 100/μL but the patient still experiences MAC and invasive CMV infection.

If the initial history, examination (including a dilated ophthalmologic study), chest roentgenogram, routine blood cultures, serum liver chemistries, and studies of induced sputa fail to explain the patient's febrile state, medications (if possible) should be discontinued (as drug-related fever can precede serious, untoward events, such as Stevens-Johnson syndrome and toxic epidermal necrolysis). Additional diagnostic studies that merit consideration include the following: pulse oximetry (as a very crude screen for PCP); assay for serum cryptococcal antigen (a rapid, sensitive, and specific test that can indicate invasive cryptococcal disease in the patient without marked meningismus—namely, headache, neck stiffness, photophobia); lysis-centrifugation blood cultures (to isolate *Bartonella henselae, Histoplasma capsulatum,* MAC, *Myco-bacterium tuberculosis*); sinus roentgenography; a gallium 67 scan ("negative" results combined with "negative" results of chest roentgenography virtually exclude PCP); and serum lactate dehydrogenase determination (a markedly elevated concentration is suggestive of PCP, tuberculosis, toxoplasmosis, disseminated histoplasmosis, or lymphoma). Persistent unexplained fever would suggest the need for computed tomography of the chest (pathologic adenopathy would suggest tuberculosis or lymphoma), abdomen (to detect MAC infection, tuberculosis, CMV colitis, hepatic abscess, splenic abscess, infectious cholangitis, visceral Kaposi's sarcoma, and non-Hodgkin's lymphoma), and brain (to detect toxoplasmosis in the patient without neurologic manifestations); analysis of the cerebrospinal fluid (to identify evidence of tuberculosis, cryptococcosis, or lymphoma); and, if the epidemiologic history is appropriate, a test for *Histoplasma* antigen in urine and serum. On occasion, biopsy for peritoneal masses or abnormal retroperitoneal lymph nodes, guided by computed tomography, will establish the cause of fever.

It is important to remember the following: It can take 2 to 6 weeks for MAC to grow in blood cultures; routine blood cultures (BACTEC culture bottles analyzed with BACTEC 860 system) appear to be comparable with lysis-centrifugation to isolate fungi (exceptions are *H. capsulatam* and *Candida glabrata*); indium 111 WBC scans can on occasion detect occult disease (colitis, sinusitis); if the test is available, examination of blood with polymerase chain reaction can suggest evidence of extracranial toxoplasmosis in patients without localizing findings who do or do not receive TMP-SMX prophylaxis.

At this stage of the diagnostic process, if the patient with FUO does not appear to be "ill" and does not manifest evidence of accelerated deterioration, it is probably prudent to await the results of the special blood cultures. On the other hand, if the patient is considered "unstable" or is losing weight, bone marrow aspiration and biopsy should be considered. Alternatively, if there is no contraindication, and particularly if the patient demonstrates abnormal liver enzymes, splenomegaly, or peripheral lymphadenopathy, the more sensitive liver biopsy might be undertaken. These procedures have the potential to assist in the diagnosis of MAC infection, tuberculosis, cryptococcosis, histoplasmosis, and lymphoma. If the patient refuses these procedures or if these tests do not provide a diagnosis, the clinician should consider initiating empiric therapy, perhaps antimycobacterial, or subjecting the patient to bronchoalveolar lavage to identify occult tuberculosis or PCP. (R.A.G.)

## Bibliography

Armstrong W, Kejenjian P. FUO in HIV. *Infect Dis Pract* 1997:21;33–36.
*An approach to the diagnosis.*

Benito N, et al. Bone marrow biopsy in the diagnosis of fever of unknown origin in patients with acquired immunodeficiency syndrome. *Arch Intern Med* 1997;157: 1577–1580.
*Bone marrow biopsy, performed in patients with persistent unexplained fever and AIDS, was a useful procedure to establish the diagnosis of disseminated mycobacterial disease, non-Hodgkin's lymphoma, and leishmaniasis.*

Bissuel F, et al. Fever of unknown origin in HIV-infected patients: a critical analysis of a retrospective series of 57 cases. *J Intern Med* 1994;236:529–535.
*This article stresses the importance of mycobacterial disease and the value of liver biopsy and thoracic computed tomography.*

Cavicchi M, et al. Value of liver biopsy for the rapid diagnosis of infection in human immunodeficiency virus-infected patients who have unexplained fever and elevated serum levels of alkaline phosphatase or γ-glutamyltransferase. *Clin Infect Dis* 1995;20:606–610.
*Liver biopsy was a valuable diagnostic procedure in patients with prolonged unexplained fever and abnormal serum liver chemistries.*

Engels E, Marks PW, Kazanjian P. Usefulness of bone marrow examination in the evaluation of unexplained fevers in patients infected with human immunodeficiency virus. *Clin Infect Dis* 1995;21:427–428.
*Bone marrow examination is indicated when a diagnosis is urgently sought or when other diagnostic studies have been unsuccessful.*

Gleckman R, Czachor JS. Assessment of fever in HIV-infected patients. *Postgrad Med* 1996;99:78–102.
*A review of the subject and a diagnostic algorithm.*

Mayo J, Collazoo J, Martinez E. Fever of unknown origin in the HIV-infected patient: new scenario for an old problem. *Scand J Infect Dis* 1997;29:327–336.
*A diagnostic approach.*

Miralles P, et al. Fever of uncertain origin in patients infected with the human immunodeficiency virus. *Clin Infect Dis* 1995;20:872–875.
*Persistent fever was caused most frequently by mycobacteria and visceral leishmaniasis.*

Ong E, Mandal BK. Tuberculosis in patients infected with the human immunodeficiency virus. *Q J Med* 1991;80:613–617.
*The chest roentgenographic findings can be negative in the febrile HIV-infected patient with tuberculosis.*

Roger PM, et al. Liver biopsy is not useful in the diagnosis of mycobacterial infections in patients who are infected with human immunodeficiency virus. *Clin Infect Dis* 1996;23:1302–1304.
*The diagnostic yield of liver biopsy is greater for the patient with splenomegaly and/or peripheral lymphadenopathy.*

Sepkowitz KA, et al. Fever among outpatients with advanced human immunodeficiency virus infection. *Arch Intern Med* 1998;153:1909–1912.
*Human immunodeficiency virus should not be considered the cause of fever in patients with AIDS, and febrile patients with advanced HIV disease merit a diagnostic evaluation.*

Tang CM, Conlon CP, Miller RF. Pyrexia of undetermined origin in advanced HIV disease. *Genitourin Med* 1997;73:308–313.
*A comprehensive diagnostic evaluation.*

Zylberberg H, et al. Prolonged isolated fever due to attenuated extracerebral toxoplasmosis in patients infected with human immunodeficiency virus who are receiving trimethoprim-sulfamethoxazole as prophylaxis. *Clin Infect Dis* 1995;21:680–681.
*Polymerase chain reaction examination of blood for evidence of* Toxoplasma gondii *genome may be useful in evaluating persistent fever, even in patients receiving TMP-SMX prophylaxis.*

## 89. PREVENTION OF OPPORTUNISTIC INFECTION IN THE HIV-INFECTED PATIENT

Until therapy becomes available to reverse the immunologic abnormalities that predispose HIV-infected patients to opportunistic infections, the standard of care will continue to consist of offering these patients combinations of antiretroviral medications and precise prophylactic compounds to decrease their risk for development of specific life-endangering infections [primary prophylaxis for *Pneumocystic carinii* pneumonia (PCP), toxoplasmosis, tuberculosis, and disseminated *Mycobacterium avium* complex (MAC) infection]. In essence, primary prophylaxis is designed to prevent initial infection or morbidity from preexisting but asymptomatic infection. Secondary prophylaxis (which consists of maintenance therapy for patients with PCP, *Toxoplasma* encephalitis, disseminated MAC infection, invasive cryptococcosis, invasive histoplasmosis, and invasive cytomegalovirus infection) is offered to prevent recurrence or reactivation of an established infection.

Although the goal of prophylaxis is to improve the quality and extend the duration of life, it is important to appreciate the concerns regarding prophylaxis (expense, side effects of the medication, potential for drug-drug interactions, difficulty of maintaining confidentiality, and perhaps modification of the manifestations of disease). Clinicians should limit prophylaxis to those disorders associated with substantial morbidity or mortality, and the consequences of the disease should outweigh those of the prophylactic regimen. Some research has also established that in addition to reducing morbidity and mortality, primary prophylaxis for PCP is cost effective and reduces the socioeconomic burden of illness. I should also stress that the prophylactic programs are not infallible, and breakthrough disease has developed following prophylactic regimens for PCP, toxoplasmosis, tuberculosis, and MAC infection, both in compliant and noncompliant patients.

Historically, the decision regarding when to initiate prophylaxis has been based on the CD4-cell count, as researchers have identified the ranges within which most opportunistic infections are manifested. It needs to be stressed, however, that numerous factors influence the quantitative CD4-cell determination, and the usual upper threshold value for an opportunistic infection can on occasion be exceeded; for example, more than 10% of cases of PCP occur in patients with a CD4-cell count above 200/μL. In addition, drug combinations that contain a protease inhibitor can on occasion elevate the CD4-cell count by 100 to 250 cells per microliter, so that the clinician acquires a false sense of security that the patient is no longer at risk and no longer a candidate for drug prophylaxis. Although this issue is "cloudy," the current recommendation is that prophylaxis be continued on the basis of the lowest CD4-cell count. In essence, once initiated, primary or secondary prophylaxis for PCP, MAC infection, and toxoplasmosis should be continued for life, regardless of the potential of antiretroviral treatment to elevate the CD4-cell count.

Before primary prophylaxis is initiated, it is essential to exclude active disease. Traditionally, this is accomplished through a combination of medical history, physical examination, laboratory tests, and chest roentgenography. As an example, special blood cultures and chest roentgenography should be performed (to exclude invasive MAC infection and tuberculosis) before a patient receives lifelong prophylaxis for MAC infection. To complement drug prophylaxis, additional preventive measures, namely vaccines, should be administered to HIV-infected patients. The vaccines to be considered are the 23-valent polysaccharide pneumococcal vaccine (to be administered as soon as HIV infection has been diagnosed) and hepatitis B vaccine [to be administered to all susceptible patients who are negative for antibody to hepatitis B core antigen (anti-HB$_c$)]. Pneumococcal immunization has been associated with a transient increase in levels of HIV-1 RNA, but most experts feel that the benefit of pneumococcal immunization outweighs the potential risk.

HIV-infected patients (including pregnant women) should receive prophylactic trimethoprim-sulfamethoxazole (TMP-SMX) as one double-strength tablet per day when the CD4-cell count is below 200/μL or the patient has had oropharyngeal candidiasis (unrelated to antibiotic or steroid therapy). Some experts would recommend TMP-SMX prophylaxis for any patient in whom an opportunistic infection develops regardless of the CD4-cell count. TMP-SMX has the potential to decrease the development of cerebral toxoplasmosis, isosporiosis, salmonellosis, and infections caused by *Nocardia* species, *Listeria* species, and *Haemophilus influenzae*. Unfortunately, however, TMP-SMX can precipitate headache, nausea, vomiting, fever, pruritus, rash, and hematologic and hepatic toxicity, and this medication can produce drug-drug interactions with oral anticoagulants, phenytoin, glipizide, and methotrexate. Myelosuppression can be enhanced when patients receive zidovudine. If a patient experiences an untoward event while taking prophylactic TMP-SMX and it is considered necessary to discontinue the medication, the clinician should (if the reaction was not Stevens-Johnson syndrome or another life-endangering adverse event) rechallenge and desensitize the patient after an interruption of 2 weeks. Some researchers have noted a relationship between an adverse reaction to TMP-SMX and rapid progression of disease.

If TMP-SMX cannot be tolerated, alternative prophylaxis should consist of dapsone (50 mg orally daily) plus pyrimethamine (50 mg orally per week) plus leucovorin (20 mg orally per week) (this regimen also prevents toxoplasmic encephalitis), dapsone (50 mg orally twice daily), or aerosolized pentamidine (300 mg daily administered with a Respirgard II nebulizer). Major adverse reactions attributed to dapsone include rash, nausea, vomiting, fever, bone marrow suppression, and transaminase elevation. The compound is contraindicated for patients with glucose-6-phosphate dehydrogenase deficiency (producing hemolytic anemia, methemoglobinemia), and it interacts with trimethoprim, rifampin, and didanosine. When dapsone is prescribed with didanosine, the absorption of dapsone is decreased, and the absorption of dapsone is impaired by achlorhydria. Pryrimethamine can cause neutropenia and thrombocytopenia.

Aerosolized pentamidine should be administered only to those patients who cannot tolerate the alternative prophylactic agents, as it is a less effective form of prophylaxis, particularly for patients with CD4-cell counts below $100/mm^3$, does not offer protection against invasive toxoplasmosis, and has been associated with the development of extrapulmonary *P. carinii* infection. Aerosolized pentamidine has induced cough, bronchospasm, pneumothorax, pancreatitis, hypoglycemia, and nephrotoxicity. Prophylactic failure with aerosolized pentamidine has resulted in atypical PCP (cysts, blebs, pneumothoraces). Before aerosolized pentamidine is offered, it is necessary to perform chest roentgenography to attempt to exclude tuberculosis. It is essential that Centers for Disease Control guidelines be followed to minimize the risk for respiratory transmission of this infectious disease.

Patients who are seropositive for *Toxoplasma* and who have a CD4-cell count below $100/\mu L$ are candidates for primary prophylaxis against *Toxoplasma* encephalitis. The recommended treatments, similar to those offered to patients to prevent PCP, consist of TMP-SMX or the dapsone-pyrimethamine combination. More research needs to be performed before azithromycin, clarithromycin, or atovaquone can be recommended for prevention of this disease. For pregnant women, if the clinician is planning to use dapsone-pyrimethamine prophylaxis, it is preferable to delay this drug combination until after the pregnancy.

Patients who have been treated and survived *Toxoplasma* encephalitis should receive lifelong secondary prophylaxis (suppressive treatment) with pyrimethamine plus sulfadiazine plus leucovorin to prevent relapse. If the patient cannot tolerate a sulfonamide, a clindamycin-pyrimethamine combination should be used. This latter combination does not, however, offer protection against PCP. Pyrimethamine is a drug with teratogenic potential; however, after a pregnant patient has been counseled, strong consideration should be given to the administration of the combination treatment because the recurrence rate of encephalitis is very high.

MAC infection prophylaxis protects patients from the disabling symptoms of a disorder that is common in severely immunosuppressed HIV-infected patients. Patients with CD4-cell counts below $50/\mu L$ should receive lifelong chemoprophylaxis against disseminated MAC infection. Three FDA-approved prophylactic regimens are currently available—azithromycin (1,200 mg orally every week), clarithromycin (500 mg orally twice a day), and rifabutin (300 mg orally every day). Azithromycin is probably the preferred prophylaxis; it is administered once a week, shares with clarithromycin the ability to prevent respiratory infections, is unsurpassed in efficacy by any other regimen, appears to be safe in pregnancy, and does not appear to have a potential for drug-drug interactions, which is a characteristic of clarithromycin. Clarithromycin has the potential to cause drug interactions with theophylline, carbamazepine, digoxin, ritonavir, cisapride, felodipine, fluconazole, warfarin, ergotamine, terfenadine, astemizole, and buspirone. Concerns with azithromycin treatment, however, include gastrointestinal adverse events, the development of reversible ototoxicity, and the possible emergence of drug-resistant MAC organisms.

Rifabutin is an effective prophylactic agent and is not associated with the development of resistant organisms. Rifabutin has caused rash, myalgias, arthralgia, nausea, headache, uveitis, thrombocytopenia, and hepatitis. A major concern with rifabutin is the potential for drug-drug interactions, such as with fluconazole, phenytoin, methadone, warfarin, oral contraceptives, dapsone, clarithromycin, phenytoin, saquinavir, indinavir, nelfinavir, ritonavir, zidovudine, beta blockers, and oral hypoglycemics.

Although absence or diminution of delayed hypersensitivity is common in HIV-infected patients with impaired cell-mediated immunity, tuberculin skin testing is the only screening method to detect tuberculosis. All HIV-infected patients who have a positive test result (skin reaction of 5 mm or greater on administration of intermediate-strength purified protein derivative) by the Mantoux method should receive a year of prophylaxis with isoniazid (300 mg daily) and pyridoxine (50 mg daily) unless they have active disease or have a history of treatment or prophylaxis for tuberculosis. In addition, HIV-infected persons who are close contacts of persons who have infectious tuberculosis should receive preventative therapy after active disease has been excluded. If there is concern that the exposure was to a patient with multidrug-resistant disease, prophylaxis should perhaps consist of pyrazinamide plus ofloxacin, but the evidence supporting this recommendation is modest, and the combination has not been well tolerated. HIV-infected patients with negative results on tuberculin skin testing should undergo repeated testing annually if they are at substantial risk for exposure to *Mycobacterium tuberculosis.*

Retrospective, case-control, and prospective studies have demonstrated the protective value of fluconazole (200 mg daily) against the development of cryptococcosis, a disseminated fungal disorder that is usually manifested when the CD4-cell count is below 50/µL. However, experts recommend that fluconazole not be routinely prescribed to prevent cryptococcosis (primary prophylaxis) because of the relative infrequency of the disease, lack of survival benefit associated with prophylaxis, potential for the development of resistant organisms, costs, and potential for drug-drug interactions (with rifampin, phenytoin, warfarin, sulfonyl urea, cyclosporine, theophylline, and rifabutin).

Patients, including those who are pregnant, who have completed therapy for invasive cryptococcosis are candidates for lifelong treatment with fluconazole (secondary prophylaxis or suppressive therapy); without suppressive therapy, 50% to 60% of patients suffer a relapse, and research studies have established the benefit of fluconazole in preventing relapse. Presumably, some of these relapses result from a persistent focus in the prostate.

Oral ganciclovir is FDA-approved for the prophylaxis of cytomegalovirus retinitis in patients with a CD4-cell count below 50/µL, although the data for efficacy are conflicting, the medication is prohibitively expensive, a cumbersome quantity of pills must be taken each day, and there are concerns regarding safety (the drug causes neutropenia, thrombocytopenia, and anemia) and the potential for drug-drug interaction (zidovudine, antimetabolites, alkylating agents). Initial research suggests that polymerase chain reaction testing may indicate which patients are at risk for development of cytomegalovirus disease, so that clinicians will have an opportunity to prescribe prophylaxis for specific patients. (R.A.G.)

## Bibliography

Brosgart CL, et al. A randomized, placebo-controlled trial of the safety and efficacy of oral ganciclovir for prophylaxis of cytomegalovirus disease in HIV-infected individuals. *AIDS* 1998;12:269–277.
  *Oral ganciclovir decreased the risk for CMV disease in patients not prescribed didanosine.*

Centers for Disease Control. 1997 USPHS/IDSA guidelines for the prevention of opportunistic infections in persons infected with human immunodeficiency virus. *MMWR Morb Mortal Wkly Rep* 1997;46:1–46.
*A comprehensive guide to reduce opportunistic infections.*

Freedberg KA, et al. The cost effectiveness of preventing AIDS-related opportunistic infections. *JAMA* 1998;279:130–136.
*An analysis of the cost effectiveness of prophylaxis against HIV-related opportunistic infections.*

Fuller JD, Stanfield LED, Craven DE. Rifabutin prophylaxis and uveitis. *N Engl J Med* 1994;330:1315–1316.
*Rifabutin-induced uveitis.*

Selik RM, Karon JM, Ward JW. Effect of the human immunodeficiency virus epidemic on mortality from opportunistic infections in the United States in 1993. *J Infect Dis* 1997;176:632–636.
*Most HIV-associated mortality is caused by opportunistic infections.*

Sepkowitz KA. Effect of prophylaxis on the clinical manifestations of AIDS-related opportunistic infections. *Clin Infect Dis* 1998;26:806–810.
*Prophylaxis can affect the clinical presentation of opportunistic infections.*

Sepkowitz KA. Effect of HAART on natural history of AIDS-related opportunistic disorders. *Lancet* 1998;351:228–230.
*An unanticipated (undesired) consequence of highly active antiretroviral therapy (HAART) may be exuberant inflammation of infection because of improved immune function.*

## 90. ANTIRETROVIRAL THERAPY

A dramatic decline in AIDS mortality was noted in 1996, when deaths dropped 21%. This trend has continued into 1997, with AIDS deaths down 44%. This dramatic advance occurred because of a better understanding of HIV pathogenesis, the ability to measure and monitor HIV RNA (viral load), and the development of new antiretroviral therapies. With treatment, HIV infection has become a chronic disease. As of April 1998, 11 drugs have been approved to treat HIV infection. The drugs can be classified into three groups: nucleoside reverse transcriptase inhibitors (NRTIs), non-nucleoside reverse transcriptase inhibitors (NNRTIs), and protease inhibitors (PIs) (Tables 90-1, 90-2).

Antiretroviral therapy began in 1986, when zidovudine first became available. Zidovudine monotherapy was the standard treatment for patients with a CD4-cell count of less than 500/mm³. When this treatment was not tolerated or failed, another NRTI, such as didanosine or zalcitabine, was substituted for zidovudine. The development of resistance is the major problem with monotherapy, and the Concorde Trial findings, presented in 1993, pointed out this lack of efficacy when zidovudine was used alone over time. A new era in antiretroviral therapy began in late 1995, when the results of ACTG 175 and the European-Australian Delta trials showed increased survival with combination therapy for both symptomatic patients and asymptomatic patients with a CD4-cell count below 500/mm³. This new approach, presented in 1996 at the International AIDS Conference, has been termed highly active antiretroviral therapy (HAART). Guidelines for implementing this "hit-early, hit-hard" approach have been issued by the International AIDS Society U.S.A. and by the Department of Health and Human Services and the Henry J. Kaiser Family Foundation (Table 90-3). The recommendations contained in each document regarding initiation of therapy are almost identical.

The recommended antiretroviral agents for starting therapy are listed in Table 90-4. For the patient naive to antiretroviral therapy, one should begin with a regimen that uses two NRTIs and one PI. An alternative regimen consists of ritonavir and saquinavir (soft-gel formulation) plus one or two NRTIs.

Table 90-1. Antiretroviral drugs: generic and trade names, characteristics

| Generic name | Abbreviation | Trade name | Manufacturer | Usual dosage | Common side effects (comments) |
|---|---|---|---|---|---|
| **Nucleoside RT inhibitors** | | | | | |
| zidovudine | AZT,ZDV | Retrovir | Glaxo Wellcome | 300 mg bid or with 3TC as Combivir 1 tablet bid | Bone marrow suppression, GI upset, headache, myopathy, insomnia |
| didanosine | ddI | Videx | Bristol-Myers Squibb | 200 mg bid* (125 mg bid if <60 kg) or 400 mg daily | Peripheral neuropathy, pancreatitis, diarrhea (take on empty stomach) |
| zalcitabine | ddC | HIVID | Roche | 0.75 mg tid | Peripheral neuropathy, pancreatitis, oral ulcers |
| stavudine | d4T | Zerit | Bristol-Myers Squibb | 40 mg bid (30 mg bid if <60 kg) | Peripheral neuropathy |
| lamivudine | 3TC | Epivir | Glaxo Wellcome | 150 mg bid | Anemia, GI upset |
| **Non-nucleoside RT inhibitors** | | | | | |
| nevirapine | NVP | Viramune | Roxane | 200 mg qd × 14 d, then bid | Rash, elevated liver enzymes |
| delavirdine | DLV | Rescriptor | Upjohn | 400 mg tid | Rash, headache |
| efavirenz | DMP-266 | Sustiva | DuPont Merck | 600 mg qd | Dizziness |
| **Protease inhibitors** | | | | | |
| saquinavir | SQV-SGC | Fortovase | Roche | 1,200 mg tid | GI upset, headache (take with meal or up to 2 h after meal) |
| indinavir | IDV | Crixivan | Merck | 800 mg q8h | Kidney stones, hyperbilirubinemia (take on empty stomach) |
| ritonavir | RTV | Norvir | Abbott | 600 mg bid | GI upset, circumoral paresthesias (refrigerate medication) |
| nelfinavir | NFV | Viracept | Agouron | 750 mg tid or 1,250 mg bid | Diarrhea (take with food), hyperglycemia*, Fat distribution and lipid abnormalities*, Possible increased bleeding in patients with hemophilia* |

RT, reverse transcriptase.
* All protease inhibitors.

Table 90-2.  Other antiretroviral drugs

| Generic name | Trade name | Class | Dosage | Side effects |
|---|---|---|---|---|
| abacavir | Ziagen | Nucleoside RTI | 300 mg bid | GI upset, hypersensitivity, reaction (life-threatening if readministered) |
| adefovir | Preveon | Nucleoside RTI | 60 mg qd (with 500 mg carnitine) | GI upset, abnormal liver enzymes, nephro-toxicity |
| efavirenz | Sustiva | Non-nucleoside RTI | 600 mg qd | Dizziness, induces CYP 3A4, night-mares |
| amprenavir | Agenerase | Protease inhibitor | 1,200 mg bid | Nausea, vomiting, large number of pills, each pill = 150 mg, 16 pills/day |

Reaction: high fever, myalgias, malaise

The National Institutes of Health sponsored a panel to define the principles of therapy for HIV infection. Eleven principles were defined as follows:

1. Active replication of HIV results in immune system damage and progression to AIDS in 98% of patients. For adults in industrialized countries, it takes about 10 years for AIDS to develop after the initial infection in the absence of therapy. In about 20% of persons, disease will progress rapidly, with development of AIDS within 5 years of infection.

Table 90-3.  Indications for initiation of antiretroviral therapy

| Clinical category | CD4+ T-cell count and HIV RNA | Recommendation |
|---|---|---|
| Symptomatic (AIDS, thrush, unexplained fever) | Any value | Treat. |
| Asymptomatic | CD4+ T cells <500/mm$^3$ or HIV RNA >10,000 (bDNA) >20,000 (RT-PCR) | Treatment should be offered. |
| Asymptomatic | CD4+ T cells >500/mm$^3$ and HIV RNA <10,000 (bDNA) <20,000 (RT-PCR) | Some experts would delay therapy and observe: however, some experts would treat. |

bDNA, branched-chain DNA; RT-PCR, reverse transcriptase-polymerase chain reaction.
Adapted from the Department of Health and Human Services *1998 Guidelines for the use of antiretroviral agents in HIV-infected adults and adolescents* (draft).

Table 90-4.  Recommended antiretroviral agents for treatment of HIV infection

**Preferred:** Strong evidence of clinical benefit and/or sustained suppression of plasma viral load. One choice each from column A and column B. Drugs are listed in random, not priority, order:

| Column A | Column B |
|---|---|
| indinavir | ZDV + ddI (NRTI) |
| nelfinavir | d4T + ddI |
| ritonavir | ZDV + ddC |
| saquinavir SGC* | ZDV + 3TC‡ |
| ritonavir + | d4T + 3TC‡ |
| saquinavir SGC or HGC** | |
| efavirenz | |

**Alternative:** Less likely to provide sustained virus suppression.

1NNRTI (nevirapine or delavirdine) + 2 NRTIs† (column B, above).

**Not generally recommended:** Strong evidence of clinical benefit but initial virus suppression is not sustained in most patients.

2 NRTIs (column B, above)

**Not recommended§:** Evidence against use, virologically undesirable, or overlapping toxicities.

All monotherapies
d4T + ZDV
ddC + ddI
ddC + d4T
ddC + 3TC

---

NRTI, nucleoside reverse transcriptase inhibitor; NNRTI, non-nucleoside reverse transcriptase inhibitor; SGC, soft gel capsule; HGC, hard gel capsule (Invirase). For abbrerrations in column B, see Table 90-1.
\* Virologic data and clinical experience with saquinavir SGC are limited in comparison with data for other protease inhibitors.
\*\* Use of ritonavir 400 mg bid with saquinavir SGC (Fortovase) 400 mg bid results in similar areas under the curve (AUC) of drug and antiretroviral activity as use of invirase 400 mg bid in combination with ritonavir.
† The only combination of 2 NRTIs + 1 NNRTI that has been shown to suppress viremia to undectectable levels in the majority of patients is ZDV + ddI + nevirapine. This combination was studied in antiretroviral-naive patients.
‡ High-level resistance to 3TC develops within 2–4 weeks in partially suppressive regimens; optimal use in 3-drug antiretroviral combinations that reduce viral load to <500 copies per milliliter.
§ ZDV monotherapy may be considered for prophylactic use in pregnant women with low viral load and high CD4+ T-cell counts to prevent perinatal transmission.
Adapted from HHS *1998 Guidelines.*

2. Levels of HIV RNA (viral load) indicate the magnitude of HIV replication and the risk for disease progression. The viral load is usually measured by two techniques: branched-chain DNA (bDNA) and RNA reverse transcriptase-polymerase chain reaction (RT-PCR). To convert the number of copies of virus per milliliter obtained by the bDNA method, multiply the result by two to obtain the number of copies per milliliter for the RT-PCR method. The viral load can increase with an acute illness and after an immunization, so that testing of HIV RNA should be deferred for 1 month under these circumstances. It is preferable to retest the viral load in the same laboratory and with the same assay. The threshold of detection with the newer, ultrasensitive assays is as few as 20 copies per milliliter. A significant change in viral load is at least a threefold or a .5 log change. Before initiation of therapy, two specimens should be obtained for HIV RNA determination within 1 to 2 weeks to provide a baseline. It is recommended that the viral load be measured again 4 to 8 weeks after initiation or change of therapy. Measurement of CD4-cell counts is critical to determine the status of the immune system. Susceptibility to opportunistic infections correlates with CD4-cell levels, and recommendations for prophylaxis are based on threshold CD4-cell levels. At present, prophylactic drugs should be continued even when CD4-cell counts increase above the levels considered to be a threshold for prophylaxis.

3. Treatment decisions to initiate or change therapy should be based on the results of viral load tests and CD4-cell counts. A decrease in viral load of 1 log is associated with an increase in CD4-cell count of about 85/mm$^3$.

4. The goal of combination therapy is to suppress the HIV RNA (viral load) to below levels of detection by the most sensitive assays. Drug resistance is likely to be present when HIV RNA levels are at or above 5,000 copies per milliliter.

5. The most effective means to achieve sustained suppression of HIV replication is to use combinations of antiretroviral drugs. Monotherapy is associated with a high risk for the emergence of viral resistance to the agent and the potential for development of cross-resistance to the drug class. For example, suppression of HIV replication is best accomplished by using two NRTIs in combination with a PI. An alternative combination regimen for antiretroviral-naive patients is two NRTIs combined with an NNRTI, such as nevirapine.

6. Antiretroviral drugs should be prescribed according to the recommended schedules and doses. Underdosing should be avoided to prevent the development of drug resistance. Also, combination therapy should be started simultaneously; the drugs should not be added sequentially. Because patient adherence to the drug regimen is critical to the success of therapy, select drugs and schedules taking into consideration the patient's circumstances and lifestyle.

7. When antiretroviral drugs are changed, cross-resistance between drugs in a class must be considered. When a failing regimen is changed, it is important never to change a single drug. Because the number of drugs is limited and cross-resistance occurs commonly, it is important not to abandon a drug prematurely. When it is necessary to change therapy for reasons such as drug toxicity or intolerance, then one drug can be substituted for another while the other components of the regimen are continued.

8. Pregnancy is *not* a contraindication for antiretroviral therapy. Women already receiving antiretroviral therapy should continue therapy if they become pregnant. For patients who are pregnant and need to begin antiretroviral drugs, it is recommended that therapy be delayed until 14 weeks of gestation. Zidovudine has been shown to reduce perinatal HIV transmission and should be offered to all pregnant women regardless of their viral load.

9. The same principles of antiretroviral therapy apply to children and infants, although certain drug formulations and pharmacokinetic data are lacking for these groups.

Table 90-5. Regimens for patients who have failed antiretroviral therapy

| Prior regimen | New regimen (not listed in priority order) |
| --- | --- |
| 2 NRTIs + | 2 new NRTIs + |
|    nelfinavir |    RTV; or IDV; or SQV + RTV; or NNRTI* + RTV; or NNRTI + IDV |
|    ritonavir |    SQV + RTV; NFV + NNRTI; or NFV + SQV |
|    indinavir |    SQV + RTV; NFV + NNRTI; or NFV + SQV |
|    saquinavir |    RTV + SQV; or NNRTI + IDV |
| 2 NRTIs + NNRTI | 2 new NRTIs + a protease inhibitor |
| 2 NRTIs | 2 new NRTIs + a protease inhibitor |
| | 2 new NRTIs + RTV + SQV |
| | 1 new NRTI + 1 NNRTI + a protease inhibitor |
| | 2 protease inhibitors + NNRTI |
| 1 NRTI | 2 new NRTIs + a protease inhibitor |
| | 2 new NRTIs + NNRTI |
| | 1 new NRTI + 1 NNRTI + a protease inhibitor |

RTV, ritonavir; IDV, Indinavir; SQV, saquinavir; NVP, nevirapine; NFV, nelfinavir; DLV, delavirdine.
* Of the two available NNRTIs, clinical trials support a preference for nevirapine over delavirdine based on results of viral load assays. These two agents have opposite effects on the CYP-450 pathway, and this must be considered in combining these drugs with other agents.
Adapted from HHS *1998 Guidelines.*

Table 90-6. Methods to achieve optimal adherence

Clarify the regimen by discussing therapy with the patient.
Provide written instructions, including a description of possible adverse effects.
Select regimens based on the patient's lifestyle and preferences.
Teach the patient how to keep a medications diary and use timers.
Simplify regimens.

10. Persons with acute primary HIV infection should be given combination anti-retroviral therapy. Some experts recommend that by "hitting the HIV hard and early" with combination therapy, the HIV viral load will be reduced and the immune system preserved, with a lower HIV set point. It has been suggested that reduction of the viral set point is associated with a more favorable subsequent clinical course. There is no evidence that initiating therapy in a patient with acute seroconversion will lead to eradication of the virus. In the absence of treatment, the viral load declines by less than 1 log per month, and the viral set point is attained at about 4 months. With standard triple-drug therapy, HIV loads decline about 1 log per week.
11. All HIV-infected persons, even those with undetectable viral loads, should be considered infectious and should be counseled on how to avoid transmitting this virus.

Recommendations have been issued for changing an antiretroviral drug regimen in cases of suspected drug failure based on a significant increase in viral load and/or a declining number of CD4 cells. When the decision to change regimens is based on the determination of an increasing viral load, it is advisable to confirm the data with a repeated viral load test. Generally, it is recommended not to change a single drug or add a single drug to a failing regimen, but rather to use at least two new drugs or an entire new regimen. Although data are limited, it is probably of little use to restart a drug that the patient has previously received because resistance recurs rapidly. Also, avoid changing from ritonavir to indinavir or vice versa for drug failure because cross-resistance is likely. For the same reason, avoid switching from nevirapine to delavirdine or vice versa for drug failure. Table 90-5 lists some regimens for patients who have failed antiretroviral therapy. Clearly, more clinical trials are needed regarding selection of drugs for failing regimens or salvage therapy.

Resistance to antiretroviral agents develops because of the rapid replication rate of HIV and the high error rate of HIV reverse transcriptase. This leads to frequent mutations and loss of antiretroviral effect. Genotypic testing is commercially available and relatively inexpensive. Phenotypic testing is not standardized and is expensive and time-consuming. Genotypic testing may help distinguish between treatment failure and nonadherence by showing that the virus present is still wild-type (susceptible). Phenotypic testing indicates how the virus interacts with various antiretroviral drugs. At present, both genotypic and phenotypic analysis have only limited use in the care of HIV patients.

The introduction of PIs has made HIV a chronic disease. The various antiretroviral regimens are complex, and failure to adhere to them results in viral resistance and drug failure. Adherence is defined as the extent to which a patient's behavior corresponds to the medical recommendations. The term adherence has replaced the term compliance because it is considered less pejorative. Measures to increase adherence are listed in Table 90-6. (N.M.G.)

### Bibliography

Bartlett JA, Benoit SL, Johnson VA. Lamivudine plus zidovudine compared with zalcitabine plus zidovudine in patients with HIV infection. A randomized, double-blind, placebo-controlled trial. *Ann Intern Med* 1996;125:161–172.
  *Use of lamivudine (300 mg/d) plus zidovudine (600 mg/d) was as effective and better tolerated than higher-dose lamivudine plus zidovudine.*
BHIVA Guidelines Co-ordinating Committee. British HIV Association guidelines for antiretroviral treatment of HIV-seropositive individuals. *Lancet* 1997;349:1086–1092.
  *Guidelines for therapy. Always add at least two new drugs.*

CAESAR Coordinating Committee. Randomised trial of addition of lamivudine or lamivudine plus loviride to zidovudine-containing regimens for patients with HIV-1 infection: the CAESAR trial. *Lancet* 1997;349:1413–1421.
*A significant reduction in progression to AIDS and death in patients given lamivudine plus zidovudine compared with zidovudine alone.*
Carpenter CC, et al. Antiretroviral therapy for HIV infection in 1997. Updated recommendations of the International AIDS Society USA Panel. *JAMA* 1997;277:1962–1969.
*Treatment guidelines of the International AIDS Society USA Panel. Treat all symptomatic HIV-infected persons and asymptomatic persons with a viral load greater than 5,000 copies per milliliter.*
Carpenter CC, et al. Antiretroviral therapy for HIV infection in 1998. Updated recommendations of the International AIDS Society USA Panel. *JAMA* 1998;280:78–86.
*Guidelines for when to initiate therapy, monitor response, and change drugs.*
Centers for Disease Control and Prevention. Report of the NIH panel to define principles of therapy of HIV infection and guidelines for the use of antiretroviral agents in HIV-infected adults and adolescents. *MMWR Morb Mortal Wkly Rep* 1998;47 (RR5):1–82.
*Guidelines (see also* Ann Intern Med *1998;128:1057–1100, republished from* MMWR*).*
Collier AC, et al. Treatment of human immunodeficiency virus infection with saquinavir, zidovudine, and zalcitabine. *N Engl J Med* 1996;334:1011–1017.
*Use of two nucleoside analogs plus saquinavir was effective in reducing viral loads and increasing CD4-cell counts.*
Concorde Coordinating Committee. Concorde: MRC/ANRS randomised double-blind controlled trial of immediate and deferred zidovudine in symptom-free HIV infection. *Lancet* 1994;343:871–881.
*Monotherapy with zidovudine was not effective.*
Condra JH, Emini EA. Preventing HIV-1 drug resistance. *Sci Med* 1997;4:1–11.
*Mutations occur about once in every 10,000 nucleosides copied, or about once every time a viral genome is copied.*
Delta Coordinating Committee. Delta: a randomised, double-blind, controlled trial comparing combinations of zidovudine plus didanosine or zalcitabine with zidovudine alone in HIV-infected individuals. *Lancet* 1996;348:283–291.
*Use of zidovudine plus didanosine or zalcitabine improved survival and delayed disease progression in comparison with zidovudine alone.*
Eron JJ, et al. Treatment with lamivudine, zidovudine, or both in HIV-positive patients with 200 to 500 CD4+ cells per cubic millimeter. *N Engl J Med* 1995; 333:1662–1669.
*A combination of zidovudine and lamivudine was better than either drug alone.*
Finzi D, et al. Identification of a reservoir for HIV-1 in patients on highly active antiretroviral therapy. *Science* 1997;278:1295–1300.
*A reservoir of latent virus in CD4 cells was found in patients responding to highly active antiretroviral therapy.*
Flexner C. HIV-protease inhibitors. *N Engl J Med* 1998;338:1281–1292.
*Review.*
Gulick RM, et al. Treatment with indinavir, zidovudine, and lamivudine in adults with human immunodeficiency virus infection and prior antiretroviral therapy. *N Engl J Med* 1997;337:734–739.
*Ninety percent of the group on triple therapy including indinavir had undetectable HIV-1 RNA (<500 copies per milliliter) at 24 weeks, compared with 43% of the group on indinavir monotherapy and none of the group on the lamivudine-zidovudine regimen.*
Hammer SM, Katzenstein DA, Hughes MD. A trial comparing nucleoside monotherapy with combination therapy in HIV-infected adults with CD4-cell counts from 200 to 500 per cubic millimeter. *N Engl J Med* 1996;335:1081–1090.
*Improved survival in patients with CD4-cell counts of 200 to 500/mm³ given zidovudine plus didanosine, ziduvudine plus zalcitabine, or didanosine alone.*
Hammer SM, et al. A controlled trial of two nucleoside analogues plus indinavir in persons with human immunodeficiency virus infection and CD4-cell counts of 200 per cubic millimeter or less. *N Engl J Med* 1997;337:725–733.

*A three-drug combination containing indinavir was superior to two nucleoside drugs in patients with AIDS (ACTG 320).*

Hughes MD, Johnson VA, Hirsch MS. Monitoring plasma HIV-1 RNA levels in addition to CD4+ lymphocyte count improves assessment of antiretroviral therapeutic response. *Ann Intern Med* 1997;126:929–938.
*Disease progression was noted in patients who had less than a 2.5-fold decrease in HIV-1 RNA levels from baseline at 8 weeks after the start of treatment.*

deJong MD, et al. High-dose nevirapine in previously untreated human immunodeficiency virus type 1-infected persons does not result in sustained suppression of viral replication. *J Infect Dis* 1997;175:966–970.
*Adverse effects with nevirapine included rash (25%) and fever (20%). Twenty percent of patients discontinued treatment.*

Kovacs JA, et al. Controlled trial of interleukin-2 infusions in patients infected with the human immunodeficiency virus. *N Engl J Med* 1996;335:1350–1356.
*CD4-cell counts increased in patients given interleukin-2 if their initial cell counts were above 200/mm³.*

Luzuriaga K, et al. Combination treatment with zidovudine, didanosine, and nevirapine in infants with human immunodeficiency virus type 1 infection. *N Engl J Med* 1997;336:1343–1349.
*A three-drug regimen of zidovudine, didanosine, and nevirapine was effective and well tolerated in maternally infected infants and children.*

Mayaux MJ, et al. Maternal virus load during pregnancy and mother-to-child transmission of human immunodeficiency virus type 1: the French Perinatal Cohort Studies. *J Infect Dis* 1997;175:172–175.
*HIV-1 was transmitted during pregnancy in 12% of cases with a viral load below 1,000 copies per milliliter, and in 29% of cases with a viral load above 10,000 copies per milliliter.*

Medical Letter. Drugs for HIV infection. *Med Lett* 1997;39:111–116.
*Review.*

Mellors JW, et al. Prognosis in HIV-1 infection predicted by the quantity of virus in plasma. *Science* 1996;272:1167–1170.
*HIV-1 RNA load is the best surrogate marker of disease progression and death.*

Montaner JSG, et al. A randomized, double-blind trial comparing combinations of nevirapine, didanosine, and zidovudine for HIV-infected patients. *JAMA* 1998;279:930–937.
*Fifty-eight percent of patients taking nevirapine plus two nucleoside analogs (zidovudine plus didanosine) had undetectable viral loads (<400 copies per milliliter) at 1 year (see also Gulick RM. HIV treatment strategies [Editorial]. Planning for the long term. JAMA 1998;279:957–959).*

Montaner JSG, et al. A pilot study of hydroxyurea among patients with advanced human immunodeficiency virus (HIV) disease receiving chronic didanosine therapy: Canadian HIV Trials Network Protocol 080. *J Infect Dis* 1997;175:801–806.
*Viral load decreased when hydroxyurea (1,000 mg/d) was given with didanosine.*

O'Brien WA, et al. Changes in plasma HIV-1 RNA and CD4+ lymphocyte counts and the risk of progression to AIDS. *N Engl J Med* 1996;334:426–431.
*Useful markers to predict progression to AIDS and death are viral load (significant increase is above threefold or >.5 log) and CD4-lymphocyte count.*

Palella FJ, et al. Declining morbidity and mortality among patients with advanced human immunodeficiency virus infection. *N Engl J Med* 1998;338:853–860.
*The death rate declined (from 29.4/100 person-years in 1995 to 8.8 in 1997) and the number of opportunistic infections decreased in patients treated with combination therapy containing a protease inhibitor.*

Panel on Clinical Practices for Treatment of HIV Infection. *Guidelines for the use of antiretroviral agents in HIV-infected adults and adolescents.* Department of Health and Human Services and the Henry J Kaiser Family Foundation, December 1, 1998:1–46.
*Guidelines for therapy.*

Saravolatz LD, et al. Zidovudine alone or in combination with didanosine or zalcitabine in HIV-infected patients with the acquired immunodeficiency syndrome or fewer than 200 CD4 cells per cubic millimeter. *N Engl J Med* 1996;335:1099–1106.

*In patients with AIDS, combination therapy with zidovudine and either didanosine or zalcitabine is not superior to zidovudine alone.*

Volberding PA, et al. A comparison of immediate with deferred zidovudine therapy for asymptomatic HIV-infected adults with CD4-cell counts of 500 or more per cubic millimeter. *N Engl J Med* 1995;333:401–407.

*Zidovudine was of no benefit in asymptomatic HIV-infected patients with a CD4-cell count above 500/mm³.*

## 91. DRUG INTERACTIONS IN PATIENTS WITH HUMAN IMMUNODEFICIENCY SYNDROME

Within the past decade, numerous agents have been marketed to treat patients with HIV/AIDS. Antiretrovirals include nucleoside reverse transcriptase inhibitors (NRTIs), protease inhibitors (PIs), and non-nucleoside reverse transcriptase inhibitors (NNRTIs). Other classes of agents are soon to be marketed. In addition to virus-specific drugs, agents to prevent or treat opportunistic infections, wasting, depression and anxiety, or neoplasia are often given to patients with HIV/AIDS. As a result, it is common for these patients to be maintained on polypharmacy that often involves five to nine medications. Many of these are known to interact with other drugs or food, such that the effects of the medications involved may be either enhanced or negated. This problem is exacerbated by the current inability to determine drug levels for most of these agents. The incidence of drug interactions in patients taking few agents has been estimated at about 5%. With polypharmacy, this can be expected at least to quadruple. Selected interactions may be life-threatening. The clinician managing the care of patients with HIV/AIDS must be aware of the potential for drug interactions, and in many cases an inordinate amount of time may be spent in determining appropriate management. Before new medications are prescribed for a patient with HIV/AIDS, both prescription and nonprescription agents being taken by the patient must be assessed. The following discussion focuses on mechanisms of drug interactions and depicts many of the most common. It is not meant to be inclusive. A caveat, however, is that with the large number of drugs that many patients ingest, interactions not heretofore known may be uncovered.

The mechanisms for drug-drug and drug-food interactions are multiple. For an agent to perform therapeutically, it must be successfully ingested and absorbed from the gastrointestinal tract. Many products are transported through the circulation by plasma proteins. Then, depending on mechanism of excretion, a drug will be metabolized and excreted by either the kidney or liver. The majority of antiretrovirals are metabolized by the liver, and it is within the liver that most problems with interactions occur. However, such problems may develop at any location along the metabolic pathway. As an example, selected agents require a specific pH for absorption, and agents that cause a change in pH (e.g., antacids, histamine₂ antagonists) may significantly interfere with absorption. Many antiretrovirals and other AIDS-related medications are excreted through the liver. Most are metabolized by the cytochrome P-450 system, for which there are several gene families and subfamilies. Three of these (CYP1, CYP2, and CYP3) are associated with the metabolism of most medications. Table 91–1 depicts substrates, inducers, and inhibitors for each of these.

Drug interactions may be either "pharmacokinetic" or "pharmacodynamic." Pharmacokinetic interactions alter blood levels of specific agents (and thus have the potential to render the product either toxic or clinically ineffective). Such alterations may be based on changes in absorption or excretion. Phamacodynamic interactions are related to toxicity or activity. Examples would include the simultaneous use of several nephrotoxic agents, or the use of products that bind to the same site (and thus may prove antagonistic).

### Nucleoside Reverse Transcriptase Inhibitors

Table 91–2 summarizes the major interactions for products within this class, which are more limited than those for other classes of antiretrovirals. Only in the case of

Table 91-1.  Major cytochrome P-450 enzymes

| Enzyme | Selected substrates | Inducers | Inhibitors |
|---|---|---|---|
| 1A2 | caffeine<br>theophylline | ritonavir<br>omeprazole | ciprofloxacin |
| 2C9 | phenytoin<br>ibuprofen | rifampin | ritonavir<br>delavirdine<br>fluconazole<br>sulfamethoxazole<br>metronidazole |
| 2C19 | omeprazole<br>phenytoin<br>propranolol | unknown | ritonavir<br>delavirdine<br>fluoxetine |
| 3A4 | saquinavir<br>indinavir<br>ritonavir<br>nelfinavir<br>nevirapine<br>delavirdine | rifampin<br>nevirapine<br>phenytoin<br>carbamazepine<br>phenobarbital | ritonavir<br>indinavir<br>nelfinavir<br>delavirdine<br>erythromycin<br>clarithromycin<br>ketoconazole<br>itraconazole<br>fluconazole<br>cimetidine |

Adapted from *J Respir Dis* 1998;19:24.

didanosine is absorption affected by gastric pH or by other products metabolized in the liver. All antiretrovirals within this class must be absorbed and metabolized by cells (intracellular phosphorylation).

Intracellular phosphorylation of zidovudine is inhibited by ribavirin, whereas both zidovudine and stavudine compete for the same intracellular enzymes (and thus inhibit each other). Didanosine is unstable in gastric acid and is therefore manufactured with buffers. Medications that are acidic (indinavir) may alter the bioavailability of didanosine, and those that require acid for absorption (ketoconazole, itraconazole) should not be administered at the same time. The buffering agents in didanosine interfere with the absorption of tetracycline and fluoroquinolones. Stavudine may cause peripheral neuropathy and should be cautiously employed with other agents capable of inducing this adverse reaction. Nevertheless, the combination of stavudine and didanosine appears to be well tolerated.

### Protease Inhibitors

PIs are major components of most intensive regimens for the management of HIV/AIDS, but they can be associated with major, life-threatening drug interactions. Agents to avoid with most PIs include astemizole (Hismanal), cisapride (Propulsid), and terfenadine (Seldane). Others to use with extreme caution with at least some of these (especially ritonavir) include amiodarone, clozapine, diazepam, flurazepam, meperidine, midazolam, ergot alkaloids, quinidine, rifabutin, triazolam, and zolpidem. Table 91–3 provides data on some of the most important of these but is not meant to be inclusive. In general, medications that enhance by-products that inhibit the cytochrome system, especially CYP 3A4, must be avoided or else utilized with extreme caution. Such a product is ketoconazole; effects of itraconazole have not been well studied. Alternatively, agents that increase the metabolic rates of PIs (rifampin, barbiturates, phenytoin) may

Table 91-2.  Major interactions for nucleoside reverse transcriptase inhibitors

| Agent | Interacting drugs | Mechanism | Result |
|---|---|---|---|
| zidovudine (AZT) | TMP-SMX dapsone ganciclovir pyrimethamine | pharmacodynamic | additive toxicity, typically hematologic |
| | probenicid fluconazole methadone | pharmacokinetic | ↑ levels of zidovudine |
| | rifampin | pharmacokinetic | ↓ levels of zidovudine |
| didanosine (ddI) | itraconazole, ketoconazole, indinavir, delavirdine | pharmacokinetic | ↓ fungal agent/delavirdine absorption; indinavir decreases didanosine absorption |
| | fluoroquinolones, tetracycline | pharmacokinetic | ↓ antibiotic absorption |
| | cisplatin, ddC, d4T, isoniazid, vincristine | pharmacodynamic | ↑toxicity |
| zalcitabine (ddC) | cisplatin, ddI, d4T, isoniazid, vincristine | pharmacodynamic | ↑toxicity |
| | ddI | pharmacodynamic | cross-resistance |
| stavudine (d4T) | cisplatin, ddI, d4T, vincristine, isoniazid | pharmacodynamic | additive toxicity |
| lamivudine (3TC) | TMP-SMX | pharmacokinetic | ↓3TC excretion |
| | ddI, ddC | pharmacokinetic | cross-resistance |

TMP-SMX, trimethoprim-sulfamethoxazole.
Adapted from Cretton-Scott E, Sommadossi JP. *Northwestern University Reports on HIV/AIDS* 1998;2:1–11.

substantially lower the effective concentrations of PIs. Rifampin is the most potent of these and generally should not be coadministered with PIs. Potentially fatal interactions between PIs and terfenadine or astemizole may occur because of enhanced levels of these histamine receptor antagonists. Quinidine and cisapride may be rendered esssentially inert when coadminsitered with PIs.

The bioavailability of saquinavir, even in its newer soft-gel form (Fortovase), is tenuous in comparison with that of other PIs. Agents associated with CYP 3A4 induction may decrease saquinavir levels to the extent that the drug is rendered impotent. In contrast, agents such as ritonavir, which are potent inhibitors of CYP 3A4, enhance the bioavailability of saquinavir by about 50 to 100 times, making this dual PI combination therapeutically viable.

Ritonavir causes numerous and conflicting interactions within the cytochrome systems. Thus, it is difficult to understand intellectually how it interfaces with other

Table 91-3.  Major interactions with protease inhibitors

| Drug | Interacting agent | Result |
|------|-------------------|--------|
| saquinavir (Fortovase, Invirase) | ritonavir | ↑saquinavir levels |
| | rifampin | ↓saquinavir levels |
| ritonavir (Norvir) | oral contraceptives, theophylline | ↓levels of interacting agent |
| | rifampin, cisapride, astemizole, terfenadine, oral antifungals, sedatives, indinavir, saquinavir, selected antiarrhythmics | ↑levels of interacting agent (some cases may be life-threatening) |
| | rifampin | ↓levels of ritonavir |
| indinavir (Crixivan) | didanosine | ↓indinavir absorption |
| | rifampin | ↓levels of indinavir |
| | astemizole, cisapride, terfenadine, triazolam, clarithromycin, trimethoprim | ↑levels of interacting agent (may be life-threatening) |
| | ketoconazole | ↑levels of indinavir |
| | ritonavir | cross-resistance |
| nelfinavir (Viracept) | rifampin | ↓levels of nelfinavir |
| | terfenadine | ↑levels of terfenadine |
| | ketoconazole | ↑levels of nelfinavir |

Adapted from Cretton-Scott E, Sommadossi JP. *Northwestern University Reports on HIV/AIDS* 1998; 2:1–11.

agents, and it should be used with caution when other products with hepatic metabolism are coadministered. In addition to being the most potent inhibitor of CYP 3A4, it has the capacity either to inhibit or to induce other isoenzymes within the system. It is also likely that interactions may exist that have yet to be fully investigated. Examples of agents to be used with great caution include serotonin reuptake inhibitors, tricyclic antidepressants, anticonvulsants, antiarrhythmics, lovastatin and simvastatin, and rifabutin.

Nelfinavir and indinavir are less potent inhibitors of CYP 3A4 than is ritonavir. Selected agents that include terfenadine, astemizole, and cisapride are contraindicated. Indinavir requires acid for absorption and cannot be taken on a full stomach. Nor can it be coadministered with didanosine.

## Non-nucleoside Reverse Transcriptase Inhibitors

Like the PIs, these agents are metabolized by the cytochrome P-450 system. Delavirdine is an enzyme inhibitor, whereas nivirapine is an inducer. Interactions with other agents are complex and incompletely studied. In general, astemizole, terfenadine, cisapride, midazolam, triazolam, rifampin, ergot alkaloids, and phenytoin should be used with caution. Levels of agents that include quinidine, warfarin, dapsone, and clarithromycin will be enhanced if they are administered with delavirdine. Delavradine will enhance the levels of selected PIs that include indivavir and saquinavir. Table 91–4 summarizes selected available data. (R.B.B.)

91. Drug Interactions in HIV Syndrome 497

Table 91-4. Interactions with non-nucleoside reverse transcriptase inhibitors

| Agent | Interacting drug | Effect |
|---|---|---|
| nevirapine (Viramune) | oral contraceptives, indinavir, saquinavir | ↓levels of interacting drug |
| | rifampin | ↓levels of nevirapine |
| | ketoconazole, itraconazole, clarithromycin, erythromycin | ↑levels of nevirapine |
| delavirdine (Rescriptor) | indinavir, saquinavir, erythromycin | ↑ levels of interacting drug |
| | rifampin | ↓levels of delavirdine |
| | ketoconazole, itraconazole, clarithromycin, erythromycin, ritonavir | ↑levels of delavirdine |

Adapted from Cretton-Scott E, Sommadossi JP. *Northwestern University Reports on HIV/AIDS* 1998; 2:1–11.

## Bibliography

Cretton-Scott E, Commadossi JP. Drug interactions in HIV therapy. *Northwestern University Reports on HIV/AIDS* 1998;2:1–9.
*This article is concise and readable. Charts are clear and not intended to be encyclopedic. The authors counsel care givers of AIDS patients to be thorough in obtaining drug histories and to be alert to drug interactions not yet reported.*
McDonald CK, Gerber JG. Avoiding drug interactions with antiretroviral agents [Parts 1 and 2]. *J Respir Dis* 1998;19:24–25,103–113.
*An extensive two-part review of drug interactions in HIV-infected patients. The authors provide contemporary information concerning mechanisms of potential interactions and depict interactions by class of antiretroviral.*
Piscitelli SC, et al. Drug interactions in patients infected with human immunodeficiency virus. *Clin Infect Dis* 1996;23:685–693.
*One of several excellent recent overviews detailing problems with drug interactions in patients with HIV/AIDS. The authors assess mechanisms of drug interactions and provide several tables outlining important examples of significant interactions. Some of the tables provide information about the potential severity of selected interactions.*

# Subject Index

## A

Abacavir, 487

Abdominal pain
  in amebic abscess, 79
  in *Mycobacterium avium* complex
    infection, 475

Abscess
  amebic, 78–80
  brain, 172–173
  ovarian, 134–138
  perinephric, 115
  peritonsillar, 4–5
  prostatic, 112
  pyogenic liver, 95–96

Acalculous cholecystitis, 93, 95

Acid-fast bacilli smear
  in *Mycobacterium avium* complex
    infection, 475
  in pleural effusion, 30

Acidification of urine, 102

Acquired immunodeficiency syndrome,
    447–497
  acquisition and transmission of, 449–452
  acute bronchitis in, 22
  acute facial paralysis in, 165
  AIDS-related dementia, 469–470
  antiretroviral therapy, 485–493
  antiviral susceptibility testing, 399
  central nervous system infections,
    167–168, 466–474
    encephalopathy, 469–470
    meningitis, 466–468
    space-occupying brain lesions,
      468–469
  drug interactions in therapy, 493–497
  fever in, 246, 478–481
    prolonged with generalized
      lymphadenopathy, 253
    of unknown origin, 290
  hepatobiliary tract infections in, 95
  HIV-mononucleosis syndrome, 452–455
  microbiologic associations, 43
  *Mycobacterium avium* complex infection,
    474–478
  needlestick injury and, 328, 329
  pharyngitis and, 3, 7
  *Pneumocystis carinii* pneumonia in,
    455–460

prevention of opportunistic infections,
    482–485
  septic arthritis in, 198
  sinusitis and, 10
  syphilis and, 131, 460–466
  toxoplasmosis in, 172
  travel-acquired, 357
  tuberculosis with, 377, 460–466

*Actinobacter* bacteremia, 385

*Actinomyces*
  alternate antibiotics when beta-lactams are
    contraindicated, 305
  in central nervous system infection, 178
  in pelvic inflammatory disease, 134
  in pyogenic liver abscess, 78

Acute bronchitis, 21–24

Acyclovir
  in acute facial paralysis, 164, 165
  for genital herpes, 139–140
  for infectious mononucleosis, 17
  in shingles, 216–217

Adefovir, 487

Adenosine deaminase test, 176–177

Adenovirus, 7

Adult acute asthmatic bronchitis, 21

Aerobic bacteria
  in animal bite wound, 346
  in necrotizing soft tissue infection, 207

Agenerase; *see* Amprenavir

AIDS; *see* Acquired immunodeficiency
    syndrome

Alanine aminotransferase, 337, 338

Alcoholism, microbiologic associations, 43

Alkaline phosphatase
  in amebic abscess, 79
  in ascending cholangitis, 94
  granulocytopenia and, 286
  in hydatid disease, 80

Alkalinization of urine, 102

Allograft rejection, renal, 265

Alpha-blockers in prostatitis, 113

Alpha toxin of *Clostridium perfringens,* 206,
    207

Amebiasis, 393

Amebic abscess, 78–80

Amikacin, 475–476

Aminoglycosides
  in animal bite, 346

Trimetrexate, 456, 457
Trophozoite, 393
Trovafloxacin, 436
  in bacterial peritonitis, 89
  for urethritis, 127
Trovan; *see* Trovafloxacin
Tuberculin skin test, 365–370
Tuberculosis, 363–381
  chemotherapy of, 376–381
  fever of unknown origin and, 289
  granulomatous hepatitis and, 82
  in human immunodeficiency virus
      infection, 460–463
  isoniazid chemoprophylaxis, 370–376
  meningitis with, 171, 176
  pleural effusion in, 31
  tuberculin skin test, 365–370
  vertebral osteomyelitis and, 191
Tuberculostearic acid, 177
Tuberculous pleurisy, 32
Tumor, hepatic, 80–81
Tumor necrosis factor, 226–227
Typhoid fever, 272
Tzanck smear
  in genital herpes, 139
  in rash, 256

### U
Ulcer
  decubitus, 217–218
  in genital herpes, 138–139
Ultrasonography
  in acute cholecystitis, 93
  in amebic abscess, 79
  in ascending cholangitis, 94
  in pyogenic hepatic abscess, 77
Upper respiratory tract, 1–18
  infectious mononucleosis, 13–18
  sinusitis, 8–13
  tonsillopharyngitis in adult, 3–8
*Ureaplasma urealyticum*
  in pelvic inflammatory disease, 134
  in prostatitis, 112
  in urethritis, 125
Urethral discharge, 125–129
Urethritis, 125–129
Urinary $\beta^2$–microglobulin, 104
Urinary frequency
  in bacterial prostatitis, 111
  in cystitis, 103
Urinary lactate dehydrogenase assay, 104
Urinary tract
  infection of, 99–121
    after renal transplantation, 266
    asymptomatic bacteriuria, 106–109
    basic principles of therapy, 101–103
    candiduria, 119–121
    catheter-related, 316–322
    complicated, 115–118

  cystitis *versus* pyelonephritis,
      103–106
  gram-negative bacteremia, 223, 385
  postoperative fever, 311–312
  prostatitis, 111–115
  pyuria, 109–111
  urethritis, 125–129
  procedures inducing endocarditis through,
      69–70
Urinary urgency in cystitis, 103
Urine, acidification and alkalinization of,
    102
Urticaria, 303

### V
Vaccination
  after animal bite, 345–346
  in chronic bronchitis, 23
  hepatitis B, 331–333
  pneumococcal, 26
  before traveling abroad, 272, 358–359
Vaginal discharge
  in bacterial vaginosis, 145
  in pelvic inflammatory disease, 135
  in vaginitis, 143
Vaginitis, 143–148
  bacterial vaginosis, 145–146
  candidiasis, 143–144
  trichomoniasis, 144
Valacyclovir, 139–140
Valve infection
  coagulase-negative staphylococci in, 235
  gram-positive bacteremia in, 389
Valvular insufficiency, infective
      endocarditis and, 64–68
Vancomycin
  antibiotic-resistant pneumococci and, 26
  in bacterial meningitis, 170
  for coagulase-negative staphylococci, 235
  in continuous ambulatory peritoneal
      dialysis-related peritonitis, 90
  in endocarditis prophylaxis, 71, 72
  in granulocytopenia, 285
  for methicillin-resistant *Staphylococcus
      aureus,* 230–231
  in native valve infective endocarditis, 66
  in nosocomial pneumonia, 39
  relapse after therapy, 418–419
  serum levels of, 401
Vancomycin-resistant enterococci, 237–241
Varicella-zoster virus, 165
Vasopressors, in toxic shock syndrome, 259
Venereal Disease Research Laboratory, 130,
    464, 467
Vertebral osteomyelitis, 189–192
Vesicle, conditions inducing, 257
*Vibrio vulnificus,* 215–216
  in travel-acquired diarrhea, 360
Videx; *see* Didanosine

Viracept; *see* Nelfinavir
Viral infection
  acute bronchitis, 21
  after renal transplantation, 265
  antiviral susceptibility testing, 398–399
  encephalitis, 154–155, 172
  hepatitis C, 335–341
  herpes simplex virus
    in encephalitis, 154–155, 172
    in facial paralysis, 163
    in genital herpes, 138–142
    in pharyngitis, 7
    travel-acquired, 357
  herpes zoster, 216–217
  infectious mononucleosis, 13–18
  meningitis, 171
    acute, 153–154
    chronic, 178
  rash in, 246
  septic arthritis, 198
  sinusitis, 8–13
  tonsillopharyngitis, 3–8
Viral load in HIV infection, 487–488
Viramune; *see* Nevirapine
Volume expansion, in gram-negative
    bacteremia, 227
Volume of distribution of antimicrobials,
    407
Vomiting
  in central nervous system infection, 167
  in toxic shock syndrome, 258
von Reyn classification of infective
    endocarditis, 57, 58

**W**
Water-borne disease, fever in traveler, 272
Western blot
  in genital herpes, 139
  in Lyme disease, 210
Wheezing, 21

Whipple's disease, 254
White blood cell count
  in cerebrospinal fluid analysis, 152
  in cystitis, 103
  in fever in HIV-positive patient, 479
  in Legionnaire's disease, 46
  in prostatitis, 112
  in prosthetic joint infection, 193
  in pyuria, 110
  in septic arthritis, 199
Wound care in animal bite, 345
Wound healing, hyperbaric oxygen therapy
    and, 208
Wound infection
  perioperative prophylaxis, 421–426
  postoperative fever in, 311–312
  prosthetic joint, 193

**X**
Xanthogranuloma, 115
*Xanthomonas maltophilia,* 385

**Y**
Yeast infection, chronic fatigue syndrome
    and, 295
Yellow fever vaccine, 358
*Yersinia enterocolitica,* 83

**Z**
Zagam; *see* Sparfloxacin
Zalcitabine
  drug interactions, 494–496
  generic and trade names, 486
Zerit; *see* Stavudine
Ziagen; *see* Abacavir
Zidovudine
  drug interactions, 495
  generic and trade names, 486
  in HIV-mononucleosis syndrome, 454
Zoonoses, 343–348